Proactive Approaches in Psychosocial Occupational Therapy

Proactive Approaches in Psychosocial Occupational Therapy

Rita P. Fleming Cottrell, MA, OTL

Occupational Therapy Program Director
Dominican College
Orangeburg, NY

SLACK
INCORPORATED

6900 Grove Road · Thorofare, NJ 08086

Publisher: John H. Bond
Editorial Director: Amy E. Drummond
Design Editor: Lauren Biddle Plummer

The work SLACK Incorporated publishes is peer reviewed. Prior to publication, recognized leaders in the field, educators, and clinicians provide important feedback on the concepts and content that we publish. We welcome feedback on this work.

Cottrell, Rita P. Fleming.
   Proactive approaches in psychosocial occupational therapy/Rita P. Fleming Cottrell.
      p. cm.
   Includes bibliographical references and index.
   ISBN 1-55642-455-8 (alk. paper)
      1. Occupational therapy--Practice--United States. 2. Occupational therapy--Philosophy. I. Title.

   RC487 .C68 2000
   615.8'515--dc21

                                                    00-029178

Printed in the United States of America.
Published by: SLACK Incorporated
                6900 Grove Road
                Thorofare, NJ 08086-9447 USA
                Telephone: 856-848-1000
                Fax: 856-853-5991
                World Wide Web: http://www.slackbooks.com

   Contact SLACK Incorporated for more information about other books in this field or about the availability of our books from distributors outside the United States.

   Authorization to photocopy items for internal or personal use, or the internal or personal use of specific clients, is granted by SLACK Incorporated, provided that the appropriate fee is paid directly to Copyright Clearance Center, 222 Rosewood Drive, Danvers, MA 01923 USA, 978-750-8400. Prior to photocopying items for educational classroom use, please contact the CCC at the address above. Please reference Account Number 9106324 for SLACK Incorporated's Professional Book Division.

   For further information on CCC, check CCC Online at the following address: http://www.copyright.com.

Last digit is print number: 10 9 8 7 6 5 4 3 2 1

DEDICATION

To my brother, Kevin Michael Fleming, whose life underscored the vital need for a holistic therapeutic approach, regardless of clinical diagnosis, and the inherent value of meaningful, purposeful occupation in one's daily life. May his legacy live on and be commemorated in my teachings and in the reader's active pursuit of a fulfilling occupational therapy career.

To the occupational therapy practitioners who continued to practice and promote authentic, holistic occupational therapy, resisting the precipitous slide into dichotomous, reductionistic practice.

To past, current, and future occupational therapy scholars, educators, practitioners, and students who refuse(d) to accept the demise of mental health practice in the profession of occupational therapy and who dare(d) to ponder, propose, and implement occupational therapy practice to holistically meet the needs of persons with mental illness and their loved ones.

CONTENTS

ACKNOWLEDGMENTS

I would like to thank my collegues and students who have challenged and enriched my professional development; and my best friends; my husband, Michael who continues to provide me with loving support for all of my multiple endeavors (even the non-profit ones!) and my son, Christopher Michael, who fills my life with creativity, laughter, a wonderful mix of classic and alternative rock, and a teen's unique blend of cynicism and optimism.

A special thanks to Gail Fidler, one of our profession's most provocative voices for questioning the status quo and the viability of fighting for our profession's core philosophical beliefs. Gail has generously shared her unwavering vision, persistent passion and uncompromising spirit in her quest to preserve "authentic" occupational therapy.

I would also like to extend my deep appreciation to the staff of SLACK Incorporated who have made this publication possible. To John Bond, Publisher, and Amy Drummond, Editorial Director, who both generously embraced the concept of the text as it was initially proposed, and to Lauren Biddle Plummer, Design Editor, and Debra Toulson, Managing Editor, who each completed their respective production tasks in an efficient and helpful manner in bringing this work to fruition, a heartfelt thank you. It has been a pleasure working with everyone on the SLACK team.

About the Editor

Rita P. Fleming Cottrell, MA, OTL, is the Program Director of the occupational therapy program at Dominican College of Blauvelt in Orangeburg, NY. Ms. Cottrell received her Baccalaureate and post-professional master's degrees in occupational therapy from New York University. Since 1987, she has held a number of academic positions at New York University, Dominican College, and other OT and OTA programs. Prior to entering academia, Ms. Cottrell worked as an occupational therapist in practice settings across the mental health continuum of care, from inpatient acute psychiatry to community day treatment and transitional living programs. She has published and presented nationally on the role of OT in mental health practice, COTA to OTR career mobility and professional development, nontraditional models for OT professional education, contemporary psychosocial OT practice and case management. She also coordinates and lectures in Dominican College's biannual review course for the NBCOT Certification Examination for the Occupational Therapist.

She has edited several textbooks and authored a number of journal articles. In 1994, Ms. Cottrell was awarded an AOTA "Award of Achievement" for her publications and contributions to the profession. She serves on the editorial board of the American Journal of Occupational Therapy and is an Education Liaison for the Hudson-Taconic District of the New York State OT Association coordinating their grant projects.

Ms. Cottrell's professional experience in mental health practice and in academia, along with her personal experience as a long-term caregiver for a beloved family member, has resulted in a strong, unwavering commitment to the inherent value of authentic OT. Her goal is to ensure that all OT students and practitioners recognize that mental health is relevant to everyone, not just persons with a psychiatric diagnosis, so that the complete potential of occupational therapy is realized by all. in addition, Ms. Cottrell is most interested in the promotion of OT to the public and to policy-makers as the profession most suited to intervene holistically to meet societal needs.

PREFACE

This text, *Proactive Approaches in Psychosocial Occupational Therapy* can essentially be considered a second edition of *Psychosocial Occupational Therapy: Proactive Approaches* which was published by the American Occupational Therapy Association (AOTA) in 1993. Due to AOTA's desire to prioritize resources, it was mutually agreed upon by AOTA and myself that a second edition of *Psychosocial Occupational Therapy* would not be published by AOTA; hence, this text's publisher is SLACK Incorporated. To eliminate potential confusion between the two publications, it was also mutually decided to rename this text *Proactive Approaches in Psychosocial Occupational Therapy*. Regardless of the name change, the intent of this text remains the same as the first. My aim in completing a compilation of professional literature related to mental health occupational therapy practice has been and remains four-fold. My goals were and are:

First, I wanted to counter the often negative view of psychosocial practice, and the sad but strong societal stigma against persons with mental illness, by providing literature that was humanistic, respectful, dignified, and hopeful for each individual and his/or her potential.

Second, I sought to expose readers to the reality that excellence, creativity, commitment and change prevails in psychosocial practice and that there exists a wealth of practice opportunities to be seized and role models to be emulated.

Third, I strove to provide literature that would foster an appreciation of the efficacy and relevance of psychosocial occupational therapy practice, regardless of the reader's selected practice area. Most important, I wanted to emphasize that mental health approaches are not just for persons with psychiatric illnesses. Rather, mental health is relevant and vital to all, regardless of diagnosis; therefore, the study and application of psychosocial occupational therapy approaches are pertinent to every area of occupational therapy practice.

Finally, on a practical level I sought to provide practitioners, educators, and students with a virtual library of the "best of the best" in professional literature related to psychosocial practice. Since the contents of this text cover a broad range of psychosocial issues and concerns; practice models and intervention programs; and professional and health care trends, it can eliminate many cumbersome copyright release procedures and serve as an efficient starting point for a literature search.

In reviewing past and current literature to determine what should be included in this text to ensure that the above goals were achieved; the refrain "everything old is new again" kept recurring in my thoughts. As I read and re-read the chapters of the 1993 text, it became clear that many of the proactive approaches described in this work had not been seized upon by occupational therapy practitioners. Since the majority of these program initiatives were originally developed and written about in the 1980s, I became saddened by the number of practice opportunities that were lost to occupational therapy over the past 15 to 20 years. I wondered why more occupational therapists did not move into Employee Assistance Programs (EAPs) as described by Maynard (see Chapter 28) or develop psychoeducational programs as proposed by Crist (see Chapter 19) or design residential programs as presented by Wilberding (see Chapter 18) or lead day centers as described by Woodside (see Chapter 10). The list of lost opportunities for occupational therapy in mental health practice seemed almost endless. The reality that occupational therapists had remained largely institutionalized; that other professionals had seized these opportunities in community practice and psychiatric rehabilitation; and, that occupational therapy had become increasingly more reductionistic over this time period was one that I had been acutely aware of; but this review of "older" literature painfully emphasized the significance of this loss.

Conversely, as I read "newer", more recent literature I was struck by the strong (albeit small) group of occupational therapists who had maintained their commitment to mental health practice and who had not only survived but thrived as psychosocial occupational therapists. In addition, I was heartened by the consistent call in the current literature for the development of community-based services, wellness and prevention programs and other practice initiatives that are not based on the medical model. Hence, the refrain "Everything old is new again!" and the inclusion of both older (but still highly relevant) literature and newer encouraging works. This extensive literature review has given me a renewed (yet cautious) optimism that more current and future occupational therapists may finally seize the opportunities afforded in mental health practice as envisioned in the late 1970s and early 1980s and as kept alive by dedicated psychosocial occupational therapy practitioners.

My hopeful outlook is supported by several trends in health care that will be discussed in detail in Sections I and VI of this text. The consumer and family advocacy movement, and an increased emphasis on functional outcomes, community integration and quality of life clearly support occupational therapists' assumption of leadership positions within the evolving health care system. In addition, managed care and the Prospective Payment System (PPS) has uprooted many traditional practice areas, resulting in "re-engineering" of systems, "downsizing" of departments, "realignment" of resources, and a balancing of the economic playing field among speciality areas. These major changes have lead many occupational therapists to reevaluate their practice, reestablish their professional priorities, and hopefully reaffirm their commitment to the core values of occupational therapy.

While a resurgence of holistic, psychosocial occupational therapy is clearly possible, it is also strongly needed. Many professionals from other disciplines are promoting their ability to provide quality, holistic functionall interventions in areas that are largely within occupational therapy's domain of concern (Wood, 1998). In addition, recent publications in other fields have raised serious questions about the value and efficacy of occupational therapy for persons with mental illness (Kopelwicz,

Wallace & Zarate, 1998, Liberman; et al, 1998). Although these studies were flawed in many respects (Bair, 1999) they were published in reputable, juried journals with large readerships.

If occupational therapists cannot articulate and demonstrate their unique role in today's professionally competitive, market-driven care environment others will readily take our place. Therefore, it is essential that all occupational therapists develop an acute awareness of the external forces that impact on our profession and the personal attributes and practice skills needed to effectively manage the significant challenges brought on by a rapidly changing health care system. It is my hope that the readings in this text will support this professional renewal by providing thought-provoking analysis of current and evolving trends, strong models for program initiatives, and pragmatic guidelines for professional development. In addition, I encourage the reader to consider the below suggested actions and to purposely pursue those that are relevant to their level of professional development.

Subscribe to, and publish in, non-occupational therapy journals and newsletters. *Psychiatric Services, Psychosocial Rehabilitation,* Haworth Press publications and many others provide a wealth of literature relevant to occupational therapy; and most importantly, their readership needs to learn about the value and efficacy of occupational therapy.

Join consumer, family and professional organizations that support quality health care services and advocate for necessary changes within the current systems of care. Several major resources are provided at the end of this preface.

Use the "50 simple things you can do to promote occupational therapy in mental health" on a daily basis (See Appendix B).

Contact the American Occupational Therapy Association and state occupational therapy associations to identify occupational therapists who have attained and maintained viable psychosocial occupational therapy practices and/or assumed leadership positions within the mental health system of care. Seek out these individuals to explore developing a mentorship relationship with them.

Explore job opportunities that are outside of the field of occupational therapy but that are within the expertise of an occupational therapy practitioner. Occupational therapists can consider positions as team leaders, program directors, consultants, and/or case managers. Once a leadership position is obtained, occupational therapists can hire occupational therapy assistants as staff to provide direct service. Occupational therapy assistants can also consider "non-OT" positions that are within their area of expertise such as activities director, mental health technician and/or residential program counselor.

Present guest lectures, inservices and workshops to consumer and family groups, professional organizations and occupational therapy education programs.

Develop and provide fieldwork opportunities for occupational therapist and occupational therapy assistant students for they are the future of our profession.

In conclusion, occupational therapists who act proactively to increase their knowledge and skills, nurture future practitioners, advocate for quality care, develop and lead model programs, and promote our profession will recapture the full potential of occupational therapy. As Jerry Johnson advised in 1981, "Our traditional values when supplemented and supported by knowledge, offer us the potential to become a powerful presence in our society–powerful in that we provide a resource that enables individuals to live their lives as they want, to become what they want to be" (Johnson, 1996, p 585).

This power of occupational therapy has deep personal meaning to me for when its potential was not realized, my brother Kevin's life of living with a disability was one of empty survival. Whereas, when the powerful potential of occupational therapy was fully engaged, his life achieved purpose and meaning (Cottrell, 1996). As I reflect upon the past 10 years since Kevin's death in 1989, I am struck by how critically urgent his life's lessons have become. I truly hope that the year 2000 begins a rebirth of our profession's tradition of using meaningful occupations and purposeful activities to promote function and achieve a quality life. As Adolf Meyer reflected on the "real needs and real opportunities" (1996, p 640) of the time–; in a 1937 address in honor of Eleanor Clarke Slagle, occupational therapists have "the opportunity to find similarly minded forces and the spirit of action that has to go with knowledge and vision to make it both fertile and practical...From reveling in thoughts of eternity, we now have the great task to inject again the joys of activity of the day" (Meyer, 1996, p 640).

REFERENCES

Bair, J. (1999). Letter to the editor. *Psychiatric Services, 50,* 419-420.

Johnson, J. A. (1996). Old values–New directions: Competence, adaptation, integration. In R. P. Cottrell (Ed). *Perspectives on purposeful activity: Foundation and future of occupational therapy* (pp 577-586). Bethesda, MD: AOTA.

Kopelwicz, A.; Wallace, C. J. & Zarate, R. (1998). Teaching psychiatric in-patients to reenter the community: A brief method of improving the continuity of care. *Psychiatric Services, 49,* 1313-1316.

Liberman, R. P., Wallace, C. J., Blackwell, G., Kopelwicz, A., Vaccaro, J., & Mintz, J. (1998). Skills training versus psychosocial occupational therapy for persons with persistent schizophrenia. *American Journal of Psychiatry, 155,* 1087-1091.

Meyer, A. (1996). Address in honor of Eleanor Clarke Slagle. In R. P. Cottrell (Ed.), *Perspectives on purposeful activity: Foundation and future of occupational therapy* (pp 639-641). Bethesda, MD. American Occupational Therapy Association.

Wood, W. (1998). Nationally speaking: Is it jump time for occupational therapy? *American Journal of Occupational Therapy, 52,* 403-411.

SELECTED RESOURCES

The below list of select national organizations is provided to help the reader obtain educational literature and up-to-date information. More extensive resource listings are available in *Perspectives on Purposeful Activity: Foundation and Future of Occupational Therapy*. (Cottrell, 1996). These resources can also assist the therapist by providing an excellent referral base for individuals and their families. While therapists cannot personally address all areas of concern for all persons, they can easily supply patients with the names and addresses of relevant resources. Readers are encouraged to contact national organizations to identify local resources and to join those organizations related to their areas of professional interest. Readers are also urged to contact their state divisions of mental health and offices for persons with disabilities, as these state agencies can provide vital information on resources, services, and policies unique to each state. Readers who actively utilize national, regional, and local resources will enhance their professional career development, improve the relevance of their occupational therapy programs, and empower clients and their families with vital information and appropriate referrals to enhance the quality of their lives.

Alzheimer's Disease and Related Disorders Association (ADRDA)
919 North Michigan Avenue
Suite 1000
Chicago, IL 60611
800-621-0379
www.alz.org

Association for Children and Adults with Learning Disabilities
4156 Library Road
Pittsburgh, PA 15234
412-881-2253
www.donline.org

Association for Retarded Citizens (ARC)
National Headquarters
500 East Border Street
Suite 300
P.O. Box 300649
Arlington, TX 76010
817-261-6003
www.thearcatmetronet.com

Autism Society of America
8601 Georgia Avenue
Suite 503
Silver Spring, MD 20910
301-565-0433

Children of Aging Parents (CAP)
1609 Woodbourne Road
Woodbourne Office Campus
Suite 302-A
Levittown, PA 19067
215-945-6900
www.careguide.net

Compeer, Inc
Monroe Square Suite B-1
259 Monroe Ave.
Rochester, NY 14607
716-546-8280
www.compeeratfrontiernet.net

Disability Resources Monthly
Disabilities Resources, Inc.
4 Glyter Lane
Centereach, NY 11720
516-585-0290
www.disabilityresources.org

International Association of Psychosocial Rehabilitation Services
10025 Governor Warfield Parkway
Suite 301
Columbia, MD 21044-3357
410-730-7190
www.iaprs.org

Job Accommodation Network
West Virginia University
P. O. Box 6080
Morgantown, WV 26506-6080
800-526-7234
www.janatjan.lcdi.wvu.edu

Life Services for the Handicapped, Inc.
352 Park Avenue South
Suite 703
New York, NY 10010-1709
212-532-6740

National Alliance for the Mentally Ill
200 N. Glebe Road
Suite 1015
Arlington, VA 22203-3754
www.nami.org

National Association for the Dually Diagnosed (NADD)
132 Fair Street
Kingston, NY 12401-4802
800-331-5362
www.thenadd.org

The National Council on Aging, Inc. (NCOA)
409 Third Street, S.W.
Suite 200
Washington, DC 20024
202-479-1200
www.ncoa.org

National Organization for Rare Disorders (NORD)
P.O. Box 8923
New Fairfield, CT 06812-1783
203-746-6518
www.orphanatraredisease.org

National Organization on Disability (NOD)
910 16th Street, N.W.
Suite 600
Washington, DC 20006
202-293-5960
800-248-ABLE
www.nod.org

Recovery, Inc.
802 North Dearborn Street
Chicago, IL 60610
312-337-5661
www.recoveryline.com

NOTE TO READERS

Due to the need to comply with copyright laws, all of the chapters in this text were reprinted as originally published. While editorial efforts were made to ensure current relevance, grammatical accuracy, and gender-neutral language, readers will note some inconsistencies in several chapters. These chapters contain pertinent content, but their formats do not always adhere to the American Psychological Association's (APA) publication guidelines. Areas of concern include various styles of referencing and nongender-neutral language.

In addition, readers will note that the terms patient, client, and consumer are all used in the text to designate the individual with whom the occupational therapist is working. While determining the best word to identify the person involved in therapeutic services has been a frequent topic of debate in many fields, there has not yet been a satisfactory, definitive agreement as to what one word best defines this role. Therefore, the term selected is often the one that is used the most in a given service delivery model. For example, "patient" is used in a medical model, "client" is used in a community health model, "consumer" is used in an empowerment model, and "member" is used in a clubhouse model. Given the diversity of models and settings presented in this text, readers are advised to consider the designation used to describe the individual in occupational therapy within its social, cultural and temporal contexts. In my own writings, I strive to use the words individual or person in most contexts. Whatever word is selected to indicate the person involved with occupational therapy, readers are cautioned to always remember that the individual is a person first–with multiple roles, values, interests, and goals–regardless of an external lable.

In conclusion, readers are advised to review all chapters critically—recognizing the strengths of each while acknowledging their limitations according to current professional standards.

Sociopolitical Issues and Policies Influencing Mental Health Practice

EDITOR'S NOTE

Occupational therapy has been significantly influenced by sociopolitical issues throughout its professional history. The founders of occupational therapy were very concerned with the contemporary issues of their time, and these societal forces largely shaped occupational therapy's heritage (Peloquin, 1996). Over the ensuing years, the development of occupational therapy continued to be responsive to changes in sociopolitical thought, values, and policies (Kielhofner & Burke, 1977; Wood, 1998). Since the 1980s, occupational therapists have been confronted with many challenges, including decreased lengths of stay, increased demands for cost-containment and accountability, and a diminished mental health occupational therapy manpower pool. Today, managed care and a growing competition among health care professionals for limited reimbursement dollars are new challenges faced by occupational therapists (Wood, 1998). Therefore, it is vital that occupational therapists are informed about these issues, as societal trends and public policies directly influence our practice. Many health care professionals (psychiatrists, physical therapists, psychologists, nurses, and social workers) are now advocating and implementing functional approaches to treatment in response to these sociopolitical trends (Ascher-Svanum & Krause, 1991; Frese, 1998).

While some therapists may view this movement as a threat to our profession, others will view it as an opportunity as great as the one that led to the initial founding of the profession of occupational therapy (which was also led by doctors, nurses, and social workers) (Peloquin, 1996). Occupational therapists who are skilled in the evaluation and intervention of functional performance and who are knowledgeable about sociopolitical issues can seize this opportunity to become leaders in contemporary and emerging mental health care practice arenas. Our models of practice and intervention approaches are highly congruent with current demands for cost-effective, quality, consumer-oriented treatment emphasizing community integration, functional outcomes, and quality of life.

The chapters in this section emphasize the unique ability of occupational therapists to respond constructively and in a proactive manner to sociopolitical trends and professional challenges influencing the mental health care system. Donalda Ellek begins this section with an historical review of mental health public policy. She discusses the economic, social, and political factors that influenced major mental health care policy initiatives. Institutionalization, deinstitutionalization, community-based care, and community support programs are the four major policies defined and discussed. Ellek provides a thoughtful analysis of the values, benefits, and limits of each of these historical public policy initiatives.

Changes within current models of care and organizational structures are explored in the next chapter by Marie Gage. As Gage notes, traditional roles within the administrative structures of many hospitals have been disrupted with positions being lost, renamed, and/or reengineered. New management structures and new models of care are continually evolving. The effects of this evolution on occupational therapy is a frequent topic of discussion with its future implications being the source of great debate. Gage analyzes these changes and concludes that the paradigm shift in health care is actually pushing the system towards models of care that are more congruent with occupational therapy philosophy and practices than those of the traditional medical model. She provides a persuasive argument that occupational therapy can not only survive these changes but actually thrive because occupational therapists can best provide what the "new" system is seeking; that is, holistic client-centered care which improves function. The opportunity for occupational therapists to provide professional leadership during this change process is great for we have a wealth of experience in client-centered practice. We can use our knowledge and skills to design and develop new systems of care that support holistic care. Gage provides clear, concise, and specific suggestions for action and urges occupational therapists to "recruit" these professional development opportunities and not wait to be asked!

A positive perspective on the potential for occupational therapists to respond effectively to the changing health care system by expanding our roles beyond traditional medical models is also presented in Chapter 3. Gail Fidler argues that the current, shorter lengths of inpatient treatment stays require occupational therapists to expand their professional view beyond the hospital walls into the community. She poses a series of questions that challenge therapists to assess their values, opinions and practice in response to the demands of the changing health care system. Suggestions for ensuring continuity of care, multidisciplinary team collaboration, and role clarification are provided to assist readers in effectively meeting "the challenge of change."

Strategies for effectively meeting the immediate and pressing challenges resulting from the implementation of managed care in mental health are provided in the next chapter by Betsy Van Leit. She begins by reviewing the historical development and evolution of managed mental health care. Issues specific to societal stigma and the chronicity of pervasive mental illness and the subsequent client reliance on public sector care are discussed. Concerns regarding the similarities between the stated goals of managed care and the failed realities of deinstitutionalization are realistically explored. The challenges and opportunities of this evolving and rapidly changing mental health system of care are presented. Her discussion focuses on the importance of measuring functional outcomes and the effectiveness of intervention, the need to identify and develop guidelines for best practice, the use of interdisciplinary teams, and the ethical dilemmas presented by managed care practice. Although these issues present many challenges to the future of occupational therapy practice, Van Leit contends that occupational therapists who are visible, accountable and assertive in defining and developing a continuum of services and who are vocal and vigorous advocates for health care reform can be effective innovators for quality mental health care.

The development of proactive roles for occupational therapists working in the evolving mental health care system is a theme that is explored further in this text. In-depth presentations on program development, implementation, and evaluation across the entire mental health continuum of care are provided in subsequent chapters. Readers are encouraged to analyze their own views about the challenges of the current health care system and their effect on the profession of occupational therapy. It is hoped that readers will adopt the proactive stance of this section's authors and seize the opportunities that the current health care system is affording occupational therapy practitioners. Our profession's traditional emphasis on the holistic development of functional living skills enables us to become leaders in the provision of quality mental health services now, and well into the 21st century (Fine, 1996; Frese, 1998; Peloquin, 1996).

QUESTIONS TO CONSIDER

1. How have policy initiatives influenced the nature and scope of mental health service delivery? What are the implications of the different sociopolitical value systems identified by Ellek on patient care and occupational therapy practice?

2. What are current trends and issues affecting the mental health care system? How do these trends and issues impact the role of occupational therapy in acute care settings? In community mental health? In long-term institutions? In home care? In school settings?

3. How can occupational therapists effectively adapt to these health care trends and professional role changes in a manner that is consistent with occupational therapy frames of reference/models of practice? What professional knowledge and skills can occupational therapists uniquely offer to develop proactive roles for themselves in the changing mental health care system?

4. What are the implications of current issues and trends in mental health practice for occupational therapy evaluation and intervention? How can occupational therapy's evaluation procedures and intervention methods be realistically adapted within the context of these changes and in a manner congruent with occupational therapy's philosophical base?

5. How will occupational therapy be viewed in the 21st century? What steps can occupational therapists take to ensure that our profession attains and maintains a leadership role in the provision of quality care across the mental health continuum?

REFERENCES

Ascher-Svanum, H., & Krause, A. A. (1991). *Psychoeducational groups for patients with schizophrenia.* Rockville, MD: Aspen Publishers.

Baum, C. (1991). Professional issues in a changing environment. In C. Christiansen & C. Baum (Eds.), *Occupational therapy: Overcoming human performance deficits* (pp. 805-817). Thorofare, NJ: SLACK Incorporated.

Fine, S. (1996). The future of mental health practice. In M. Brinson & K. Kannenburg (Eds.), *Mental health service delivery guidelines.* Bethesda, MD: American Occupational Therapy Association.

Frese, F. J. (1998). Occupational therapy and mental illness: A personal view. *Mental Health Special Interest Section Quarterly, 21*(3), 1-3.

Kielhofner, G. & Burke, J. P. (1977). Occupational therapy after 60 years: An account of changing identity and knowledge. *American Journal of Occupational Therapy, 31,* 675-689.

Peloquin, S. (1996). Occupational therapy service: Individual and collective understanding of the founders. In R. P. Cottrell (Ed.), *Perspectives on purposeful activity: Foundation and future of occupational therapy* (pp. 5-26). Bethesda, MD: American Occupational Therapy Association.

Woods, W. (1998). Nationally speaking: Is it jump time for occupational therapy? *American Journal of Occupational Therapy, 52,* 403-411.

CHAPTER ONE

The Evolution of Fairness in Mental Health Policy

Donalda Ellek

This chapter was previously published in the American Journal of Occupational Therapy, 45, *947-951. Copyright* © *1991, The American Occupational Therapy Association, Inc.*

Anyone who is involved in health policy, whether as a patient, a health professional, a payer, or an administrator, has at some time experienced feelings about the fairness of a policy. Policies stir intense controversy about who is getting what benefits from a policy, and why. The purpose of this (chapter) is to examine fairness in mental health policy as it has evolved over several decades. Because the mental health system has been heavily dependent on public funds and public policy, especially for those persons with the most chronic and severe mental illness, this discussion will be limited to public policy in mental health.

States differ in the quality of mental health care and the amount of money earmarked for mental health, but the intent of mental health policy from one state to another is strikingly similar. Thus, the fairness of mental health policy can be discussed as a national issue. Those policies that have been applied in every state throughout the United States are broadly described as institutionalization, deinstitutionalization and community-based care, and the community support program.

Many groups of people have a role in the development of policy, as well as a personal stake in its outcome. Professionals in the mental health field have traditionally been advocates for patients' interests, but also have spoken for the economic and political interests of their various professions. The government must advocate for the interests of society as a whole, consider the effect of policies on persons with mental illness as a particular group within society, and be responsive to particular lobbies. In recent years, persons with mental illness and their families have formed organizations and have begun to advocate for their interests in mental health policy. Rarely do all interested parties benefit equally from a policy; often, benefits are realized by one group over another, and some groups may suffer a loss.

The fairness of the allocation of benefits can be viewed from the perspective of theories of social justice, which present reasons for, or explanations of, how the benefits and losses that occur in a society should be allocated and, most importantly, why they should be allocated in a particular way. As might be expected, the why reflects a value system of what is important in society (Veatch, 1981). These value systems are very different from one another, and I think they are the crux of controversy about health policy.

An analysis of major mental health policy initiatives (i.e., institutionalization, deinstitutionalization and community-based care, and the community support program) shows that mental health policy does not share one common underlying theory of justice. Rather, policy development has been an evolutionary process in which the particular interests of persons with mental illness have been addressed differently at various stages.

INSTITUTIONALIZATION

Prior to the 20th century, there was widespread belief that mental illness was due to possession by the devil or to immorality. In either case, it was viewed as an uncontrollable phenomenon to which the individual's own weakness contributed. People were fearful that the person with mental illness would cause physical harm to others or in some way negatively influence their morality. This fear was perhaps the most basic reason why persons with mental illness were extruded from society and locked in poorhouses and jails against their will. In essence, institutionalization was viewed as a method of protecting society from the physical harm and moral wrongdoing of persons with mental illness (Mechanic, 1969).

Around the mid-1800s, social reformers began advocating that persons with mental illness be treated more humanely, pointing out that the state could provide care more efficiently in large institutions than communities were providing it in poorhouses and jails. Thus, by 1900, state governments had assumed responsibility for persons with mental illness (Greenberg & Archer, 1979).

Institutionalization of persons with mental illness provided several benefits:

a. society was protected from the physical harm it was feared persons with mental illness would inflict;

b. treatment offered the potential of a cure along with the potential future economic benefits of a healthy and productive member of society; and

c. economies of scale could be realized through the provision of care in large institutions where it could be handled en masse with personnel working to their fullest capacity.

The fairness of institutionalizing persons with mental illness can be best explained by a utilitarian concept of justice. Utilitarian theory evaluates social actions strictly in terms of their impact on general human welfare (Veatch, 1981). If society is happier or has increased "utility," the policy is fair. Certainly, the general society seemed to benefit from institutionalization. From its perspective, it was being protected from the dangerousness of persons with mental illness.

However, utilitarianism also generally places a great value on individual liberty; thus, institutionalization seems to conflict with utilitarianism. While society was protecting its safety, it was depriving persons with mental illness of liberty. But the utilitarian doctrine accounts for this. John Stuart Mill, a utilitarian philosopher, wrote:

> The sole end for which mankind are warranted, individually or collectively, in interfering with the liberty of action of any of their number is self-protection.
>
> That the only purpose for which power can be rightfully exercised over any member of a civilized community, against his will is to prevent harm to others. (Mill, 1956, pp. 72-73)

Thus, if members of society believed they were in danger from persons with mental illness, they were just in depriving those persons of their liberty.

The harm principle is a widely accepted principle to limit liberty, but its extensive applicability to persons with mental illness is doubtful. In some cases, it is true that persons diagnosed as mentally ill are dangerous and present a serious threat of physical harm to others. It does not follow, though, that every mentally ill person poses a threat to others. Studies have shown either that mentally ill people, as a group, are no more dangerous than others or that, if they are, the differences are so small that they allow little success in predicting dangerousness.

This harm principle, then, has limited applicability to persons with mental illness, at least in the present day. It might be asked if it was fair to apply the harm principle in previous times, when society believed that persons with mental illness were dangerous. Because society had to decide based on the information available at that time, it was fair to apply the harm principle. It did not conflict with the principle of liberty as explained under utilitarianism.

In later years, the perceived dangerousness of persons with mental illness diminished somewhat, but institutionalization remained with the argument that persons with mental illness could not care for themselves and often were not rational enough to determine their own best interests. This protec-

tion of persons with mental illness fits within fairness under the utilitarian concept because mentally ill persons are not able to look after themselves. In assigning a high value to individual liberty, the utilitarians also define instances in which paternalistic intervention is appropriate, in order to bring the greatest good to the greatest number.

Another factor that figured into the welfare of society is the economic cost of providing care for persons with mental illness. These costs were paid by society through taxes. However, society attached great value to having the objectionable behavior of persons with mental illness removed from society's view. In this respect, while institutionalization generated cost, it also generated benefits equal to the value of the non-pecuniary cost no longer imposed on society by the behavior of persons with mental illness. Thus, institutionalization was just, according to utilitarian doctrine, because it protected society, provided certain economic gains over the non-system of care in communities, and benefited society overall.

DEINSTITUTIONALIZATION AND COMMUNITY-BASED CARE

During the 1950s, several factors coincided, beginning a policy of deinstitutionalizing seriously mentally ill (then called chronically mentally ill) patients, discharging them to live in the community and receive care on an outpatient basis. An important factor that spurred this policy change was the burgeoning population of mentally ill people and the increasing economic strain on the states to maintain psychiatric patients in state hospitals (Rose, 1979). Also, the development of psychotropic medications was advancing, making it possible to better control the overt symptomatology of mental illness. This made it more possible for patients to live in the community. Another important factor was that the federal government became aware of a national problem presented by psychiatric illness when 1.75 million Americans were rejected for service during World War II (Greene, 1984). This prompted Congress to pass the National Mental Health Act of 1946 (Pub. L. No. 79-487). This act established the National Institute of Mental Health (NIMH), which served as a major advocate of mental health care on a national level (U.S. Department of Health and Human Services, 1980).

For several years, there was controversy over government's role in mental health care and whether federal funds should be directed toward preventive, acute, or chronic care. In 1961, President Kennedy appointed a committee to study the federal role in mental health care. The committee came up with the community mental health plan, which led to the Community Mental Health Centers Act of 1963 (Pub. L. No. 88-164). Through this act, the federal government provided funding to establish community mental health centers (Bachrach, 1983).

Pub. L. No. 88-164 was enacted with a wide base of support and seemed to have the potential to give something to everyone. It was expected to increase the accessibility and availability of mental health services to the public; expand the professional area of psychiatrists and other mental health professionals into primary prevention; and decrease the costs associated with state hospital care (Rose, 1979). It also was expected to benefit persons with serious mental illness by reintegrating them into the community where they could, with the aid of medication, live more independently and participate meaningfully in community life. The community mental health centers and the state hospitals were expected to function together to provide a broad array of services (Bachrach, 1983).

In a short time, many problems began to surface. Because of the funding structure of Pub. L. No. 88-164, community mental health centers could be federally funded and operate independently of state hospitals and state mental health authorities. Because no economic link existed between them, no communication link developed (Clarke, 1979). Patients were discharged from state hospitals, but their linkage to a community mental health center was tenuous. Even when seriously mentally ill patients were linked to a community mental health center, few services were designed to meet their needs.

In addition to the lack of community-based services for seriously mentally ill patients, legal issues further tested the treatment of these persons. Legal cases were increasingly concluding that serious deprivation of liberty (i.e., hospitalization) could only be justified if adequate treatment was given. This principle was known as the "right to treatment." The economic implication was that more effective demand (by the courts) for better quality care, with no shifts in available supply, raised the costs of care to the states. Along with the right to treatment, another ruling essentially said that a person should be deprived of liberty only to the extent absolutely necessary. Thus, patients hospitalized either voluntarily or involuntarily could demand to be treated in the least restrictive environment. All of these legal rulings created an effective demand for community-based care.

As a result of these political and legal developments, it became increasingly apparent that the state hospitals had not developed after-care services and that community mental health centers were focused on prevention and acute care. This meant that chronic patients being discharged into the community were not receiving necessary services.

In reviewing the long, complicated history of the deinstitutionalization and community-based care policy initiative, one is faced with the question of who benefited from the policies and whether their benefit was fair. The state governments seemed to have benefited economically overall. Several studies suggest that, after considering all costs (i.e., cost shifting between levels of government, the cost of supporting community inpatient services, and state hospital back-up care), the cost of deinstitutionalization was less than that of inpatient care provided through the hospital alone (Buck, 1984; Nash & Argyle, 1984; Rose, 1979). Additionally, the census in state hospitals decreased.

The general public also seemed to benefit in that more psychiatric services were available for persons who needed psychiatric care but were not necessarily severely or chronically mentally ill. Also, mental health professionals grew in number and kind and had opportunities to expand their roles and professional skills.

People with serious mental illness, however, were in a questionable position. Although they gained their liberty, it became clear that many of them were mentally disabled to the extent that they could not provide for their own basic human needs. After-care services were sparse and often did not address their special needs. As a result, some patients had frequent rehospitalizations, some lived in unhealthy or unsafe conditions, and others were in the dubious circumstance of depending entirely on their family members. Persons with serious mental illness essentially traded security for liberty.

The fairness of the deinstitutionalization and community-based care policy initiative can best be explained from the perspective of the Pareto doctrine (Pareto, 1935), which considers an action, or policy, to be fair if no one is worse off. Another important element of the Pareto doctrine is that each person is the sole determiner of his or her own welfare. However, this concept is based on the premise that all rational people seek to maximize their welfare.

Persons with mental illness clearly did not express any particular interests to spur the policy initiative, and it is debatable whether they would be considered rational enough to do so. However, advocates for these persons served as spokespersons, advocating liberty as the goal. Liberty was achieved. Persons with serious mental illness received the benefit of liberty, but gave up some security. The fact that they benefited the least of all interested parties is insignificant under the Pareto doctrine.

COMMUNITY SUPPORT PROGRAM

The NIMH developed the community support program in 1977 as a policy initiative aimed specifically at improving the quality of life for the chronically and severely mentally ill people who were deinstitutionalized and living in the community. The community support program provided funding for states to set up a community support system, which was intended to address the comprehensive needs of persons with serious mental illness and drew on elements from the medical rehabilitation and social support models of care (Stroul, 1984).

The 10 essential components of a community support system were as follows:

1. Identification of the target population
2. Assistance in applying for entitlements
3. Crisis stabilization in the least restrictive environment
4. Psychosocial rehabilitation services
5. Supportive services of indefinite duration
6. Medical and mental health care
7. Backup support to families, friends, and community members
8. Involvement of concerned community members

9. Protection of clients' rights
10. Case management (Turner & Ten Hoor, 1978).

The community support system model was flexible in that implementation was not prescribed; every state was expected to implement it according to their own particular needs, circumstances, and resources (Stroul, 1984).

Legal rulings, coupled with public moral outrage, seemed to have prompted the community support program initiative. As mentally ill people lived in the community, the public could see the deplorable living conditions of many of them. The public media also began to expose the plight of persons with mental illness. The low level of benefits received by persons with serious mental illness, in comparison to the much greater benefits received by others, was obviously unjust, and public opinion was that the deinstitutionalization and community-based care policy was unsatisfactory.

Another factor might be at least equally important in explaining how interest in the community support program initiative was generated. The legal rulings regarding civil commitment, the right to treatment in the least restrictive setting, and the right to refuse treatment all stood as rights to be asserted by persons with serious mental illness. These rulings provided a legal mandate to the public sector to develop services that respect patients' rights.

The Omnibus Reconciliation Act of 1981 (Pub. L. No. 97-35) combined formerly categorical grant programs and established block grants to states (Nash & Argyle, 1984). This resulted in a reduction of the federal contribution to mental health care by approximately 25% (Buck, 1984). However, state mental health departments did not abandon their commitment to provide service to persons with serious mental illness as a priority population (Jerrell & Larsen, 1985).

The disappointment with the community mental health center concept and its failure to provide service to persons with serious mental illness, as contrasted with the community support program and its particular attention to persons with serious mental illness, raises an interesting issue. Community mental health centers were equally available and accessible to all categories of mentally ill people. That is, any mentally ill person who went to a community mental health center and requested service could theoretically receive service (assuming he or she lived in the catchment area and was able to use the services that were offered). In this sense, there was equal access and availability. What really seemed to hinder the provision of services to persons with serious mental illness was a lack of consideration for their special needs. For example, these persons often were not capable of following the intake procedures of the community mental health center, such as making and keeping an appointment. They also spent a great deal of effort attending to their basic needs, which could preclude their ability to participate in traditional therapeutic regimens. In this sense, access and availability were equal but not equitable, because persons with serious mental illness did not have the same capacity as the general population to seek services in a community mental health center.

The Rawlsian concept of justice (also referred to as the egalitarian concept of social justice) accounts for inequities of opportunity (Rawls, 1971). The Rawlsian concept of justice is that those persons with the greatest need should benefit the most, and the allocation of benefits should be available in consideration of equal opportunity, or ability, to seek potential benefits. Those persons not able to seek benefits should be given additional help. Thus, a policy such as the community support program, which gives special consideration to persons with serious mental illness, would be fair under the Rawlsian concept of social justice.

In contrast to the Rawlsian theory of justice, the Pareto theory, which could explain deinstitutionalization and community-based care, does not consider the individual's initial level of welfare, or his or her ability to use established procedures.

CONCLUSION

The mental health policy initiatives have been formed by interdependent economic, social, and political factors. Social factors that have affected mental health policy have sometimes been specific to mental health, such as perceptions and public attitudes toward mental illness and definitions of mental illness. However, these social factors usually operate in tandem with broader social factors. The decade of Pub. L. No. 88-164 (late 1960s and early 1970s) illustrates this point because it was marked by public disappointment in and distrust of government and a movement toward social change across many aspects of society. During that time, systems changed to promote public welfare. The Social Security Amendments of 1965 (Pub. L. No. 89-97) were enacted, and court decisions affirmed the rights of persons with mental illness. The mental health system, by advancing the rights of persons with mental illness, participated in the activism to promote social change.

Once social change is in the air, the political process responds. Special interest groups want to be sure that their best interests are considered during a time of change; often, public interest takes a secondary position to the narrower interests of politicians and others in the policy-making arena as they pursue economic benefits and personal power. Thus, the political process shapes an idea for change to suit the diverse needs of the most powerful segments of society. In this way, social factors can lose some of their strength in creating change.

Economic factors also enter into the mental health care policy-making process as either constraints or opportunities. The crisis in state hospital care that led to deinstitutionalization was presented as an economic problem created by a rising census and overcrowding. The economy of scale of large institutions was outstripped. The solution to this economic problem was either to allocate more funds to state mental hospitals, and thus increase the supply of services, or to decrease the use of services (i.e., decrease demand), and so decrease the cost of mental health care to the states. The choice was made to decrease the use of state mental hospital services.

Social justice reflects the values of society at a given point in time. These values are most directly expressed as public opinion and social movements for change. The political process responds to these values but tempers them and determines the specifications of policy.

The fairness of mental health policy has evolved with these social, political, and economic factors. It evolved from the institutionalization policy of the mid-1800s, when society's idea of fairness was providing the greatest good to the greatest number of people, through the deinstitutionalization and community-based care era of the 1960s and 1970s, when society thought everyone could benefit to some degree and fairness meant that no one should lose, to the 1980s, when society began dealing with perceived limitations in resources and designated special populations to receive greater benefits. This latter policy perspective aims to address issues of equity in addition to issues of equality.

Whether or not a policy is fair is still a matter of values at a particular point in time, in the context of social, political, and economic factors. One particular social justice theory cannot always be fair under all circumstances. However, social justice theories are useful in explaining the most common perspectives on fairness. Society has appeared to formulate mental health policy within social justice theories of one kind or another as society's values and circumstances have evolved.

REFERENCES

Bachrach, L. (1983). An overview of deinstitutionalization. *New Directions for Mental Health Services, 17*, 5-14.

Buck, J. (1984). Block grants and federal promotion of community mental health services, 1946-65. *Community Mental Health Journal, 20*(3), 236-247.

Clarke, G. (1979). In defense of deinstitutionalization. *Milbank Memorial Fund Quarterly/Health and Society, 57*(4), 461-479.

Community Mental Health Centers Act of 1963 (Public Law 88-164).

Greene, B. (1984). Evolving mental health policy. *Journal of Health Administration Education, 2*(2), 193-220.

Greenberg, E., & Archer, J. (1979). Abandonment of responsibility for the seriously mentally ill. *Milbank Memorial Fund Quarterly/ Health and Society, 57*(4), 485-505.

Jerrell, J., & Larsen, J. (1985). Policy and organizational changes in state mental health systems. *Administration in Mental Health 12*(3), 184 -191.

Mechanic, D. (1969). *Mental health and social policy.* Englewood Cliffs, NJ: Prentice Hall.

Mill, J. S. (1956). *On liberty.* New York, NY: Liberal Arts Press.

Nash, M., & Argyle, N. (1984). Services for the mentally ill: A reversal in federal policy. *Administration in Mental Health, 11*(4), 263-276.

National Mental Health Act of 1946 (Public Law 79-487).

Omnibus Reconciliation Act of 1981 (Public Law 97-35). 42 U.S.C., §1396.

Pareto, V. (1935). *The mind and society: A treatise on general sociology.* New York, NY: Dover.

Rawls, J. A. (1971). *A theory of justice.* Cambridge, MA: Harvard University Press.

Rose, S. (1979). Deciphering deinstitutionalization: Complexities in policy and program analysis. *Milbank Memorial Fund Quarterly/ Health and Society, 57*(4), 429-459.

Social Security Amendments of 1965 (Public Law 89-97).

Stroul, B. (1984). *Toward community support systems for the mentally disabled.* Rockville, MD: National Institute of Mental Health.

Turner, J., & Ten Hoor, W. (1978). The NlMH community support program: Pilot approach to a needed social reform. *Schizophrenia Bulletin, 4*(3), 319-344.

U.S. Department of Health and Human Services. (1980). *Toward a national plan for the chronically mentally ill.* Washington, DC: U.S. Government Printing Office.

Veatch, R. M. (1981). *A theory of medical ethics.* New York, NY: Basic.

CHAPTER TWO

Reengineering of Health Care: Opportunity or Threat for Occupational Therapists?

Marie Gage

This chapter was previously published in the Canadian Journal of Occupational Therapy, 62, *197-207, and is reprinted here with permission of CAOT Publications ACE © 1993.*

The health care system is responding to a paradigm shift from the industrial era to the knowledge society. The rapidly changing administrative structures of some hospitals and increasing numbers of proposals for new models of care are disconcerting for therapists who are used to working in traditional organizational structures and models of care. However, with a broader understanding of the shift that is occurring, it becomes apparent that this paradigm shift is pushing the system toward care practices that are more consistent with occupational therapy practices than those of the traditional medical model. This (chapter) describes the factors influencing the direction of the paradigm shift, the major emerging models of care and organizational structures associated with the paradigm shift, and then discusses the issue of whether the paradigm shift presents a threat or a challenge to occupational therapists.

"We are beginning to see a return to large scale thinking, to general theory, to the putting the pieces back together again. For it is beginning to dawn on us that our obsessive emphasis on quantified detail without context, on progressively finer and finer measurement of smaller and smaller problems leaves us knowing more and more about less and less" (Tofler, 1981, p. l46).

Organizational changes in health care settings are becoming a common phenomenon; a phenomenon that is creating stress for many therapists and is the subject of much debate and discussion. The traditional management model where members of a given discipline are clustered in a department directed by a member of that discipline is fast falling out of favor. In addition, the health care literature is full of articles suggesting new ways to design health care delivery systems, some of which advocate for crosstraining or for the development of generic health care workers. The changes in health care are being made in response to a global paradigm shift,

from the industrial era to the knowledge society (Drucker, 1993). The nature of this shift is captured by Tofler's quote (Drucker, 1933; Tofler, 1981).

The changes in organizational structure and care delivery systems, which are a direct result of this paradigm shift, may at first appear to threaten the integrity of the discipline of occupational therapy. However, with a better understanding of the factors that are driving these changes it becomes clear that the system is adopting practices that are consistent with long standing occupational therapy practice patterns. Thus, rather than presenting a threat, the health care paradigm shift presents an opportunity for occupational therapists to provide professional leadership in the change process.

In this (chapter) the factors that are driving the changes in health care are examined. Subsequently, four major models of care that are emerging in response to these factors and the rebound effect that these models of care are having on organizational structures will be examined. Finally, the issue of whether these changes present an opportunity or threat to occupational therapists will be discussed.

The health care literature contains four different descriptors, of the recipient of health care services, which are often used interchangeably: patient, client, consumer, and customer. For the sake of consistency the term *client* will be used throughout this (chapter) even when the source documents contain the term patient, customer, or consumer. It is beyond the scope of this (chapter) to attempt to resolve the ongoing debate about which term is the best choice, however, the interested reader is referred to Herzberg (1990) and Patterson and Marks (1992) for examples of competing positions.

Please note that the one exception to the use of the term client is when the term *patient* is used as a proper noun (i.e., the name of a model of care).

INFLUENCING FACTORS

Historical

Prior to the 17th century, the manner in which an individual experienced an illness was the major source of information for the physician prescribing the treatment (Reiser, 1993). In the 17th century an English physician, Thomas Sydenham, began to notice patterns to the symptoms of his clients. Thus began the process of categorizing illness into diagnostic groupings. As the process of classification became more entrenched in medical practice, over the ensuing centuries, the idiosyncratic symptoms experienced by some clients were virtually ignored. The client's personal experience with the disease was no longer an important variable in the prescription of a management program.

The technological revolution of the 19th and 20th centuries provided a means by which the physician's diagnosis could be objectively confirmed (Reiser, 1993). As diagnostic technology improved, the reliance on objective data became the norm and what could not be confirmed through testing procedures was virtually ignored or considered to be psychosomatic. "Developing a portrait of a medical problem was increasingly less the province of the [client] and more the prerogative of the physician (Reiser, 1993, p. 1013)." As the practice of medicine became more bound by the rules of scientific inquiry, the art of healing began to fall by the wayside (Buckman & Sabbagh, 1993). Clients became dissatisfied with medicine's emphasis on curing through science and began seeking clinicians who practiced healing through alternative forms of medicine.

The same technological revolution, which enabled objective measurement of disease, gave physicians the power to prolong life through the use of advanced technology. Beginning in the 1950s, health workers began to be faced with ethical decisions that could not be answered by the application of their diagnostic tools. Some of these ethical dilemmas related to an inability to offer new technology to all clients due to funding shortfalls, while other dilemmas related to the prolongation of life when quality of life could not be guaranteed. Ethicists discovered that public opinion and the clients' experience of their illnesses were two important factors for the resolution of these ethical dilemmas (Reiser, 1993).

Parallel to the medical ethics movement, the consumer and human rights movements began to change the public's expectations of its role in health care decision-making, their rights to give informed consent, and their right to act as autonomous beings (Reiser, 1993). These expectations further enhanced the need for health care workers to attend the individual's experience of illness and led in the 1980s to the proliferation of measures of client expectations and client satisfaction.

The technological revolution has also given today's health care client better access to health care information than ever before (Drunker, 1993). This information enables the client to question the knowledge of health care professionals in a way that was unheard of a mere 30 years ago.

Thus, today's health care client is often well informed, expects to be privy to health care information and to be a part of the decision-making process, understands his or her rights as a consumer, and is dissatisfied with the discrepant information received from various health care professionals. There is a growing expectation that clients will be treated as individuals and that their individual experience of their condition will be understood. There is a growing demand that health care services meet the needs of health care clients, as defined by the health care client. Thus, work reporting the needs of the health care client is beginning to appear in the literature.

Client Needs

It is surprisingly difficult to find literature that examines the needs of health care clients from the perspective of the client rather than that of the professional. This gap in our knowledge base reflects the historical assumption that the professional is the expert and knows what is best for the client. Thus, needs have always been defined by the professional, not the client (Silberman, 1992).

In response to a recognized need for information about the needs of clients, as perceived by the client, the Picker/Commonwealth Program for Patient Centered Care began a systematic exploration of client needs. Beginning in 1987, researchers associated with this group ran focus groups, developed a survey based on the expressed needs of focus group participants, applied this survey across the United States, and visited facilities that scored well and those that scored poorly. The results of this work are now available in a book titled *Through the Patient's Eyes* (Gerteis, Edgman & Levitan, Daley, & Delbanco, 1993).

Essentially, the Picker/Commonwealth Program found that clients do not focus on prettier rooms and better hotel services (Delbanco, 1992), as is suggested by some reengineering experts. Instead, what is important to clients is that they are treated like individuals, can trust that their providers are competent and that their care is coordinated effectively, receive meaningful information, have their pain controlled, and receive emotional support to help them deal with their fears. They want their families involved in their care and decision-making, and finally, expect their needs for information and care post-discharge to be met (Gerteis et al., 1993).

Another source of information about client-defined needs comes from a review of client accounts of their journey through the health care system. These accounts validate the Picker/Commonwealth list of client needs. Stories such as that of Little Mountain, an Indian child who suffered massive damage after receiving her immunization at 2 months, serve to illustrate the failings of a system that is provider-centered (Goodwater, 1993). Little Mountain's parents were forced to become advocates for her care due to a system that failed to recognize the different needs of a family living on an Indian reserve; a system that did not recognize the individual values and beliefs of the client and failed to provide integrated services. Comfort was received only through a ceremony conducted by the tribal medicine man. Similar stories are found in the books *Laugh, I Thought I'd Die* (Kaye, 1993) and *The Body Silent* (Murphy, 1990), along with many others.

Summary

The factors that are influencing the emergence of a new health care paradigm have already begun to have an impact on the design of services, as is evidenced by the sheer number of articles appearing in the health care literature that are related to new models of care. Understanding the factors that are influencing change in the health care system results in a better understanding of the desired outcome of the health care change process. It is concluded that to be successful, a new health care model must result in a new, more balanced relationship between the health care professional and client, must emphasize healing rather than science, and must recognize the needs, values, and beliefs of each client, from the perspective of the client, as central to the design process. In addition, the model must be structured to facilitate outcome measurement related to the total process of care, not the outcome of each separate discipline.

The traditional way of organizing professionals into departments is considered to be a barrier to the development of outcome measures that go beyond the scope of practice of each separate discipline. Thus the next sections of this (chapter) will review both the new models of care that are emerging and the changes in organizational reporting relationships associated with these new models of care.

EMERGING MODELS OF CARE

Client-Centered Care

There has been a proliferation of articles dealing with the implementation of client-centered care. However, the term client-centered is not consistently used to describe one homogeneous form of provider/client relationship. The term is broadly applied to any model that centers care around what are believed to be the client's needs. In fact, this term has been used to describe:

- changing the physical environment so that it is more welcoming or home-like for the client (Lumsdon, 1993);
- changing the roles and responsibilities of workers so that the clients receive good "hotel" services during their admission (O'Malley, 1992; Stewart-Amidei, 1992);
- paying more attention to what the client has to say (Kerr & Birk, 1988; Smith & Hoppe, 1991)
- forming relationships with clients that could be described as partnerships (Ahmann & Bond, 1992; Braddy & Gray, 1987; Friesen & Koroloff, 1990; Roter, 1987)

- putting the client in charge of the decision making (Brown & Ringma, 1989; Larrson, Svardsudd, Wedd, & Saljo, 1992; Leviton, Mueller, & Kauffman, 1992; Wilson, 1985)

Thus, the term client-centered has many different meanings and a different model of care associated with each meaning.

When examining the client-centered literature, it is interesting to note that literature dealing with models of care for children is quite different from that which deals with client-centered adult care. The pediatric literature, often labeled family-centered care, advocates for empowering models of service delivery that create partnerships or place control in the hands of the family of the minor child. Family-centered care articles never suggest that the new model of care should concentrate on improving the appearance or "hotel" services of the facility: family-centered care articles always emphasize the change in the balance of power between the client and provider.

Moloney and Paul (1993) provide some insight into the difference between the pediatric and adult literature. They state that it is a product of the expectations of the baby boom generation who are the parents of the children receiving services. They state: "The formative experiences of the baby boom generation have been the civil rights movement, feminism, the Vietnam War, Watergate, and the information explosion" (p. 285). As a result, this generation has an expectation of control and involvement and less respect for authority and conformity.

The health care needs of the baby boomers have been predominantly related to giving birth or caring for their children. The vast changes in birthing practices and pediatric units reflect the impact of this generation's lobbying on the design of health care services. In general, obstetric and pediatric health care systems empower clients to form partnerships with health care professionals in the design of health care. As the baby boomers age and begin to require adult health care services, the same impact is likely to be felt. Hence, it may be reasonable to assume that the term client-centered, when applied to adult services of the future, will consistently refer to the empowerment of the client through partnerships and client control. However, the current differential use of the term client-centered has rendered the term meaningless. The number of distinct uses of the term client-centered makes it impossible to present evaluation information on any one client-centered model of practice.

Patient-Focused Care

The term patient is being used in this section due to its use in this model as part of the proper name of the model. While the term patient-focused may appear to be just another form of client-centered care, it is important to note that Patient-Focused Care Units are a unique type of unit that is quickly infiltrating many organizations, resulting in major changes to organizational reporting relationships and staff job functions. Patient-Focused Care Units were first developed by

Booz Allen Health Inc. due to a recognition that hospitals must focus on the needs of patients if they are to survive (Lathrop, Seafert, MacDonald, & Martin, 1991). An analysis of current hospital operations led to the following findings:

- only 16% of the hospital budget went to direct patient care
- documentation activities accounted for 30% of clinical time
- it was not uncommon for 10 or more staff to interact with a patient without the patient even leaving his/her room
- caregivers were often forced to compete for the patient's time in order to deliver services
- many procedures occur because they have always been done that way rather than as a result of rational thought
- booking patients for routine procedures was an operational nightmare with many steps in the procedure where errors that cause delays could occur

Thus the patient-focused model of care was developed with the following operating principles:

- documentation procedures must be streamlined and simplified
- routine services would be placed closer to the patient even if this meant duplication of equipment and space
- caregiver qualifications would be broadened through cross–training in order to decrease the number of different people the patient must interact with and to decrease the chance of error, or service delay, due to the complex process of communication
- processes would be simplified
- variability in the patient population would be decreased by grouping like patients on one unit

Decreasing the number of personnel involved with each patient and increasing the skill set of each employee through cross-training appears to make intuitive sense to health administrators, as is evidenced by the proliferation of literature documenting the implementation of Patient-Focused Care Units (Bowers & McNally, 1983; Brider, 1992; Curran, 1992; Sherer, 1993; Stewart-Amidei, 1992). In addition, Lathrop, et al. (1991) indicates that there is high staff and patient satisfaction with this model. However, once again the studies are not scientifically rigorous and there is no evidence that the satisfaction level of patients is greater than previous satisfaction levels, although decreases in staff turnover rates do indicate increased staff satisfaction (Brider, 1992; Lathrop et al., 1991). Curran (1992) cautions interested administrators to consider the high cost of implementing this system of care. He credits the high cost of implementing Patient-Focused Care Units, estimated to be 1 million dollars per unit, to the need to install diagnostic equipment on each unit and cross-train staff. The cost of cross-training the personnel is also an ongoing expense to the organization. One facility notes that staff of the new unit had to be relieved of their normal duties for 6 to 8 weeks to participate in cross-training that would allow nurses to perform lab and diagnostic procedures. Due to the low volume of each of the cross-trained procedures per nurse quarterly, updates and enhanced quality monitoring

procedures became necessary (Brider, 1992). It is important to note that the issue of cross-training of professional functions has not been addressed in this model. The cross-training recommended by Lathrop, et al. (1991), deals only with support and technical diagnostic procedures. It must be understood that this model emerged from a management review, not in response to expressed patient needs.

Case Management Model

Finding one's way through the health care system and gaining access to needed services can be a difficult and sometimes impossible task for a person suffering from an illness. The Case Management Model emerged in response to the need for a client advocate: someone who will help the client define his or her needs and access appropriate services in a timely fashion (Kerr & Birk, 1988; Rose, 1991; Weinstein, 1991).

There is not just one case management model. The underlying principle of one primary person interacting with the client is consistent for all models. From there the process of care begins to vary. In some Case Management situations the case manager determines the client's needs and seeks services required. The client is only required to comply with the program established, if he or she wishes to continue to benefit from the program (Kerr & Birk, 1988; Weinstein, 1991). In other case management situations the client plays a more active role in defining his or her needs (Rose, 1991). Once the case manager understands the client's desired outcomes, the case manager investigates available solutions and presents all options to the client with the risks and benefits of each option defined in a way that does not reflect the case manager's personal bias. The client chooses from the available alternatives and the case manager facilitates the initiation of the selected services.

Regardless of the specific process of case management being used there are benefits derived from having a knowledgeable health care worker advocate for the client's needs. It is this success that is leading to a proliferation of uses of case management in a variety of different health care settings. While the roots of the Case Management approach lie in community care, where the client needs to interface with many different agencies, its success has resulted in its application to single agency situations. For example, it is being used to improve the quality of care of complex clients in acute care facilities. Complex acute care clients often move from unit to unit and interface with many different team members. The assignment of a case manager to complex acute care clients provides the client with a consistent person to advocate for their needs as they encounter new health care professionals (Andre et al., 1994). Thus, the process of case management is likely to be a common part of many new models of care.

Client-Driven

The term client-driven, as a descriptor of a model of care, appeared in the literature for the first time in 1986 and with growing frequency in the 90s (Gage, 1994; Gage & Polatajko,

1995; Jenna, 1986; Moxley & Freddolino, 1990; Prehn, 1990; Rose, 1991). Client-driven practice is described as a relationship between the professional and client that places decision-making control in the hands of the client. Operationalization of this intervention model is based on a philosophy of client empowerment and a belief that the perception of the client is the only reality that matters. Assessment procedures in a client-driven setting are different from the traditional assessment model. In a traditional model the client is assessed by the professional, the professional analyzes the data, prepares a treatment plan, and presents it to the client for approval. In a client-driven model, the provider spends time with the client determining what the client expects to achieve through the interaction with the provider and eliciting ideas the client may have about the manner in which this outcome can be achieved. The professional assessment addresses the areas identified by the client and omits areas that may have been automatic parts of the traditional assessment protocol. If the provider believes the client has missed significant areas of concern, this observation is discussed with the client or the client's representative in the case of an incompetent client. The Planetree model is the first example of client-driven practice to appear in the literature.

The Planetree model of health care delivery emerged from the vision of one woman, Angelica Thieriot (Jenna, 1986). Jenna suggests that Thieriot's experiences with the health care system as a client, and as a close relative of two other clients left her frustrated and seeking a better solution. To this end, she gathered a group of resourceful people together who eventually created Project Planetree: a model medical-surgical unit in one San Francisco hospital that is designed to marry humanistic medicine and technology (Orr, 1987). Planetree is the tree under which Hippocrates taught that the melding of mind and body was essential to health.

On the Planetree unit, the degree to which clients assist in their care and participate in decisions about their care is self-determined. A client's decision to be a passive recipient of care is respected. The family is considered to be the client's most valuable resource and thus, they receive encouragement and support as they learn to assist in the physical and emotional care of the client.

The unit functions with an open chart policy and clients are encouraged to add comments to the chart themselves. Sometimes clients are willing to write things they are unable to gain the courage to say. Thus, the staff get to know the client in a way which is not always possible on a more traditional unit.

The Planetree model includes beliefs that food choices should be respected and that a pleasant, home-like environment is conducive to faster recovery. However, the foundation of the Planetree Model is the belief in active client participation, not cosmetic changes to the environment.

Rigorous scientific evaluation of the Planetree unit has not been reported in the literature. However, it is reported to be inexpensive to implement and to be well received by the clients (Jenna, 1986; Orr, 1987). One indicator of client satisfaction is that physicians are being asked by their clients to send them to the Planetree unit. The number of physicians referring clients to the Planetree Unit has grown from 15 to 120 two years after its implementation in 1985 (Orr, 1987). Orr quotes one physician as saying "sharing the responsibility with the client not only made my job more pleasurable but actually improved the quality of care delivered" (Orr, 1987, 39).

Overall, the outcomes associated with client-driven models of care are not yet well-documented in the literature. However, the preliminary findings support the need for further research into the efficacy of client-driven service delivery systems. There is data in the literature related to the efficacy of client control that adds additional support to the belief that client-driven practice is efficacious (England & Evans, 1992; Levine & Greenlick, 1991; Morris & Royle, 1988; Schulman, 1979). Further support for client-driven practice is found in articles that report that clients have different needs than those that health care workers articulate on their behalf (Bartholome, 1992; Batavia & Hammer, 1990; Delbanco, 1992).

Moloney and Paul (1993) in the final chapter of the book *Through the Patient's Eyes* state that the push toward client administered and monitored treatment could "usher in a system in which the patient's values regarding risks and rewards are central to determining the 'appropriate' course of treatment, one in which a treatment's value is gauged in terms of such 'soft' measures as the ability to improve patients' functioning or to relieve pain, anxiety, or depression (p. 296)." Thus, client–driven models of care may be the wave of the future.

Summary of Models of Care

While it may appear that there has been a proliferation of new models of care, they can really be categorized into four types: client-centered, patient-focused, case management, or client-driven. The major thrust of all models is to improve the care for the client; however, each model developer has interpreted the needs of the client differently and has developed a different model to meet the perceived needs of the client. Table 2-1 contains a summary of the four models of care.

ORGANIZATIONAL STRUCTURE

The viability of the traditional departmental organizational structure of health care facilities, where members of a given discipline report to a member of that discipline, is thought to be a barrier to implementation of more holistic health care models (Hassen, 1993). Within the departmental structure, outcome is measured on a discipline by discipline basis with no one being assigned responsibility for ensuring that the total care resulted in the best outcome for the client. New organizational structures, thought to be more in line with models of care that emphasize the meeting of all needs of the client, are becoming popular. Before examining the various new organizational structures one should first understand the history of the current structure.

Table 2-1
Summary of Emerging Models of Care

Item	Client-Centered	Patient-Focused	Case Management	Client-Driven
Perceived need of client	• varies according to the specific use of the term • could be a perceived need for better hotel services, perceived need to center care around identified needs of client, or perceived need to leave control in the hands of the client	• belief that the client should come in contact with fewer different employees during the course of the stay	• belief that the client requires assistance accessing and in some cases identifying the services required	• belief that leaving decision control in the hands of the client will result in better health outcomes
Benefits	• varies according to the specific use of the term • if term is used to indicate a need to explore client perception of need, there is more likely to be beneficial outcome	• client sees fewer new faces and thus, is not as confused about who is who • multiskilling results in less duplication for the patient • good client satisfaction • good staff satisfaction	• client has an advocate that knows his/her particular needs and understands the context of the client's life • if client is encouraged to be active in the assessment and decision making roles he/she is more likely to perceive his/her needs are being met	• client sets and evaluates the outcome of care and thus, is more likely to believe he/she has derived the desired benefit from the interaction •• increased control has been found to be related to better health outcomes
Weaknesses	• depending on application of term, may not meet the health care needs of the client any better than the medical model due to the concentration on environmental factors other than health care needs	• it is still possible to work within the medical model in a patient-focused environment • although there are fewer contacts with different providers, the providers who are in contact with the patient may not interact any differently with the patient than previously	• some forms of case management are still based on the paternalistic medical model and thus, may not change the ability of the system to meet the perceived needs of the client	• some clients may not be ready or able to be responsible for health decisions

The design of the present day health care system was influenced by the industrial era (Goldsmith, 1989). The application of production line thinking, so much a part of the industrial era, to the provision of health care, resulted in the proliferation of health care workers specialized to deal with a narrow area of focus, such as neurologists, neurosurgeons, art therapists, music therapists, respiratory therapists, etc. Although the proliferation of health care specialties facilitated the development of expert knowledge within each specialty, the difficulty coordinating the services of many independent specialists resulted in problems meeting the needs of clients (Gerteis, et al., 1993; Lathrop, et al., 1991).

As society moves into a more holistic era, the importance of understanding the interaction between all of the pieces of specialist knowledge is recognized (Drucker, 1993; Toiler, 1981). There is a move toward organizing work around the holistic needs of the client rather than the individual fields of specialists who are needed to meet these needs. The business literature refers to this as a product or service-line orientation (Van Pelt, 1985). As stated previously, the traditional organizational structure of departments of specialists, each contained within their autonomous department, is falling out of favor and new organizational structures are evolving. A major challenge in the redesign of reporting relationships is the need to maintain the gains brought about by expert knowledge while promoting new working relationships. Drucker (1993) states that the earlier thinking about organizational redesign concentrated on the promotion of generalist rather than specialist knowledge. However, he states that it soon became apparent that you still needed the neurosurgeon who was an expert at tying the right knot if you wanted to succeed in the field of neurosurgery. The following briefly describes the major types of new reporting relationships appearing in the health care literature:

- *Program Management:* All members of the team required to treat a given type of client report to a program director. There is no distinct department for each discipline (Van Pelt, 1985; Baker, 1993).
- *Matrix Management:* All members of the team required to treat a given type of client report to a program director and report in a matrix relationship on issues of professional concern to a discipline leader (Knight, 1980; Seaby, 1993). The reverse can also be true, where the discipline leader is the strong reporting relationship with a matrix relationship to a program manager.
- *Rehabilitation Division:* All members of rehabilitation disciplines (occupational therapy, physical therapy, speech pathology, and sometimes recreation) report to the same manager. There is often a discipline leader for each discipline who is responsible for professional issues. This is not a model specifically articulated in the literature but is a model implemented in many facilities known to the author.
- *Self-Directed Work Teams:* Members of the team of professionals treating the client form a work group. Administrative roles are divided between group members and reporting occurs through a committee structure (Dumaine, 1990).

The common objective of all of these reporting relationships is to improve the communication between service providers at the level of the care of each individual client, in an attempt to ensure that client's, rather than profession's, needs are being met. There are problems with each of these organizational structures (Seaby, 1993; Baker, 1993; Van Pelt, 1985). The program management structure is wrought with problems due to the loss of the discipline connections that have historically ensured that advances in the body of knowledge of the profession are integrated into practice. The matrix structure creates workload issues associated with attending both team and departmental meetings. The rehabilitation department creates problems with professional identity and, because the combined department does not include all health providers, communication issues between providers are not resolved by this change in organizational design. Lastly, the self-directed work team can be wrought with internal problems associated with power struggles. Thus, management experts are still experimenting with new organizational designs for health care organizations. For instance, the Sunnybrook Hospital in Toronto, Ontario has combined facets of different models in an attempt to maximize the benefits of each (Moffat & Prociw, 1992).

The future evolution of organizational relationships is unclear. Drucker (1993) predicted that organizational structures would increasingly become concentric, over-lapping coordinated rings. Helgesen (1990) uses the analogue of a cobweb to assist the reader in understanding how such an organization would look. Just as the spider operates from the center of the cobweb, the administrator is positioned in the center of the organizational structure with communication lines flowing in both directions to and from the center. Such models are only just beginning to appear in the health care literature (Hassen, 1993).

If the needs of the client are to be met and the expert knowledge of the professional used to its best advantage, a design that incorporates linkages to the health care team and the discipline, without increasing non-client care time, must be created.

THREAT OR OPPORTUNITY FOR OCCUPATIONAL THERAPISTS?

The reengineering of health care could be viewed as a threat to the profession of occupational therapy.

After all, there is much talk of cross-training and the training of multiskilled health care workers. In addition, new management models are resulting in occupational therapists being dispersed between programmer, or work groups, rather than consolidated in a department. There is fear that without the unifying structure of a department the system will cease to recognize the unique value of occupational therapy and that occupational therapy functions will be assumed by multiskilled caregivers.

The reengineering of health care could also be viewed as an opportunity for the profession of occupational therapy. The changes are pushing the system toward holistic, client-centered care that is based on meeting the needs of the client, as expressed by the client; an approach that has a goodness of fit with occupational therapy practice. Goldsmith acknowledges that "managing the cause of chronic illness and restoring the already compromised client to improved functioning is the emerging mission of the health care system" (1989, p. 107). Cleary, Edgman, Levitan, Walker, Gerteis, & Delbanco (1993) indicate that there is a need to develop treatment systems that facilitate and encourage clients' active participation and that ensure the needs of the client are met. Occupational therapists have a wealth of experience with client-centered practice and understand how to engage clients as active participants in their care (Crist & Stoffel, 1993/1996; Peloquin, 1993/1996; Pollock, 1993; Schlaff, 1993; Woodside, 1991). This knowledge base could be used by occupational therapists to provide leadership in the design of new care systems.

Experts in the field of reengineering are calling for tools that measure outcome from the perspective of the client (Moloney & Paul, 1993). Canadian occupational therapy leaders have already risen to that challenge and created the Canadian Occupational Performance Measure (Law, et al., 1991). This is an instrument that is a model for all health care workers to follow and has already been proposed in an adapted format as a means to facilitate better interdisciplinary care planning (Gage, 1994).

The changes that are occurring in organizational structures could also be considered a threat to the profession. The traditional departmental structure facilitates the growth and development of the profession and thus, the growth and development of the occupational therapists working within this structure. However, changes in organizational reporting relationships do not necessarily need to threaten the growth and development of the profession. Some models, the matrix model for instance, leave a discipline structure in place with the express intent of ensuring that the therapists in the matrix structure have an opportunity to benefit from one another's skills. The fact that health care administrators are still searching for an ideal organizational design for the new paradigm provides an opportunity for occupational therapists to have input in this process. Organizational structures that hamper the development of expert clinical skills will not thrive due to the negative effect on quality of client care. Occupational therapists need to stop resisting changes in organizational structure and instead join forces with health care administrators in the search for a design that will both support holistic, client-centered care and enable professional growth.

Occupational therapists can position themselves for the coming changes in practice and organizational structure by:

- learning to clearly articulate their unique contribution to the meeting of client needs
- reading about the reengineering of health care so that they will be the resident experts when decisions about new models of care or organizational structures are being made
- making it apparent that they have expertise in holistic, client-centered practice that predates the current paradigm shift to client-centered practice; information that can be used to assist others in the change process
- paving the way for a new era of client-driven practice by developing effective techniques that empower clients to make effective choices that maximize health outcomes.

SUMMARY

The current transition to models of care that meet the needs of a more knowledgeable health care consumer is far from complete. Proposed new models continue to appear in the literature and are likely to continue to appear as the system develops a better understanding of the needs of the clients it is serving. As the knowledge base grows, new organizational reporting relationships will also be proposed due to the strong influence that reporting relationships have on the quality of the output of any system. Occupational therapists must begin to seek opportunities to help design new organizational reporting relationships.

The expertise gained from years of client-centered practice will serve the profession well in the new paradigm. However, occupational therapists must continually seek opportunities to demonstrate the leadership potential that this body of knowledge provides. These opportunities will be different in each practice situation, but are likely to include a need to have occupational therapists:

- sit on committees within health care institutions and the community at large
- respond to health care briefs
- participate in focus groups that seek an understanding of the needs of health care clients
- provide education sessions that share information about specific client-centered strategies that will be useful to other professions

If occupational therapists wish to act as leaders in the change process they must actively seek opportunities to participate in work groups that are exploring new models of care and organizational structures. It is important that occupational therapists not sit and wait to be asked, but instead actively recruit opportunities to be part of the design process.

REFERENCES

Ahmann, E., & Bond, N. (1992). Promoting normal development in school-age children and adolescents who are technology dependent: A family centered model. *Pediatric Nursing, 18,* 399-405.

Andre, C., Hartigan, E., Smith, J., Light, C., Kinnear, C., Balbierz, J., O'Connor, D., & Beck, S. (1994, October). *Program to improve patient care at the University of Utah hospital and clinics.* Paper presented at: Strengthening Hospital Nursing: A program to improve patient care, Portland, OR.

Baker, G. R. (1993). The implications of program management of professional and managerial roles. *Physiotherapy Canada, 45,* 221-224.

Bartholome, W. G. (January 1992). A revolution in understanding: How ethics has transformed health care decision-making. *Quality Review Bulletin, 6-11.*

Batavia, A., & Hammer, G. (1990). Toward the development of consumer-based criteria for the evaluation of assistive devices. *Journal of Rehabilitation Research, 27,* 425-436.

Bowers, J., & McNally, K. (1983). Family-focused care in the psychiatric inpatient setting. *Image, 15,* 26-31.

Braddy, B., & Gray D. (1987). Employment services for older job seekers: A comparison of two client-centered approaches. *The Gerontologist, 27,* 565-568.

Brider, P. (September 1992). The move to patient-focused care. *American Journal of Nursing, 26-33.*

Brown, C., & Ringma, C. (1989). New disability services: The critical role of staff in a consumer-directed empowerment model of service for physically disabled people. *Disability, Handicap, & Society, 4,* 241-256.

Buckman, R., & Sabbagh, K. (1993). *Magic or medicine?* Toronto, Canada: Key Porter Books.

Cleary, P., Edgman-Leviton, S., Walker, J., Gerteis, M., & Delbanco, T. (1993). Using patient reports to improve medical care: A preliminary report from 10 hospitals. *Quality Management in Health Care, 2,* 31-38.

Crist, P. A. H., & Stoffel, V. C. (1993). The Americans With Disabilities Act of 1990 and employees with mental impairments: Personal efficacy and the environment. *American Journal of Occupational Therapy, 46,* 434-443. (Reprinted in Cottrell, R. P. (1996). *Perspectives on purposeful activity: Foundation and future of occupational therapy* (pp. 217-228). Bethesda, MD: AOTA.)

Curran, C. (1992). Patient-centered care is not enough. *Nursing Economics, 10,* 164.

Delbanco, T. (1992). Enriching the doctor-patient relationship by inviting the patient's perspective. *Annals of Internal Medicine, 116,* 414-418.

Drucker, P. (1993). *Post-capitalist society.* New York, NY: Harper Business.

Dumaine, B. (May 7, 1990). Who needs a boss? *Fortune,* 52-60.

England, S., & Evans, J. (1992). Patients' choices and perceptions after an invitation to participate in treatment decisions. *Social Science and Medicine, 34,* 1217-1225.

Friesen, B. J., Koroloff, N. (1990). Family-centered services: Implications for mental health administration and research. *The Journal of Mental Health Administration, 17*(1), 1325.

Gage, M. (1994). The patient-driven interdisciplinary care plan. *Journal of Nursing Administration, 24*(4), 2635.

Gage, M., & Polataiko, H. (1995). Naming practice: The case for the term client-driven. *Canadian Journal of Occupational Therapy, 62,* 115-118.

Gerteis, M., Edgman-Levitan, S., Daley, J., & Delbanco, T. (1993). *Through the patient's eyes.* San Francisco, CA: Jossey-Bass.

Goldsmith, J. (May/June 1989). A radical prescription for hospitals. *Harvard Business Review,* 104-110.

Goodwater, D. (1993). Little Mountain: A mother's story. *Abilities, 17,* 69-70.

Hassen, P. (1993). *Rx for hospitals: New hope for Medicare in the nineties.* Toronto, Canada: Stoddart.

Helgesen, S. (1990). *The female advantage.* New York, NY: Doubleday.

Herzberg, S.R. (1990). Client or patient: Which term is more appropriate for use in occupational therapy? *The American Journal of Occupational Therapy, 44,* 561-564.

Hudson & AJ.Cox (Eds.) *Dimensions of state mental health policy* (pp. 138-154). New York, NY: Praeger.

Jenna, J. (May/June 1986). Toward the patient-driven hospital. *Healthcare, 3,* 8-18.

Kaye, D. (1993). *Laugh, I thought I'd die.* Toronto, Canada: Viking-Penguin.

Kerr, M., & Birk, J. (1988). A client-centered management model. *Quality Review Bulletin, 14,* 279-283.

Knight, K. (1980). Matrix organization: A review. In H. Koontz, C. O'Donnell, & H. Weihrich. *Management: A book of readings* (pp. 307-312). New York, NY: McGraw-Hill.

Larsson, U., Svardsudd, K., Wedel, H., & Salp, R. (1992). Patient involvement in decision-making in surgical and orthopedic practice. *Scandinavian Journal of Caring Science, 6*(2), 8796.

Lathrop, J., Seufert, G., MacDonald, R., & Martin, S. (1991). The patient-focused hospital: A patient care concept. *Journal of the Society of Health Systems, 3*(2), 3350.

Law, M., Baptiste, S., Carswell-Opzoomer, A., McColl, M. A., Polatajko, H., & Pollock, N. (1991). *Canadian Occupational Performance Measure.* Toronto, Canada: CAOT Publications ACE.

Levine, S., & Greenlick, M. (1991). Removing barriers to the empowerment of the elderly in health programs. *Gerontologist, 31,* 581-582.

Leviton, A., Mueller, M., & Kauffman, C. (January 1992). The family-centered consultation model: Practical applications for professionals. *Infants and Young Children, 18.*

Lumsdon, K. (February 1993). Form follows function: Patient-centered care needs strong facilities planning. *Hospitals,* 22-26.

Moffat, M., & Prociw, M. (1992). Case mix management education in a Canadian hospital. *Health Care Management Forum, 5*(4), 40 44.

Moloney, T. W., & Paul, B. (1993). Rebuilding the public trust. In M. Gerteis, S. Edgman-Levitan, J. Daley, and T. Delbanco (Eds.), *Through the patient's eyes.* San Francisco, CA: Jossey-Bass.

Morris, J., & Royle, G. T. (1988). Offering patients a choice of surgery for early breast cancer: A reduction in anxiety and depression in patients and their husbands. *Social Science and Medicine, 26,* 583-585.

Moxley, D., & Freddolino, P. (1990). A model of advocacy for promoting client self-determination in psychosocial rehabilitation. *Psychosocial Rehabilitation Journal, 14,* 69-82.

Murphy, R. (1990). *The body silent.* New York, NY: W. W. Norton.

O'Malley, J. (1992). Redesigning roles for patient-centered care: The hospitality representative. *Journal of Nursing Administration, 22* (7/8), 30-34.

Orr, R. (1987). A new design for modern health care: The Planetree project. *World Hospital, 23*(3-4), 38-40.

Patterson, J. B. & Marks, C. (1992). The client as customer: Achieving service quality and customer satisfaction in rehabilitation. *Journal of Rehabilitation, 58*(4), 16-21.

Peloquin, S.M. (1993). The patient-therapist relationship: Beliefs that shape care. *American Journal of Occupational Therapy, 47,* 935-942. (Reprinted in Cottrell, R. P. (1996). *Perspectives on purposeful activity: Foundation and future of occupational therapy* (pp. 217-228). Bethesda, MD: AOTA.)

Pollock, N. (1993). Client-centered assessment. *American Journal of Occupational Therapy, 47,* 298-301.

Preen, R. (1990). Developing a client-driven quality assurance program. *International Journal of Partial Hospitalization, 6,* 15-20.

Reiser, S. (1993). The era of the patient. *Journal of the American Medical Association, 269,* 1012-1017.

Roter, D. (1987). An exploration of health education's responsibility for a partnership model of client-provider relations. *Patient Education and Counseling, 9,* 25-31.

Rose, S.M. (1991). Strategies of mental health programming: A client-driven model of case management. In C. G. Hudson & A. J. Cox (Eds.), *Dimensions of state mental health policy* (pp. 138-154). New York, NY: Praeger.

Schlaff, C. (1993). Health policy: From dependency to self-advocacy: Redefining disability. *American Journal of Occupational Therapy, 47,* 943-948.

Schulman, B. A. (1979). Active patient orientation and outcomes in hypertensive treatment. Application of a socio-organizational perspective. *Medical Care, 17,* 267-280.

Seaby, L. (1993). From matrix management to pure program management: An evolution or a revolution? *Physiotherapy Canada, 45,* 226-228.

Sherer, J. (February 1993). Putting patients first: Hospitals work to define patient-centered care. *Hospitals,* 14-18.

Silberman, C. (1991). Providing patient-centered care. *Health Management Quarterly,* fourth quarter, 12-16.

Smith, R., & Hoppe, R. (1991). The patient's story: Integrating the patient and physician-centered approaches to interviewing. *Annals of Internal Medicine, 115,* 470-477.

Stewart-Amidei, C. (1992). Redesigning the system. *Journal of Neuroscience Nursing, 24,* 179-180.

Toiler, A. (1981). *The third wave.* Toronto, Canada: Bantam Books.

Van Pelt, G. (1985). Program management and matrix reporting. *Hospitals, 59*(24), 83-84.

Weinstein, R. (1991). Hospital case management: The path to empowering nurses. *Nursing, 17,* 289-293.

Wilson, R. (1985). Patient-centered health education: A chance for provider change. *Family and Community Health, 7*(4), 14.

Woodside, H. (1991). The participation of mental health consumers in health care issues. *Canadian Journal of Occupational Therapy, 58,* 35.

CHAPTER THREE

The Challenge of Change to Occupational Therapy Practice

Gail S. Fidler

This chapter was previously published in Occupational Therapy in Mental Health, *11(1), 111. Copyright © 1991, Haworth Press. Reprinted by permission.*

It has been evident for some time that the health care system is in the process of significant change. Increasing medical and social problems, accelerating development of complex technology, reductions in federal funding, spiraling health care costs and public demand for increased accountability have all contributed to the reordering of priorities and alterations in the system. These are evident in the cost containment efforts of governments and insurance companies and in the shift of responsibility for monitoring care from professionals to third party payers. The resulting change from the provision of long-term hospital care to short-term care, efforts to develop alternatives to hospitalization such as case management and mobile care units, and the establishment of productivity standards all significantly impact the practice of occupational therapy. There are drastic changes in the context of our practice. Such change challenges us to examine the validity of occupational therapy, demonstrate its effectiveness, and reexamine our professional values, ethics and motivations.

What is the nature of this challenge? The challenge is in the rethinking, in confronting what it is we do and why we do it. It is in sitting out and in clarifying the core focus of occupational therapy, how this then defines the nature and parameters of hospital practice and how we conceptualize and plan for post hospital services. The challenge is in reassessing professional standards, values, expectations, roles, functions, and priorities.

When the length of a hospital stay is open-ended, one can rely on time for sorting out essentials, time for the process itself to evolve a direction and focus. When time is limited, the early clarity of purpose becomes critical and there are necessary shifts in priorities. It is not so much the length of time as it is how that time is used that makes the difference.

This challenge then of scrutiny, reassessment, and analysis should address at least four major questions:

- What adaptations will need to be made in how the delivery system is viewed?
- What adaptations will need to be made in the content of the treatment/remedial process? In other words, what should our in-hospital practice look like?
- What alterations will need to be made in our patterns of communication?
- What adaptations will need to occur in our values, attitudes and expectations?

With a shortened hospital stay, in-patient treatment can no longer be viewed as a self-contained system, responsible for providing the full spectrum of treatment. Reliance on community-based services becomes essential. A continuity of treatment and rehabilitation requires a range of intact community-based services well beyond the traditional out-patient psychotherapy. Out-patient clinics, partial care programs, day treatment centers, and the family all become significant agents and must be viewed as sharing with the hospital and the patient responsibility for treatment outcomes. It becomes a partnership! Thus, the meaning of discharge is altered. Rather than signaling an end to a comprehensive treatment regimen, it marks the beginning of a next level in the continuity of care and treatment.

Development of a collaborative working relationship between occupational therapists, other hospital staff, and the staff of community agencies becomes crucial. Furthermore, experience has demonstrated that at this time, much of such relationship building is still up to the occupational therapist. Traditional attitudes and role expectations change slowly and change initiatives such as these require a persistence, a sensitivity, and practice, practice.

The challenge then is to come to understand and define the role of occupational therapy within these changed perspectives so that remediation plans with the patient extend beyond the here and now of the hospital setting. It is necessary to ensure that information sharing and recommendations for the focus of post-hospital remediation programs are clearly provided and that these are supported by dialogue with the relevant external persons or agency. And finally, it is imperative that such functions are conceptualized as an inherent role responsibility of an occupational therapy staff.

One of the challenges to the broader system is to come to understand the system as a system and to provide services to patients accordingly. Although the "delivery system" is a frequently used term, what often exists in reality is not a system but rather a number of services in competition with one another for the diminishing dollar. Organizationally and functionally there is, traditionally, a clear line separating hospital services and community services. Funding practices furthermore reinforce such separation in both public and private enterprises. For example, it was disturbing to learn recently that the New Jersey Governor's Advisory Council was charged with making recommendations for a plan for mental health services. Not for a mental health system, but for services! The separations, the fragmentation is at risk of continuing. In such models, a shortened hospital stay can indeed pose problems for the patient and hospital staff. Many of our values, attitudes and territoriality get in the way of evolving a truly comprehensive system with interdependent parts. The question then is how do we describe our role within this context? As you critique your system's operations, what adaptations will need to be made?

What plans and initiatives will need to be generated in order to facilitate such change? In terms of the functions of occupational therapy? In relation to the roles of colleagues, and the role of the patient? Internalizing the belief that patient care extends beyond the hospital, that it is not necessarily a short term of care but a shorter time in the hospital will, like all attitudinal change, take work and time.

The second question to be examined is, *What adaptations will need to be made in the content of our remedial process?* Addressing this question requires, first of all, taking a second, very critical look at the principal focus of how we define the core concern of our discipline.

Short-term care brings the reality of time and priorities clearly to the fore. It is indeed the time of "when push comes to shove"! The questions are: what stays, what goes? what needs to be done now? what later? To use time efficiently and effectively, in the best interest of the patient, requires a clarity of focus and well-organized, incremental steps for getting there.

A reexamination of one's frame of reference, one's treatment model or paradigm and how it is being operationalized should be undertaken periodically. When faced with a shortened timeframe, such scrutiny is essential. To sustain the quality of care while accommodating to a shortened hospital stay, requires a truly critical assessment and consensus about fundamentals. It is only from such a base that adaptations can be made. To do otherwise places quality at risk. There is no viable short cut for such a process. Without this step there is great risk that time pressures will force structural and/or technologic changes without the support of conceptual substance. Such a dichotomy dooms most initiatives to failure! At the very least it erodes quality. What must now be asked is: What is your fundamental core focus and how does this determine decisions? What gets relinquished and what are established as top priorities?

For example, my perspective is that as occupational therapists, as specialists in the rehabilitation process, our fundamental focus is performance. Thus the content of intervention relates directly to the patient's ability to perform those roles and tasks of daily living that are relevant to their age, to their social/cultural norms and interests, and to the social/cultural norms and expectations of the social structure in which they live: their family and the community. The explicit purpose of such a focus is to enable the patient to evolve a lifestyle, a way of living that is more satisfying than not to self and to the significant others with whom he or she lives.

How do you articulate your frame of reference? Your core focus? What consensus have you established?

If my thesis is tenable, then it follows that all assessments and rehabilitation plans will address four very basic questions:

- What is it that the patient must be able to do? What performance skills are essential for this patient at this time and at what level?
- What can the patient do? What are the strengths, abilities, and interests of the patient, what are the resources of the external environment?
- What can the patient not do? What internal/external factors interfere?
- What interventions, what remedial activity must be taken and in what order of priority so that the patient will be able to move toward fulfilling relevant lifestyle performance expectations?

Are such questions relevant to your formulations? What factors determine the parameters of your assessments, of your plans of intervention? What questions are the organizers for your assessment and planning?

The process of clarifying what the content of interventions should be and thus what adaptations will be needed, involves taking a look at several additional factors. If indeed occupational therapy is in the business of making it possible for the individual to evolve a lifestyle more satisfying than not to the person and to his or her society, then it becomes necessary to come to closure with regard to identifying and categorizing what is considered to be the major roles and tasks of daily living. What are the components of a lifestyle? How should these be categorized so that relevant functional skills can be defined and measured? Without a model that sets such criteria, assessment and treatment initiatives with patients risk hanging in limbo without context, without meaning or relevance to the patient or to others. Credibility is at high risk and time becomes poorly used.

A second issue is related to what criteria should be used to determine what are relevant functions and a relevant lifestyle for a given patient. What are the interdependent variables among the resources, the expectations, the potential of the community, of the family, and of the patient which help to define relevance? With whom does one collaborate in addressing such questions? Without such a formula, it is unlikely that a truly individualized rehabilitation plan will be designed, especially under the pressures of time. Assessment is critical and should not be short-changed. Designing a rehabilitation plan that extends into the community requires some very solid and complex information. Obviously, in a short hospital stay more information must be gathered in a shorter period of time. Knowing what to look for and how to obtain and use the information reduces time. The use of a comprehensive (and comprehensive must be emphasized), functional skills assessment instrument is an extremely valuable organizing, data collection procedure. When there are limits on time, the use of such an instrument is essential. It must, however, accommodate to age and cultural variations and have a clear relevance to the definition of one's focus and frame of reference. A functional skills assessment instrument facilitates consensual planning, concertizes goals and progress, measures and documents outcomes and provides an M.I.S. base for quality assurance and program evaluation. One needs to be regularly reminded that treatment and assessment are interrelated. There is no treatment without assessment and no information gathering without therapeutic gain. Our action-oriented groups and activities are rich laboratories for simultaneous remediation and assessment. This reality maximizes the effective use of time to the benefit of the patient.

The patient's participation in the design of his/her rehabilitation plan takes on added significance in a short term setting. Shared planning and reaching consensus more frequently than not generate a sense of ownership on the part of the patient. Such investment pays dividends during hospitalization and is more likely to make a difference in the incentive to follow through after hospitalization. Furthermore, the shared planning, the negotiating, compromise and consensus regarding plans and priorities is an important learning opportunity. It is an exercise in volition, an experience in assessing one's alternatives, making decisions, and planning for follow through. It is learning about being one's own agent and having some influence over one's life, an essential ingredient in a satisfying lifestyle.

Content adaptations will require a new look at community resources. Not only in terms of their role in post hospital programs but their significance as part of in hospital programming. The use of community resources while the patient is still hospitalized provides an important bridge to the community. What educational, vocational, recreational resources, what peer support groups exist in the patient's community? What can they provide and what can be done to foster their involvement? This kind of bridging is so important to the young borderline and substance abuse patient. For the schizophrenic patient, it compensates for problems with generalizing function and provides some essential mapping.

A hospital environment with fluid boundaries between itself and community resources is an environment that maximizes the potential of the patient to cope with the community and can reduce the need for continued stay. An experience early in my career in a small psychoanalytic hospital with remarkable collaborative relationships with and use of community resources, was a lesson I will always remember. I have since viewed the self-contained or total hospital with self-contained programs and services, with at least a jaundiced eye.

Scrutiny of the content of occupational therapy practice should also address our intervention strategies and methodologies. These are related to both the expeditious use of time and to the critical variable within time of role clarification. Although the temptation to embark on a discourse regarding the importance and meaning of activities is great, it is acknowledged that this is not the purpose of this paper. Suffice it to say that the use of purposeful activity (or occupation if you prefer) is without question our intervention of choice. It is purposeful action, the process of doing as remediation, which is the essence of our expertise, in contrast to the expertise and technologies of verbal expression and dialogue. Implicit in this thesis is the tenet that feelings, perceptions, and behaviors are shaped and changed as the result of action experiences. Psychomotor activity is a fundamental learning process. In these respects we are different from other traditionally recognized health professionals.

A second and related point of differentiation is our primary attention to the strengths, capacities, intact skills, and interests of the patient. Ours is an over-riding concern for the discovery of such assets and their use in the process of successful doing. Our principal focus is maximizing the healthy aspects of the patient in contrast to a focal concern about pathology or disease. We are different and our difference brings a critical dimension to conceptualizing and implementing the curative process.

Time and again there is evidence of the on-going risk of our getting lost, of losing our unique identity in the practice setting. The risk increases in environments where strong leadership and role modeling comes from outside of our profession. Upward mobility is the hallmark of a mobile society such as our western culture. The incentive to assume, to emulate the characteristics and behaviors of those who occupy a more privileged status, is a universal phenomenon. The health care system is no exception. The psychologist strives to emulate the physician; the occupational therapist tries to emulate the psychologist and so on. As a newcomer to the hospital system, the occupational therapist's white uniform was no small effort to be seen as more like the influential registered nurse than like ourselves. Today, several rungs up the ladder, we take on testing behaviors and the clinical white coat! Abandonment of the ubiquitous uniforms in psychiatric hospitals seems to have had more to do with the politics of social class and power than patients' needs.

To be more like others rather than different is a strong social pull. However, when we lose our purposeful activity focus, we resign our responsibility and fail the patient. It is differences in perspectives, methodologies and expertise that best and most expeditiously serve the patient. That is the value of the interdisciplinary team, it provides a wide angle lens and a diversity of focus and methods!

For many years I have understood a functional difference in the meaning of treatment and the meaning of rehabilitation. In practice, treatment most characteristically references those interventions, those processes which are directed toward the reduction or elimination of pathology. Rehabilitation by contrast most generally connotes relearning, redevelopment, as Webster states, "to restore to suitability." The focus is on function. The coin has two sides, each different, distinguishable, but integrated to form the whole. So it is with treatment and rehabilitation—each different and distinguishable, each interrelated and essential to form the whole.

Ongoing role clarification is critical, particularly when hospital stay is brief. It relates to time, efficiency and the comprehensive quality of care. Knowing who does what well, having different expertise available makes it possible to expeditiously use special expertise, as well as to share some roles and functions without threat to the integrity of care to the patient.

No one needs to be convinced that communication is vital to the life of any organization, any endeavor, any group or dyad. Over time institutions develop their own unique patterns of communication. These generally relate to the mission of the institution and in particular to its organizational and operational philosophy. Communication patterns reflect an institution's values, locus of power, and influence and thus how it goes about achieving its mission. Who talks to whom about what is the mirror of operations and philosophy of care. Thus, for example, the typical long-term psychoanalytic hospital has its unique patterns of communication which reflect, support, and reinforce its psychoanalytic values, standards, ethics, and beliefs. Within this context, communication around patient care and treatment decisions generally tend to be exploratory, speculative, thoughtful, and without the pressure of time. It is understood that there is always time to work things through, and this process (the working through) is viewed many times as more significant than the coming to closure.

When hospital stays are shortened, when there are the inevitable alterations in the delivery system, when priorities are necessarily resumed, many of the traditional patterns of communication no longer support the goals of the institution. Some, because of changed circumstances, become counterproductive.

Clearly any change calls for a reexamination of patterns of communication. In light of the adaptations that you identify as needing to occur in your delivery system, and in the content and focus of your interventions, what should your communication network look like? Among yourselves, with patients, with other staff, and with the community? What should be the content of each of such dialogues? How do you facilitate and/or bring about the needed change and adaptations?

Values clarification is perhaps such an over-used phrase that hearing it no longer elicits a sense of challenge. Nevertheless, it seems evident that most of the issues that have been raised here for consideration involve values, beliefs, ethics, and sets of expectations. Our values set the stage for our decisions and for our performance. Getting clear on one's own values and beliefs is a first and necessary step in addressing response and adaptations to the complex and challenging issues of short-term hospitalization. A critical reassessment of your values and beliefs is fundamental to coming to grips with the challenge.

Finally, meeting the challenge means confronting the threat of change. We have learned to explain the resistance to change as a response to the threat to one's power, influence, and control to the bureaucratic investment in the status quo, to job security, and the like. The constructs are so generalized and have become such cliches that frequently they are of only limited help to us in understanding why in the face of pending change we feel as we do and thus what might be done to reduce our anxiety and free us to act. Over the years, I have come to understand how resistance to change is caused not so much by the fear of change itself but rather, by the threat of change. It is the uncertainty, the numerous, open-ended possibilities, the ambiguities that are frightening and that threaten to unlock the "ghosts" in our closet.

With many unknown possibilities, with untested waters, our ability to predict is threatened. Familiar cause and effect formulas no longer seem so reliable. Our ghosts of questionable competence, adequacy and validity of our practice begin to stir. The old fears of being able to cope and to manage begin to reemerge and urge us to reaffirm that indeed a bird in the hand is preferable to two in a bush. In her impressive book *The Change Masters*, R. K. Kantor suggests that the threat of change implies loss of control when it is assumed that one does not have the resources to make the transition possible. Furthermore, she goes on to say that "the threat of change arouses anxiety when it is still a threat, not an actuality." Certainly, my experience has shown that when we confront the threat by planning, our resources and capabilities are disclosed and reaffirmed. In the process of scrutinizing the challenge and in planning for change, we assume control over events and the "too many possibilities" become known and manageable. The threat of change then becomes the challenge of opportunity.

I have raised more questions than suggested solutions. First, because I have always believed that understanding the question is the essence of resolution. Additionally, and more important perhaps, my purpose has been to provoke analytic dialogue among you, knowing that through this process you are capable of making those decisions that will maximize the potential inherent in each of you, in the patient, and in the system.

CHAPTER FOUR

Managed Mental Health Care: Reflections in a Time of Turmoil

Betsy Van Leit

This chapter was previously published in the American Journal of Occupational Therapy, 50, *428-434. Copyright © 1996, The American Occupational Therapy Association, Inc.*

The topic of managed care has stimulated emotional discussion among occupational therapy practitioners. When therapists in general get together, our talk turns to the short lengths of stay, the impossibility of providing effective treatment, the hassles of paperwork and bureaucracy, and the seeming loss of control over professional decision making. Anger, frustration, loss, and grief are the dominant feelings about a changing health care system that we no longer recognize.

In mental health, occupational therapists are not the only professional group feeling the changes. For example, one article recently and dramatically described psychiatry departments as though under assault:

"...countless Indians [managed care companies] have seemingly come out of nowhere on fast horseback to assault a slow, self-absorbed wagon train...Most of the surviving senders psychiatrists] are in shock trying to redefine their goals. A few are self righteous, angry, and some are incapacitated by depression" (Summergrad, Herman, Weilburg, & Jeillinek, 1995, p. 215).

Some authors are concerned that mental health clinicians have become so absorbed in their own emotional issues concerning professional identity, self-esteem, and even survival that our clients have been forgotten (Backlar, 1995; Lipsitt, 1995). Others have suggested that in all the turmoil, clinicians are losing their perspective:

"There is an unfortunate trend for mental health professionals to become hypnotized by certain phrases or slogans that become affectively laden even though there may be little agreement about the meaning of the words. We then judge systems and initiatives in the cortex of these value-laden terms. Thus systems with "case management" and "assertive community treatments" are judged favorably without reference to the actual implementation of these concepts, and "privatized" systems are summarily dismissed because they evoke the notion of profit (Hoge, Davidson, Griffith, Sledge, & Howenstine, 1994, p. 1088)."

To sort out affective distortion from fact, I will discuss the effect of managed care on mental health care and the opportunities and challenges that occupational therapy professionals must address assertively and immediately in this time of confusion and concern.

THE DEVELOPMENT OF MANAGED MENTAL HEALTH CARE

Over the past few decades, deinstitutionalization and consumers' growing acceptance of the value of mental health and substance abuse treatment have accelerated demands for services (Jonas, 1986; Mechanic, Schlesinger, & McAlpine, 1995). Unfortunately, the costs of mental health and substance abuse services have been outpacing costs in other areas of medicine in both the public and private sector (Bevilacqua, 1995; Mechanic, 1987). For example, Medicaid expenditures (an important source of funding for public mental health services) have been growing exponentially in recent years. Total state government budgets used for Medicaid rose from 8.1 % in 1987 to 18.4% in 1993 and have now surpassed higher education as the largest category of state spending.

From the private insurer's perspective, unmanaged fee-for-service for mental health and substance abuse was a disaster. Bartlett (1994) identified concerns about rapidly increasing costs, wide variability of treatment for the same psychiatric diagnoses, lack of accountability on the part of providers who blamed patients for lack of progress, and treatment planning decisions that seemed to be determined according to benefit design. For example, length of in-patient stay and number of outpatient visits consistently corresponded to available reimbursement. In response, the majority of mental health and substance abuse benefits are now managed via utilization review and case management, and the use of behavioral care vendors that specialize in managing mental health care benefits is increasingly common (Bartlett, 1994;

Mechanic, et al., 1995). In the public sector, the use of managed care has also been growing rapidly (Steinwachs, Kasper, & Skinner, 1992).

Ironically, in spite of increased usage of services, there is strong evidence that considerable unmet need for mental health and substance abuse treatment remains. The Epidemiological Catchment Area Survey of the National Institute of Mental Health (Myers, et al., 1984) reported a 6-month prevalence rate of 15% for major psychiatric disorders and a lifetime prevalence of 25%. The frequency of unrecognized or inappropriate treatment for these illnesses in the primary care setting is disturbingly high (Eisenberg, 1992). In addition, in spite of escalating costs, mental health and substance abuse services continue to lag other medical services in terms of available reimbursement (Mechanic, 1987).

SIMILARITIES OF MENTAL HEALTH TO OTHER TYPES OF MANAGED CARE

Currently, managed care means many things to many persons. Different authors have emphasized varying definitions, depending on their point of view about the appropriateness of managed care and their role as provider, insurer, administrator, or recipient of services.

Some authors emphasized the attempt of managed care to balance resources, cost, and quality of services (Bevilacqua, 1995; Wood, Bailey, & Tilkemeir, 1992). Schreter, Sharfstein, and Schreter (1994) suggested that

"managed care is not a solution, but a framework for a process... [that] involves answering some very basic questions such as 1) how much money is needed, 2) where the money should) who should pay, 4) who should use mental health services, and 5) who should decide these questions" (p. 214).

Clinicians often highlight the loss of provider control over clinical decision-making (Goodman, Brown, & Deitz. 1992). Finally, quality of care under managed care is seen as a sham by some; that is, they believe that the sole intent of managed care in psychiatric services is cost control (Wells, Astrachan, Tischler, & Unutzer, 1995).

Managed care systems as described in the literature may include preferred provider organizations, health maintenance organizations (HMOs), or independent managed care firms. Managed care processes used in mental health and substance abuse services, as well as in other types of medicine, may include pre-certification (reimburser preauthorization to treat), concurrent review (on-going reimburser evaluation of the appropriateness of treatment), gatekeepers and case management, provider selection, clinical guidelines and protocols, benefit definition and redefinition, general budget constraints, and financial incentives for providers, such as capitation (Mechanic, et al., 1995; Wells, et al., 1995). However, because mental health and substance abuse benefits and services are different from other types of medical services in many ways, they are often managed separately by companies specializing in these types of services (Wells, et al., 1995).

MANAGED CARE ISSUES SPECIFIC TO MENTAL HEALTH

Mental illness and substance abuse differ from other types of medical needs in ways that affect the application of managed care practices (Mechanic, et al., 1995). Although many persons requiring mental health or substance abuse treatment have acute episodes that resolve quickly, others experience chronic mental illness and may require on-going support services to cope effectively in the community. Persons with serious mental illness may have major social and functional deficits that persist or recur. A restrictive managed care system that refuses to address issues such as housing, employment, and supportive rehabilitation efforts for persons with long-term mental illness may force families and the community to bear the burden of providing necessary services that the system will not allow. A 1991 survey of National Alliance for the Mentally Ill (NAMI) members reported that more than 60% of them indicated that the primary residence for their relatives with mental illness is the family home and that families serve as the safety net and constant case manager for the adult with mental illness (Flynn, 1994).

Another concern is stigma, which is still prevalent and peculiar to mental health and substance abuse. For instance, the executive director of NAMI asks, "Would managed care companies try to discharge cancer patients from the hospital before they have completed their chemotherapy? Do they deny life-saving medications to people with heart disease? I wonder why mental illness is so often targeted for cost-containment?" (Flynn, 1994, p. 203). Because of stigma and the attitudes that it engenders, there continues to be discrimination against persons with mental illness and fewer available benefits for treatment than for non-psychiatric medical conditions. In addition, prevailing stigma can easily discourage persons with mental illness or substance abuse problems from seeking care or can lead to concerns about confidentiality. Further, stigma may negatively affect the ability of clients and families to advocate for the services they need (Mechanic, et al., 1995).

Another issue pertinent to mental health and substance abuse treatment because of chronic effects of long term mental illness is the importance of the public sector. Downward mobility may occur as persons with serious, persistent mental illness become unable to obtain or maintain employment and eventually depend on the state for health care and basic living expenses. Gerson (1994) suggested that termination of private behavioral health care coverage typically occurs for persons with baseline chronic psychosis; chronic mental illness who are non-compliant with treatment; major depressive illness who are chronically suicidal; severe personality disorder; organic brain syndrome; conduct disorder; and serious, long-term chemical dependency. In fact, persons with chronic mental illness have always had to rely on the public sector for care (Mechanic, et al., 1995) in the form of state-run psychiatric institutions or community-based services financed by Medicaid.

Health care reform is not new to mental health providers. Historically, deinstitutionalization and the community mental health movement in the 1960s and 1970s offered the great promise for less expensive care that simultaneously provided better quality of services. The promises of managed care sound similar to the promises of the deinstitutionalization movement; however, mental health care providers also know that the consequences of deinstitutionalization were unlike the promises. Many of our clients who needed care and services ended up in the street with no follow through or other assistance. The resultant mental health system was fragmented and unmanaged and was characterized by an absence of accountability and follow-up for individual clients; difficulty in clients finding and accessing services; poor coordination among providers and discontinuity in treatment planning; reimbursement disincentives for community-based rehabilitation treatment; and inadequate systems for monitoring necessity, appropriateness, or effectiveness of care (Hoge, et al., 1994). Some of the current anger and depression of mental health service providers may be in response to hearing the same promises again. Is it a surprise that a promise of better care for less money is met with cynicism? Cynicism will not assist clients with mental illness or shepherd a positive evolution in mental health practices. Mental health service providers must identify and fight for changes that lead toward a system of care that is not only effective but also mindful of cost.

GENERATIONS OF MANAGED CARE IN MENTAL HEALTH

Perhaps some of the confusion about the meaning of managed care results from the fact that it is evolving. In mental health, its tools and tactics are changing, and one can identify three generations of managed care (Bartlett, 1994). First generation approaches (still evident in many plans and organizations) focus on extensive utilization review by reimbursers who may lack mental health experience or expertise. To make matters worse, reviewers often have used clinical criteria that were kept secret from clinicians. As can be imagined, first generation managed care was and is coercive, adversarial, and the source of tremendous distrust, paranoia, and hostility between managed care companies and providers, and clients have often been caught in the middle of their battles.

First generation managed care has sometimes cut costs, but it has not improved quality of care. It has alienated providers and clients and has the potential to project an uncaring or greedy image that could discredit managed care

organizations. In response, some companies have evolved to second generation approaches that are more collaborative and flexible. Second generation managed mental health care may use networks of providers, often shifts financial risks (e.g., through capitation) from reimbursers to providers, focuses on measurement of outcomes, and encourages sharing of clinical criteria and standards of care. Managed care agents using second generation approaches may actually serve as part of the treatment team to de-emphasize the belief that "outsiders" are the decision-makers (Olsen, Rickles, Travlik, 1995). The intent is to include providers in the quest for cost-effective mental health care to overcome the barriers created by first generation approaches to managing care. Second generation managed care not only maintains the focus on cost-containment but also attempts to reinsert the concept of quality and effectiveness of care.

According to Bartlett (1994), third generation managed care approaches are just beginning to develop. These approaches go beyond mechanisms of control to development of optimal mental health care that truly provides flexible, comprehensive, cost-effective care in a continuum of settings. It remains to be seen whether third generation managed care becomes a reality or remains as wishful thinking. In the meantime, a number of challenges and opportunities arise for occupational therapists to address as health care systems continue to develop and change.

CHALLENGES AND OPPORTUNITIES IN AN EVOLVING SYSTEM OF CARE

Measuring Outcomes and Effectiveness of Care

Managed mental health care is emphasizing the importance of measuring the outcomes of service delivery. Although occupational therapists have known for years that outcome measures are the only way to calculate the impact of treatment and improve the quality of the services provided (American Occupational Therapy Association [AOTA], 1995; Stoffel & Cunningham, 1991/2000; Thien, 1987/1993), the economic incentive to become more cost-effective is what is driving the widespread measurement of outcomes.

It is critical to systematically gather a broad range of data to understand the results of treatments and the meaning of outcome studies. For example, the client's baseline status, sociodemographic factors, clinical factors, and treatment are all pertinent to understanding outcomes (Kane, Bartlett, & Potthoff, 1995). The International Association for Psychosocial Rehabilitation Services (IAPSRS) has identified a number of domains of outcome measurement for psychosocial rehabilitation programs, including frequency of rehospitalization, employment status, independent living status, educational status, income, program of attendance, and accomplishment of rehabilitation goals (Lacayo, 1995). Additionally, IAPSRS has identified that more research is needed on complex outcome domains, including social activities and skills, level of functioning, quality of life, and client satisfaction with services. Occupational therapists can contribute important information to the measurement of many of the outcomes associated with these domains. In particular, occupational therapists can contribute their expertise in the use of observation of performance versus self-report and the effect of measurement of occupational performance in the natural environment versus the clinical setting.

Measuring effectiveness of care will allow occupational therapists to determine clinical guidelines or protocols that outline appropriate clinical decision-making. Mental health professions have avoided taking the lead in identifying appropriate parameters of practice or clinical guidelines partly because of fear of losing control of treatment decisions and concern that reimbursement will become even more restricted (Ellek, 1995). It is true that clinical decision-making must remain flexible, reflecting the complexities of mental health and substance abuse issues, but refusal to identify treatment guidelines has put occupational therapy professionals at great risk. By continuing to demonstrate wide variability in clinical decision-making, occupational therapy practitioners appear subjective and lacking in professional expertise. In response to lack of identified protocols, managed care companies have taken the lead, announcing that if professionals cannot identify dimensions of cost-effective care, then the insurers will. It is paramount that practitioners regain control of the clinical process by clearly articulating the processes and outcomes of mental health services.

Because outcome measurement is complex, there is the danger that cost-effectiveness may be evaluated from a perspective that focuses exclusively on cost as opposed to one that addresses effectiveness (Wells, et al., 1995). The business goal of cost-containment in managed mental health care has been demonstrated in a number of studies, although the results have sometimes been inconsistent (see Mechanic, et al., 1995). However, questions about the quality and effectiveness of services have not yet been answered with any precision. It is clear that cost-cutting by reducing use, but doing so in a manner that maintains quality, is a greater challenge (Mechanic, et al., 1995). In evaluating the effects of managed care, it is necessary to describe specifically which managed care mechanisms were used and what outcomes were measured. For example, a study examining the practices of managed care programs for mental health, alcohol abuse, and drug abuse during the late 1980s found that large variations in utilization review programs were common (Garnick, Hendricks, Dulski, Thorpe, & Horgan, 1994). Review personnel, clinical criteria to authorize care, the use of mental health "carve-outs" (in which psychiatric services are managed separately from other medical benefits), integration of employee assistance programs, penalties for not following plan procedures, and the type and amount of outpatient review varied considerably among managed care companies. The authors concluded that the diversity seemed to be growing into the 1990s and that this will make it difficult to ascertain which aspects of managed care actually work to control costs while protecting quality of care. Similarly, another research team reviewed what is known about the effects of managed care on mental health and substance abuse services (Mechanic, et al., 1995). These authors found the task difficult given the wide heterogeneity of managed care plans.

Generally, they found that there was cost savings through decreased use of in-patient days, but that decreased in-patient time was not always accompanied by increased out-patient or partial hospitalization use, suggesting that cost-containment merely reflected more unmet need or a shifting of the burden of care to the family and community. By assertively becoming involved in outcome research, providers, including occupational therapists, may be able to focus more directly on cost-*effectiveness* as opposed to cost-*control* of services.

Best Care Practices

As outcome measurement occurs, we will be able to identify which types of mental health and substance abuse practices are best. Currently in the private sector, managed care emphasizes brief, focused therapies for persons with *mild* to *moderate* psychological difficulties. Budman (1992) characterized the dominant values of brief and long-term therapists. Brief therapists prefer pragmatic solutions, emphasize client strengths and resources, and see being in the world as more important than being in therapy. Long-term therapists focus on seeking changes in the client's basic character, assume that presenting problems are always indicative of underlying pathology, and view being in therapy as the most important part of the client's life. It is my impression that most occupational therapists would actually agree with many of the values espoused by the brief therapist and already apply them in practice. More research is needed to determine when brief therapies are appropriate.

In the public sector, some long-term empirical studies have been completed concerning the outcomes of programs for clients with complex and chronic psychosocial problems. The most effective tested approaches to date include assertive community treatment for adults with severe mental illness and multi-systemic therapy for adolescents with serious emotional disturbances (Santos, Henggeler, Burns, Arana, & Meisler, 1995). In both approaches, several operant principles were at work, including the use of:

- a socioecological model of behavior that emphasizes the importance of context to support functional capacity
- pragmatic treatment that focuses on action-oriented, well-specified interventions and careful monitoring of treatment outcomes
- field-based services that occur in the client's natural environment
- individualized treatment that addresses flexible, collaboratively developed goals
- accountability in which staff members are discouraged from blaming clients for lack of progress and encouraged to focus on the use of creative solutions to problems.

Both assertive community therapy and multi-systemic therapy are congruent with basic occupational therapy beliefs and principles. The roles and tasks in these descriptions of best mental health practice for clients with chronic psychosocial problems include therapy that is collaboratively determined, is functionally oriented, and takes place in the client's natural home and community settings (e.g., Nielson, 1993; Quinn, 1993). If increasing numbers of empirical studies demonstrate the cost-effectiveness of comprehensive, intensive, community-based practice, then occupational therapy practitioners will have strong ammunition to argue for reimbursement of these services. It may be hard for professionals struggling with first generation approaches to managed care to envision more extensive coverage for services, but it is important to advocate for these types of programs and assist in the process of demonstrating efficacy and cost-effectiveness. The current emphasis on an inpatient medical model for mental health practice needs to be examined and preparations made for the transition into flexible, integrated, community-based practice (AOTA, 1995).

Interdisciplinary Teams

Interdisciplinary teams have been around for a long time in mental health practice, (e.g., Greenberg, et al., 1986) but managed care is emphasizing them even more as a cost-effective way to deliver care. An interdisciplinary focus is encouraging to occupational therapists who may envision themselves as part of the core team. Recent descriptions of managed care teams, however, do not identify occupational therapists as possible members. Of even more concern is the importance of master's level providers in assuring quality team care (Goodman, et al., 1992; Olsen, et al., 1995; Schuster, Kern, Kane, & Nettleman, 1994). The assumption seems to be that only master's level training is adequate to successfully perform the skilled tasks required in a managed mental health care setting. My own experience as a clinician providing mental health and substance abuse services in an HMO is congruent with this observation, because the advertisement for my job stated that only occupational therapy practitioners with a master's degree were eligible to apply.

Ethical Considerations

Sabin (1994) identified a credo for ethically-managed mental health care in which he suggested that clinicians must learn how to care for clients while acting as stewards of society's resources; must recommend less costly treatments, unless there is strong evidence that a more expensive intervention is clearly superior; and must advocate for justice in the health care system in addition to advocating for clients. Can we apply this credo in occupational therapy? Backlar (1995) highlighted the dilemma of concern for the individual client versus the larger needs of the mental health care system. It is difficult to envision what it means to act as "stewards for society" while meeting obligations to clients. In addition, until more outcome research is completed, the efficacy of various interventions is controversial. Finally, as long as the perception exists that any cost-savings go into the pockets of large managed care companies as profit instead of being funneled back into the development of a just and fair health care system, the concept of stewardship is false (Sabin, 1994). In that case, I believe that our responsibility is to fight the inappropriate care-rationing and unfair profit-making that occur at the client's expense.

MOVING FORWARD

Occupational therapy may be in particular danger of being lost in the turmoil of mental health care system changes. We are currently a small part of the mental health treatment picture because there are few occupational therapy practitioners in mental health and substance abuse practice settings (AOTA, 1991; Bonder, 1987). Occupational therapists need to be visible, proactive, and accountable in the process of defining and developing a cost-effective continuum of programs and services that emphasizes the community over the in-patient setting as appropriate, identifies effective methods to measure outcomes, and develops clinically reasonable and flexible guidelines and protocols. While the occupational therapy profession struggles over its role in mental health and continues to refer to community-based mental health practice as non-traditional (AOTA, 1995), other providers have already recognized the critical nature of function for clients with mental illness, are addressing community living skills (Farms & Anthony, 1989; Liberman, 1988), and are actively developing guidelines and measuring outcomes for these services (Andrews, Peters, & Teeson, 1994; Lacayo, 1995).

Lazarus (1994) described a number of reasons why psychiatrists may dislike managed care. Many of those reasons probably also apply to occupational therapists, including under-funding for services, new practice patterns, turf wars, demand for proof of value of services, bureaucratic hassles, and moral dilemmas. But occupational therapy professionals cannot ignore the evolving mental health care system or pretend the past few decades have been a golden era. Empirical support for alternatives to in-patient hospitalization (e.g., partial hospitalization, community-based programs) has existed for years, but recommended programs were never implemented because they were not reimbursed by traditional indemnity insurance (Bartlett, 1994). Occupational therapists must vigorously advocate for appropriate mental health services and assist in moving beyond the most negative attributes of first generation managed care that emphasize cutting costs and care. At its best, managed care may actually support innovations and diversity of treatment approaches as long as empirical evidence supports the effectiveness and efficiency of those approaches. It is even possible that mental health and substance abuse practices and outcomes may be improved.

References

American Occupational Therapy Association. (1991). *1990 member data survey: Summary report*. Rockville, MD: Author.

American Occupational Therapy Association. (1995). *Mental Health SIS Education Task Force report*. Bethesda, MD: Author.

Andrews, G., Peters, L., & Teeson, Al. (1994). *The measurement of consumer outcome in mental health: A report to the National Mental Health Information Strategy Committee*. Sydney, Australia: Clinical Research Unit for Anxiety Disorders.

Backlar, P. (1995). Health care reform: Will the subject fall out of the topic. *Community Mental Health Journal, 31,* 297-301.

Bartlett, J. (1994, Fall). The emergence of managed care and its impact on psychiatry. *New Directions for Mental Health Services, 63,* 25-35.

Bevilacqua, J. (1995, Summer). New paradigms, old pitfall. *New Directions for Mental Health Services, 66,* 19-31.

Bonder, B. R. (1987). Occupational therapy in mental health: Crisis or opportunity? *American Journal of Occupational Therapy, 41,* 495-499.

Budman, S. (1992). Model of brief individual and group psychotherapy. In J. Feldman & R. Fitzpatrick (Eds.), *Managed mental health care: Administrative and clinical issues* (pp. 231-248). Washington, DC: American Psychiatric Press.

Eisenberg, L (1992). Treating depression and anxiety in primary care. *New England Journal of Medicine, 326,* 1080-1084.

Ellek, D. (1995). Health Policy—Managed competition: Maintaining health care within the private sector. *American Journal of Occupational Therapy, 49,* 468-472.

Farms, M., & Anthony, W. (Eds.). (1989). *Psychiatric rehabilitation programs: Putting theory into practice*. Baltimore, MD: Johns Hopkins University Press.

Flynn, L. (1994). Managed care and mental illness. In R. Schreter, S. Sharfstein, & C. Schreter (Eds.), *Allies and adversaries: The impact of managed care on mental health service* (pp. 203-212). Washington, DC: American Psychiatric Press.

Garnick, D., Hendricks, A., Dulski, J., Thorpe, K., & Horgan, C. (1994). Characteristics of private sector managed care for mental health and substance abuse treatment. *Hospital and Community Psychiatry, 45,* 1201-1205.

Gerson, S. (1994, March/April). When should managed care firms terminate private benefits for chronically mentally ill patients? *Behavioral Healthcare, 40,* 42-43.

Goodman, M., Brown, J., & Deitz, P. (1992). *Managing managed care: A mental health practitioners survival guide*. Washington, DC: American Psychiatric Press.

Greenberg, L., Fine, S., Cohen, C., Larson, K., Michaelson-Baily, A., Rubinton, P., & Glick, I. (1986). An interdisciplinary psychoeducational program for schizophrenic patients and their families in an acute care setting. *Hospital and Community Psychiatry, 39,* 277-282. (See Chapter 55 in this text.)

Hoge, M., Davidson, L, Griffith, E., Sledge, W., & Howenstine, R. (1994). Defining managed care in public sector psychiatry. *Hospital and Community Psychiatry, 45,* 1085-1089.

Jonas, S. (1986). *Health care delivery in the United States* (3rd Edition). New York, NY: Springer.

Kane, R. Bartlett, J., & Potthoff, S. (1995). Building an empirically based outcome information system for managed mental heath care. *Psychiatric Services, 46,* 459-461.

Lacayo, J. (1995, August). IAPSRS proposed "tool-kit" for measuring PSR outcomes. *La Voz,* 5-8.

Lazarus, A. (1994). Ten reasons why psychiatrists may dislike managed competition. *Hospital and Community Psychiatry, 45,* 496-489.

Liberman, R. (Ed.). (1988). *Psychiatric rehabilitation of chronic mental patients*. Washington, DC: American Psychiatric Press.

Lipsitt, D. (1995). Managed care: A catalyst for integrated medicine. *General Hospital Psychiatry, 17,* 243-245.

Mechanic, D. (1987). Correcting misconceptions in mental health policy strategies for improving care of the seriously mentally ill. *Milbank Quarterly, 65,* 203-230.

Mechanic, D., Schlesinger, M., & McAlpine, D. (1995). Management of mental health and substance abuse services: State of the art and early results. *Milbank Quarterly, 73,* 1956.

Myers, J., Weissman, M., Tischler, G., Holzer, C., Leaf, P., Orvaschel, H., Anthony, J., Boyd, J., Burke, J., Kramer, M., & Stolzman, R. (1984). Six-month prevalence of psychiatric disorders in three communities. *Archives of General Psychiatry, 41,* 959-967.

Nielson, C. (1993, September). Occupational therapy and community mental health: A new and unprecedented turn. *Mental Health Special Interest Section Newsletter, 16*(3), 12.

Olsen, D., Rickles, J., & Travlik, K. (1995). A response team model of managed mental health care. *Psychiatric Services, 46,* 252-256.

Quinn, B. (1993, June). Community occupational therapy in Canada: A model for mental health. *Mental Health Special Interest Section Newsletter, 16*(2), 14.

Sabin, J. (1994). A credo for ethical managed care in mental health practice. *Hospital and Community Psychiatry, 45,* 859-860.

Santos, A., Henggeler, S., Burns, B., Arana, G., & Meisler, N. (1995). Research on field-based services: Models for reform in the delivery of mental health care to populations with complex clinical problems. *American Journal of Psychiatry, 152,* 1111-1123.

Schreter, R., Sharfstein, S., & Schreter, C. (Eds.). (1994). *Allies and adversaries: The impact of managed care on mental health service*. Washington, DC: American Psychiatric Press.

Schuster, J., Kern, E., Kane, V., & Nettleman, L. (1994). Changing roles of mental health clinicians in multidisciplinary teams. *Hospital and Community Psychiatry, 45,* 1187-1189.

Steinwachs, D., Kasper, J., & Skinner, E. (1992). Patterns of use and costs among severely mentally ill people. *Health Affair, 11,* 178-183.

Stoffel, V., & Cunningham, S. (1991). Continuous quality improvement: An innovative approach applied to mental health programs in occupational therapy. *Occupational Therapy Practice, 2*(2), 52-60. (See Chapter Nine in this text.)

Summergrad, P., Herman, J., Weilburg, J., & Jeillinek, M. (1995). Wagons ho: Forward on the managed care trail. *General Hospital Psychiatry, 17,* 251-259.

Thien, M. H. (1987, December). Demonstrating treatment outcomes in mental health. *Mental Health Special Interest Section Newsletter, 10*(4), 23. (Reprinted in Cottrell, R. P. (1996). *Psychosocial occupational therapy: Proactive approaches* (pp. 361-364). Bethesda, MD: AOTA.)

Wells, K., Astrachan, B., Tischler, G., & Unutzer, J. (1995). Issues and approaches in evaluating managed mental health care. *Milbank Quarterly, 73*, 57-76.

Wood, R., Bailey, N., Tilkemeir, D. (1992). Managed care: The missing link is quality improvement. *Journal of Nursing Care Quality, 6*, 55-65.

Strategies for Program Development, Management, and Evaluation

EDITOR'S NOTE

To respond proactively to the issues and trends identified in the preceding section, the occupational therapist must have a solid foundation in program development, management, and evaluation. The knowledge and skills that occupational therapists use to provide direct care (ie: evaluation, clinical reasoning, treatment implementation, and reevaluation) can be naturally extended to the development of occupational therapy programs. Competent program planning and development is essential for ensuring that occupational therapy is available to a diversity of populations across the entire health care continuum.

Effective program planning in today's complex and changing health care system requires occupational therapists to collaborate with other professionals to ensure comprehensiveness and excellence in their provision of professional services. Adequate knowledge and understanding of the roles and functions of other professionals are essential to the development of close collaborative relationships that will result in the most comprehensive program plan and the best possible outcome for the client. The therapist who collaborates with other professionals to plan and implement programs must have a solid foundation in occupational therapy philosophy, theories, frames of reference, and models of practice and an understanding as to how their occupational therapy knowledge fits into the practice models of other professions.

The chapters in this section support the development of excellence in program planning and management based upon a strong foundation in occupational therapy theory and philosophy. In Chapter 5, Judy Grossman and Jody Bortone present a four-step model for program development. Each step is systematically and comprehensively described. The provision of practical suggestions and methodologies for clinical application of this program development model makes the process understandable and manageable.

The ability of occupational therapists to develop and implement program changes and to assume leadership roles within their settings, is often dependent upon their communication skills. In this section's next chapter, Susan C. Robertson and Susan C. Schwartz define strategic communication and explore this vital link between occupational therapy and the practice setting. Environmental, organizational, and professional factors that influence communication and clinical decision-making are analyzed. Strategies for developing effective communication skills are described. A practice-oriented framework for utilizing strategic communication within a clinical setting is presented. The efficacy of applying strategic communication principles to clinical practice is highlighted by two relevant examples.

Another powerful tool that occupational therapists can use to position themselves as leaders in a rapidly changing health care care system is strategic planning. In Chapter 7, Teri L. Shackleton and Marie Gage describe the strategic planning process that was implemented in their department to provide a consensual framework for addressing identified obstacles to occupational therapy leadership, while positioning occupational therapists to seize the role opportunities offered by emerging health care trends. The concepts and benefits of strategic planning and a selected strategic planning process are presented. Clear, relevant examples from the authors' departmental experience are provided for all eight elements of this strategic planning process. Readers are encouraged to use Shackleton's and Gage's shared experiences to apply the strategic planning process to their practice setting. At this time of limited resources, professional competition, and required accountability, the use of the strategic planning process is essential for occupational therapy program development.

One of the most frequent outcomes of strategic planning and occupational therapy program development is the formation and implementation of therapeutic groups. Susan Haiman reviews pertinent health care issues that influence the use of groups in occupational therapy practice in Chapter 8. According to Haiman, effective, relevant groups are selected and designed based on a needs assessment and they consistently use clinical reasoning throughout their development and implementation (in contrast to a cookbook approach). Based on these principles, Haiman presents a group protocol selection system that readers will find applicable to any setting and client population that uses groups for evaluation and intervention.

One cannot assume that a program will automatically maintain its excellence, no matter how good the initial development process. Population characteristics change, goals are met (or unmet), and new needs arise. To respond proactively to these changes, the therapist must view program evaluation as an essential component of program development. As Grossman and Bortone emphasize in their chapter on program development in this section, program evaluation is the last stage in the program development cycle.

Program evaluation ensures that consumers are receiving the highest quality of professional services. This assurance of quality of care is essential in today's health care system. Increased demands for accountability and cost-effectiveness, the growth of the consumer movement, and the rise of competition within the health care market all require the occupational therapist to become fluent and skilled in program evaluation principles and methods. By evaluating treatment efficacy, occupational therapists can modify and adjust their programs, as needed, to increase the effectiveness and relevance of their interventions. The accumulation of treatment efficacy data can also be used to market model programs, obtain increased funding, expand program services, recruit and employ additional staff, maintain program accreditation, and increase staff pride and consumer satisfaction.

Occupational therapy programs are frequently successful in their outcomes; however, the profession has not produced sufficient research to document this success (Wood, 1998). Consequently, in some areas of practice, the professional image of occupational therapy has been diminished due to this lack of outcome studies. The acquisition of program evaluation skills can empower occupational therapists with the knowledge and skills to do their jobs better, and to demonstrate this enhanced effectiveness to consumers, administative bodies, regulatory agencies, policy makers, and third-party payers.

The role of the occupational therapist in program evaluation is examined in this section's next chapter by Virginia Carroll Stoffel and Susan M. Cunningham. These authors present the continuous quality improvement (CQI) approach of evaluating and improving the quality of patient care in mental health. The relevance of the CQI approach to current trends in mental health practice is explored. CQI concepts and principles are described, with relevant clinical examples given to illustrate the application of CQI to current occupational therapy practice. Suggestions and references for the implementation of CQI are provided. According to the authors, the utilization of this consumer-oriented, interdisciplinary, systems approach to program evaluation will result in substantial benefits for treatment settings, patient populations, and the profession of occupational therapy.

The relevance and efficacy of using a CQI approach to program planning is presented in this section's final chapter by Mary Hostetler Brinson. She presents a strong rationale for implementing CQI to develop programs, based on the current constraints in mental health care and the realistic concerns of consumers. Brinson describes the process of change that occurred on an acute psychiatric unit when an interdisciplinary team used CQI to develop a therapeutic milieu. The major role occupational therapists played in shaping this meaningful, structured, and well planned milieu program is a strong example of the leadership role occupational therapists can assume in program development, management, and evaluation.

While many program development projects and evaluation studies are implemented solely to meet administrative requirements and accreditation standards, therapists are often pleasantly surprised by the energizing momentum that arises from their efforts. Documenting the efficacy of their treatment can empower therapists to challenge themselves to be their professional best. The resulting increase in quality of care and improvement of consumer outcome can enhance professional image, decrease stagnation, and prevent burnout. Readers are urged to use these chapters and the references provided to develop their program development, management, and evaluation skills; and to ensure quality of care in their provision of occupational therapy services.

The ability of occupational therapists to utilize their unique professional knowledge, along with their effective communication and clinical reasoning skills, to plan intervention programs and assume leadership roles in today's health care system is also strongly supported by this section's authors. These issues are further emphasized and expanded upon in Section Three, which discusses the practice of occupational therapy along the mental health continuum of care.

QUESTIONS TO CONSIDER

1. How can occupational therapists apply their knowledge and skills to the development of intervention programs? What are important differences between client-centered treatment planning and population-focused program planning?

2. What are current issues and trends that influence program planning? What are the essential steps to developing an effective occupational therapy program?

3. How does an occupational therapist's frame of references influence program planning? Which frames of references are compatible with the intervention program needs of today's health care system? Which frame(s) of reference would you use in developing an occupational therapy program for an acute, in-patient unit? An out-patient, day treatment program? A long-term residential facility? A wellness and prevention program?

4. What are current issues and important factors for occupational therapists to consider when designing group interventions? How can the clinical decision-making process facilitate the development and selection of relevant group protocols? What clinical reasoning skills are vital to utilize in the implementation and evaluation of therapeutic groups?

5. What are the issues and factors that influence effective communication within today's health care system? What principles and methods can an occupational therapist use to develop strategic communication skills? How can these strategies be applied in a practice setting to enhance the role of occupational therapy?

6. How do current health care issues and trends impact occupational therapy program evaluation? What effect may cost-containment and accountability demands have on program evaluation?

7. What are the areas of occupational therapy intervention most relevant for program evaluation studies? What can the occupational therapist uniquely offer to interdisciplinary program evaluations? How can the occupational therapist maximize a collaborative, client-centered approach to program evaluation?

8. How can the outcomes of program evaluations be used to benefit the consumer? The treatment setting? The occupational therapy profession? What are the marketing implications of program evaluations?

9. Imagine you have recently been hired as the director of a community day treatment program for persons with chronic mental illness. The program's primary goal is to develop community living skills through the provision of case management and theraputic activity groups. The program's population totals 35; however, daily attendance averages between 8 and 12 clients. Your clinical staff includes an Occupational Therapy Assistant, a nurse, and a mental health aide. You are designing your program evaluation plan. Which approach will you use? What are potential implications of your study for program development?

REFERENCES

American Occupational Therapy Association. (1996). *The occupational therapy manager* (Revised Edition). Bethesda, Md: Author.

American Occupational Therapy Association. (1991). *Quality assurance in occupational therapy: A practitioner's guide to setting up a QA system using three models.* Rockville, MD: Author.

Hoffman-Grotting, K., & Ralph, V. J. (1991). Enhancing the program's image and performance by comparing and using quality assurance and program evaluation information. *Occupational Therapy in Practice, 2*(2), 16-25.

Schwartz, S. C. (1988) Service management strategies for occupational therapy. In S. C. Robertson (Ed.), *Mental health FOCUS: Skills for assessment and treatment.* (pp. 137-143). Rockville: MD: American Occupational Therapy Association.

Smith, G. R., Fisher, E. P., Nordquist, M. A., Mosley, C. L., & Ledbetter, N. S. (1997). Implementing outcomes management systems in mental health settings. *Psychiatric Services, 48,* 364-368.

Smith, S. R., Manderscheid, R. W., Flynn, L. M., & Steinwacks, D. M. (1997). Principles for assessment of patient outcomes in mental health care. *Psychiatric Services, 48,* 1033-1036.

Wood, W. (1998). Nationally speaking: Is it jump time for occuaptional therapy? *American Journal of Occupational Therapy, 52,* 403-411.

CHAPTER FIVE

Program Development

Judy Grossman and Jody Bortone

To provide mental health services in occupational therapy, the program manager must develop competencies on several levels, grouped under the broad "micro" and "macro" levels of planning. The micro level represents clinical management issues for a patient. The macro level represents programmatic issues for a population. The micro and macro levels actually parallel each other in the sequencing of problem identification, planning, implementation, and outcome. Both patient treatment and population-focused planning require good clinical judgment and analytical skills for assessment and intervention. They differ, however, in some important respects that will be discussed in this chapter.

Micro—Patient	Macro—Population
Screening and evaluation	Needs assessment
Treatment planning	Program planning
Treatment intervention	Program implementation
Reevaluation	Program evaluation and quality assurance

The changing nature of mental health services delivery, the needs of chronic mentally ill patients, and the acute staffing shortage are all driving forces behind the need for increased competencies in program development. Good planning skills will have an effect on patient care and career mobility in occupational therapy.

The most critical step in program development is the shift to population-based planning. The objective in developing an occupational therapy program is to design the most effective program for the most people.

There are four basic steps in program development:

1. Needs assessment
2. Program planning
3. Program implementation
4. Program evaluation

Step I—Needs Assessment: This step involves data gathering and problem identification, including a description of the population to be served and an assessment of the treatment needs and the resources available to meet these needs.

Step 2—Program Planning: This step integrates the treatment needs and resources with theoretical frame(s) of reference. It also establishes goals and objectives for problem-focused planning.

Step 3—Program Implementation: This step focuses on documentation, communication, and coordination with other providers. It also requires the appropriate selection of assessments and interventions for each patient/client.

Step 4—Program Evaluation: This step involves systematic review and analysis of the program based on the established goals and objectives.

Program development is a progressive and cyclical process in which the therapist continually monitors and adjusts the program to meet the needs of the target population. This process is depicted graphically in Figure 5-1.

NEEDS ASSESSMENT

Needs assessment is very important, yet is often the most overlooked step in program development. Collecting appropriate information about the target population is necessary in order to design an effective program. This step deserves adequate time and attention.

Needs assessment takes place on several levels from the patient/client level (micro) to the community at large level (macro), as shown in Figure 5-2.

For example, the occupational therapist will first want information on an identified patient/client. The therapist who is implementing a treatment program will put the most effort into assessing the individual patient/client and the target clinical population of which the patient is a member (for example, a young adult chronic patient in a transitional unit). The therapist will then want to obtain information about the target population in the community in order to locate resources or develop programs for continuity of care (for example, day treatment programs for deinstitutionalized

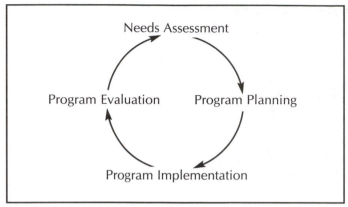

Figure 5-1. Program development.

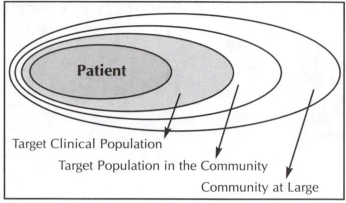

Figure 5-2. Levels of needs assessment.

chronically mentally ill patients/clients). Finally, the therapist will want information about the community to which the patient/client will return (the expected environment) and the functional skill requirements that the community will demand. To develop a program in which any patient/client will participate, information must be gathered on all these levels using micro and macro perspectives.

Needs assessment requires a systematic approach to data gathering. The steps in this systematic approach include (a) describing the community, (b) describing the target population, (c) identifying needs, and (d) identifying resources.

Describing the Community

This first step in gathering data for needs assessment is important for planning relevant programs and developing realistic discharge plans. A sensitive therapist should understand the patient's/client's natural environment and the daily routines of community residents. This step involves both quantitative and qualitative data gathering. The following information will be helpful to the therapist during this stage:

1. Sociodemographic Data on Community Residents

These data may include information on age, sex, family structure, religious and ethnic background, education, income, occupational level, and employment.

2. Community Description

A community description provides information on the physical, social, cultural, and economic factors that are relevant for mental health planning. The physical description of the community should include the boundaries of the geographic area or catchment area, physical landmarks, and the location of essential services. This information relates to the utilization and accessibility of essential services and community resources. The social and cultural description provides information about attitudes, beliefs, expectations, proscribed roles, and standards of behavior. It is critical to appreciate the value system of community residents and the patterns of work and leisure time activities. An economic description provides information on the power structure in the community, support for essential services, and the economic livelihood of residents.

3. Community Trends and Populations at Risk

It is often helpful to have information on community trends, such as the stability or transitional nature of different neighborhoods. While conducting the needs assessment, it is possible to identify populations at risk in the community that may need additional services and resource development. At-risk populations can be defined according to developmental status (e.g., geriatric, adolescent), life crises (e.g., divorce, hospitalization of family member), or chronic strains (e.g., multi-problem families). The identified population for occupational therapy programming may or may not be recognized as one of the high-risk groups.

Describing the Target Population

The second step in gathering information for needs assessment is to define the target population, that is, those people for whom an occupational therapy program is to be designed.

Demographic data must also be gathered on the target population, and it is often helpful to compare these data to the community data. The targeted population may constitute a distinct subgroup in the community or be representative of a particular culture or socioeconomic strata in the community. To conduct population-focused planning, it is helpful to categorize the target population in a way that will emphasize the similarities of the targeted group, such as the diagnosis or prognosis of the illness or disorder, or perhaps the level of function. Other useful information that may be collected from medical records is the average length of stay, number of hospitalizations, and level of pre-morbid functioning.

To develop programs for the target population, it is important to be familiar with the clinical description of the disability. It is necessary to review the theoretical and research literature to understand each disorder and to be alert to significant manifestations, associated signs and symptoms, prognosis, and functional abilities and disabilities.

Identifying Needs

The third step in gathering information for needs assessment is to identify the specific needs of the target population. In many cases, specific treatment needs appear obvious, but a more systematic approach is warranted.

There are different levels of needs. First are the felt needs of the patients/clients. While these are not always realistic, they provide the basis for collaboration between the therapist and patient. Within this context, felt needs can be modified or shaped. Occupational therapy personnel should always ask patients about what they need to work on or what they want to get out of the program.

Second are the perceived needs reported by others. Occupational therapy personnel may wish to interview or survey department staff, treatment providers in both the present system and the expected environment, or significant others, such as family members or teachers. It is important to consider patient/client needs from the perspective of other people.

Third are the real needs that describe the true functional abilities and disabilities of the population, as measured by objective evaluation instruments. Therapists must systematically use a battery of evaluation instruments to determine if the patient/client population has a deficiency. For example, 60% of the people may be deficient in work skills, whereas only 20% may not be independent in activities of daily living. It is important to understand the actual and full range of abilities and disabilities of the target population. This information is usually gathered for individual patients/clients and must be synthesized in aggregate form for use in planning occupational therapy programs.

Once needs are assessed, it is helpful to determine any discrepancy between felt and real needs. This process is important to communicate goals and objectives to all people concerned, including the consumer, providers of service, and family members.

The purpose of the needs assessment is to identify unmet needs and to categorize them in priority order for planning. To establish priorities, it is necessary to assess how the needs match the expectations of the general population. For example, the feasibility of vocational training in a given job market or the value placed on certain social activities will influence the emphasis placed on meeting certain population needs.

Identifying Resources

The last step in gathering information for needs assessment is to evaluate the resources available for implementing the program. Resources can be categorized as both formal and informal sources of support. Formal, or institutional, resources include administrative support: staff, supplies and equipment, space, time, and money. Staff support includes occupational therapy staff, as well as other professional staff.

In evaluating institutional resources, it is important to know what programs exist and whether they are meeting real needs. Some services are offered on an in-patient basis, and others are available after discharge. Analysis of the services provided by the institution should encompass not only those delivered by occupational therapy personnel but also those delivered by other team members.

Some questions to consider in assessing resources are whether services are available, accessible, and effective. The full range of services currently available should be analyzed to determine what real needs have not yet been met. Any gaps in services should become apparent, and these will enter into the formulation of goals and objectives for the occupational therapy program.

It may also be appropriate to identify formal resources in the community, such as educational, recreational, health, and social services. Occupational therapy personnel should become familiar with community programs: the referral process, expectations of the agency, and, most important, the ways the program is addressing real needs.

It is also essential to identify informal resources to support the program itself or the population it serves. These resources may be either institutional- or community-based. They may be advocates of occupational therapy in the hospital, or support personnel who will help implement the occupational therapy program. Social supports such as family, friends, religious and cultural figures, and self-help groups may be identified in the community. The various contributions of informal caregivers should also enter into the program planning done by occupational therapy personnel.

Needs Assessment Methods

There are many ways to assess needs. A good place to start is the sociodemographic and descriptive information that is readily available in communities. This information may be found in documents and reports from the U.S. Census Bureau, state and local government, health departments, health planning agencies, community planning boards, mental health associations, research departments of community mental health centers, and universities. These sources can be located through the town hall, local library, and telephone directory. Specific program information may be obtained by contacting facilities directly or the state mental health agency.

Objective information on the community should be supplemented with subjective information. The occupational therapist's personal experience and conversations with community residents, community caregivers, social service agencies, and school personnel, for example, may provide a perspective that complements or reinforces the objective assessment.

Objective methods include the use of surveys, key informants, community forums, rates under treatment, and social indicators.

The *survey method* is a reliable and comprehensive way to collect a great deal of information. The survey can involve interview or self-report, and it may be directed to any group, such as the target population, the providers of service, or community residents. For this method, it is important to select a representative sample and to develop a relatively reliable survey.

The *key informant* approach is a method of surveying key people who are in a position to perceive patterns of needs, rather than sampling the entire population. It is simple, less expensive, and less time-consuming than the survey method. There may, however, be bias in the sampling or in the interviewing technique.

The *community forum* is a method that achieves broad representation through panels or public meetings. This approach is most applicable to problems that affect the entire community or significant subgroups. A potential disadvantage of this method is that these groups may not be representative of the community at large and that their opinions may represent a bias.

The *rates under treatment approach* is really a measure of service utilization gathered through records and reports. Caution should be exercised in relying on this approach, since statistics reflect those in treatment and not necessarily those in need.

Social indicators are actually indirect measures of need. Social indicators are social and environmental factors that correlate with mental health problems and are therefore used to predict problems or derive inferences about a population. This type of analysis can be conducted through statistics available through such sources as the U.S. Census Bureau.

PROGRAM PLANNING

After needs have been assessed, the second step in population-based program development is program planning. Program planning uses the information obtained in the needs assessment about the needs of the population and the present resources available to address those needs. To plan a program, one must integrate this information with appropriate frames of reference to establish the program's goals and objectives.

A comprehensive plan for any program will also include the establishment of standards for the program's outcome, a timetable, methods of integrating the program with the existing system, the definition of roles, and the establishment of a referral system that details how people enter and leave the program.

The program planning step is a systematic integration of factual information with theoretical frames of reference in order to define a comprehensive program plan designed to address the needs of the target population in a prescribed sequence. The steps for developing a program plan follow:

1. Defining a focus
2. Adopting frame(s) of reference
3. Establishing goals and objectives
4. Establishing methods to integrate the program into the existing system
5. Developing referral systems

Defining a Focus

The ability to define a focus for a program depends on an analysis of the needs assessment results. The needs assessment will yield a massive amount of information that the program planner must categorize and establish priorities for, so that a focus for the program can be determined.

The content focus of a program can be determined by first categorizing the needs (felt and real) identified according to the various occupational performance areas and component skill functions, and then identifying those areas and skills that are deficient for a specific percentage of the target population. Since the intent of program development is to address the unmet needs of the target population, only those skill areas that are deficient for the majority of the target population will be given priority in content focus.

By comparing the functional skill deficit areas with the skill demands of the expected environment, the therapist can identify occupational performance areas and component skill functions that are crucial for the program to address. This list of priorities may then be further refined by evaluating available resources and patterns of use. If the therapist identifies needs that are already being addressed by other resources, it will not be necessary to duplicate those services. Close coordination of services is, however, essential. Occupational therapy should focus the program on needs deficits and skills deficits that are not adequately addressed and that could not be addressed by other resources.

The level of difficulty of the occupational performance and component skills addressed in the program must be incorporated into its design. The level of any program is not static, but includes a range of levels so that a larger percentage of the target population can be served. The program can thereby include a coherent sequence by which people can progress through the program with increasing challenge.

The range of levels should begin at the current lowest level of functioning of the clear majority of the target population. The lower, or minimal, functional level of a program is the set of minimal expected behaviors and skills that people must have to enter the program. This level of the program is determined by assessing the real needs of the target population, using assessment and evaluation instruments.

The upper, or maximal, functional level of the program is the set of maximum or most difficult skills and behaviors that can be offered by the program. Again, this level of the program is obtained by assessing felt and perceived needs and is determined by the level of functional skills demanded by the expected environment. The program's content addresses only the needs or functional skills of the target population that are considered deficient in relation to the skill functions at the level demanded by the expected environment.

Adopting Frames of Reference

Frame(s) of reference give the therapist the criteria by which findings of the needs assessment can be categorized into content areas and levels. In the context of the program planning stage, however, the therapist must now evaluate and choose the frames of reference that are most likely to be successful in addressing and resolving the needs that constitute the program's focus.

Reevaluating and selecting alternative frames of reference can be systematically completed by paying attention to three basic considerations. First, therapists must consider their own experiences and familiarity and comfort with the various occupational therapy frames of reference. Second, therapists must be familiar with relevant clinical and research literature that will offer guidelines about those frames of reference found helpful in addressing specific functional needs of specific populations. Finally, it is essential that the therapist have a thorough understanding of the frames of reference that are used and emphasized in the institution or treatment system.

It is important for the occupational therapist to be familiar with a variety of frames of reference. For example, therapists who develop a program based only on a frame of reference with which they are familiar may indeed develop a perfectly balanced program according to that frame of reference. But this program may not specifically address the needs of the target population, or it may include treatment approaches that have been found to be ineffective with the target population. It may also be a program that, by its very design, constantly conflicts with the rest of the treatment system.

A review of the clinical and research literature may validate the therapist's choice of a particular frame of reference and/or may pinpoint new frames of reference that the therapist should understand and incorporate into the program design.

The occupational therapist must consider the frames of reference used and considered primary by the institutional system. It is important to select a frame of reference for the occupational therapy program that is compatible with those of the institutional system. Each profession has its own frames of reference. Compatible definitions of a functional or dysfunctional state may differ among professions, and treatment goals and methodologies differ. Major conflicts in the system's and program's frame of reference may place the program and its therapists in a difficult position.

Establishing Goals and Objectives

Establishing goals and objectives is the next step in developing a program plan. The goals and objectives of the treatment program are specifically related to the focus of the program. The goals should be problem-oriented and should be described in behavioral terms, specifying the level of performance expected at the outcome. Goals should paint a clear picture of what patients/clients will be able to do once they complete the program.

When establishing treatment goals for patients/clients in the program, it is also important to establish standards for the program as a whole. In this way, quality assurance becomes an integral part of the overall program plan. Standards should project the acceptable percentage of the target population that is served by the program, the percentage of patients/clients who enter and complete the program, and the percentage of patients/clients who actually reach the goals. Such standards need to be set during the program planning stage. By establishing standards ahead of time, the therapist will have guidelines for documenting information

in order to evaluate the efficacy and efficiency of the program over an extended period. Goals and standards are crucial to any program evaluation and must therefore be established in the planning phase.

Establishing Methods to Integrate the Program

The next step in program planning describes exactly how the program will be integrated into the existing treatment system. It involves the establishment of timetables and the definition of therapists' roles and areas of collaboration with other professionals. The identification of potential obstacles to the implementation of the program and of key resources that could be helpful in implementation is also essential.

The first part of this integration process is the establishment of a realistic timetable. This timetable should show when the program will be implemented and in what sequence. In establishing this timetable, it is desirable to involve professional groups within the system who are key to the success or failure of the program.

Definition of the roles of various disciplines is the second part of this integration process. Roles should be defined in accordance with professional competencies and affiliations. The success or failure of a program depends on appropriate staff assignments.

Definition of roles may well include areas of collaboration with other professionals when appropriate. Consultation among professionals and coleadership of program components should be considered carefully and should be formally established only when suited to the program's focus. For example, one component of a program for alcohol abusers might be to help them develop more appropriate parenting skills with their children. An occupational therapist and a social worker might collaborate on this process. The social worker provides expertise in family therapy and the occupational therapist provides expertise in interpersonal skill development through purposeful activities with their children.

The final consideration in integrating a program is identifying potential obstacles to implementation. Conflicts over professional turf and competition for patients'/clients' time could interfere with the implementation of the best planned program. Once obstacles have been identified, program developers should then find ways to deal with these obstacles before the program is implemented. Once again, collaboration with other professional groups is beneficial.

Developing Referral Systems

The final step in designing a new program is the development of patient/client referral systems. Mechanisms must be designed that establish how people enter a program, how they move through the program, and how they will be discharged from the program. Referral systems require the integration of the micro and macro levels of planning. A referral system must account for the needs of each person and must offer a mechanism by which each patient/client is able to have a complete program suited to his or her own needs and goals.

Referral systems include four basic components: evaluation protocols, criteria for entry into the program, criteria for entering and leaving each level of the program, and exit or discharge criteria.

Evaluation protocols include all evaluation instruments and procedures that will be completed for each patient/client. The purpose of having a standardized protocol is twofold: (1) to standardize the kinds of information obtained, and (2) to determine the appropriate treatment program for each person.

Criteria for entry into the program may include some procedural prerequisites as well as minimum expected behaviors and functional skill levels. Criteria for entering and leaving each level of the program will also be necessary so that both the patient/client and therapist know when advancement through the program is appropriate.

Finally, exit or discharge criteria are necessary to determine when the maximum gain has been achieved. Exit criteria are defined by the goals of the program. Usually, when a person has achieved the goals described for the program, he or she has met the exit criteria.

Program Implementation

Program implementation is the third step in developing a program. It includes not only the actual implementation of the program plan but also the documentation, communication, and coordination.

Implementation of the program plan involves starting the program and its components according to the timetable and sequence described in the planning stage.

An important part of program implementation is documentation of what is going on in the program and how the program is being used. Documentation leads to program evaluation. To document the program, the therapist will have to gather statistics to assess the efficacy and efficiency of the program and to evaluate whether the program goals and standards have been achieved. Specific guidelines on what and how to document are fully discussed in the literature on quality assurance. Items that may be documented include the following:

1. The total number of patients/clients evaluated
2. The percentage of the target population referred into the program
3. The percentage of patients/clients referred into the program who remained until discharge (vs. those who dropped out before discharge)
4. Use of the therapists' time: hours in direct patient/client care, hours in indirect patient care, and so forth
5. Administrative and supervisory time
6. The percentage of the target population served by the program

To maintain a program, communication and coordination are required within the occupational therapy department and among other parts of the institutional system. Those who develop and implement the program must continually monitor and identify obstacles as they occur, communicate about them internally, and coordinate problem-solving efforts.

Program Evaluation

The aim of program evaluation is to measure the effects of a program against the goals it is designed to accomplish. The objective is to improve programming. Program evaluation guides the decision-making process by providing data that will help determine if programs should be continued, discontinued, or changed. The purpose of program evaluation is to answer program-related questions, such as what the best intervention is, who benefits from the program, what the optimum program duration is, and what the best format is for the program.

The initial stage of program evaluation begins with the development of clear, specific, and measurable goals and objectives. In stating goals, it is critical to be specific rather than general and to state goals in terms of behavioral change. Determination of the measures for the goals and objectives of the program occurs early in the development process and must be directly aligned with the program itself.

Program goals are actually measures of outcome, such as improved functional capacity, improved role functioning, or improved coping or social skills. The most common outcome measures in mental health are recidivism and employment figures, but these are gross indications of function. Other measures of outcome cited in the literature include the degree of independent living, level of symptomatology, social behavior, skill gain, patient/client satisfaction with services, and cost-effectiveness. A good program evaluation study typically includes multiple outcome measures.

Several specific steps for conducting program evaluation are described below:

1. Description of program goals and objectives. Differentiation between short- and long-term goals should be the first step in deciding on meaningful outcome criteria.
2. Description of program inputs that include, for example, the type of program or intervention, staff, population served, location, and length of treatment.
3. Design of the evaluation study. All forms of research design are appropriate depending on the nature of the study, such as descriptive, quasi-experimental, case study, or time-series design.
4. Selection of methods of collecting information, such as the interview, the questionnaire, the observation, tests, and the record review. The method selected will depend on the nature of the study and the characteristics of the sample.
5. Analysis and reporting of the results and limitations of the study. The results may be used to support the efficacy of occupational therapy intervention.

CONCLUSION

The four basic steps of program development, as described in this chapter, constitute a working model for occupational therapy personnel employed in institutional or community-based settings. Program development is an ongoing process, each step of which contributes to overall program effectiveness. Inherent in this process is a clear and well-defined view of the role of occupational therapy in the selected setting. It also requires appropriate collaboration with other service providers to create well-designed and specifically targeted programs. This model of program development can be used by all occupational therapy personnel to improve existing programs and/or to create new programs.

RESOURCES

Anthony, W. A., Cohen, M. R., & Vitalo, R. (1978). The measurement of rehabilitation outcome. *Schizophrenia Bulletin, 4,* 365-383.

Bachrach, L. (1984). Principles of planning for chronic psychiatric patents: A synthesis. In J. Talbott (Ed.), *The chronic mental patient: Five years later.* New York, NY: Grune and Stratton.

Braun, P., Kochansky, G., Shapiro, R. (1981). Overview: Deinstitionalization of psychiatric patients: A conical review of outcome studies. *American Journal of Psychiatry, 138,* 736-749.

Cubie, S. H., Kaplan, K. L., & Kielhofner, G. (1985). Program development. In G. Kielhofner (Ed.), *A model of human occupation* (pp. 156-176). Baltimore, MD: Williams and Wilkins.

Frey, W. R. (1985). Planning is a continuous process. *Occupational Therapy Forum, 1*(23), 2021.

Kamis. (1981). Sound of target compassion: Assessing the needs of and planning services for reinstitutionalized clients. In *Planning for deinstitutionalization: A review of principles, methods, and applications.* Human Services Memorgraph No. 28, 23-33.

Morrissey, J. P., & Goldman, H. H. (1984). Cycles of reform in the care of the chronically mentally ill. *Hospital and Community Psychiatry, 35,* 785-792.

Suchman, E. A. (1968). *Evaluative research: Principles and practice in public service antisocial action programs.* New York, NY: Russell Sage Foundation.

Strauss, J. S., & Carpenter, W. T. (1977). Prediction of outcome in schizophrenia. *Archives of General Psychiatry, 34,* 159-163.

Struening, E. L, & Guttentag, M. (Eds.). (1975). *Handbook of evaluation research* (Vol. 2). New York, NY: Sage Publications.

Weiss, C. H. (1983). Evaluation research in the poetical context. In E. Struening & M. Brewer (Eds.), *Handbook of evaluation research* (pp. 31-43). New York, NY: Sage Publications.

Weiss, C. (1972). *Evaluation research: Methods of assessing program effectiveness.* Englewood Cliffs, NJ: Prentice Hall.

Williamson, J. W., Ostrow, P. C., & Braswell, H. R. (1981). *Health accounting for quality assurance: A manual for assessing and improving outcomes of care.* Rockville, MD: American Occupational Therapy Association.

CHAPTER SIX

Strategic Communication for Occupational Therapy Practitioners in Mental Health

Susan C. Robertson and Susan C. Schwartz

This chapter was previously published in S. C. Robertson (Ed.), Mental health focus: Skills for assessment and treatment *(pp. 162-168). Rockville, MD: The American Occupational Therapy Association, Inc. (AOTA). Copyright © 1988, AOTA.*

Communication is a highly complex human activity. It can be verbal, written, or non-verbal. Having effective communication skills in all three areas is essential for occupational therapy practitioners. It is not enough, however. Occupational therapy practitioners today must also have effective strategic communication skills to strengthen their position in the marketplace and to develop additional resources for optimal patient/client care.

This chapter explores the essence of strategic communication and its use in occupational therapy practice. The focus here is on verbal communication patterns and content. It is assumed that the reader is practiced in non-verbal communication and its therapeutic and non-therapeutic uses. For this reason, non-verbal communication is not dealt with separately but is integrated into the discussion of verbal communication.

STRATEGIC COMMUNICATION

Strategic communication takes place in an organizational setting and effectively mobilizes resources, accurately conveys departmental accomplishments and contributions, and positions the department to achieve internal and organizational goals. It is a complex but learnable skill that requires an understanding of the dynamics of the environment, organization, and profession.

Strategic communication is a means of linking program needs and goals to the patient/client, the organizational context, and the greater environment. Whereas effective communication is essential for relating assessment results to the patient/client, family, and treatment team, strategic communication is necessary for integrating occupational therapy services with other services provided in the setting. It strengthens team contributions in the organizational environment. Without strategic communication, patient care and client services may be compromised or be less than optimal. Strategic communication requires skill in organizational decision-making that affects individuals and large and small groups in the system.

FACTORS THAT INFLUENCE COMMUNICATION

Both external and internal factors influence the effectiveness of communication. Some external factors are found in the environment, others in the organization, and still others in the profession. Communication is also influenced by the experiences and skills of individual practitioners.

Psychosocial, political, legal, economic, and cultural issues from the external environment have an impact on the content of communication and the way in which it is delivered. By analyzing these forces, practitioners can specify both the content and style of their communications. Strategic communication can shape these external factors and, thereby, influence service delivery.

There is also a parallel set of psychosocial, political, legal, economic, and cultural influences in all organizational settings. By understanding the internal environment of these settings, a practitioner can effectively contribute to the informal communication of the team network and the more formal written and oral presentations needed by the organization. By defining the corporate culture (i.e., the values, norms, and habits of administrators and service providers), a practitioner can enhance the clarity, specificity, and relevance of all occupational therapy communication. Understanding other elements of the system helps define the receptiveness of the receiver of communication.

The occupational therapy profession itself influences communication among occupational therapy personnel. There are guidelines for the use of terminology in the profession, standards of behavior, and recommended formats for documentation. The defined domain of responsibility in the field also dictates how occupational therapy practitioners communicate with colleagues and others outside the profession.

Looking at the art of communication from another vantage point, the form, style, and type of communication are also influenced by the unique experiences and attributes of the individual who is sending information and the knowledge of the person who receives the information. Individual communication patterns can be assets or liabilities to effective communication. Each practitioner must adjust his or her personal style in order to be responsive to the demands of the individual patient/client, organization, or environment.

AN ENVIRONMENTAL SCAN

The practice of occupational therapy must be well integrated within the organization and environment to be a viable and desirable component of the service delivery network. There are many elements in an environmental scan; only some of them are presented below. You will want to explore others that are unique to your particular setting.

On the national level, federal laws and regulations affect the delivery of mental health services nationwide. These include Medicare legislation, regulations for Medicare prospective payment, and the Community Mental Health Centers Act. Other national groups affect the practice of occupational therapy, including professional associations, such as the National Association of Private Psychiatric Hospitals, and accrediting organizations, such as the Joint Commission on the Accreditation of Healthcare Organizations. Both of these types of groups can have broad effects on service design and accountability.

Similar organizations exist on the state level and will be designated differently by each state. Each practitioner will want to examine the structure of service delivery within the state and identify groups that directly and indirectly affect the design of occupational therapy services and communication about them. There may be an office for statewide health planning, a department of health services, state and county commissions for health facilities, or an association of county mental health directors. There also may be medical associations, social service departments, and psychiatric societies on both the state and local levels.

An environmental scan consists of two activities: identifying external factors that influence the practice of occupational therapy in a particular setting and state, and analyzing the roles, functions, and procedures of the external factors as they relate to the goals and structure of the occupational therapy service. Because the set of external influences is very complex and always changing, it is important to scan the environment regularly. Once you have conducted one scan, it is relatively easy to update it on an ongoing basis. All practitioners should know which factors affect the delivery of occupational therapy services in general and in their own setting. Only by understanding the larger context can occupational therapy services be designed to maximize the use of resources.

AN ORGANIZATIONAL ANALYSIS

A similar analysis is also conducted at the organizational level, where numerous economic, political, social, and cultural influences are assessed within the practice setting. This internal analysis is conducted for the in-patient unit or outpatient center, for example, and for the occupational therapy department and the institution as a whole.

The challenge facing every practitioner is to determine which unique set of factors affects the way occupational therapy services are designed in a given setting. One of the most critical factors in evaluating an organization is to determine how economic decisions are made and enforced. Finances always govern service delivery mechanisms, and, thus, it is critical to know how budgets are developed and approved and to understand what sources of income are available to the institution. Practitioners should also know how occupational therapy services bring revenue into the organization and how the occupational therapy department allocates expenses. With this understanding of the flow of authority and accountability, a practitioner will be able to ascertain how to access the system successfully.

The practitioner must also be aware of the internal communication patterns followed within the organization. The type of planning methodology used within the organization will indicate how decisions are made and who has the power to effect change. There may only be downward communication or a combination of downward, upward, and lateral communication. These patterns will have a major influence on how the organization plans for progress, plans to minimize crisis, or plans for stability.

External communication patterns are also important for the organizational analysis. The marketing methodology used by the organization will indicate how its administrators wish to present the organization to consumers, third party payers, and the community. An understanding of these concerns will be key to selecting the type of communication patterns that occupational therapy personnel will use to support the organization's efforts. The goals and philosophy of the organization are typically reflected in its marketing approach.

Lastly, the practitioner will need to consider how personnel in the in-patient unit communicate internally and externally. An objective exploration of communication in the occupational therapy department then follows. Communication patterns will suggest the political, psychosocial, and cultural forces within an organization. These forces, coupled with economic factors, will point to the critical resources and constraints within the organization that support or inhibit occupational therapy services.

CURRENT ISSUES IN OCCUPATIONAL THERAPY

Besides the environmental and organizational factors mentioned above, there are equally important and influential factors within the profession of occupational therapy that shape what practitioners need to do, can do, and should do.

Occupational therapy has a culture of its own. Although we are part of a larger health care system, we have a set of values, beliefs, norms, and expectations to which we are responsible as members of the profession. The educational process, from academic preparation to field work and supervision, guides our behavior in accordance with this professional culture.

National and state associations collaborate on defining the professional culture and disseminating information about the values, beliefs, norms, and expectations to its members. Policy-making bodies (the Representative Assembly and State Executive Boards) address such concerns as the philosophical base of the profession, the definition of occupational therapy, the national stance on licensure, and responsibility for career development. The American Journal of Occupational Therapy and other publications of the AOTA convey the results of these policy deliberations and the direction of growth of the profession. Individual occupational therapy practitioners use this information along with their environmental and organizational understanding to decide how to provide services to patients and clients.

One example may help to illustrate the influence of the profession on practice. The occupational therapy practitioner needs to define the existing and potential roles and status of occupational therapy in the health care system and in the specific practice setting. The profession has defined uniform terminology and standards of practice, and position papers have been written on various approaches to service delivery. These describe the norms for occupational therapy nationwide. There is also another set of guidelines and expectations imposed on the practitioner by the organization and the environment. The practitioner must weigh all these many forces and determine how to present occupational therapy in a given setting.

DECISION-MAKING AND COMMUNICATION

Decision-making and reasoning are integral elements of strategic communication. They enable the practitioner to respond to the needs and qualifications for interaction dictated by the environment, system, and profession in the same way that they enable the practitioner to respond to a patient's/client's needs and to interact with him or her effectively.

Identifying the information that needs to be communicated is a component of the environmental, organizational, and professional analysis. The practitioner isolates which economic or political factors, for example, affect the

services that can be provided to each patient/client. Knowing that a patient/client is covered by Medicare, for example, dictates what needs to be communicated to ensure reimbursement. Administrators in the practice setting have additional strategies for ensuring reimbursement and designing cost-effective services; these must also be considered when defining interventions for a patient/client. The occupational therapy profession also has guidelines for quality intervention which, if not followed, could result in negative consequences. All these factors are computed as the practitioner determines what to say and how to communicate with the patient/client, department personnel, organization administrators, and external agencies. They influence how the occupational therapy practitioner plans, delivers, and markets his or her services.

Disregard for the principles of decision-making limits the influence that occupational therapy can have on patient/client care, the department, and the organization. Adopting and improving skills in this area gives each occupational therapy practitioner an opportunity to give better service to the patient/client population.

HOW TO DEVELOP STRATEGIES FOR COMMUNICATING EFFECTIVELY

Many skills are helpful in improving strategic communication (Figure 6-1), including listening, concept formation, organization, negotiation, and conflict resolution. The degree of skill each practitioner can gain in these areas has an impact on his or her degree of comfort in verbal and non-verbal communication.

There are numerous forms and styles of communication useful for the demands of the practice setting. The reasoning process helps practitioners decide on the best pattern choice. The following questions may help determine the content and format of strategic communication:

- What needs to be said?
- What could be said?
- What should be said?
- Who will hear it?
- Who will say it?
- When should it be communicated?
- Where should it be communicated?
- Why should it be communicated?
- How should it be communicated?
- How may it be received?
- What resistance could be anticipated?

In occupational therapy practice settings across the country, many influences affect how these questions are answered. The language of the practice setting is based on shared values, as is the conceptual model of the corporate culture. Within this culture, there are built-in patterns of communication—who talks with whom, when, where, how, and why are influenced by the value system and norms of the organization. How the patterns are adjusted is often the result of

Issue	Environmental Resources/ Constraints	Organizational Resources/ Constraints Communication	Goal(s) of Occupational Therapy	Content of Strategic Communication	Pattern of Strategic Communication
Occupational therapy budget is limited to 5% of unit costs	Reduced funds for mental health services in the form of prospective payment system JCAHO HCFA DRR Regional legal factors	Budgeting process Financial officer values constraint and compliance Administration threatened by overspending and resistance to requests for additional funds Quality assurance standards for facility	To increase budget for occupational therapy because program requires additional materials and supplies To negotiate increase in operating budget for occupational therapy To use information about occupational therapy to promote the department and the services offered to the organization To use identified network of power to influence change	Revenue-produced occupational therapy for department Range of services provided by occupational therapy Write budget Costs associated with various programs Number of patients/ clients seen in each type of occupational therapy service Anticipate benefits to organization of additional expense Survey of referral sources regarding satisfaction with occupational therapy	Negotiate with unit supervisor, institution financial officer Plan agenda and place of negotiation Compile survey results of patient satisfaction Perform outcome studies Establish reciprocal relationships and maintain informal communication Keep up with literature to support your position

Figure 6-1. Strategic communication in practice: budget.

specific alliances that are formed between key personnel. The occupational therapy practitioner's ability to build alliances with support figures, such as the service chief, financial officer, and team members, plays a critical role in successful strategic communication.

Understanding the organization and environment enables occupational therapy personnel to integrate their services into the full range of service offered. It also has an impact on how well occupational therapy services will be funded. But understanding the system is only half of the expertise needed. The other half is related to the personal communication style of the practitioner. The degree of conflict and resistance, or the support received for occupational therapy services, has a great deal to do with the practitioner's mastery of strategic communication.

APPLYING STRATEGIC COMMUNICATION IN PRACTICE

Figures 6-1 and 6-2 present a framework for developing the content and pattern of strategic communication within a particular practice setting and give specific examples of issues often confronted by occupational therapy personnel. The framework includes several factors, the analysis of which will increase the likelihood of achieving desired outcome(s).

These factors include:
- Issues
- Environmental Resources/Constraints
- Organizational Resources/Constraints
- Goal(s) of Occupational Therapy Communication
- Content of Strategic Communication
- Pattern of Strategic Communication

All kinds of issues, from management issues in the department to economic issues dictated by the environment, can be evaluated within this framework. It can be used to evaluate strategic communication in the various roles occupational therapy personnel perform in support of service delivery. The final selection of strategic communication patterns must be determined by the resources and constraints in the unique practice setting You are urged to use this framework to analyze the factors that affect communication within your own practice setting. As with any action, it is important to assess the results of the strategic communication and its effect on reaching desired goals. Adaptations based on assessment results will influence later communication strategies.

RESOURCES

Bair, J., & Gray, M. (1986). *The occupational therapy manager.* Rockville, MD: American Occupational Therapy Association.

Issue	Environmental Resources/ Constraints	Organizational Resources/ Constraints Communication	Goal(s) of Occupational Therapy	Content of Strategic Communication	Pattern of Strategic Communication
Discharge placement of patient/client	Community settings have unique culture and are affected by economic, political, legal, and social variables. Each setting is different Management techniques differ in the same facility and between facilities	Discharge planning is staff team responsibility led by chief physician Occupational therapy manages placement in school, work, volunteer job, or other prevocational setting Nursing staff manages placement in residential setting	To improve reliance of physicians and nursing staff on OT assessment of functions To negotiate expanded role of occupational therapy in self-care, work, leisure assessment, and placement To use information about patient's/ client's functional abilities to promote department and services provided To use identified network of influence to increase team collaboration in the unit	Survey satisfaction of patient/client and referral source with occupational therapy Define role and contribution that occupational therapy is able to make in the area of human function Correlate outcome of occupational therapy with success of placement for previously discharged patients (length of stay in discharge placement, time between hospitalizations) Define patterns of coordination with other members of the treatment team	Negotiate with unit chief, nursing staff Write definition of role of occupational therapy in functional assessment Survey patients/clients, referral sources Perform outcome studies Establish reciprocal relationships with team members and maintain informal communication

Figure 6-2. Strategic communication in practice: discharge placement.

Donnelly, J., Gibson, J., & Ivanchevich, J. (1978). *Fundamentals of management* (3rd Edition). Dallas, TX: Business Publications, Inc.

Esman, M. J. (1972). The elements of institution building. In J. Eaton (Ed.), *Institutional building and development.* Beverly Hills, CA: Sage Publications.

Fox, E., & Wunwick, L (1977). *Dynamic administration. The collected papers of Mary Parker Follett.* New York, NY: Hippocrene Books, Inc.

Jacobs, K. (1987). Marketing occupational therapy. *American Journal of Occupational Therapy, 41,* 315-320.

Miyake, S., & Trostler, R. (1987). Introducing the concept of a corporate culture to a hospital setting. *American Journal of Occupational Therapy, 41,* 310-314.

Naisbitt, J., & Elkins, J. (1984). The hospital and megatrends. *Hospital Forum,* May-June, 9-17.

Schulz, R., Peterson, R., & Greenley, J. (1984). Management, costs and quality of acute in-patient psychiatric services. *Medical Care, 21,* 911-928.

Tosi, H., & Carroll, S. (1976). *Management: Contingencies, structure, and process.* Chicago, IL: St. Clair Press.

Zaloccu, R., Joseph, W. & Doremus, H. (1984). Strategic marketing planning for hospitals. *Journal of Health Care Marketing, 4*(2), 19-28.

CHAPTER SEVEN

Strategic Planning: Positioning Occupational Therapy to be Proactive in the New Health Care Paradigm

Teri L. Shackleton and Marie Gage

This chapter was previously published in the Canadian Journal of Occupational Therapy, 62(4), *188-196, and is reprinted here with permission of CAOT Publications ACE © 1995.*

In the mid 1990s, Canadian health care was in the midst of a revolution. A review of the literature identifies the economic, social, and political environmental factors influencing this shift (Carswell-Opzoomer, 1990; Gage, 1995/2000; Stan, 1987). These factors encompass: 1) decreasing governmental spending, with increased focus on maximizing existing or decreasing resources; 2) increasing consumer demand for health services, coupled with increasing expectations for accountability, with emphasis on meeting the consumer's needs; 3) 20 years of national initiatives advocating a new health paradigm, one where health promotion, the process of enabling people to increase control over their health, complements and strengthens the existing health care system (Epp, 1986; Lalonde, 1974).

These are exciting times for the evolving profession of occupational therapy. Our visionary leaders have highlighted the affinity that exists between the profession's philosophical base and the paradigm shift that is occurring in health care (Carswell-Opzoomer, 1990; Gage, 1995/2000; Stan, 1987), proclaiming that occupational therapists "have the knowledge and skills to be in the forefront of that revolution" (Carswell-Opzoomer, 1990, p. 197).

Has the profession of occupational therapy evolved sufficiently to become positioned to seize the opportunities offered in this new health paradigm? In 1992, the occupational therapy department staff, comprised of 15 occupational therapists (including the authors), four assistants, and one secretary, of an acute care university-affiliated institution, were not able to answer this question with a whole hearted "yes." Major obstacles identified included:

- the diversity of occupational therapy's clinical foci making it difficult to articulate a clear statement of what "business we are in"
- blurred professional image
- philosophical ambivalence resulting in inconsistencies between our philosophy and current practice
- stretched resources
- geographical boundaries created by the department being located on three different sites
- political flux including uncertainty about administrative decisions regarding structural changes within the hospital
- discrepancies between the foci of hospital-based care and occupational therapy's concern for community reintegration

In 1995, members of this same department believed that they are better positioned to seize the opportunities offered by the emerging health care paradigm. A strategic planning process, implemented in 1992, provided a consensual framework for action. A framework that 1) evokes enthusiasm and commitment, 2) enables negotiation of the obstacles identified above, and 3) has been successful in positioning members of this department to act as leaders in the new health paradigm.

The purpose of this chapter is to highlight the importance of strategic planning as applied to the profession of occupational therapy; to present the model for our strategic planning process; and to focus on the benefits of this process for the department.

BACKGROUND

Historically, the word strategic derives its meaning from the military. It refers to designing a plan for action based on an analysis of internal strengths and weaknesses, of anticipated changes in the environment, and contingent moves by opponents (Ostrow, 1985). While present day strategic planning theory encompasses a similar analytical approach, the key to success is the incorporation of a process that is consistent with participative management principles. Strategic planning has been defined as "a rational method for building consensus for participation, commitment urgency, and action" (Burkhart & Reuss, 1993). Although modern conceptualization originated in the business sector, strategic planning has become recognized as an essential process for the health care industry, in an age when accountability is required and competition for dollars is either directly or indirectly a challenge (Brockett & Kuretzky, 1992; Ostrow, 1985).

Strategic Planning—The Benefits

The general overall benefits of strategic planning are highlighted in the literature, as follows:

1. Given the rapidly evolving health care environment, strategic planning provides *a way to anticipate and adapt to changes in its environment* (Espy, 1986; Hrebiniak & Joyce, 1984; Ostrow, 1985). Environmental scanning, with its inherent analysis of external opportunities and threats, is a fundamental process to the creation of a trend or an innovation that will change the future (Ostrow, 1985).

2. A *common framework* is created which matches environmental conditions with internal distinctive competencies (Hrehiniak & Joyce, 1984). Such a framework provides a *consensual basis* for problem-solving, decision-making, integrating organizational actions, and coordinating resources (Ostrow, 1985; Robert, 1988; Spencer, 1989), resulting in increased effectiveness and efficiency (Spencer, 1989).

3. Strategic planning is important for being postured to take advantage of critical opportunities, termed *positioning*. Positioning, a function of possessing a clear purpose, adequate resources, enthusiasm and commitment, is considered a prerequisite for long-term organizational success (Burkhart & Reuss, 1993).

The team-building effects of the participative process, inherent in today's conceptualization of strategic planning, have been identified as follows:

1. Increased *cohesiveness and commitment* of staff (Espy, 1986; Spencer, 1989). A higher level of staff commitment results from their increased understanding of the needs and goals of the organization (or department, or program, etc.) and from their active participation in establishing goals, objectives and actions.

2. Enhanced *innovation* results from the cross-fertilization of ideas of staff from diverse backgrounds. Staff demonstrate an enhanced ability to challenge traditional assumptions and define new possibilities (Spencer, 1989).

3. Heightened *enthusiasm and initiative* (Espy 1986; Spencer, 1989). Staff are more likely to feel a sense of ownership for their part in the organization.

4. Increased formal and informal *communication* between staff members, which endures long after the planning process is completed (Spencer, 1989).

Strategic Planning—A Strategy

While involvement in a strategic planning process was mandated by the Victoria Hospital administration, the advantages afforded by implementing such a process quickly became apparent. The benefits of the strategic planning process, as outlined above, were considered to be worth pursuing in efforts to overcome the obstacles facing the authors and their colleagues. Staff expressed the following personal desired gains:

- achieving consensus/cohesiveness,
- possessing a clear identity,
- determining "what is important to us,"
- gaining a sense of direction,
- recognizing our commonalties, and
- being at the head of the wave of change in health care.

STRATEGIC PLANNING—A MODEL FOR THE PROCESS

Overview

The selected strategic planning process (refer to Figure 7-1) comprised the interaction of eight elements: Environmental Analysis, Purpose and Philosophy Statements, Our Vision, Obstacles to Our Vision, Strategic Directions, Stakeholder Consultation, Systematic Actions, and Implementation Timeline. The outcome of the process is a *living* document that must be updated to meet changing environmental demands. It does not result in a document that simply sits on the shelf. This process was adapted to meet our needs, from the model proposed by the Institute of Cultural Affairs (ICA) (Spencer, 1989). All staff approved its use prior to its implementation.

A steering committee, comprising clinical and management representation, was struck to coordinate the planning process. While the chair of this committee could be the director, in this case, a delegate assumed the responsibility of overseeing the coordination of the strategic planning process.

Environmental Analysis

The context for our strategic planning process was provided by an examination of historical data, the occupational therapy department current profile, and environmental trends. The implications of provincial, regional, hospital, and professional trends were considered. The data collected were used in the analysis of the department's strengths, weaknesses, opportunities and threats, termed a SWOT Analysis. In our experience, the SWOT Analysis proved to be a valuable tool for facilitating productive problem solving in the exploration of critical issues.

An important part of this environmental analysis was the one which examined the strengths and weaknesses of the

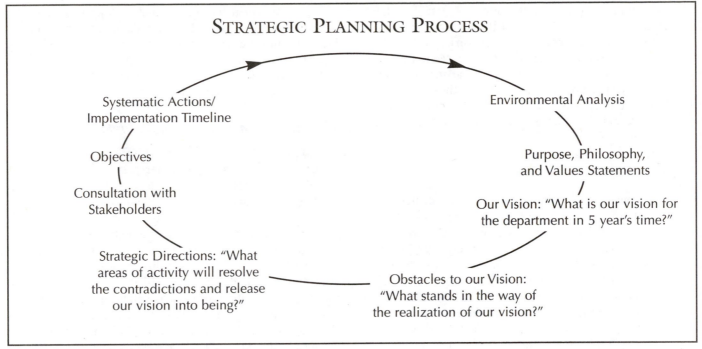

Figure 7-1. Model for strategic planning process.

occupational therapy profession with respect to the emerging health care paradigm. Excitement over the shifts in thinking, characteristic of this paradigm, has been expressed in our professional literature (Carswell-Opzoomer, 1990; Stan, 1987). In this new perspective, health ceases to be measurable strictly in terms of illness and death; it is considered "a basic and dynamic force in our daily lives, influenced by our circumstances, our beliefs, our culture and our social, economic and physical environments" (Epp, 1986). Consequently, health promotion is considered "the process of enabling people to increase control over, and to improve, their health" (Epp, 1986).

An affinity exists between this perspective of health and the philosophical base of occupational therapy (Carswell-Opzoomer, 1990; Stan, 1987). Our professional philosophy and values highlight the individuals' dignity and worth, their unique capacity to interpret, mediate, act on, and to be influenced by physical, social, and cultural environmental factors (Canadian Association of Occupational Therapists (CAOT), 1991; Polatajko, 1992). Thus, in practice the individual is considered an active participant in the therapeutic relationship (CAOT, 1991), essential for the empowerment of that individual to influence the state of his/her own health.

Our philosophical base is obviously considered a strength, one which we should build on as we meet the challenges provided by the changing health care environment. But what are the profession's weaknesses or obstacles in meeting these challenges? A perusal of our professional literature reinforces the issues identified by the members of this department. Occupational therapy, as a diverse profession, has been plagued by difficulties in articulating its importance and unique contribution to client care (Bell, 1980; Bruhn, 1991;

O'Shea, 1977; Polatajko, 1997; Stan, 1987; Tompson, 1989). Instead of assuming a proactive stance in determining the focus of practice, occupational therapists have been vulnerable to the expectations and demands of others, especially those in the medical profession, in establishing a professional role (O'Shea, 1977). The result has been inconsistencies between the profession's endearing philosophy and its present day actions (Stan, 1987). Sequalae have included a general lack of confidence about our role and a lack of respect from other health care professionals (Tompson, 1987).

Statement of Purpose

With the analysis of environmental factors completed, the authors and colleagues were able to revisit the Departmental Statement of Purpose. Efforts were directed toward exploring the questions: "Why are we in existence?" and "What do we do to fulfill our purpose?" In answering these questions it was possible to articulate occupational therapy's contribution to the mission and goals of Victoria Hospital; in general, clinical practice, education, and research.

Philosophy and Values

An attempt was made to capture the philosophical base for the practice of occupational therapy in the department's Philosophical and Value Statements. Philosophy refers to a set of values, beliefs, truths, and principles that guide the actions of the profession's practitioners (Hopkins, 1988) Thus, in order to articulate our philosophical basis answering the question, "Why do we do what we do the way we do," we referred to the *Occupational Therapy Guidelines for Client-*

Centered Practice (CAOT, 1991) and to Polataijko's (1997) Values Statement. The authors of the present chapter were involved in the Conceptual Framework Group at the University of Western Ontario that contributed to the formulation of these values. As a result, the department did not try to create its own list of values, but adopted those presented by Polataijko's (1992). Thus, with solidarity in our professional fundamental beliefs we were ready to progress to the creation of our vision.

Our Vision

An empowering participative process was adopted for the creation of our vision, and for the subsequent steps of identifying obstacles and strategic directions. All staff attended two half-day brainstorming workshop sessions, facilitated by Polataijko, then Assistant Professor, Department of Occupational Therapy, the University of Ontario. To provide a common destination for the planning efforts, all staff were asked to consider the question, "What do we want our department to look like in five years?" After generating ideas in small groups, the whole group participated in a consensual process of gathering common ideas together and carefully naming the themes that emerged. These themes became our vision statements and Our Vision was entitled "Building on Our Strengths." The characteristic themes we arrived at are outlined in Figure 7-2.

The reaction to this process was very positive. There as almost an "ah-ha" experience as staff realized that what had been implicit in each of their minds was non–explicit, and was embraced by all staff.

Obstacles to Our Vision

Next, the staff was directed to answer the question, "What stands in the way of our vision?" This step has been advocated by some authors (Spencer, 1989) as an in between step to goal setting in that it allows groups to work at removing roadblocks with a clear focus on what obstacles exist. Once again, brainstorming was conducted in small groups with the whole group reflecting on the ideas generated, identifying common themes that became the Obstacles to Our Vision. These themes were presented in the introduction of this (chapter). All staff appeared exhausted at the end of this step. As has been suggested in literature (Espy, 1986; Spencer, 1989), this activity can result in depression, as staff see more clearly the obstacles that stand before them. However, relief can also result as staff identify the obstacles, thus objectifying them so that they can be viewed as opportunities ready to be dealt with.

Our Strategic Directions

With our vision and obstacles articulated, attention was then directed toward answering the question, "What areas of activity will resolve the contradictions and release our vision into being?"

Ideas were brainstormed in small groups as before, with the whole group reflecting on the ideas, grouping common ideas together and articulating common themes that became Our Strategic Directions. Refer to Figure 7-3 for a diagrammatic representation of Our Strategic Directions, entitled "Towards Excellence in Practice."

Consultation with Stakeholders

Stakeholders are, quite literally, those persons who have a stake in the department, whether past, present or future. Stakeholders in this case included Victoria Hospital physicians/surgeons, applied health disciplines, nursing, administration, research department, patients and volunteers of the department, and University of Western Ontario's Department of Occupational Therapy. Stakeholder feedback was collected on our vision and our strategic directions by circulating the draft document and through an invitation to a stakeholder meeting. The meeting format has helpful in gaining a broad base of support from within Victoria Hospital and the University of Western Ontario. With the strategic directions affirmed by the stakeholders and stakeholder feedback collected, the next stage was to plan objectives and specific actions.

Action Implementation Timelines

The strategic directions served departmental goals, providing a consensual grounding upon which to develop objectives and actions for the next year. In a one-day action planning workshop, each strategic direction was analyzed with respect to strengths, weaknesses, opportunities, and threats. At least one specific accomplishment, stated as an objective, was established for the next year for each strategic direction. Special attention was paid to whether the objective was worded in a way that would ensure movement toward our vision, but be attainable in the next year. Group brainstorming was then used to identify possible actions, which would be effective in achieving the objective.

IMPLEMENTAION OF STRATEGIC PLAN

Although the department had a five committee quality assurance structure in place as per Shimeld's (1982) Five Star Approach to Quality Assurance, it was agreed that there was a need to design a new committee structure that would most effectively deal with the Strategic Directions. The Strategic Directions were examined, grouping similar themes together to arrive at a three committee structure, namely: Quality Improvement and Research, Unique Clinical Contributions, and Resource Management. Membership on these committees has determined by staff interest in the respective directions. The activities, previously carried out under the old committee structure, were reanalyzed to determine which activities required committee involvement. While activities considered essential for the department and requiring committee involvement were delegated to the new committee structure,

Our Vision
"Building On Our Strengths"

Our Vision for Occupational Therapy provides the common focus and direction for our Strategic Plan. Based on our analysis of departmental strengths we created a Vision which reflects our commitment to the ideals of patient care, education, and research at Victoria Hospital, London, Ontario. Entitled "Building On Our Strengths," Our Vision for Occupational Therapy is characterized by:

FOCUS ON CLIENTS' NEEDS

Quality Patient Care
Continued emphasis on the quality of patient programmes which include:
- patient education
- programme development
- monitoring of intervention outcomes

Client-Centered Approach
Leadership in client-centered issues which includes:
- the inclusion of the client's perspective in the evaluation of occupational performance and in the setting of intervention goals
- the enablement of competence in occupational performance
- the empowerment of individuals to maintain and improve their state of health

Community Reintegration
Leadership in community reintegration which includes:
- the provision of services which enhance the continuity of care received by our clients
- advocacy for community health promotion and disability prevention efforts

Empirically Based Practice
Clinical practice based on empirical data through:
- collaborative relationships with colleagues at Victoria Hospital and the Department of Occupational Therapy at the University of Western Ontario

OPTIMAL SERVICE DELIVERY

Productive Partnerships
Recognized contributions to clinical care education and research through productive partnerships:
- among our colleagues and with other health care professionals at Victoria Hospital
- in the provision of clinical education experiences for undergraduate Occupational Therapy students

Optimal Resource
Optimal use of resources through:
- the provision of comprehensive cost-effective services to clients who will most benefit
- the rationalization of services based on the results of efficacy studies

PROFESSIONAL COHESION

Clear Professional Identity
Clear professional identity portrayed through:
- our unique contributions to clinical care at Victoria Hospital
- clinical competence of staff and Occupational Therapy students

Increased Professional Status
Increased professional status due to:
- recognition of our unique contributions to clinical care by our clients, their families, other health care professionals at Victoria Hospital, and the community at large
- our research contributions recognized across North America

Figure 7-2. Our vision statement.

Towards Excellence in Practice	Preparing for the future	Enhancing Quality of Patient Care Increasing Expertise in Client-Centered Practice Promoting ReIntegration into Community Enhancing Research Development	Focus on Client Needs
		Facilitating Productive Partnerships Streamlining Clinical Services	Optimal Service Delivery
	Growing Together	Facilitating Staff Development Promoting Our Unique Strengths	Professional Cohesion

Figure 7-3. Our strategic directions—towards excellence in practice.

those activities not requiring committee involvement were delegated to appropriate personnel. Some of the activities performed by the old committee structure were found no longer necessary, given the evolution of the strategic planning process.

It was the responsibility of the new quality improvement committees to discuss ideas generated at the Action Planning Workshop, refine the actions, and decide how the actions would get done by whom and when. Once the detailed actions were drafted by the committees, they were presented to the Senior Quality Improvement Committee (which includes in this case a chair, the director, supervisory staff, and the chairs of the quality improvement committees). A reality check is an important part of the process at this stage. It is important to ask if the actions support the spirit of the agreed upon objective and if the resources are available to implement the action. The refined action implementation timeline is then presented to all staff for approval before implementation.

ANNUAL REVIEW

As stressed earlier it is important to consider a Strategic Plan to be a *living document,* where review on a regular basis is conducted at an Action Planning Workshop. At these Action Planning Workshops the progress made toward Our Vision is reviewed, environmental trends considered, the Strategic Directions are reaffirmed, objectives for the coming year are decided, and actions are brainstormed.

Recycling through the process is an important aspect of strategic planning (refer to Figure 7-1). All staff are encouraged to remain flexible in the annual review process so that assumptions made previously can be challenged, internal and external developments can be considered, and modifications made to Our Vision and/or Our Strategic Directions as found appropriate.

STRATEGIC PLANNING—EVALUATING THE BENEFITS

There are many indicators that the strategic planning process has begun to bear fruit for this department. There has been recognition at the senior and middle management level of the hospital that members of the Occupational Therapy Department are experienced in client-centered practice and that there is a wealth of experience to share with peers in other departments. One senior manager remarked that there has been a noticeable increase in cohesiveness among the members of the department and an outward appearance that the staff are happier. Staff within the department have confirmed this observation and remarked on how important this change is given the tough economic times and the resultant pressure on staff to see more patients. Feeling a commitment to the Vision seems to provide some shelter from the emotional impact of the changes due to fiscal restraint.

Immediately upon articulation of the Vision before the plan was even set, the director of the department began to notice opportunities that were consistent with the collective vision and was able to capture these opportunities knowing they would be embraced by the staff. Since completion of the plan, it has guided the selection of administrative activities within the department and provided a focus for success. The following is a list of benefits articulated by members of the Senior Quality Improvement Committee:

- Staff, as a group, are much more positive about their strengths and contribution to clinical care, education, and research.
- During the first year, much more was achieved toward our vision, than the actions which had been delineated. As soon as Our Vision was on paper, it became a selffulfilling prophesy, in that staff involvement in hospital activities became oriented in the areas of our Strategic Directions.
- The areas of Our Vision that were the boldest tended to elicit the most informal activity, that is, activity not specifically planned at the Action Planning Workshop.

- There was an increase in visibility throughout the organization. Staff members were asked to sit on committees that dealt with issues related to the Strategic Directions.
- Communication issues within the department had historically been discussed at length at each Annual Planning Day without successful resolution. A multi-site operation was a major barrier considered to be insurmountable. One year postimplementation of the strategic plan, staff no longer felt the need to address this issue.
- Committee meetings were more productive. They were much more action and project-oriented than had been the case in the past. Staff found that the responsibility was much more equally shared within the committees, with staff more willing be involved.

In an effort to ensure that they were representing the opinion of all, the authors surveyed staff to gain their insight into the strategic planning process. All therapists indicated that they were excited about our Vision, committed to its operation, had an increased awareness of the department goals, and viewed the department as better positioned to be at the head of the wave of health care change. Staff opinions differed with respect to the areas of progress toward our Vision, effectiveness of the new committee structure, and the possession of a clear sense of professional identity. The results of the survey also suggested a general agreement that the inconsistencies between the occupational therapy philosophy and current clinical practice have not yet been resolved and that there is a need to develop strategies for dealing with stretched resources. These perceived areas for further development could be viewed as appropriate, given the early developmental stage of the implementation of the Strategic Plan.

For new members of staff, those who were not employed at Victoria Hospital when our Vision was set, it has been a slow process of understanding what our Vision really meant. The Action Planning Workshop was felt to be a key event in exciting them about our Vision but there is a suggestion that more should be done to inspire this excitement earlier in the employment process.

Overall there is general agreement both externally and internally that although the work has only just begun the department has made a strong start on the path toward our Vision. Continued collective problem solving is required to maximize Individual staff contribution and commitment to the operation of Our Vision over the next five years.

SUMMARY

Strategic planning has enabled the members of this department to build on their strengths thus positioning occupational therapists at Victoria Hospital to demonstrate leadership in the rapidly evolving health care environment. It is hoped that by sharing this experience occupational therapists faced with similar obstacles will be able to apply participative strategic planning principles to their organizations.

O'Shea (1997) posed the question, "Do occupational therapists recognize their individual potential for directing their own futures?" (p. 102). It is the hope of the authors that occupational therapists embrace the motto, "What the future holds for us depends on what we hold for the future" (Forbes, 1992, p. 494). As Bruhn (1991) suggested, "We each have maps in our head of the way things are and the way things could be. The more we are aware of our maps, the more we can take responsibility for shifting our thinking. To shift from one way of seeing the world to another creates powerful change, which we can direct and master" (p. 780).

ACKNOWLEDGMENTS

The authors would like to acknowledge the collective contributions of colleagues at Victoria Hospital in the creation of Our Vision and Strategic Directions and throughout the strategic planning process.

REFERENCES

Bell, E. B. (1980). Muriel Driver Memorial Lecture: Directions for the decade. *Canadian Journal of Occupational Therapy, 47,* 147-153.

Burkhart, P. J., & Reuss, S. (1993). *Successful strategic planning: A guide for nonprofit agencies and organizations.* Newbury Park: CA: Sage.

Brockett, M., & Kuretzky, E. (1992). Strategic planning for occupational therapy. In T. Sumsion (Ed.). *Guidelines for occupational therapy manager: A resource manual* (pp. 5-9). Toronto, ON: CAOT Publications.

Bruhn, J. G. (1991). Occupational therapy in the 21st century: An outsider's view. *American Journal of Occupational Therapy, 45,* 775-780.

Canadian Association of Occupational Therapists. (1991). *Occupational therapy guidelines for client-centered practice.* Toronto, ON: CAOT Publications.

Carswell-Opzoomer, A. (1990). Muriel Driver Memorial Lecture: Occupational therapy: Our time has come. *Canadian Journal of Occupational Therapy, 57,* 197-203.

Epp, J. (1986). *Achieving health for all: A framework for health promotion.* Ottawa, ON: Health and Welfare Canada.

Espy, S. N. (1986). *Handbook of strategic planning for nonprofit organizations.* New York: Praegar.

Forbes, M. (1992). *The Forbes scrapbooks of thoughts on the business of life.* Chicago, Ill: Triumph.

Gage, M. (1995). Reengineering of health care: Opportunity or threat for occupational therapy. *Canadian Journal of Occupational Therapy, 62,* 197-207. (See Chapter Two in this text.)

Hopkins, H. L. (1988). Current basis for theory and philosophy of occupational therapy. In H. L. Hopkins, & H. D. Smith (Eds.). *Willard and Spackman's occupational therapy* (7th ed.) (pp. 38-42) Philadelphia, PA: J. B. Lippincott.

Hrebiniak, L. G., & Joyce, W. F. (1984) *Implementing strategy.* New York, NY: Macmillan Publishing.

Lalonde, M. (1974). *A new perspective on the health of Canadians.* Ottawa, ON: Health and Welfare Canada.

O'Shea, B. J. (1997). Muriel Driver Memorial Lecture. Pawn or protagonist: International perspective or professional identity. *Canadian Journal of Occupational Therapy, 44,* 101-108.

Ostrow, P. C. (1985). Strategic planning: In J. Blair, & M. Gray (Eds.), *The occupational therapy manager.* Rockville, MD: American Occupational Therapy Association.

Polatajko, H. J. (1992). Muriel Driver Memorial Lecture: Naming and framing occupational therapy: A lecture dedicated to the life of Nancy B. *Canadian Journal of Occupational Therapy, 59,* 189-199.

Robert, M (1988). *The strategist CEO: How visionary executives build organizations.* New York, NY: Quorum Books.

Shimeld, A. (1982). A five point approach to staff development for quality assurance. *Canadian Journal of Occupational Therapy, 49,* 53-56.

Spencer, L. J. (1989). *Winning through participation: Meeting the challenge of corporate change with the technology of participation—The group facilitation methods of the Institute of Cultural Affairs.* Iowa: Kenndal/Hunt Publishing.

Stan, L J. (1987). Muriel Driver Memorial Lecture: Making our mark in the marketplace. *Canadian Journal of Occupational Therapy, 54,* 165-171.

Tompson, M. (1989). Muriel Driver Memorial Lecture: Ripples to tidal waves. *Canadian Journal of Occupational Therapy, 56,* 165-170.

CHAPTER EIGHT

Selecting Group Protocols: Recipe or Reasoning?

Susan Haiman

This chapter was previously published in Gibson, D. E. (Ed.). Group protocols: A psychosocial compendium (pp. 114). New York, NY: Haworth Press. Copyright © 1990, Haworth Press. Reprinted by permission.

The health care delivery systems of the 1990s promise to be more demanding of evidence that occupational therapists provide essential services in psychosocial settings. Mandates to demonstrate predictable outcomes, relevance and efficiency require more research around theory and clearer definitions of practice. We can no longer justify reimbursement for occupational therapy by relying on the conventional wisdom. Instead, we must substantiate the efficacy of the various groups and programs we select as tools for intervention. We must take time from routinized methods of program planning to look anew at the use of occupational therapy's philosophy, domain of concern and theoretical basis for making sound clinical judgments. Refining our use of clinical decision-making and clinical reasoning enables us to determine which groups best integrate our frames of reference/practice models; which groups are indicated for specific patients; when in the course of illness the groups are appropriate interventions; and in what settings groups should occur, e.g., acute or long-term settings.

Using this opportunity to move slowly through the steps in the process of group protocol design or selection allows us to set the parameters within which occupational therapists can use reasoning, not recipes, to enhance practice. Of course, there are critical ingredients common to all groups, but let us take the time to blend them from scratch, rather than taking the shortcut of using a mix!

The first step is to look at group activities as interventions evolving from particular historical and environmental contexts. Next we will look at how to use the process of clinical decision-making, thus producing protocols that truly reflect our critical thinking around the techniques we believe to be effective (Parham, 1987; Pelland, 1987; Mattingly, 1988; Neuhaus, 1988). Finally, a case example will highlight some of the issues addressed in the more theoretical aspects of this (chapter).

ESTABLISHING THE CONTEXT

It is not the purpose of this (chapter) to review the history of the role of groups in the era of moral treatment during the nineteenth century, or during the evolution of occupational therapy practice. Suffice it to say, that although patients were engaged frequently in tasks within group settings, it was not until the 1950s that theories of group dynamics and group process emerged, fostering the concept of groups as agents of change in addition to the traditional view of groups as vehicles for social interaction. During the 1950s group activity was used for skill building to enhance functioning. From [the] 1950s to [the] 1970s the focus was on intrapsychic or ego skill building, while in the 1980s the focus was on performance in occupational roles and activities of daily living (Howe & Schwartzberg, 1986; Mosey, 1979; Fidler, 1984).

As we move forward, and look prospectively at group activity as a viable intervention, we must consider the environmental context in which our current practice occurs and the environmental context in which future practice will occur. None of us could be strangers to the crisis in health care, as it has an impact on every mental health care delivery system (Bonder, 1987; Fine, 1987). The reality is that resources are diminishing while costs rise; consumer demands for quality care intensify in the face of increased pressure to shorten lengths of stay. These factors have forced practitioners in acute care settings to consider "reevaluation of the objectives and methods for short lengths of stay... and rehabilitation interventions to provide a basic foundation for post hospital adjustment" (Fine, 1987, p. 9). Similarly, occupational therapists in longer term inpatient and community settings must reassess their program goals and objectives in order to assume the task of working with patients who may be increasingly acutely ill, less stabilized on medications, and more chronically impaired than those in past years.

In addition to the impact of increased accountability and decreased resources, what are other environmental factors to bear in mind when designing group interventions? Some critical ingredients to consider include the facility's location and the relationship between the facility and the socioeconomic level of the community. For example, the skills required to be a functional member of the community in New York City are not the same as those required in rural North Dakota. For example, negotiating crowded subways to get to work in New York City is quite different than relearning how to drive a tractor. Thus, group protocols dealing with independent living skills will have to be designed quite differently for those two geographical locations. In addition, knowing what resources are available to patients in the community is essential, in order that the objectives of groups designed to integrate patients into the outside world are relevant to the realities encountered. One must be careful about encouraging patients' participation in community center social activities, when their lack of social skills will only result in failure at being integrated into a group.

Consideration of the population's demographics served by the facility is important. For example, ages, ethnicity, educational levels, premorbid functioning, diagnoses, and prognoses of the patients must be considered when designing a group which is relevant to its context. Other important considerations are the average length of treatment and other intervention services available to the patients at the facility or in the outside community (Grossman, Bortone, 1986). Occupational therapy interventions should be appropriate, necessary, and unique, when balanced against the efforts of other members of the multidisciplinary team; they should meet patient needs, and needs identified by functional assessment, rather than meeting perceived needs of the staff (Grossman & Bortone, 1986/2000). One example is of the psychiatrist who wouldn't allow the wife of a blue collar worker to go home until she could identify and explain her feelings, despite the fact that she could again cook for her family (Gibson, 1989).

Other questions to consider when designing group interventions are financial and legal constraints or mandates. Therapists should be aware of how facilities are funded and how occupational therapy services are reimbursed, i.e., per diem, as part of a set bed rate, or fee-for-services. Differences in reimbursement methods can influence how services are managed and whether or not groups are a cost-effective method of delivering care. For instance, fee-for-service departments might not support coleadership of groups, while departments whose services are part of the per diem rate might be less concerned about the increased cost of coleadership of group activities. Whether or not the department is able and encouraged to generate income is certainly a factor to weigh in designing programs or groups. Caseload size, session length, frequency of visits and reimbursement rates also contribute to the feasibility of implementing certain activities.

Finally, as therapists, we must ask ourselves what are the "legal" constraints on our group or programs. Every setting, whether public or private, large or small, acute or custodial, institutional or community based, must answer to the regulations imposed by federal, state and local governments, the courts and patients' rights organizations. Consider, for a moment, the impact of Medicare and the impact on reimbursement of Diagnostic Related Groups (DRGs). Other regulating bodies, such as Joint Commission on Accreditation of Health Organizations (JCAHO), licensure boards and peer review agencies also have the power to influence, and, at times control our practice. Even the American Occupational Therapy Association, representing our own professional standards, ethics and practice with uniform terminology, certification and registration procedures has policies we all incorporate into our daily role functioning in the field.

Narrowing the focus to occupational therapy services/departments, we can determine whether or not they will, or can, support particular group interventions. Is the department organized around a particular frame of reference? What level of staff experience is required to lead a new group? What special skills or training is required? Does the department have support from the facilities administration to engage in quality of life and rehabilitation efforts or is the setting strictly biomedical (Cynkin, 1979)?

When the issues and questions raised above have been addressed, we are free to engage in the "ethics, science and art" (Rogers, 1983, p. 601/1996, p. 327) of clinical decision-making and clinical reasoning. By employing clinical decision-making and clinical reasoning we prevent occupational therapy from becoming "cookie cutter therapy," we individualize the treatment of our patients and we specifically address the functional problems they face (Parham, 1987).

CLINICAL DECISION-MAKING AND CLINICAL REASONING

Clinical decision-making and clinical reasoning about development and/or selection of group protocols is a dynamic interactive systems process which for academic purposes will be divided into two phases. The descriptions of these phases are adapted from the work of Rogers (1983), Pelland (1987), Barris (1987) and Mattingly (1988), all of whom have written extensively on the subject. (See Figure 8-1.)

Clinical Decision-Making

Clinical decision-making, a four step process, represents the first phase, the one that occurs while sitting in the office, with the luxury of time to reflect on the results of the environmental analyses and assessments which precede group design. Step one in this phase is to *identify a frame of reference or practice model* which sets the framework for all of the planning to follow. A critical aspect of identifying a frame of reference/practice model is that it be consistent, or at least consistent with that of the department and of the institution. Imagine selecting a Cognitive Disabilities frame of reference (Allen, 1988) in a setting where psychoanalytic approaches are endorsed! That would be like submitting wok recipes to a French cookbook.

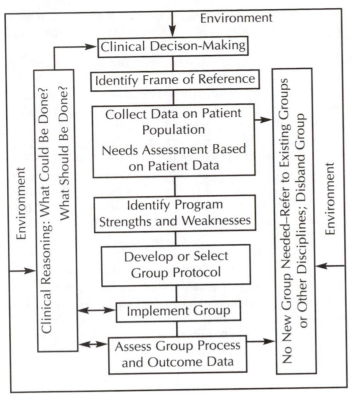

Figure 8-1. Group protocol selection system. Adapted with permission from Pelland (American Journal of Occupational Therapy, 41(61), p. 353).

It is the frame of reference which delineates the continua of function and dysfunction, and defines the postulates for change (Demon, 1987; Robertson, 1988), thereby moving us to step two, that of *clarifying what specific data we need about our population,* and how to analyze activities for the best fit between patient and group design. For example, if a patient is given the Allen Cognitive Level Test, and achieves level 4 or below (Allen, 1988), it would be inconsistent with the Cognitive Disabilities frame of reference to place the patient in a group activity requiring the ability to think abstractly (Denton, 1987; Pelland, 1987).

Step three in the decision-making process is *program assessment* of existing groups and individual intervention possibilities. This assessment is intended to identify strengths and weaknesses in departmental services as well as strengths and weaknesses in the services provided by other disciplines throughout the facility. Once again, the frame of reference/practice model helps identify ways in which occupational therapists can either offer unique services, or refer patients to other disciplines who share concerns, rather than duplicating services (Denton, 1987). In this instance the choice is not to develop a new group at all.

The fourth step in decision-making about groups is *selection or design of an appropriate protocol.* Required at this juncture is a return to the art and science of activity analysis, along with knowledge about group process and the critical elements of a group plan. As defined by Howe and

Schwartzberg (1986, p. 141), these elements are structure and content. The structure includes: group name; time and length of meeting; place; whether group is open or closed; goals and outcome criteria for goal attainment stated in behavioral terms; criteria for patient selection; leadership roles and functions; nature of the group contract; and methods and procedures. Content refers to the medium used in the groups.

Group structure and content must be considered vis à vis the frame of reference as we develop the rationale for the activities we choose and establish goals and objectives for our group (Kaplan, 1988). The importance of clarity around these issues lies in the reality that occupational therapists must begin to produce observable, measurable evidence that demonstrates the link between our theory and practice; replicates and validates our interventions; and substantiates the strength of our clinical decision-making and clinical reasoning skills. Setting observable, measurable outcome criteria makes the task of quality assessment and/or research easier to manage. For example, specificity in group structure can be compared to the need for specificity in learning to cook! I remember asking my great-grandmother how to make chicken soup. Her response was, "First you take a chicken!" While some of us cook by intuition, others rely on recipes to insure our success each time we cook. So, too, there are those of us who run groups according to protocols, defining clear goals and objectives, and with a significant amount of preparation, while others make decisions about group design only moments before the arrival of the patients.

Clinical Reasoning

The transition from clinical decision-making to clinical reasoning occurs at the moment we take the step to *implement* the group and *begin to evaluate it,* both as the group process emerges and as outcome data is generated. Mattingly (1988) has written about clinical reasoning in occupational therapy as a patient-centered approach which relies on the patient's perception and interpretation of his illness. In the clinical decision-making process, theory is linked to group process skills, activity analysis, and generalized patient needs. In the clinical reasoning process, the focus is on applying theories in a very specific context, with specific patients, who bring their own symbolic and concrete meanings to the activities we offer in occupational therapy group. How many of us have had to do a fast reshuffling of group plans when the patients proclaim, "We hate that activity, it's boring!"?

The essence of clinical reasoning is its dependence on patients' active participation in their choice of goals and definition of the methods for achieving them. "Efficacious treatment in occupational therapy relies on mobilizing patient commitment to the treatment process" (Mattingly, 1988, p. 1: 86). When starting a group, clarifying "what therapeutic intervention would most effectively propel the patient in a positive direction (Mattingly, 1988, p. 1:87) is as important as awareness about the context in which treatment occurs. Working with the patient requires us, as occupational therapists, to be conscious of therapeutic use of self, and to utilize the capacity to think on our feet or "reflect in action," when with the group (Shon, 1983; Mattingly, 1988).

Ongoing *assessment* of the group interaction and *evaluation of outcome data* is the step following implementation. This phase is also directly linked to both the clinical decision-making and clinical reasoning process. While the group is in progress, the therapist must continually use effective leadership skills to interact with patients and to respond to the ever changing nature of the individuals (Mosey, 1979; Kaplan, 1988); the nature of the environment and the nature of the activity. Neuhaus (1988) refers to this as constantly generating hypotheses and revising them to find the best fit between patients and activities.

The question of the efficacy of the group, as demonstrated by outcome data, is the last phase in the decision-making reasoning cycle. Results at this point might suggest these possible options: continue the group as established; acknowledge the need to return to the decision-making phase; or end the group. Whichever choice is made depends on the consequences of each preceding phases.

To better demonstrate the principles described above, let us look at a case example. Bear in mind that real life rarely fits perfectly into diagrams. Thus, the stages depicted in Figure 8-1 are somewhat obscured by demands of a brief narrative. Furthermore, this case represents clinicians' thought processes. The content related to actual content of clinical decisionmaking and clinical reasoning will vary from occupational therapist to occupational therapist and depends upon the chosen frame of reference/practice model.

*   *   *

Clinic A is a private, voluntary, nonprofit, acute care psychiatric hospital. It is part of a university medical center located in the urban northeast. Of the 104 beds, a maximum of 16 are available to adolescents in scatterbed fashion, spread among three 24 bed general psychiatry units. Census ranges from zero to sixteen, depending on fluctuations in admissions.

The Department of Rehabilitation Services consists of occupational therapists, music, dance and recreation therapists and teachers. Services offered to adolescents are part of the per diem rate and are conceptualized from a biopsychosocial frame of reference/practice model.

Adolescents, ranging in age from 13 to 18, are admitted for a full range of psychiatric and behavioral disorders, including major depression, acute psychotic disorders and conduct disorders. After a period of evaluation and observation on their units, patients are referred to a centralized adolescent rehabilitation program including school, occupational therapy, recreational therapy and dance therapy. In this way, patients from three units were gathered into peer groups which better replicate life outside the institution.

Clinic A is a tertiary care facility in which patients often come from great distances and from a variety of living situations including residential treatment centers and other social agencies. Third party payers, both public and private, bear the cost of hospitalization. Adolescents are from a wide spectrum of socioeconomic backgrounds, from homeless to extremely wealthy; and attend public or exclusive private and parochial schools.

Patients perform at all levels of scholastic achievement, task, and interpersonal functioning as demonstrated through the Barth Time Construction evaluation. Wide variation exists on Axis IV and V diagnosis. At the time of this case example, most patients demonstrated the capacity to engage in peer group interaction despite the wide range of DSM III-R Axis I diagnoses and variability on Axis II diagnoses.

Patients were able to use multiple task group activities to practice social skills and gain mastery over new functional skills within the context of a setting that enhanced their capacity to cope with and adapt to the normative developmental tasks and roles of adolescence. Almost uniformly, patients spoke of and behaviorally demonstrated their difficulties with transition to increased autonomy/independence. Often the concept of separation from home was the focus of individual psychotherapy and family therapy. This led to the development of intense attachments to co-patients and hospital staff, as hospitalization represented a crisis time in the transitional periods between early, middle and late adolescence.

As a result, there was a long history of patients staying in touch with co-patients after discharge, and of some even returning to the hospital cafeteria to meet for coffee and to touch base with the inpatient friends they left behind. Patients' return visits demonstrated the need to establish some mechanism for easing the transition from hospital to home, family and school. Even those who were discharged to residential treatment settings or long-term hospitalization seemed to need an arena to deal with concerns about separation from the hospital. Discharge to the community for inpatients often meant return to school, friends and family, with some constellation of therapy at other agencies, but with no transitional intervention around reintegration into peer groups. That gaps were created by discharge from centralized adolescent programs seemed obvious.

One solution to this service gap was to establish a transitional group, designed around the old concept of "rap groups" for high school students. The biopsychosocial frame of reference provided the theoretical foundation for the group, as it is consistent with departmental and institutional frames of reference, and pays particular attention to environmental issues. The "rap group" was to meet once weekly for one and a half hours (from 4:00 to 5:30 p.m.) in the department kitchen.

Led by an occupational therapist, this open-ended group is available to inpatients nearing discharge and outpatients who return to the clinic for approximately ten sessions. The rationale for the group is to provide a therapeutic forum in which issues around the difficult transition to life outside the hospital can be addressed, and thereby making it easier to separate from the inpatient experience at this hospital. This structured environment is intended to replace the informal "coffee klatches" in the hospital cafeteria.

Goals of the group include patients demonstrating the ability to loosen inpatient ties while tightening ties to post hospital dispositions, especially to follow-up therapy. Evidence for this ability is decreasing interest in attending the "rap group" and the patients' increasing ability to describe evidence of integration into other treatments and appropriate school community or peer groups.

Roles and functions of the group leader are to: assess and monitor interpersonal skills, aid in the development of increasingly adaptive capacities to separate successfully from the hospital, encourage independence rather than dependence, and monitor patients' ability to utilize disposition resources. In the face of failure to integrate post-discharge plans, the occupational therapist intervenes to facilitate integration or seeks consultation regarding whether or not plans could or should be altered.

Group methods include spending one half hour in preparation of snacks, drinks, coffee, etc. and informal "hellos," after which everyone is expected to settle into the more formal group discussion for approximately 45 minutes. Especially important to formalize is saying "hello" to new members and "goodbye" to departing members. Psychoeducation methods such as continually reeducating patients to group goals is an important aspect of this process. The final 15 minutes of the group are used for clean-up, planning for snacks the next week, informal goodbyes and individual intervention, when necessary.

Establishment of the transitional "rap group" emerged from the process of sound clinical reasoning and clinical decision-making. It also emerged from an environmental analysis which both identified the absence of services to aid in the transition out of the hospital and enabled occupational therapy to formally become part of the services offered through the Child/Adolescent Outpatient Clinic. The addition of services by occupational therapists to this clinic increases the capacity of the clinic to generate essential revenue through fee-for-service billing. Thus the group provides a good marketing strategy as well as a sound clinical service.

*   *   *

With these thoughts in mind, I invite you to consider whether a "cookbook" approach to group protocol selection is the recipe we, as professionals, want to follow. Or, is it time to build scientific inquiry into our practice, by establishing group protocols which represent the use of critical thinking in occupational therapy (Barris, Keilhofner, & Watts, 1983)? It is time to be reflective practitioners, designing and implementing treatment groups in collaboration with our patients, and with constant awareness of the fluid nature of the treatment environment. It is our professional obligation to continually reassess and revamp our practice, both from the "safety" of our offices, as in clinical decision-making, and from the moment to moment context of groups in progress, through the clinical reasoning process (Parham, 1987; Robertson, 1988; Shon, 1983; Rogers, 1983).

REFERENCES

Allen, C. (1988). Cognitive disabilities. In S.C. Robertson (Ed.). *Mental health focus: Skills for assessment and treatment*. Rockville, MD: The American Occupational Therapy Association, 318-334.

Barris R. (1987). Clinical reasoning in psychosocial occupational therapy: The evaluation process. *The Occupational Therapy Journal of Research, 3*, 148-162.

Barris, R., Keilhofner, G., & Watts, J. H. (1983). *Psychosocial occupational therapy: Practice in a pluralistic arena*. Maryland: RAMSCO.

Bonder, B. (1987). Occupational therapy in mental health: Crisis or opportunity? *American Journal of Occupational Therapy, 41*(7), 495-499.

Cynkin, S. (1979). *Occupational therapy: Toward health through activities*. Boston, MA: Little, Brown, & Co.

Denton, P. L. (1987). *Psychiatric occupational therapy: A workbook of practical skills*. Boston, MA: Little, Brown, & Co.

Fine, S. B. (1987). Looking ahead: Opportunities for occupational therapy in the next decade. *Occupational Therapy in Mental Health, 7*(4), 3-11.

Gibson, D. (1989). *Personal Communication*.

Grossman, J., & Bortone, J. (1986). Program development. In S.C. Robertson (Ed.). *Mental health scope: Strategies, concepts and opportunities for program development and evaluation*. Rockville, MD: The American Occupational Therapy Association, 91-100.

Howe, M. C., & Schwartzberg, S. L. (1986). *A functional approach to group work in occupational therapy*. Philadelphia, PA: Lippincott.

Kaplan, K. L. (1988). *Directive group therapy: Innovative mental health treatment*. Thorofare, NJ: SLACK Incorporated.

Mattingly, C. (1988). Perspectives on clinical reasoning for occupational therapy. In S. C. Robertson (Ed.). *Mental health focus: Skills for assessment and treatment*. Rockville, MD: The American Occupational Therapy Association, 181-188.

Mosey, A. C. (1979). *Activities therapy*. New York, NY: Raven Press.

Neuhaus, B. (1988). Ethical considerations in clinical reasoning: The impact of technology and cost containment. *American Journal of Occupational Therapy, 42*(5), 288-294.

Parham, D. (1987). Toward professionalism: The reflective therapist. *American Journal of Occupational Therapy, 41*(9), 555-561.

Pelland, M. J. (1987). A conceptual model for instruction and supervision of treatment planning. *American Journal of Occupational Therapy, 41*(6), 351-359.

Robertson, S. C. (1988). Reasoning in practice. In S. C. Robertson (Ed.). *Mental health focus: Skills for assessment and treatment*. Rockville, MD: The American Occupational Therapy Association, 1, 48-150.

Rogers, J. C. (1983). Eleanor Clarke Slagle Lectureship 1983: Clinical reasoning, the ethics, science and art. *American Journal of Occupational Therapy, 37*(9), 601-616. (Reprinted in Cottrell, R. P. (1996). *Perspectives on purposeful activity: Foundation and future of occupational therapy* (pp. 327-339). Bethesda, MD: AOTA.)

Shon, D. A. (1983). *The reflective practitioner: How professionals think in action*. New York, NY: Basic Books.

CHAPTER NINE

Continuous Quality Improvement: An Innovative Approach Applied to Mental Health Programs in Occupational Therapy

Virginia Carroll Stoffel and Susan M. Cunningham

This chapter was previously published in Occupational Therapy Practice, *2(2), 52-60. Copyright © 1991 Aspen Publishers. Reprinted by permission.*

A value intrinsic to health care professionals is the desire to influence improvement in patients. For occupational therapists, the guiding objective that propels our day-to-day activities is facilitating optimal patient functioning. Yet how do we really know that we have, indeed, contributed to improvement in function? Frequently, we only hope that we have used appropriate treatment techniques and, consequently, that we will see visible results in the patient's behavior. If we have used the appropriate treatment techniques correctly and have obtained the desired result, then we may subjectively feel confident in our ability to provide quality patient care. In many mental health settings, however, we still do not have a systematic means by which to focus our review of patient care, to collect meaningful data, to determine how we can improve occupational therapy mental health services, and, consequently, to improve patient outcomes.

The issues of professional accountability and making determinations about effectiveness have been germane to all health care professionals. The need for a formal process to review and evaluate the quality of patient care provided was an important issue for the American College of Surgeons in 1917. At that time, the minimum standard was established for review of medical staff performance in hospitals. The minimum standard contained the first formal requirements for the review and evaluation of the quality of patient care for physicians.[1] Since that time there has been a proliferation of standards through organizations such as the Joint Commission on Accreditation of Healthcare Organizations (Joint Commission). Mechanisms for evaluating the quality and appropriateness of care have evolved from retrospective audits to the hospital-wide, systematic, problem-focused monitoring and evaluation approach to quality assurance. Occupational therapists, particularly those working in hospital-based settings, should be familiar with the current quality assurance mechanisms for evaluating processes and outcomes care.

This (chapter) describes a practical approach to evaluating and improving the quality of patient care in mental health occupational therapy programs. Clinical examples are provided for clear illustration of the continuous quality improvement (CQI) process. We suggest that each and every registered occupational therapist and certified occupational therapy assistant be actively involved for the CQI process to be effective under the direction of a supportive, facilitative supervisor or director. When such activities become an integral part of the daily activities of each occupational therapy staff member, CQI will become a reality.

CQI, as developed by Deming[2,3] and Juran[4,5], may be seen as the evolving approach to quality monitoring in health-care in the 1990s. This approach espouses development of a system to measure, direct, and improve the quality of services on a continuous basis. Such an approach can be used by occupational therapists in all settings. In mental health settings, occupational therapists may find CQI to be a particularly helpful process. Frequently, the mental health environment is not conducive to clear articulation of the occupational therapist's role and to demonstration of the outcome of occupational therapy services to consumers and other professionals because of the various functions performed by the occupational therapist and the other mental health professionals.

Because CQI is formulated on an interdisciplinary systems approach to the quality of care, the contributions of all professionals working in the system are examined to identify opportunities for improved patient outcomes. As the CQI approach takes hold throughout the health care industry, the occupational therapist in mental health will probably spend less time trying to explain his or her rationale for treatment and more time demonstrating contributions through group problem-solving techniques and other improvement approaches inherent in CQI.

Trends in Mental Health Occupational Therapy Practice

In the 1990s, the role of occupational therapy personnel working in mental health settings was in a state of flux. Numerous concerns have been reported in the literature. Bonder[6] and Kielhofner and Barris[7] reported shortages of occupational therapy personnel in mental health. The report of the Ad Hoc Commission on Occupational Therapy Manpower[8], further clarified by Silvergleit,[9] noted a decline in the percentage of registered occupational therapists and an increase in the percentage of certified occupational therapy assistants working in mental health between 1973 and 1982.The reasons behind such a shift in personnel have not been fully explored. Possible contributing factors may include better utilization of both levels of occupational therapy personnel, cost-saving measures, and the flow of therapists into other practice arenas. A CQI approach could provide data, more systematically measure outcomes in care, and lead to action that could affect the utilization of human and material resources in mental health settings.

The Ad Hoc Commission's reports[8] also noted other factors influencing changing practice trends in mental health. They include the continued movement of mental health consumers from institutions into the community, the increase of occupational therapy personnel in case manager roles, and continued emphasis on skilled and accountable clinical management. Given these trends, the need to gather data to analyze systematically the impact of community-based care compared to institutionally-based care for specific mentally ill groups is indicated. Monitoring the outcomes of case management programs staffed by occupational therapists lends support to this emerging role. CQI is a tool for clinical management that will enhance program accountability as well as improve patient care.

Given the state of change in the mental health practice arena, Cottrell[10] examined the level of perceived competence among occupational therapists practicing in mental health. She reported that 90% of the respondents perceived their ability to adapt to their role changes and changes in the mental health system as being good to excellent. Additionally, 97% reported that they felt good to excellent about their ability to describe the occupational therapy role in psychiatry to multidisciplinary staff. When asked about their ability to conduct a quality review of their mental health program, however, one of four saw their competence as fair to poor. CQI could offer occupational therapists a philosophy and methodology for systematically collecting data, analyzing information, and making decisions regarding opportunities to improve care.

Definition of Terms

How can CQI and quality assurance be distinguished? Essentially, the distinction lies in a philosophic shift from seeking out the bad apples to promoting quality and excellence. Quality assurance, as practiced during the last decade, assumes that there will be defects and that ongoing inspection will identify these defects so that the service can be restructured to eliminate defects or problems. For example, in quality assurance typically we conduct audits of medical records to determine whether all the essential elements are documented rather than assess the data to identify opportunities for improvements in the quality of care provided.

The attitude toward customers (patients) approach, as suggested by Berwick[11], differs as well. The mindset of the supplier (in this case, the health care provider) toward the customer has traditionally been "I know what the customer wants," and the resources are allocated toward remaking or redoing the product to match the supplier's perception of what the customer wants. Applying this concept to occupational therapy, a therapist may say "Mr. Jones needs assertiveness and relaxation training. I will place him in these groups." Instead of the patient being involved in the program development and selection process, he or she is slotted into existing programs on the basis of the resources or convenience of the staff.

CQI acknowledges that there may be defects in the products or services. This approach, however, is highly sensitive to customer needs and constantly strives to receive customer input to improve and to meet the customer expectations. For example, the therapist could ask "Mr. Jones, what would you like to do in occupational therapy today?", "How can I help you meet your goals?", or "What are your suggestions for improving the assertiveness training program?"

CQI, rather than honing in on an individual practitioner's deficiencies, emphasizes improving systems, which lessens the employee's defensiveness and negativity toward the self-assessment process. Berwick[11] suggests that by focusing on systems all personnel can continuously seek ways to improve rather than seek out the bad apples in the inspection-oriented approach. Additional differences in the approaches or mindset between quality assurance and CQI are illustrated in the example below.

Sally, a registered occupational therapist working on a day hospital unit, has a history of not monitoring potentially dangerous tools such as scissors and knives in her task groups. Given the nature of the client tasks and the fact that the clients go home each day, she feels justified in having her clients take responsibility for keeping track of their own tools and materials. Because the occupational therapy program also serves acute inpatients who may be suicidal, Sally's approach to this issue is clearly at odds with that of her coworkers, who see her as being irresponsible and unsafe.

An inspection-oriented approach might identify Sally's behavior as not reaching the 100% standard of providing a safe and secure environment, and Sally might be dealt with by her supervisor in a disciplinary manner. Sally could feel coerced and misunderstood and that her professional integrity is being challenged.

A CQI approach might ask "How is Sally facilitating individual responsibility with her clients? What are the risks in expecting clients to monitor tools? How can the task group be run in a safe and secure manner while responsibility is promoted on the part of the client?" With this approach, Sally and her coworkers can grow from their collective wisdom and arrive at a decision that demonstrates respect for their professional concerns while at the same time recognizing the different needs of the different patient groups. The supervisor now acts in a facilitative manner.

In other words, a focus for monitoring is determined by identifying the important functions of the service being provided, describing how these key functions should be performed in a quality situation, and measuring the difference between what is and what should be on an ongoing basis.

Understanding CQI can be enhanced by further examination of its concepts. Continuous means an ongoing and planned approach. This is accomplished through monitoring. Monitoring is the systematic and ongoing collection and organization of data related to the indicators of quality and appropriateness of important aspects of care and the comparison of cumulative data with thresholds for evaluation related to each indicator.[1] Quality addresses two components: process and outcome.[1] Quality as related to process answers the question "Am I doing the appropriate thing effectively?" In other words, is the occupational therapist providing the appropriate therapeutic approach or technique in a correct manner? For example, when working with a manic patient, is the therapist following appropriate protocols for dealing with stimulus-sensitive patients? Quality as related to outcomes addresses the results of care. That is, what is the patient able to do as a result of the therapeutic interventions provided? Processes and outcomes are related by virtue of the fact that appropriate and effective application of processes will probably have an impact on outcomes.[12] Improvement is defined by Juran[4] as the organized creation of beneficial change or the attainment of unprecedented levels of performance. He likens improvement to breakthrough.

In summary, CQI provides the philosophic framework for designing systems to improve care by systematically monitoring the quality of the processes and the outcomes of care.

WHERE TO BEGIN

Here are several suggestions that might help create the environment that is necessary for CQI to flourish:

- Make a commitment to educating yourself and your staff about CQI.
- Attend CQI workshops, train your staff and coworkers in CQI techniques (e.g., Pareto analysis and fishbone diagrams) and use them regularly in your department (see the reference list at the end of this chapter).
- Be sensitive to the overall organization. Take care to control what you can control by integrating this approach in your own department. The ideal environment is for the total organization to espouse the CQI climate.
- Involve all staff.
- Provide encouragement to one another, and foster teamwork.
- Become adept at setting up data collection systems so that the data can be translated into meaningful information.
- Hone in on what you are doing well in your program, and celebrate your successes as a group.

Additionally, staff can build on their current quality assurance activities. Two resources, The Joint Commission Guide to Quality Assurance[1] and "Getting Started: Perspectives on Initiating a Quality Assurance Program,"[13] provide information to carry out the 10-step, data-driven monitoring and evaluation process suggested by the Joint Commission. The 10 steps for monitoring and evaluation used in quality assurance are applicable to the CQI process as well. The 10-step process in CQI will shift to a more internal continuous improvement mindset rather than being used to fulfill requirements for meeting quality assurance standards as the primary objective.

CASE EXAMPLE

The following case example illustrates how the data-driven process can help in making decisions that will lead to CQI.

An occupational therapy department meeting was initiated to identify important aspects of care that could be the focus for improved patient care. The staff generated a list of items that included patient assessment, treatment planning, timely initiation of therapy, attendance, safety issues, patient satisfaction with the treatment program, and matching the occupational therapy groups with the patients' functional abilities.

The staff decided that they were concerned about patient assessment because they were uncomfortable with the timelines and availability of assessment information in the medical record. Questions were generated that would help identify specific activities carried out by the therapists that could be systematically reviewed as they related to quality assessment. They asked the question, "What needs to take place in the patient assessment for quality care to occur?" The following activities were identified and correlated with the existing department standards for patient assessment:

1. The patient is assessed within 48 hours of admission.

2. The assessment is conducted by a registered occupational therapist.

3. The assessment is conducted with the department protocol for initial assessment battery.

4. Results of the assessment are documented in the patient's medical record within 72 hours of admission.

5. Appropriate referrals to other disciplines are made for additional testing (e.g., psychologic testing, chemical dependency consultation).

A system was designed for data collection; for the purposes of this discussion, we will assume that data had been collected and aggregated over a 3-month period. A total of 30 patients were monitored, and the following characteristics emerged:

1. In 50% of the cases the patient was assessed within 48 hours.

2. All assessments were conducted by a registered occupational therapist.

3. In 5% of the cases the assessment was not conducted with the department-specific protocol.

4. In 30% of the cases the results were documented within 72 hours of admission.

5. Only two cases indicated a need for referral, and the referrals did occur in both cases.

When evaluating this information, it would be easy to conclude that the therapists are not doing their jobs and that irresponsibility is at the root of the situation. A CQI mindset will focus on the system to explain the problems and the opportunities for improvement. The staff would again meet to engage in a group problem-solving process. With the data noted above, the group identified numbers 1 and 4 as priority issues because these two aspects of the evaluation process fell significantly below the norms for the established protocol.

The next step was to identify possible contributing factors that might lead the group to potential solutions. Possible contributing factors for number 1 included the following:

1. The referral was written after 5 pm on Friday and not received until Monday morning.

2. A record number of admissions occurred within a 2-day period (Monday and Tuesday).

3. Because the department protocol for the initial assessment battery takes 2 hours for each patient, the therapists were not able to complete it within 48 hours.

4. There may be workload problems (i.e., balancing scheduled treatment groups with limited assessment time.)

5. Patients could have refused to do the assessment.

6. Patients could have been unavailable during the 48 hours because of scheduling conflicts with other disciplines conducting their assessments.

Possible contributing factors generated by the group for number 4 included all the points listed for number 1 plus the following:

1. Therapists may not see the written assessments as priorities in comparison to other job tasks.

2. Therapists may value verbal more than written reporting.

3. Therapists may find written documentation cumbersome.

4. Therapists may experience difficulty in gaining access to the patient's medical record.

Once the group felt that they had identified all the contributing factors, they rank ordered the factors that they felt were most significant to the issue. For example, the highest ranked contributing factors for number 1 included the record number of admissions on Monday and Tuesday and the fact that the assessment process was too long (conclusions). Potential solutions (recommendations) to these problems included reallocating the personnel resources so that a registered occupational therapist could devote time exclusively to the evaluation team, flexibility to allow for admission rates, streamlining the assessment to a 30-minute screening or small group process, and changing the 48-hour standard to reflect more accurately the ability of the available staff.

For number 4, the highest ranked factor was that the therapists found the documentation system cumbersome (conclusion). Possible solutions (recommendations) could be providing inservice training about the importance of written and verbal assessment reports for team communication, reimbursement, and accreditation; building in a reward system for timely completion of documentation; and experimenting with other documentation formats such as checklists, dictation of assessments to a dedicated stenography pool, or computerized documentation. The group noted that some improvement could occur with number 4 if the solutions for number 1 were put into place because the two factors interrelate.

Once a solution is identified, there is a tendency to implement it and to assume that it will alleviate the problem and improve the situation. It is important, however, to proceed to the next step in the CQI process, which is to continue to monitor on the basis of the actions to improve, so that it can be determined whether the improvement actually occurs. This process can continue to be fine-tuned until the team feels comfortable with the assessment and its level of efficiency and effectiveness, having evaluated the results of the action taken. The acronym CRAE (conclusion, recommendations, action, evaluation) is helpful for remembering the steps toward improvement (Table 9-1).

CQI is dependent on the involvement of all staff. By being involved, each staff member will experience greater improvement in his or her own work process, which in turn positively affects the quality of care provided to patients.

CQI offers a systematic process by which occupational therapists can measure, direct, and improve the quality of patient services. To date CQI has been integrated into several well-known hospitals, such as Hospital Corporation of America; Humana, Inc; Massachusetts General Hospital; and New England Medical Center.[14] CQI is in the planning stages for inclusion in future Joint Commission standards. CQI is practical, useful, and powerful, as evidenced by its success in Japanese industry and more recently in American industry.[15]

The potential for affecting constructive change can take many forms. Occupational therapists who incorporate the CQI approaches may find that they can enhance productivity by focusing on priority activities through team efforts. Department cohesiveness may be fostered. Mental health patients will be encouraged to take more responsibility for their own care in a service environment where their input will be more respected and will have more impact, thus reinforcing their own ability to function. Staff time can be spent

Table 9-1
Format Used in Making Improvements (Acronym: CRAE)

Important Aspects of Care Monitored: Timely Documentation of Patient Assessment

Information element 1: In 50% of cases, the patient was assessed in 48 hours.

Conclusion (result of information analysis)
- Record numbers of admissions on Monday and Tuesday.
- Assesment process too long.

Recommendations (proposed conclusions)
- Reallocate personnel resources (e.g., OTR doing assessments only).
- Streamline assessment to 30 minutes.
- Conduct assessments in small groups.
- Change 48-hour standard to a more realistic time frame based on resource availability.

Information element 4: In 30% of cases, the results were documented within 72 hours of admission.

Conclusions
- Documentation too cumbersome

Recommendations
- Inservice training about importance of documentation for communication, reimbursement, and accreditation.
- Reward for timely completion.
- Design more efficient assessment formats (e.g., checklists).
- Dictate assessments to a dedicated stenography pool.
- Use computerized documentation.

Actions (solution implementation)

Choose proposed solution(s) from above and implement until enough data are collected to make judgments regarding effectiveness of actions.

Evaluation

Evaluate results of action taken and determine whether to accept solution (conclude monitoring) or try another proposed solution until acceptable improvement is evidenced.

---

more effectively on a focused approach to improving services and systems rather than the staff feeling out of control or lacking ability to solve problems.

Clinical and administrative decisions will be based on objective data rather than on hunches and speculation. Most important, a CQI approach promoted in the occupational therapy mental health setting will equip occupational therapists to improve and upgrade continually the quality of services provided.

CQI as a management style that values data for the purpose of continuous improvement will evolve over time. By incorporating CQI approaches now, occupational therapists will proactively prepare themselves for the inevitability of CQI being implemented in health care organizations throughout America. One benefit of adopting interdisciplinary group problem-solving for quality improvement endeavors is that occupational therapists will enhance their credibility in the mental health arena.

REFERENCES

1. Joint Commission on Accreditation of Healthcare Organizations. (1988). *Joint commission guide to quality assurance.* Chicago, IL Joint Commission.

2. Deming, W. E. (1982). *Quality, productivity, and competitive position.* Cambridge, MA: Massachusetts Institute of Technology Center for Advanced Engineering Study.

3. Deming, W. E. (1982). *Out of the crisis.* Cambridge, MA: Massachusetts Institute of Technology Center for Advanced Engineering Study.

4. Juran, J. M. (1989). *Juran on leadership for quality: An executive handbook.* New York, NY: Free Press.

5. Juran, J. M., Gryna, F. M., Jr, Bingham, R. S., Jr, Eds. (1979). *Quality control handbook.* New York, NY: McGraw-Hill.

6. Bonder, B. R. (1987). Occupational therapy in mental health: Crisis or opportunity? *Am J Occup Ther, 41,* 495-499.

7. Kielhofner, G., Barris, R. (1984). Mental health occupational therapy: trends in literature and practice. *Occup Ther Ment Health, 4,* 35-49.

8. Masagatani, G., Olson, T., Reed, K., et al. (1985). *Occupational therapy manpower: A plan for progress.* Rockville, MD: American Occupational Therapy Association.

9. Silvergleit, I. T. (1987). Clarifies figures from manpower commission. *Am J Occup Ther, 41,* 759. Letter.

10. Cottrell, R. F. (1990). Perceived competence among occupational therapists in mental health. *Am J Occup Ther, 44,* 118-124.

11. Berwick, D. M. (1989). Sounding board: continuous improvement as an ideal in health care. *N Engl J Med, 320,* 53-56.

12. *The joint commission 1991 accreditation manual for hospitals.* Oakbrook Terrace, IL: Joint Commission; 1990.

13. Brinson, M. H. (1987). Getting started: perspectives on initiating a quality assurance program. *Ment Health Spec Interest Sect Newsletter,* 104.

14. James, B. C. (1989). *Quality management for health care delivery.* Chicago, IL: Hospital Research and Educational Trust.

15. Walton, M. (1986). *The Deming management method.* New York, NY: Dodd, Mead.

CHAPTER TEN

Continuous Quality Improvement: Developing a Therapeutic Milieu in an Acute Psychiatric Hospital

Mary Hostetler Brinson

This chapter was previously published in the Mental Health Special Interest Section Newsletter, 12, 5-6, 8. *Copyright © 1989, The American Occupational Therapy Association, Inc.*

Quality is becoming one of the most frequently addressed issues in health care today. Most occupational therapists are familiar with the concept of quality assurance and now use monitoring techniques to gauge treatment effectiveness. Quality assurance as it has been practiced in the last decade has typically been departmentally focused, with an emphasis on finding the defects or bad apples. A typical example of this method in occupational therapy is the chart audit, in which criteria are developed that detail essential elements for an initial occupational therapy assessment or an activities of daily living (ADL) evaluation. Medical records are audited to determine whether the essential elements are present, with a goal of increasing the number of documents in which all elements are represented. Improperly documented or missing elements are attributed to practitioner error (Stoffel & Cunningham, 1991/2000). Although this method of quality assurance may produce better or at least more complete records, it does not necessarily lead to improved quality of care for patients. Quality assurance too often becomes a task done to satisfy accrediting bodies rather than a system that truly affects patient care.

Quality assurance methods are now shifting from retrospective, departmentally-focused audits to hospital-wide, systematic, ongoing, problem-focused monitoring and evaluation. This approach is called continuous quality improvement (CQI). The CQI concepts are based on the work of W.E. Deming, a statistician and management expert who is credited with revolutionizing Japanese industry by introducing management methods based on the principles of continuous quality improvement (Masters & Schmele, 1991). These methods have been widely applied in industry and are now being introduced into the health care field. CQI emphasizes the development of systems that measure, direct, and improve the quality of services on a continuous basis. Key elements in the CQI approach are involvement of all levels of staff, starting with top management, a systems approach, consumer participation, and continuous monitoring to evaluate the effectiveness of the program (Joint Commission on Accreditation of Healthcare Organizations, 1991).

With the multiple changes in health care, occupational therapists in mental health have had difficulty articulating their role, particularly in acute settings. This problem has grown because decreased length of stay and increasing health care costs have forced many hospitals to downsize and occupational therapy departments are a frequent target for major staff cutbacks. This trend emphasizes an even greater need for occupational therapists to clarify and modify their roles in acute care.

Traditional quality assurance methods have provided occupational therapy departments with methods for improving documentation and clarifying treatment goals. However, these methods have not encouraged occupational therapists to collaborate with other disciplines in solving system-wide problems that affect patient care. One system-wide problem that poses a challenge in the current acute psychiatric hospital is the need to develop a therapeutic treatment environment, or milieu, with decreasing resources, shortened length of stay and increased patient acuity. Traditionally, occupational therapists have given structure to the milieu through the provision of a variety of groups using verbal and activity modalities. With fewer resources, the occupational therapist must look at a more collaborative model for addressing the needs of patients in the hospital milieu. In redefining the occupational therapist's role in acute care settings, occupational therapists can be effective consultants to the milieu, can assume a leadership role in shaping and defining the therapeutic milieu, and can assist in training and supervision of other staff members.

The CQI approach to program planning provides a broad framework for the development of the milieu by (a) engaging the entire multidisciplinary team from the beginning of the project, (b) getting feedback from patients to determine levels of satisfaction, and (c) providing an ongoing mechanism for monitoring the usefulness of the interventions. The following is an account of how the CQI method was used to develop the milieu program at Butler Hospital, a private, nonprofit, acute psychiatric hospital with 117 inpatient beds serving both adults and adolescents.

BACKGROUND

Hospital care has undergone a number of changes in the last decade. Shortened length of stay, increased patient acuity, an increasing philosophical shift to the medical model, and reliance on psychopharmacological treatment have led to the dissolution of much of the group program. At Butler, occupational therapy provided the majority of the groups or activities in the milieu. However, these were generally provided in a centralized off-unit facility, which made it difficult for patients who were acutely dysfunctional to access the service. Unit staff members complained of the lack of structure and activity for patients, patients complained of having nothing to do, and referral sources believed there had been a decline in the amount of active therapeutic programming outside of physician-directed psychotherapy and medication. The lack of a clearly defined therapeutic milieu emerged as a major problem.

DEFINING THE PROBLEM

The Milieu Committee, an interdisciplinary group, was formed to enhance inpatient programming. The Director of Occupational Therapy chaired the committee, which consisted of the directors of social service, nursing, and psychology, as well as the chief of inpatient services. Staff members from every unit and discipline met in unit-based focus groups to discuss the problem.

The hospital was developing specialty units requiring that the nature of each unit milieu would be different. The units also varied in the degree of value they placed on groups and activities in the milieu. During the unit-based focus groups, some staff members expressed concern that they would be expected to perform duties (e.g., leading groups or running activities) for which they were not trained. Lack of training and knowledge and lack of time were the most frequent reasons cited for not participating in more groups. Patients were also surveyed in community meetings and through a Patient Satisfaction Questionnaire that the public relations department routinely sent to discharged patients. Many patients commented that there was too much unstructured time; the complaint was echoed by referral sources from the commu-

nity. All groups agreed that there was a problem and expressed belief that it could be addressed through careful planning, problem solving, and monitoring and that the result would be better quality of care.

IMPLEMENTING THE PLAN

Training and supervision were the next pieces of the program to be put into place. Outside trainers as well as experienced staff in the institution were used to develop four training modules: (a) an eight-session introduction to groups, (b) a six-session activity therapy module, (c) a two-session family psychoeducation module, and (d) a four-session advanced group training module. Staff members attended the modules before they began running groups. The occupational therapy department developed and implemented the activity therapy module. In addition to training, ongoing supervision was provided using a variety of models. Several units chose to eat lunch together weekly for peer supervision, and other units met on their own. Members of the Milieu Committee and senior group therapists were available for consultation and supervision.

The milieu program on each unit was developed by the multidisciplinary team. Unit philosophy, types of patients, staff mix, and patient acuity were some of the components considered. The following questions were asked to help staff members guide their thinking about program planning.

- How would you describe your philosophy of patient care?
- What do you value in the milieu?
- What are your goals?
- What is the composition of your patient population?
- What needs do you see for your patient population and your milieu program?
- What current interventions are being done on your unit?
- What interventions would you like to see added?
- Are there problems or needs in implementation, training, or supervision? If so, specify.

Units used this form in different ways. Some units asked each discipline to complete the questionnaire from their discipline perspective and then meet and develop the unit perspective. Others met to articulate and develop their unit philosophy, goals, and program.

Group proposal outlines (Figure 10-1) were developed to guide staff as they designed groups on each unit. Protocols under development were shared with other staff members, who discussed whether the proposed group fit the philosophy of the unit.

ONGOING MONITORING

Each unit meets annually with the Milieu Committee to review their milieu. A notebook is kept on each unit with updated unit milieu schedules, names of people who have

Group Proposal

I.   Format:

    A. Title:

    B. Place:

    C. Times:

    D. Leader(s):

II.   Rationale: (What patient needs will be addressed by this group? What values of the unit milieu are represented in this group?)

III.   Purpose: (What are you going to provide to clients?)

IV.   Client goals/objectives: (What specifically do you want the patient to gain from this group?)

V.   Criteria for patient selection:

VI.   Method of feedback to the treatment team:

VII.   Role and responsibilities of the leader:

VIII.   Resources:

    A. Staff members: (How many staff members will be needed to run this group?)

    B. Space: (How much space/where?)

    C. Supplies/cost:

    D. Equipment/cost:

Figure 10-1. Outline for a group proposal. (Copyright 1993 by Butler Hospital, Providence, RI. Reprinted with permission.)

completed various group training courses, descriptions of all of the groups, and copies of results from the Patient Satisfaction Questionnaire. This provides an ongoing record of the milieu program and schedules and is a readily available reference for new staff.

The Patient Satisfaction Questionnaire has been adapted and is now administered to all inpatients twice a year as well as to all discharged patients. The outpatient department also uses a satisfaction questionnaire. The admissions department developed a more focused questionnaire based on findings from the inpatient survey. In addition to the first page of the questionnaire, a second page asks patients other information (e.g., which unit they are on and the length of their stay), and leaves a space for comments. This information is then fed back to the specific units.

Several mechanisms have proved useful in transmitting and sharing information among staff members. The Milieu News, a monthly newsletter, contains brief articles of interest and updates on milieu developments. In the example shown here (Figure 10-2), one pair of group leaders developed a supervision tool that they found useful in peer supervision meetings. Results of one item from the patient questionnaire are also highlighted.

Milieu News
April 1991

Group Supervision

Group leaders on each of the in-patient units are developing supervision plans which meet the particular needs of their unit and staff. Juliet Ritter, OTR/L, and Jackie Pillay, ACSW, have developed a form to be used after a group in order to help the group leaders structure and focus the peer supervision process. In piloting this form, Ritter and Pillay feel that it stimulates relevant discussion between leaders and gives a framework to group leaders for reflecting on their work both during the group and afterwards.

Group Supervision Form

1. Who did leaders decide to include/exclude in the group and why?

2. If the leaders chose a warm-up activity, what was it and why did they choose it?

3. How did leaders handle difficult patterns both before and during the group? For example, interfacing with unit staff to encourage patients to attend group, letting staff know status of patient's ability to participate or managing difficult patients (i.e., irritable manics or monopolizers).

4. Identify two interventions you made. Describe one that was effective and one that could be improved. Discuss why you made each intervention (both from a group and a patient perspective). Was the intervention effective? If not, what would you do differently?

5. What were the therapeutic factors evident in the group (altruism, hope, universality, psychoeducation, socialization, cohesiveness, catharsis).

6. How did you facilitate interaction between patients?

Milieu Monitor

Two monitors have been completed using the revised patient questionnaire. A review of the item overall satisfaction across all six monitors that have been conducted shows a slight increase in the satisfaction that patients feel with the way they spend their time in the hospital.

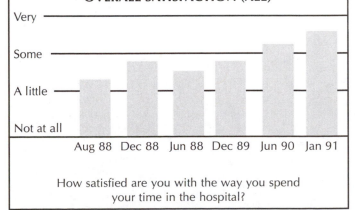

OVERALL SATISFACTION (ALL)

How satisfied are you with the way you spend your time in the hospital?

Figure 10-2. From Milieu News. Copyright 1991 by Butler Hospital, Providence, RI. Reprinted with Permission.

The process of change described in this article has taken place over years rather than months. The results, while not immediate, were the outcome of sound planning and have formed the basis of a well-planned, structured, meaningful milieu program. Occupational therapists have played a major role in shaping the therapeutic milieu, because their unique abilities in environmental demands allowed them to make important contributions as both direct care givers and consultants. As the nature of the units change, so must the milieu change. Using a CQI approach allows staff to meet the challenge of change through careful planning, monitoring, and problem-solving.

REFERENCES

Joint Commission on Accreditation of HealthCare Organizations. (1991). *Using CQI approaches to monitor, evaluate, and improve quality.* Oakbrook Terrace, IL: Author.

Masters, F., & Schmele, J.A. (1991). Total quality management: An idea whose time has come. *Journal of Nursing Quality Assurance, 5*(4), 716.

Stoffel, C. S., & Cunningham, S. M. (1991). Continuous quality improvement: An innovative approach applied to mental health programs in occupational therapy. *Occupational Therapy Practice, 12*(2), 52-60. (See Chapter 9 of this text.)

The Practice of Occupational Therapy Across the Mental Health Continuum of Care

EDITOR'S NOTE

Today's mental health care system presents numerous challenges to the provision of competent and caring occupational therapy practice. Section One of this text provided a comprehensive analysis of the sociopolitical policies, issues, and trends that impact on the quality of mental health care. Strategies and suggestions for effectively dealing with systemic barriers to quality care are also provided by several authors in Section One and in this text's last section on professional development. Many of these authors conclude that although there are undeniably real obstacles to occupational therapy practice in today's managed care environment, there are also tremendous opportunities for occupational therapists to assume leadership positions within this system of care.

The current market emphasis on the development of functional living skills and increased demands for accountability in consumer-oriented treatment enable occupational therapists to become leaders in the provision of mental health services. Occupational therapy's holistic approach is highly congruent with present calls for programs that facilitate community integration and continuity of care (Baum & Law, 1998; Foto, 1998; Frese, 1998; Schreter, Schreter & Sharfstein, 1997). Therefore, the occupational therapist is highly qualified to be at the forefront of program development and treatment implementation along the entire mental health continuum of care.

Today's mental health care system includes a variety of treatment settings—ranging from public to private, acute to long-term, institutional to community-based—with multiple combinations possible, and a diversity of client populations serviced. Therefore, occupational therapists practicing in mental health have innumerable choices for their practice settings. The opportunities for career mobility are still substantial, and areas of specialization abound. The chapters in this section provide an overview of traditional occupational therapy programs and emerging, contemporary areas of occupational therapy practice in mental health.

TRADITIONAL HEALTH CARE PROGRAMS

The role of the occupational therapist in traditional hospital-based settings is the focus of this section's first seven chapters. Robinson and Avallone begin this discussion by reviewing the current challenges affecting occupational therapy practice on acute, inpatient psychiatric units. To meet these challenges effectively, the authors developed a program that clearly defined occupational therapy's role on their unit and provided relevant evaluation and goal-oriented intervention for the inpatient, psychiatric client. Their emphasis on an activities health approach and multidisciplinary collaboration is relevant to a diversity of occupational therapy practice settings. The provision of clear practical descriptions of each step in the program development process can assist readers in the clinical application of program development principles across the mental health continuum of care.

The next chapter by Kaplan also presents an intervention program that has a strong theoretical foundation and a well-organized program design. In her presentation, Kaplan describes a three-level interdisciplinary, therapeutic group program for an acute, psychiatric unit. Primary emphasis is placed on a comprehensive description of the Directive Group. The applicability of this group approach to different treatment settings and patient populations with low functional levels is examined.

The range of functional levels among patients on a short-term psychiatric inpatient unit can be very wide; therefore, occupational therapists are often challenged to design programs to meet broad and varied functional needs. Chapter 13 describes a living skills program design that addresses the functional deficits of patients in an acute psychiatric setting. An overview of patient characteristics, evaluation procedures, program goals, group format, and treatment activities is presented.

Although acute psychiatric settings are traditionally based on the medical model, occupational therapists often use other models that are more congruent with occupational therapy philosophy to guide their practice, (e.g., Robinson's and Avallone's use of the activities health model in Chapter

11). The use of a wellness model to provide a framework for an acute psychiatric intervention program is described in this section's next chapter by Swarbrick. Given that individuals are admitted to inpatient facilities due to their difficulties in maintaining wellness, Swarbrick advocates for the use of a psychoeducational group model to foster wellness and promote health. She describes the multiple dimensions of wellness and contrasts the major characteristics of a wellness model to those of a medical model. Basic principles for implementing a program founded in a wellness model and specific content suggestions for wellness groups are provided. Supportive statements about the benefits of this holistic approach within an institutional setting are provided by clients, staff members, and administrators.

The perceived and real benefits of looking at the whole person from a wellness perspective within traditional medical settings is examined further in Chapter 15. In this chapter, Dale Y. Watanabe and Linda J. Watson present a psychiatric-consultation liaison program for an acute physical disabilities setting. This program provides multidisciplinary services to medically or surgically ill patients who are also experiencing psychological or emotional problems. Displaced anger, social withdrawal, impaired memory, poor judgment, and anxiety may become problematic for the client with physical illness and for the medical/surgical staff unaccustomed to dealing with psychosocial issues. The psychiatric-consultation-liaison team provides early detection of potential problems, educates and supports the staff, and assists the individual in developing effective coping strategies.

Hilda P. Versluys continues this theme of utilizing psychosocial methods with the physically disabled by applying role theory to occupational therapy practice in physical rehabilitation. In Chapter 16, she examines the tremendous impact a physical disability can have on a person's occupational, familial, and avocational roles. Guidelines for evaluation are provided in a comprehensive manner. The patient, the family, personal factors, and sociocultural influences are all considered in role assessment. Treatment is directed at maintaining, transforming, and/or reassigning valued roles using a practical, educational approach. A number of role-focused groups are presented by Versluys to assist the patient in acquiring and/or maintaining the functional role skills that are vital to a satisfying quality of life and a return to community living.

The need to facilitate an effective transition from an inpatient hospital to a community-based setting to decrease recidivism has become increasingly important as inpatient lengths of stays have progressively decreased. A model program that bridges the gap between inpatient and outpatient care is described in Chapter 17 by Sharon Baxley. This well-integrated program includes pre-discharge groups and supervised visits to community rehabilitation programs to develop patients' readiness for community placement. The provision of graded activities and multiple supports to effectively meet the diverse needs and address the different concerns of client populations with varying functional levels is described. Models of consultation are presented with concrete programatic examples given. The specific role of the occupational therapist within these different models and the ability of the occupational therapist to serve as an effective liason between the hospital and community is examined. A sample letter of understanding that clarifies the role of each setting in providing a continuum of care is provided and can be used by others to replicate this collaborative program design for successful community integration.

However, as Baxley notes, some individuals may find community living beyond their skill level, despite careful transitional planning. For these individuals, supportive residential programming is indicated. In this section's next chapter, Deborah Wilberding describes a quarterway house program designed to develop basic living skills in individuals with chronic mental illness. She begins with a literature review to examine the historical development of residential care, identify principles of transitional services, and define specific residential programs. Admission criteria, resident characteristics, assessment procedures, program structure, treatment goals, intervention methods, and staff roles are described for each program. The positive effect of this program on patient recidivism supports residential transitional living programs as effective models of intervention along the health care continuum for persons with chronic mental illness.

The development of functional living skills for community living is also explored in depth in Chapter 19 by Patricia Hickerson Crist. Crist reviews therapeutic models used in the treatment of patients with chronic mental illness who reside in the community. The psychoeducational model is presented as a viable form of mental health service delivery that can effectively develop community living skills. Psychoeducational concepts and principles are identified. Guidelines for program development are provided and supplemented by two program case studies. While many community mental health settings may not be able to provide "pure" psychoeducational programs, readers will find many of the psychoeducational concepts and practices described by Crist relevant to and easily implemented in a diversity of treatment programs.

The next two chapters on community day treatment services also provide information that is readily applied to diverse practice settings. In Chapter 20, the authors describe a continuum of partial hospitalization programs designed to be alternatives to institutionalization. These day treatment services focus on stabilizing and maintaining the individual within the community. Population characteristics, intake and referral procedures, program structure and therapeutic activities are described. The authors' discussion is supplemented by clear examples of a day treatment program schedule, a client contract and a relapse plan form. These items are clearly written and relevant to the realities of chronic mental illness. The role of the occupational therapist in creating a "laboratory" for learning in which clients can practice new, more functional behaviors is emphasized.

In Chapter 21, Coviensky and Buckley further explore the role of the occupational therapist in traditional community mental health by examining day activities programming for persons with chronic mental illness. Program philosophy, structure, and goals are described. The authors emphasize that a supportive structured milieu providing consistency, concreteness, and normalization in treatment programming is essential for community integration and the maintenance of a quality life for persons with chronic mental illness.

Frequently, the individual's ability to function in the community and attain a satisfactory quality of life is compromised by the social skills deficits that often accompany serious mental illness. The need for specific interventions to develop social skills for successful functioning is explored in this section's next chapter by Sisko Salo-Chydenius. She describes a social skills training group for persons with chronic mental illness that was designed to develop verbal and non-verbal communication abilities through a series of structured activities. The theoretical assumptions, goals and intervention principles of social skills training are reviewed and supported by the presentation of a case study. Salo-Chydenius provides an overview of a series of group sessions with session goals, activities and case study outcomes described. The efficacy of this social skills training program is evaluated with the author concluding that her qualitative data supports the benefits of this approach for persons with chronic mental illness.

By its very definition, chronic mental illness is a long-term, potentially lifetime condition. Therefore, it is critical that all occupational therapists who work with the elderly (whether in acute rehabilitation, a skilled nursing facility, home care, etc.) be aware of the mental health issues of elders for they will definitely encounter individuals in these settings who have psychosocial needs that must be addressed. Therefore, the next five chapters in this section will explore the role of occupational therapy in psychogeriatrics. Trace and Howell begin this discussion in Chapter 23 by describing the unique contributions occupational therapists can make to the mental health of elderly persons by utilizing our holistic approach. Preserving autonomy, enhancing integrity, and increasing the personal and community safety of the elderly are all viable outcomes of occupational therapy intervention. Relevant clinical issues and realistic barriers to optimal service delivery are analyzed with proactive suggestions and adaptive strategies provided to meet these challenges in psychogeriatric practice effectively.

Occupational therapy's role in psychogeriatric practice is further explored by Alisa Ofsevit Eilenberg in her presentation of a community-based wellness program to promote health and prevent depression in the elderly. In Chapter 24, Eilenberg reviews developmental issues pertinent to aging and provides a theoretical base for the creation of this program. Needs assessment procedures, program objectives, group format, and session activities are described with realistic case vignettes supplementing the presentation. The efficacy of this wellness program is examined, with Eilenberg advocating that occupational therapists should assume an active role in health care promotion and preventative services.

The benefits of occupational therapy services that are designed to prevent dysfunction in the elderly is strongly supported by the landmark study of Clark, et al. This research on the efficacy of preventative occupational therapy services for well elders who were living independently in the community is presented in Chapter 25. Clark, et al., describes the major aspects of this rigorous research study which found significant improvements in several dimensions of life satisfaction and perceptions of health among participants in an occupational therapy program. This preventative program was based on the fundamental occupational therapy principle of "health through occupation" to provide highly individualized intervention that enhanced the personal meaning of the treatment activities for the participants. The increased effectiveness of the occupational therapy intervention, to prevent illness and improve quality of life, as compared to a social activity control group and a non-treatment control group, is a finding that validates the provision of occupational therapy services to well elders living in the community.

The ability of an occupational therapy intervention program to support health and wellness is also discussed in Chapter 26 by Laurie Ellen Neustadt, who describes an adult day care program that provides coordinated, comprehensive health care services to elderly persons who are physically ill, medically fragile, or disabled. These supportive services enable the elderly to remain in the community, preventing premature institutionalization. Neustadt discusses program philosophy, goals, and activities. Case examples are provided to highlight the vital role day treatment plays in maintaining functional independence and increasing quality of life.

While community-based services can clearly meet the needs of many elderly persons, there is a growing necessity for institutional psychogeriatric programming to address the special needs of elderly persons with more severe illnesses. In Chapter 27, Dannielle N. Butin and Colleen Heaney describe a comprehensive psychosocial rehabilitation program used in an inpatient psychiatric setting. The program's philosophical base, assessment tools, treatment goals, and individual and group interventions are described and substantiated with practical clinical examples. The authors' emphasis on a collaborative, individualized approach to the provision of a multi-level, structured program graded according to each patient's functional abilities is consistent with occupational therapy's holistic philosophy.

WORK AND VOCATIONAL REHABILITATION PROGRAMS

As a well-established and expanding practice area, occupational therapy in geriatrics offers many opportunities for program development across the continuum of care. In the next five chapters, the authors will examine another practice area that provides occupational therapists with a wealth of opportunities to engage in innovative programming that ranges from prevention to long-term rehabilitation. These chapters focusing on work and vocational rehabilitation programs begin with Maynard's discussion on the role of occupational therapy in Employee Assistance Programs (EAPS). Maynard begins by reviewing classic occupational therapy literature on prevention and community health. She describes the philosophy and standard practices of EAPs and discusses the relevance of occupational therapy evaluation and intervention principles and techniques to the promotion of health and wellness in EAP's community-based work settings. Maynard examines the role of the occupational therapist on the EAP team and provides a sample profile of an occupational therapy EAP intervention plan. Due to the significant contribution occupational therapists can make to EAPs, Maynard advocates for expanded education and fieldwork opportunities in this area.

The need for occupational therapy students to be educated academically and clinically in the role of occupational therapy in work settings has increased greatly since the implementation of the Americans with Disabilties Act [ADA] (Crist and Stoffel, 1996). This section's next chapter describes the employment provisions of Title I of ADA and the process used to determine reasonable accommodations to overcome the limitations of persons with disabilities as defined by ADA. In this chapter, Scott also analyzes the difficult issues of stigma, fear, and ignorance that a person with mental illness may encounter if they decide to disclose their disability and try to use the protections and rights provided by ADA. The role of the occupational therapist in preparing the individual to disclose his/her mental disability, establishing qualifications for work and conducting job analyses to determine essential job functions and accommodation recommendations is comprehensively described. A case example is used throughout this discussion to highlight the pragmatic realities of seeking and maintaining competitive employment even with ADA protections. The vital role occupational therapists can play in developing the individual's ability to advocate for him or herself is strongly emphasized by Scott.

However, as Scott notes there are some individuals with mental illness with symptoms that are too severe to be able to work in the competitive marke place. For these individuals, therapeutic work programs are indicated. In Chapter 30, Palmer and Gatti present a comprehensive vocational program based upon sound theoretical principles. Program structure, evaluation procedures, treatment goals, activities, and tasks are described. An in-depth analysis of patient characteristics, treatment concerns, and environmental considerations is well integrated with occupational therapy theory. A clinical case study highlights the relevance and efficacy of the vocational principles and methods presented.

The successful outcome of vocational rehabilitation is often dependent upon the quality of the patient's transition into competitive employment. Chapter 31, by Dulay and Steichen, describes a transitional employment program (TEP) for the chronic mentally ill. The role of the occupational therapist in the development and implementation of TEP is clearly discussed. The description of TEP screening, evaluation, and training methods is supplemented with a clear work sample and a relevant case example.

While vocational rehabilitation programs and transitional employment programs can be highly successful in developing the knowledge, skills and attitudes needed to succeed at a job,

the potential employee still needs to find an employer willing to hire and work with a person with mental illness. Like all civil rights legislation, ADA has been limited in its ability to mandate attitudinal changes and end discrimination. Since most forms of discrimination are based on fear and ignorance, the need to educate the public about illness and disability remains primary. An innovative program that provides an educational group for employers to learn about mental illness and its behavioral manifestations is presented in Chapter 32. In this chapter, the authors explore the attitudes of employers towards persons with psychiatric disabilities and their concerns about hiring these individuals as employees. The demystification of mental illness and the building of collaborative partnerships with employers are primary program goals. The role of the program's employment specialist in providing a bridge between the employer and employee, learning the essentials of the job, supporting the employee and counseling other employees is clearly described. Occupational therapy's role in performing cognitive evaluations, assessing the work environment, and making accommodation suggestions to prevent problems and facilitate performance is also discussed. Employers' favorable response to occupational therapy evaluation, consultation and intervention, and their implementation of successful accommodations and proactive education and training programs for managers, supervisors and coworkers provides strong support for further program development.

CONTEMPORARY AND EMERGING PRACTICE AREAS

The grant-funded program described in Chapter 32 provides an excellent model for occupational therapy program initiatives. The ability of innovative occupational therapists to think and move "out of the box" of traditional practice settings is a tremendous resource for our profession. While occupational therapists can (and will continue to) make meaningful contributions in traditional health care programs, current realities and future constraints are indicative of the need for many occupational therapists to move into non-traditional practice areas. The next twelve chapters of this section examine contemporary and emerging practice areas that are viable in, and relevant to, the existing and changing professional marketplace.

The assumption of a nontraditional position in today's health care system requires occupational therapists to generalize and transfer their unique professional skills to a diversity of roles and settings. While occupational therapists clearly have the knowledge and skills to acquire nontraditional roles, the assumption of these roles may be deterred by a number of factors. In Chapter 33, Adams explores these potential deterrents to nontraditional practice. He provides constructive suggestions to turn these deterrents into opportunities for professional growth.

This section's next chapter by Cottrell examines the rapidly growing practice area of clinical case management. Since consumers, families, legislators, and health care providers are strongly advocating for clinical case management services to ensure individuals with mental illness receive appropriate, quality care in a cost-effective, efficient manner there has been a substantial increase in the demand for competent case managers. Cottrell offers specific information and suggestions to help the reader develop the knowledge and skills needed to provide competent clinical case management. She describes major case management models, roles and tasks. Occupational therapy principles and practice skills applicable to case management services are analyzed. Cottrell asserts that occupational therapists who expand their roles to assume case manager positions can make vital contributions to the provision of quality care in a challenging, managed, mental health care system. Realistic concerns about, and obstacles to, assuming this role are also discussed.

The importance of case management services given the limitations of current mental health care and the need for practitioners to assume nontraditional roles to provide essential care to persons with mental illness, is further explored in the next four chapters which focus on working with individuals who are homeless. While homelessness has been recognized as a major social problem in the United States; and, the mentally ill are particularly at risk for homelessness due to service delivery gaps; the ongoing debate as to the best way to deal with this crisis has often resulted in inaction. In Chapter 35, Asmussen, et al., advocate for an increase in community services for persons with mental illness who are homeless. They propose that existing community service agencies can be integrated into comprehensive systems of care designed to meet the unique needs of each person who is homeless and mentally ill. They present a system of case management as a process that enables the individual to use the services he or she needs. A model program which modified existing services within a well-established mental health care system is presented. Program changes that were initiated to meet the complex needs of persons who are homeless and mentally ill are realistically discussed. Pragmatic assumptions and practical guidelines for developing programs for this population with multiple needs are provided. The authors' research on the initial outcomes of their program initiatives demonstrated that they were effective in stabilizing individuals with mental illness and in remediating many of their problems due to homelessness.

The effectiveness of model programs in dealing with the complexities of homelessness is also examined in Chapter 36 by Kannenberg and Beyer who present a demonstration project that provided an employment program for homeless youth. The goal of this program is to develop participants' job skills to improve their employability and subsequently, their housing status. The authors also analyze the unique developmental needs of homeless youths. Since these young people have an increased incidence of a history of abuse and neglect, the impact of these traumas on their sensorimotor and psychosocial development must be considered in program plan-

ning. Kannenberg and Beyer review major developmental concepts which provide the foundation of this program's design. The rationale for occupational therapy in this setting and the role of the occupational therapist in assessing the individual's developmental stage and functional level are described. Occupational therapy interventions used to facilitate sequential mastery of normal developmental tasks and promote the acquisition of job skills in homeless youth are discussed. A case study is provided to illustrate the efficacy of occupational therapy evaluation and intervention, based on a developmental model.

The value of an occupational therapy approach in working with the homeless is supported by Barth in Chapter 37. Barth discusses how occupational therapists can apply their skills, knowledge, and training to plan and run programs and shelters for individuals who are homeless. She describes client characteristics frequently observed in homeless shelters and the multiplicity of diagnoses (i.e., mental illness and chemical addition, [MICA]) that are often present in one individual. Barth raises realistic concerns about the limitations placed on treatment when a person is classified with a MICA label. She provides relevant suggestions and practical strategies for engaging the client with a dual diagnoses into the treatment process. The importance of facilitating self trust so that the homeless individual can see his/her capacity to change and the relevance of entering the individual's life space is highlighted by a moving case example.

Another case example of a homeless woman becoming engaged in treatment through the intervention of an occupational therapist working at a homeless shelter is provided in Chapter 38. In this chapter, Kearney describes an occupational therapy program that uses structured, meaningful activities to achieve therapeutic goals for homeless women attending a dinner program at a shelter. This program, based upon a survey of potential participants' interests, uses the Model of Human Occupation [MOHO] to analyze and understand the assets and deficits of women who are homeless. Activity characteristics and the therapeutic value of parallel and shared group tasks for homeless women are explored. Kearney advocates for an expansion of occupational therapists' role in unconventional settings such as homeless shelters and provides a model for including nontraditional practice areas in occupational therapy educational curricula. Kearney also discusses the feminization of poverty and the sociocultural issues that has increased the prevalence of homelessness among women.

Since many women become homeless as a result of leaving their homes to escape domestic violence, it is critical that all health care practitioners recognize this major social problem. In Chapter 39, Helfrich describes major types of domestic abuse and examines the effects of domestic violence on its victims. Clear guidelines on how to identify victims of abuse and appropriate responses to abuse are provided. Helfrich poses a series of questions based upon the Model of Human Occupation that can be used to uncover psychological and behavioral indicators of abuse. Implications for occupational therapy intervention with victims of domestic violence are discussed. Helfrich's discussion strongly supports the absolute necessity for all occupational therapists in all practice areas to recognize and treat survivors of domestic violence.

Another social problem that is becoming increasingly important for all occupational therapists to be aware of is that of criminality. As Schindler explains in Chapter 40, the current reality of mental health care is that the number of individuals who are involved both with the mental health care system and the criminal justice system is growing significantly. Since it is likely that this trend will continue in the future, occupational therapists need to be prepared to work with individuals with criminal histories in a diversity of settings. Schindler begins with a brief history of forensic psychiatry and describes forensic settings and population characteristics. Definitions of common forensic terms are provided and the role of the occupational therapist in working with forensic populations is discussed. She provides a clear description of a well-organized occupational therapy rehabilitation program in a maximum security inpatient forensic psychiatric setting that offers a continuum of treatment to address the diverse functional needs of this population. Two case studies illustrate the complex realities of this population and demonstrate the efficacy of an occupational therapy rehabilitation program in forensic psychiatry.

Since forensic psychiatric settings are clearly nontraditional, they offer tremendous opportunities for contemporary and emerging occupational therapy practice. However, there are also traditional areas of occupational therapy practice that provide significant opportunities for the assumption of nontraditional roles by occupational therapists. The next three chapters explore opportunities for new roles in the traditional settings of school-based practice and home care. Chapter 41 by Hildenbrand describes the author's personal experience in developing a role for psychosocial occupational therapy in a school setting. The need to define and articulate the importance of a psychosocial focus in occupational therapy evaluation and intervention with children is emphasized. The steps Hildenbrand took to move her practice from a medical educational model, focused solely on sensorimotor issues, to a holistic integrative model that included the psychosocial domain, is clearly described. The need to document psychosocial occupational therapy and educate administrators, teachers, other service providers, and families about the psychosocial role of occupational therapy in educational settings is emphasized by Hildenbrand. Case studies highlight the three main areas in which she believes occupational therapy can make an impact. These include responding to psychological concerns, reframing psychosocial dysfunction and addressing psychiatric symptoms. Obstacles to, and strategies for, successful implementation of psychosocial occupational therapy approaches in a traditional school-based practice setting are presented.

The tremendous need for occupational therapists to expand their roles in school settings to include psychosocial practice is further explored in this section's next chapter by Schultz. Schultz discusses the paucity of holistic interventions in school settings and analyzes the major factors that she believes have contributed to the underutilization of occupational therapy services for students with behavioral disorders. She reviews interdisciplinary literature to examine constructs that support the value of and need for occupational therapy services for these students. Based on a synthesis of the seven interdisciplinary constructs that she discusses, Schultz presents a model for occupational therapy intervention with students who have behavioral disorders. This proposed model is designed to provide normalizing, age appropriate, school-based activities to develop the child's competencies and interests, as compared to traditional special education programs which are often limited to behavioral management. Guidelines for implementing this well-designed model are presented providing therapists with a solid framework for the development of innovative psychosocial programming in traditional school settings.

This section's next chapter also examines the expansion of psychosocial occupational therapy practice into a setting that traditionally does not address the psychosocial aspects of function, that is, home care. The authors, Azok and Tomlinson, describe a well-established psychiatric occupational therapy home care program. They explain that the use of AOTA's uniform terminology to define the parameters of occupational therapy practice enabled the home care team to understand and recognize what occupational therapists can offer in mental health home care. Population characteristics, evaluation considerations and methodology, major occupational therapy intervention goals and treatment activities, and client and caregiver education are discussed. The importance of adhering to home care documentation standards and maintaining interdisciplinary team communication is emphasized. Azok and Tomlinson present a case study that provides an overview of how psychosocial occupational therapy intervention enhanced functioning within the home and improved the quality of life for the individual and her family. They advocate for the expansion of occupational therapy mental health home care services based upon the effectiveness of this model program.

While there are many opportunities for occupational therapists to expand their roles as direct service providers of mental health care in many traditional and nontraditional practice settings, there is also a growing need for occupational therapy practitioners to explore indirect service roles. In this section's last chapter, Wittman advocates for the development and effective use of consultation skills by occupational therapists to meet the demands of a changing health care system. She argues that occupational therapists must learn new ways of providing service beyond the traditional direct care model in order to survive and grow as a viable mental health profession. She proposes that using consultation theories and techniques will enable occupational therapists to work in a diversity of practice settings. Wittman presents an overview of four main types of consultation that can provide a theoretical framework for practical application by occupational therapists. Her discussion includes a number of realistic occupational therapy practice examples supportive of the assumption of the role of a consultant.

Whether providing effective consultation, home care, school-based services, crisis intervention, long-term care, community integration, vocational rehabilitation, or psychogeriatric services, the occupational therapist makes a significant contribution to the mental health continuum of care. Readers are encouraged to review the programs presented in this section critically, and to use the information to clarify the role of occupational therapy in mental health practice.

However, readers are cautioned not to rely solely on program descriptions for their definition of occupational therapy professional roles. A solid theoretical foundation and the ability to articulate a frame of reference for practice is essential to the development of a clear professional identity. The selection of a frame of reference is a critical preliminary step in the process of providing effective occupational therapy evaluation and intervention (Cole, 1998; Hemphill-Pearson, 1999; Hinojosa and Kramer, 1998; Kielhofner, 1997; Kramer and Hinojosa, 1999; Mosey, 1986).

The relevance and value of using a frame of reference to link theory to practice is strongly supported by this section's authors, who provide clear theoretical foundations for their program descriptions. While the presentation of occupational therapy frames of reference and models of practice is beyond the parameters of this text, readers are urged to use the references provided at the end of this introduction to explore further the theoretical base of occupational therapy practice. While it is important that occupational therapy practitioners use occupational therapy frames of reference to guide their practice, it is equally essential for them to become fluent in the models of practice of other professions, for a unilateral, circumscribed view of mental health practice does not benefit the consumer or the profession (Foto, 1998; Quinn, 1993). The ability to communicate and demonstrate the value of occupational therapy in a manner that is congruent with the language and philosophy of other professions enhances occupational therapy's contribution and worth to the treatment team and leads to improved quality of care for the individual. Therefore, readers are urged to seek and use information from the literature of related disciplines. In addition, there are a wealth of continuing education and professional development opportunities available from a diversity of consumer and professional organizations. See reference and resource listings at the end of this text's preface, section introductions, and chapters for further details. The use of broad-based resources to expand professional knowledge can place occupational therapists at the forefront of current and future practice across the mental health continuum of care.

QUESTIONS TO CONSIDER

1. What services and resources are available in your community to provide continuity of care to persons with mental illness? How can an occupational therapist advocate and network with these programs to ensure quality of care and enhance community integration for the mentally ill?

2. What were the major theoretical foundations used by the programs described in this section? Which occupational therapy frames of reference/models of practice are congruent with the different practice settings that are along the mental health continuum of care?

3. What are important considerations for selecting and using evaluations along the mental health continuum of care? Which evaluation methods and tools are applicable to short-term acute units? Long-term care settings? Community mental health programs? Vocational rehabilitation? Psychogeriatric programs? Home care? School-based programs?

4. What are the primary goals of occupational therapy along the mental health continuum of care? How can the occupational therapist facilitate functional goal attainment for the diverse client populations seen in the varied treatment programs and practice settings of today's mental health care system?

5. What are the similarities and differences between the role of the occupational therapist in traditional practice settings and in forensic settings? What modifications would be needed in occupational therapy programming to meet the needs of a forensic psychiatric population while ensuring the safety of program staff and participants? What are your views regarding meeting the mental health needs of a client with a criminal history? What are your assets and limitations for assuming a position in forensic psychiatry?

6. How can therapeutic groups be employed as effective intervention methods along the mental health continuum of care? What adaptations to group structure, format, and activities may be needed to meet individual treatment goals and accommodate the different functional levels of clients and the varying practice realities of different treatment settings?

7. What are the aftercare programs and support services available to clients upon completion of their treatment programs? How can the occupational therapist ensure effective referrals to maintain functional skills, community integration, and quality of life for persons with mental illness?

8. What skills do occupational therapists possess to enable them to pursue non-traditional professional roles? What are challenges to nontraditional practice facing occupational therapists? How can occupational therapists respond proactively to these challenges to assume leadership roles within the health care system of today and the future?

9. What are the potential reasons that many occupational therapists did not seize the opportunities to expand their roles in mental health practice during the 1980s and 1990s? What are current trends supporting new roles for occupational therapists and increased opportunities for innovative programming?

REFERENCES

Baum, C. & Law, M. (1998). Nationally speaking: Community health: A responsibility, an opportunity and a fit for occupational therapy. *American Journal of Occupational Therapy, 52*, 7-10.

Cole, M. B. (1998). *Group dynamics in occupational therapy: The theoretical basis and practice application of group treatment* (2nd Edition). Thorofare, NJ: SLACK Incorporated.

Crist, P. & Stoffel, V. (1996). The Americans with Disabilities Act of 1990 and employees with mental impairments: Personal efficacy and the environment. In R. P. Cottrell (Ed). *Perspectives on purposeful activity: Foundation and future of occupational therapy* (pp. 217-228). Bethesda, MD: American Occupational Therapy Association.

Foto, M. (1998). Presidential Address: The Merlin factor: Creating our strategic intent for the future today. *American Journal of Occupational Therapy, 52*, 399-402.

Frese, F. J. (1998). Occupational therapy and mental illness: A personal view. *Mental Health Special Interest Section Quarterly, 2*(3), 1-3.

Hemphill-Pearson, B. (1999). *Assessments in occupational therapy mental health: An integrative approach.* Thorofare, NJ: SLACK Incorporated.

Hinojosa, J. & Kramer, P. (1998). *Evaluation: Obtaining and interpreting data.* Bethesda, MD: American Occupational Therapy Association.

Kielhofner, G. (1995). *A model of human occupation: Theory and application* (2nd Edition). Baltimore, MD: Williams & Wilkins.

Kielhofner, G. (1997). *Conceptual foundations of occupational therapy* (2nd Edition). Philadelphia: FA Davis.

Kramer, P. & Hinojosa, J. (1999). *Frames of reference for pediatric occupational therapy* (2nd Edition). Baltimore, MD: Williams & Wilkins.

Mosey, A. (1986). *Psychosocial components of occupational therapy.* New York, NY: Raven Press.

Quinn, B. (1993). Community occupational therapy in Canada: A model for mental health. *Mental Health Special Interest Section Newsletter, 16*(2), 1-4.

Schreter, Schreter, & Scharfstein (Eds). (1997). *Managing care, not dollars: The continuum of mental health services.* Washington, DC: American Psychiatric Press.

Wilcok, A. A. (1998). *An occupational perspective of health.* Thorofare, NJ: SLACK Incorporated.

CHAPTER ELEVEN

Occupational Therapy in Acute In-Patient Psychiatry: An Activities Health Approach

Anne Mazur Robinson and Joan Avallone

This chapter was updated by the authors in October, 1998. It was previously published in the American Journal of Occupational Therapy, *44, 809-814. Copyright © 1990, The American Occupational Therapy Association, Inc.*

The activities that we do every day provide a foundation for our lives. Psychiatric illness often interferes with a person's ability to perform the activities that are part of everyday living. When one considers the kinds of symptoms that psychiatric patients exhibit (e.g., disturbances in thinking, judgment, reality testing, and communication; social withdrawal, anhedonia, and dysphoria), problems in daily functioning are not surprising. Functional difficulties are most severe when symptoms are exacerbated to the extent that hospitalization is required.

It is a widely accepted assumption in the mental health field that psychiatric illness has an impact on day-to-day functioning. It has been observed that in the course of patient assessments professionals from virtually all of the disciplines involved in the treatment of psychiatric inpatients comment on the degree to which these patients are able to carry out daily activities. Reasons for hospitalization are often described in terms of the person's inability to function adequately in the community, and improvement in psychiatric status is often first noted in improved hygiene and grooming, improved orientation to unit routines, a greater ability to keep one's hospital room orderly, and more appropriate social interactions.

The gradual shortening of lengths of stay for psychiatric inpatients has raised important questions about the role of occupational therapy in acute, short-term hospital settings. Occupational therapists, who are concerned with the improvement of daily functioning, are often frustrated by the lack of time available for treating long-standing functional problems (Jackson, 1984/;1993; Short, 1984). Given the realities of briefer stays in inpatient settings, how can the role of the occupational therapist best be defined? What kind of program would meet the overall occupational therapy objectives for patients at the acute stage of psychiatric care?

In this chapter we will address these questions by briefly reviewing the changing patterns of service provision affecting inpatient psychiatry and by discussing the implications for the practice of occupational therapy in short-term hospital settings. We will then describe a model for occupational therapy practice in short-term acute inpatient psychiatry that is in its early stages of development at the 100-bed inpatient service of the Department of Psychiatry at St. Vincent's Hospital and Medical Center of New York. Included is a step-by-step approach to program development that can be applied to a variety of inpatient psychiatric settings.

Changing Patterns of Inpatient Hospitalization

Since the deinstitutionalization of chronic psychiatric patients began in the 1950s, there have been dramatic reductions in average lengths of stay for in-patient hospitalizations. In 1990, lengths of stay hovered at 30 days and under, requiring a shift in focus in which diagnostic assessment, control of acute symptoms, and early discharge planning assumed the greatest priority. Subsequently, the growth of managed care in psychiatry has caused further, more drastic reductions in length of stay, with averages ranging from 10 to 14 days. The in-patient milieu treatment model of the 1960s through 1980s has been replaced by a model focused on crisis intervention, management of symptoms, and discharge of patients who are often at lower levels of functioning than previously (Sargent, Scherl, & Muszynski, 1988).

It is noted in the literature that although the evidence suggests that there are advantages to briefer hospitalizations, follow-up out-patient treatment in day programs is seen as an important factor in the promotion of successful outcomes with this chronic psychiatric population (Talbott & Glick,

1988). This finding underscores the importance of careful assessment of the kinds of out-patient services the chronic psychiatric patient needs, in order to effectively address more long-term functional problems.

DILEMMAS INHERENT IN IN-PATIENT OCCUPATIONAL THERAPY PRACTICE

The acute exacerbation of chronic psychiatric illness often results in the deterioration of the patient's ability to adequately fulfill roles assumed in everyday living. Because the physical environment, socio-cultural surroundings, and pattern of activities of an inpatient psychiatric unit bear little resemblance to everyday living, and because the very nature of each activity changes when separated from its natural context, hospitalized patients lose contact with the familiar activities associated with life roles, which compounds the role dysfunction that is often triggered by the exacerbation of symptoms. Addressing issues of daily functioning in an inpatient setting therefore presents a fundamental challenge to the occupational therapist.

GUIDING PRINCIPLES AND OVERALL OBJECTIVES

The approach to inpatient occupational therapy programming presented in this (chapter) incorporates the concept of activities health, which is based on the premise that health in an activities sense (or function) is possible even in the presence of a chronic illness. Activities health has been defined as a state of being in which a person is able to perform the activities of everyday living in ways that are comfortable, satisfying, and socio-culturally acceptable (Cynkin & Robinson, 1990). The distinction between an activities health approach and more traditional approaches may be difficult to discern at the start. The primary difference lies in the degree of emphasis on diagnosis and symptoms. In a more traditional approach, the amelioration of symptoms is often a major focus of intervention. In an activities health approach, symptoms are of concern only insofar as they interfere with the patient's ability to achieve activities health. For a particular patient, for example, a traditional approach might be to identify symptom-specific needs such as increased concentration, socialization, and self-esteem. In an activities health approach the therapist would assess the patient's ability to perform activities needed for the particular roles to be assumed in particular environments after discharge in ways that are comfortable, satisfying, and socio-culturally acceptable. Thus, an activities health approach emphasizes the importance of understanding both the typical patterns of activities as they occur in the patient's everyday life and the inextricable connections that exist between the activities and the natural contexts in which they take place (i.e., time, place, and socio-cultural surroundings).

Given the hospitalized person's need to remain in contact with familiar activities associated with life roles and the limitations that are present when addressing activities-related problems out of context, the objectives of occupational therapy in acute, short-term in-patient treatment are as follows:

1. Provide the patient with a normalizing, structured routine, integrating meaningful activities from the various aspects of daily living (i.e., self-care, chores, work, leisure, sleep).

2. Provide opportunities for the patient to participate in daily simulations of activities associated with his or her roles outside of the hospital, to maintain partial contact with the roles to be resumed after discharge.

3. Monitor the degree to which treatment interventions (e.g., medication, behavioral management) are affecting the patient's ability to manage everyday activities in the milieu. The treatment team can use this information as one of many indicators of the patient's recovery from an acute episode.

4. Obtain information about the patient's roles and daily routine outside the hospital. This includes the identification (with the patient) of those aspects of his or her activities life that are in need of change.

5. Make recommendations to the treatment team regarding the kinds of services the patient will need upon discharge to improve everyday functioning, and convey assessment findings and long-term occupational therapy goals to the agency to which the patient is referred.

The in-patient occupational therapy program is viewed as a point of entry into a long-term progression toward a more desirable state of activities health—a progression that is likely to extend well beyond the inpatient stay if the goal is to be fully achieved. The patient's ability to manage activities in a hospital situation does not necessarily indicate an ability to do similar activities within the context of everyday living. Recognizing this fact helps the inpatient therapist provide more accurate functional assessments, because it brings a clearer understanding of what can and cannot be inferred from observations of patients on an inpatient unit. Once what can and cannot be accomplished in a hospital setting is understood, it becomes incumbent upon the therapist to consider and make provisions for the steps that need to be taken after discharge to help the patient integrate gains made in treatment into everyday life outside the hospital. Thus, functional assessment and participation in discharge planning are integral parts of the inpatient occupational therapist's role.

THE PROGRAMMING PROCESS

The following is a step-by-step approach to inpatient program development for an acute setting, to be followed once the objectives of occupational therapy at this level of care have been established.

Step 1: Assessing the Population and Setting

The patient population can be systematically assessed from two general perspectives: (a) characteristic lifestyles and

(b) level of functioning (i.e., the degree to which the patient's psychiatric disturbance is affecting his or her performance of everyday activities).

First, the commonalties and variations of lifestyle within the group are examined to determine what aspects are characteristic of the population as a whole. Such information can be gathered from a variety of sources, including historical information from current and previous hospital records, verbal reports from other team members, and informal or formal interviews with the patient. All of this information is used together to determine the demographics of the population, the range of roles that the patients in any given setting are likely to assume outside the hospital, the specific activities required for these roles, and the prevailing norms and expectations of the sociocultural groups to which the patients belong. The Activities Health Assessment (Cynkin & Robinson, 1990) can be adopted to provide a means of eliciting information about commonalties and variations in the patients' activities lives.

The group's clinical status must also be assessed, including range of diagnoses, severity of symptoms, and level of functional abilities. Assessments administered by other team members (e.g., psychological reports, mental status examinations, nursing and social work assessments) can be used in conjunction with occupational therapy assessments designed to measure cognitive skills (Allen, 1988), social interaction skills (Mosey, 1986), and other specific components of activities performance.

Step 2: Assessing the Clinical Setting

In addition to analysis of the patient population, the characteristics of the clinical setting are examined, so that the programs that are planned can realistically be implemented given the existing unit structure and interdisciplinary goals. The therapist specifically investigates unit routines, the potential for modifying components of the routines (e.g., mealtimes, wakeup times, and procedures), and opportunities and limitations regarding the use of a variety of hospital and community environments.

Once all of this information has been gathered, efforts can be directed toward planning a program in collaboration with other disciplines that is meaningful to the patients, socio-culturally relevant, realistic in view of the patients' levels of functioning, and feasible in view of the resources and limitations of the clinical setting.

Step 3: Determining the Overall Structure

In the context of everyday living, activities occur not as isolated events but in rhythms and patterns that are typical of each person. Therefore, to provide patients with an "orderly rhythm in the atmosphere... [to help them] become attuned to the larger rhythms of night and day" (Meyer, 1922/1996), it is critical for milieu activities to be sequenced and timed in ways that are representative of out of hospital living Similarly, it is important that opportunities be available for

patients to participate in activities both alone and with others—again, in keeping with general patterns of everyday activities.

The unit schedule is best conceptualized as a 24 hour, 7 days a week sequence of activities. Consequently, it takes into account the patient's activities around the clock, even beyond the limits of the occupational therapist's workday. Collaboration with the nursing staff in designing the unit program is therefore an essential ingredient in this programming approach. The activities program in the milieu can be seen as a simulation of a group (or sociocultural) activities pattern, in which activities are arranged in rhythms and patterns that are typical of their at-home schedules. This provides opportunities to interweave activities in socioculturally relevant sequences. Such an activities pattern can be used to restore a sense of balance, structure, and variety in the patients' daily routines, while also providing opportunities for the assessment of each person's performance of activities. Because virtually all patients carry out activities that fall into the general categories of self-care, chores, work (or its analogue), leisure, and sleep, the program can be designed so that patients are expected to carry out familiar, relevant activities from each of these areas of everyday living, timed and sequenced whenever possible in keeping with life outside of the hospital. Examples will be described later in this (chapter).

Obviously, it is impossible to create a program that is representative of the specific activities pattern for each patient. Therefore, in addition to structuring communal activities that are relevant to the population as a whole, the occupational therapy program must also include means of examining the activities life of each person, including the exploration of the degree to which and ways in which each patient's psychiatric symptoms interfere with the performance of routine activities outside of the hospital. The rapid turnover of patients that is characteristic of short-term settings requires that the methods selected be efficient ones. Examples are discussed under Step 4.

Thus, the two major components described above—providing opportunities for involvement in normalizing activities in the milieu and gathering lifestyle information from each patient—can be used together to achieve the overall occupational therapy objectives discussed earlier. Ultimately, it is the occupational therapist s job to systematically put all of this information together to make predictions about each patient's readiness to return to the demands of everyday living and to identify the kinds of supports and services that will be needed for successful functioning in the community.

Step 4: Determining Program Specifics

Once the program's overall structure has been established, appropriate activities can be selected and integrated into the schedule. Selected portions of the occupational therapy program at St. Vincent's Hospital are described as an example. These program developments are not in their final form; they represent the beginning of efforts to program activities in ways that specifically address the overall occupational therapy objectives identified. The descriptions are included for purposes of illustration and are not intended to be a blueprint for successful inpatient programming. As indicated earlier, it is important to arrive at a program design that is specific to the population of patients in each unique clinical setting.

Functional assessment. To assess each patient's degree of activities health, the occupational therapist gathers information from a variety of sources. Information presented on admission helps the occupational therapist begin to formulate a picture of the person's activities pattern, both at his or her optimal level of functioning and immediately prior to admission. As information is collected from the patient and significant others by various team members after admission, it can also be used to identify the roles that the patient has assumed by choice or necessity and the factors influencing success in carrying out these roles (Barris, Kielhofner, & Watts, 1983; Miller, 1988). From this information, the occupational therapist can then identify the performance components required for each of the activities needed for successful daily living (Mosey, 1986).

The patient is a necessary source of information for the assessment of activities health. The Activities Health Assessment provides a graphic pattern of the patient's activities life, which is used to explore the person's own perception of his or her lifestyle. The assessment begins with the graphic reconstruction of the patient's weekly activities schedule when at baseline and before admission. Once the pattern has been obtained, the patient is asked to categorize each activity (i.e., work, leisure alone, leisure with others, sleep, chores, self-care) and color code it. This graphic pattern is used as the point of reference for an interview about the patient's activities life, which culminates in the patient's rating of his or her degree of overall satisfaction, overall comfort, and sense of sociocultural fit. Thus, the Activities Health Assessment is used to (a) identify those activities that are part of everyday living, (b) explore the patient's perception of specific activities, and (c) determine his or her degree of activities health.**

THE MILIEU PROGRAM

The milieu program is conceptualized as a continuation of the assessment process and a means of helping patients to make the transition to their routine lifestyles upon discharge. Therapy groups and individual sessions focus on the categories designated in the Activities Health Assessment: home/self-care, work and leisure.

In the current health care environment, with hospitalizations averaging 10 to 14 days, it is crucial to choose those aspects of daily living that are priorities for the patient and reinforce them throughout the therapeutic program.

When possible, each patient is given a schedule at the time of admission, including all prescheduled appointments, groups, and meetings he or she is expected to attend. Staff members from other disciplines are asked to refer to the patient's schedule when discussing appointment times, thereby reinforcing the importance of the schedule. The schedules are used as a point of departure for a Time Management Group, where the patients address difficulties in organizing time in concrete, specific terms, rather than in an abstract, hypothetical way. The ability to use a daily schedule, which is actually a representation of the various appointment books on which so many people passionately rely, is one important predictor of the patient's ability to return to work or participate in a day program following discharge.

Patients' ability to care for themselves and for their environment is monitored by observing them as they carry out their sequence of self-care activities and as they perform chores to maintain order in the environment. Such observations have traditionally been part of the nursing staff's assessment. To complement the nursing assessment, occupational therapy cooking groups are used to provide opportunities for patients to participate in yet another set of activities associated with a universal activity—eating. Information obtained during cooking groups is used to assess a patient's ability to assume partial or complete responsibility for the preparation of meals after discharge. Whenever feasible, cooking groups are held at mealtime, so that they retain as much reality as possible. Cooking, like many other activities, is both preceded and followed by a sequence of other related activities, so these related activities are also incorporated to the extent possible. Meal planning, budgeting, shopping for supplies, setting the table, eating, clearing the table, and washing the dishes are some of the antecedent and consequent activities inextricably tied to the activity of meal preparation.

Depending on each patient's living situation in the community, he or she may assume anywhere from no responsibility to total responsibility for preparing meals at home. Patients who live with their families may not prepare the whole meal, but may be responsible for a related task like setting the table or cleaning up. On the other hand, a patient who lives in a group residence may not be involved in any of the meal preparation activities, but may simply be served food and be expected to eat meals with other residents. The therapist focuses on each patient's ability to engage in the activity in the way that will be required of him or her in the community.

Some of these related activities are rather easily simulated; others, like shopping, present logistical problems. More realistic activities will be substituted during the out-patient stage of treatment.

The use of leisure time is frequently an area in which dysfunction is evident. To address this aspect of everyday living, both group and individual activities are used. Supplies for individual pursuits are made available (e.g., books, needle-

---

**Some will note that the Activities Health Assessment bears a resemblance to the Barth Time Construction (Barth, 1978), in that they both use an activities configuration as a point of departure. An analysis of both instruments, however, reveals differences in purpose, design, and kind of information elicited.

crafts, stationery, games) so that the ability to plan leisure activities and follow through on such plans can be assessed. Leisure planning groups conducted by the recreational therapist are used both for the planning of leisure time while the patient is in the hospital and for formulating long-term leisure plans that the patient can pursue after discharge. To obtain accurate leisure assessment information, it is critical that the materials supplied be relevant to the patients' lives outside the hospital. The tile trivets and ashtrays that unfortunately have proliferated in psychiatric settings are, therefore, to be avoided.

Physical exercise, which is widely viewed as a valuable activity for psychological and physical well-being, is also integral to the program. For some, exercise is perceived as self-care; for others it is considered leisure; still others classify it as a chore. Regardless of individual perceptions, exercise experiences are structured and conducted in much the same format as the classes that are popular in the community, although they are markedly less physically demanding. An adapted exercise program (Avallone, 1986) can either provide an introduction to an activity that may be of benefit upon discharge or can help reacquaint a patient with an activity that is, or has been, a part of everyday living for him or her.

Patient education has assumed a greater priority as consumer rights and responsibilities are emphasized in health care. The use of a psycho-educational approach to address some of the difficulties in everyday living most frequently reported by patients, (i.e. stress management, symptom identification, relapse prevention) provides additional opportunities to identify areas of dysfunction and provides a forum for addressing coping skills needed upon discharge.

Finally, the expressed interest of some patients in returning to a previous job or seeking new employment upon discharge must be reality-tested. Assessment of vocational readiness is particularly difficult in an inpatient setting, because it is impossible to replicate in a supportive institutional setting the kinds of pressures and environments that are characteristic of the workplace. Therefore, the patient's work history is used as the primary means of predicting whether or not the person will be able to work once acute symptoms are relieved. For those patients who express the desire to work immediately after discharge, group activities (such as unit bake sales and patient-run thrift shops) can be used to supplement the examination of the patient's work history. These vocationally oriented groups are also valuable for patients for whom work is a long-term goal; they serve as preliminary work simulations for such patients and are used to monitor the patient's work-related and interpersonal skills, activities, habits, and attitudes.

SUMMARY

This approach to occupational therapy in short-term psychiatric inpatient settings has been developed in response to questions that we and other occupational therapists have grappled with regarding our role in acute settings. Many persons, both inside and outside the field of occupational therapy, have an ample knowledge base yet have difficulty articulating the contribution that can be made at this level of care.

This approach is not revolutionary; clearly, some occupational therapists have already been assuming some of these roles and functions in their practice, and some occupational therapists have included therapeutic activities similar to those we have described. What is unique about this approach, however, is its emphasis on incorporating into treatment programs an understanding of activities as phenomena in and of themselves, paying attention to when, why, where, and how they occur in the course of everyday life. Also distinctive is the lack of emphasis on psychiatric diagnosis and symptoms per se; they are of concern only as they relate to the person's capacity to achieve activities health. This kind of perspective on activities helps the therapist to design simulations of everyday activities that are representative of the context in which they naturally occur and focus individual functional assessments on the activities required to fulfill roles assumed outside the hospital. Efforts are directed toward structuring the in-patient milieu to (a) have as normalizing a routine as possible, (b) promote engagement in everyday activities, and (c) provide a means of assessing the person's ability to resume everyday life roles following discharge.

By maintaining an awareness of the inextricable connections between activities and the contexts in which they occur, the therapist can also be clear about the conclusions that can and cannot be drawn about the patient's functioning in the hospital. Functional assessment in an inpatient setting provides a valuable starting point, but it cannot be seen as a definitive predictor of functioning after discharge. Because the ultimate goal is to produce changes in patients' activities patterns, it is critical that discharge for those patients in need of further occupational therapy services includes means for assessment of actual functioning in their everyday environments and means for helping patients carry over into the community gains made in the hospital.

Thus, if occupational therapy services in acute inpatient psychiatric care are understood as the initial steps of what is often a long-term progression toward greater activities health, both the therapist and the patient can direct their efforts toward attaining objectives that are meaningful and attainable within a brief stay. The role of the inpatient occupational therapist is a vital one, because the therapeutic process sets the stage for the post-discharge phases of treatment that ultimately can help the patient achieve a better quality of everyday living, even in the presence of chronic psychiatric illness.

ACKNOWLEDGMENTS

We credit Simme Cynkin, MS, OTR, FAOTA, for many of the ideas that underlie this approach, and we thank her and Linda Silber, MA, OTR, for their valuable feedback during the writing of this article.

REFERENCES

Allen, C. K. (1988). Occupational therapy: Functional assessment of the severity of mental disorders. *Hospital and Community Psychiatry, 39*(2), 140-142.

Avallone, J. (1986). *Anybody can.* Los Angeles, CA: Framework Books.

Barris, R., Kielhofner, G., & Watts, J. (1983). *Psychosocial occupational therapy practice in a pluralistic arena.* Laurel, MD: Ramsco.

Barth, T. (1978). *Barth time construction.* New York, NY: Health Related Consulting Services.

Cynkin, S., & Robinson, A. M. (1990). *Occupational therapy and activities health: Toward health through activities.* Boston, MA: Little, Brown, & Co.

Jackson, G. (1984). Short-term psychiatric treatment: How will occupational therapy adapt? *Occupational Therapy in Mental Health, 4,* 11-17. (Reprinted in Cottrell, R. P. (1993). *Psychosocial occupational therapy: Proactive approaches* (pp. 27-30). Bethesda, MD: AOTA.)

Meyer, A. (1977). The philosophy of occupational therapy. *Archives of Occupational Therapy, 1,* 7-10. (Reprinted in Cottrell, R. P. (1993). *Perspectives on purposeful activity: Foundation and future of occupational therapy* (pp. 21-24). Bethesda, MD: AOTA.)

Miller, R. J. & Kielhofner, G. (1988). In R. J. Miller, K. Sieg, F. Ludwig, S. Shortridge, & J. van Deusen (Eds.). *Six perspectives on theory for the practice of occupational therapy* (pp. 169-204). Rockville, MD: Aspen.

Mosey, A. C. (1986). *Psychosocial components of occupational therapy.* New York, NY: Raven.

Sargent, S. C., Scherl, D. J., & Muszynski, J. D. (1988). The New Jersey experience with diagnosis-related groups. In D. Scherl, J. T. English, & S. Sharfstein (Eds.). *Prospective payment and psychiatric care.* Washington, DC: American Psychiatric Association.

Scherl, D., English, J. T., & Sharfstein, S. (Eds.). (1988). *Prospective payment and psychiatric care,* Washington, DC: American Psychiatric Association.

Short, J. (1984). Changing role expectations of psychiatric occupational therapists. *Occupational Therapy in Mental Health, 4,* 19-27.

Talbott, J. A. & Glick, I. D. (1988). The inpatient care of the chrinically mentally ill. In J. R. Lion, W. N. Adler, & W. L. Webb, Jr. (Eds.), *Modern hospital psychiatry* (pp. 352-370). New York, NY: Norton.

CHAPTER TWELVE

The Directive Group: Short-Term Treatment for Psychiatric Patients with a Minimal Level of Functioning

Kathy L. Kaplan

This chapter was previously published in the American Journal of Occupational Therapy, 40, *474-481. Copyright* © *1986, The American Occupational Therapy Association, Inc.*

Patients in short-term psychiatric inpatient units function at various levels and have a wide range of functional needs; they vary greatly in terms of their age, diagnosis, and background. This diversity presents great challenges to occupational therapy programming. There are relatively few resources published that address the problems associated with treating these patients in the limited time frame of the acute care unit. In addition, many acute care units employ only one occupational therapist so that there is no daily support from similarly trained personnel. Because the health care environment stresses accountability for staff positions, reimbursement, and professional autonomy, occupational therapy must not only offer a unique service to these patients within a limited time frame, but must also find effective ways to contribute and collaborate within an interdisciplinary team.

All inpatient psychiatric units provide some form of group therapy; their structure and content vary as determined by administrative factors and philosophical values (Yalom, 1983). Brief hospitalization has accounted for improved social functioning and decreased rates of admission in some patients (Herz, Endicott, Spitzer, 1977; Decker, 1972), but the specific forms of therapy that contribute to such benefits are not clearly defined.

Based on a review of 10 years of group psychotherapy outcome studies, Parloff and Dies (1977) recommend that clinicians resolve conceptual issues before proceeding with research questions. They suggest that the highest priority is to develop explicit definitions and descriptions of specialized forms and techniques of group psychotherapy.

This advice is appropriate for our field. Occupational therapy personnel in mental health are currently competing with many other professionals who use activities and lead groups. A survey found that 60% of the occupational therapists sampled use groups in all areas of practice (Duncombe, 1985). Our priority should be to specify what type of occupational therapy groups are best for which patients and to examine whether changes in behavior and improved functioning are due to therapists' skills, techniques employed, duration of treatment, type of instrumentation, or theoretical assumptions.

Increasingly, short-term units are admitting more chronic psychiatric and elderly patients who, along with the acutely psychotic and organically impaired patients, are difficult to involve in the ward milieu because of their extremely disorganized, dependent, or disruptive behavior. During a brief hospitalization, these patients face the difficult task of reorganizing their behavior to learn or relearn the minimal skills necessary to perform routine daily activities.

In most settings these types of patients are treated with medication, structure, and individual therapy until they are sufficiently organized to join a psychotherapy group. Although some settings offer occupational therapy or activity groups for these patients, this kind of treatment is not usually very important within the total group program. However, based on the author's experience, occupational therapists can expand their role in mental health by developing a framework for coordinating an interdisciplinary group program and taking a leadership position in treating the most disorganized patients on the unit.

This (chapter) presents an overview of a comprehensive group program developed on a short-term inpatient psychiatric unit and describes in detail the Directive Group, a specialized form of group therapy developed by the author for patients functioning the least well.

BEGINNINGS OF THE PROGRAM

The new program was developed for the 34-bed inpatient unit of The George Washington University Medical Center. The unit offers a continuum of services, including day treatment and outpatient programs. Adolescent, adult, and elderly patients are admitted for evaluation and treatment of acute emotional problems. During a 2 to 3 week stay patients participate in a wide range of therapeutic services, including individual psychotherapy, primary nursing care, psychotropic medications, family therapy, and group therapy.

Nine years ago, perceiving program fragmentation and staff isolation, several staff members revised the original program. Using a developmental approach, we reorganized the existing groups to meet the needs of the patients functioning at different levels. The Directive Group, the most innovative part of the program, was created for the patients functioning at the lowest level.

The following is a description of the program as it has evolved during the author's six years of coordinating it. Special emphasis is given to the Directive Group, which has since received public recognition (Yalom, 1983) and withstood the test of time.

RESEARCH SUPPORT

Research supports the use of group programs for the remedial treatment of the acutely ill, provided short-term treatment is part of a continuum of care. The most effective group programs and those most valued by staff members provide daily group therapy, monitor group composition, strive to decrease professional rivalry, and have an interactive focus (Yalom, 1983).

In terms of specialized approaches for the minimally functioning patient, reviews of outcome studies generally agree that there is a lack of evidence to support the value of verbal, insight-oriented group psychotherapy for psychotic and schizophrenic populations (Parloff & Dies, 1977; Bednar &, Lawlis, 1971; Meltzoff & Kornreich, 1970; Stotsky & Zolik, 1965; Moriarity, 1976; May, 1976; Mosher & Keith, 1979). Groups for this population are most effective when they rely on structured activity and reality-based approaches (Bednar & Lawlis, 1971; May, 1976). In fact, groups with intense interpersonal stimulation may be harmful (Linn et al., 1976). Furthermore, groups are more effective when combined with other forms of treatment, such as psychopharmacology and individual therapy (Parloff & Dies, 1977). However, drugs and psychotherapy alone are insufficient for developing social and occupational skills (May, 1976; Keith, 1982). This finding is important for occupational therapists promoting activity-oriented groups.

THEORETICAL FRAMEWORK

Without a theoretical framework, the clinician lacks a coherent way to organize knowledge, ascribe meaning to observations, or predict outcomes. We used the model of human occupation, which describes individuals as complex, open systems who are in constant interaction with the environment and who maintain and change their behavior through action (Kielhofner, 1985). We chose the model for several reasons. Since the model is based on general systems theory (Kielhofner, 1978; Boulding, 1956), it is congruent with interdisciplinary views. At the same time the focus on occupational behavior delineates the scope of occupational therapy services and is consistent with the short-term unit goals of improving the patient's functioning and enabling him or her to return to the community. The model allows the therapist to integrate information from other professionals pertaining to such factors as the patient's environment or support system. Finally, the model enables the therapist to specify an organized approach to the diverse patient group in acute inpatient care.

We used the model in three ways. First, the model specifies a continuum of occupational behavior represented by three levels of arousal and accomplishment: exploration, competence and achievement (Reilly, 1974; Kielhofner, 1985). Criteria for each of these levels were developed (Cubie & Kaplan, 1982) and used to organize each group in the total group program. Second, the model serves to identify the variables necessary for assessing patient behavior and specifying treatment goals (Roger & Kielhofner, 1985). Referral criteria were based on behavioral descriptions of the most typical patient problems addressed in each group and translated into the language of the model for consistency. Third, the model provides a way to conceptualize group treatment as the creation of therapeutic environments in which patients interact to learn about themselves and enact changes. The environment is created by titrating levels of arousal, enhancing internal control, stimulating interest and meaning in activities, and conveying expectations relevant to patient needs, goals, and roles (Barris, Kielhofner, Levine, Neville, 1985).

PROGRAM DESIGN

All groups in our setting are organized by three levels of arousal and demands or performance. The exploration level groups are organized at the simplest level of challenge to help severely disorganized patients develop basic process skills, perceptual motor skills, and communication/interaction skills. The group leaders select activities and organize the treatment environment: patients are required to participate in the scheduled group meetings.

Competence level groups are appropriate for patients who have basic skills but may need to integrate them into habit patterns. These groups are designed to help patients expand their skills and to identify goals, interests, and needs for meaning and action. As patients approach discharge, they begin to learn new ways to cope with problems experienced at home and in the community. Groups at the achievement level are designed to help patients integrate skills into daily life roles.

Table 12-1

Program Groups Categorized by Level and Professional Discipline

| | Professional Discipline | | |
| | Therapeutic | Occupational | Psychiatry/ |
Level	Recreation	Therapy	Psychology
Achievement	Leisure Awareness	Assertiveness Training	
Competence	Activity Planning Evening Activity	Task Group	Community Meeting Supportive Group
Exploration	Exercise Group	Directive Group	Directive Group

Table 12-1 illustrates how groups are differentiated by levels by each professional discipline. The purpose of the vertical dimension is to assure that the program has depth. Each level includes a number of groups, which are organized similarly but differ in content or focus. Therefore, groups are also planned to show variation along three horizontal dimensions (Figure 12-1). The horizontal structure of the framework prompts consideration of the balance and range of groups. Together, the vertical and horizontal dimensions build a coordinated framework in which each individually designed group contributes to the group treatment program as a whole.

REFERRAL CRITERIA

When patients are admitted to the unit, they are interviewed and evaluated by a psychiatrist and a nurse. Later, after meeting with the patients on rounds, in meetings, and informally, the interdisciplinary team members contribute to the master problem list and make referrals to groups. Each treatment group has a referral form itemizing specific referral criteria to match the patient's level of functioning with the goals of the groups. In addition, patients are referred to groups whose content is relevant. For example, a patient with depression and a workaholic lifestyle is referred to a leisure awareness group, which has an overall goal of clarifying leisure values and increasing awareness of lifestyle choices.

The occupational therapy and therapeutic recreation staff assist members of the team to think clinically about the groups and make appropriate referrals. The referral criteria serve as an individualized initial assessment of patient functioning. Identified problems are translated into short-term goals and provide a way to measure outcome. The following discussion of the Directive group provides an example of this assessment and treatment process.

THE DIRECTIVE GROUP

The Typical Patient

The Directive Group is designed for patients with varied diagnoses whose functioning is profoundly incapacitated. The group has included patients experiencing hallucinations, paranoia, catatonia, severe depression, organicity, hyperactivity, concrete thinking, or loose associations.

The model of human occupation provides a way of conceptualizing the dysfunctions of this diverse group of patients who have extreme difficulty functioning in the most basic of tasks and roles. They feel out of control, expect failure, avoid mastery experiences, and fear exploring the environment. They typically have difficulty identifying interests and goals. Their habits of selfcare and time management are markedly disrupted. Although these patients may have had adequate habits prior to the acute episode, their current situation is characterized by extremely limited interpersonal and task-oriented skills.

The Format of the Group

The term *Directive* refers to the active and supportive way in which the group leaders elicit adaptive behaviors and structure the environment to assure maximum participation of all members. The purpose of the group is to assist patients in reorganizing their behavior to a beginning level of competence. In general, patients are ready to be discharged from the group when they actively participate and can sustain minimal interaction throughout the 45-minute session.

The group, consisting of 6 to 12 members, meets 5 days a week at a routine time and place. The sessions begin and end promptly to emphasize a realistic use of and attention to time. On the average, patients attend 10 to 15 sessions, depending on the length of their hospital stay and speed of

Occupational Dimensions			
Leisure			Work
	Leisure Awareness	Activity Planning	Assertiveness Training
	Evening Activities	Supportive Group	Task Group
Interpersonal Dimension			
Social Interaction			Intimate relationships
	Directive Group	Assertiveness Training	Supportive Group
	Evening Activities	Leisure Awareness	Community Meeting
Mind/Body Dimension			
Physical Capabilities			Cognitive Abilities
	Directive Group	Task Group	Assertiveness Training
	Exercise Group	Evening Activities	Activity Planning

Figure 12-1. Occupational, interpersonal, and mind/body dimensions of program groups.

recovery. Once referred, attendance is mandatory to ensure continuity of treatment. Regular attendance depends largely on the assistance of nursing staff, since most of the patients are initially too disoriented or confused to take on this responsibility.

The relationships and activities of the Directive Group occur in a playful arena, a safe environment, which encourages risk-taking in patients who are threatened by the possibility of failure (Vandenber & Kielhofner, 1982). Patients are encouraged to move from passivity and internal preoccupation to goal-directed processes in which spontaneity and competence begin to emerge (Bertelanffy, 1966).

Content of a Typical Session

Each session of the Directive Group is complete within itself to accommodate the level of function and short stay of the patients. A session has four parts: orientation and introductions, warm-up activities, selected activities and wrap-up.

The first few minutes are usually spent reviewing the purpose of the group and specific treatment goals. Members who have been in the group are relied on to explain the purpose of the group and give examples of activities they have enjoyed and found useful. Introductions are conducted to make patients realize that their presence is valued.

For example, a group session typically begins with a co-leader asking a relatively experienced group member to help fill in the blanks on the blackboard. The board includes questions about the date, name of the group, its meeting time, its purpose, and the activities of the day before (or the previous weekend). Asking patients to call out the answers to the questions encourages them to focus on the activity and participate actively. This is usually followed by a balloon game in which each patient says the name of the person to whom he or she is throwing the balloon. The game is adapted by asking patients to choose a category, like cars or hobbies, and then to name items in that category.

The warm-up phase generally consists of 10 minutes of physical activity, the complexity and vigor of which are based on individual capacities. Movement provides a simple, familiar, and shared experience without the stress of verbal interactions. Exercises also allow for participation in simple rule behaviors such as taking turns and following instructions. For example, in a low energy group, members seated in a circle are told to move as little as possible. The leader slowly lifts one finger and moves it up and down. As the members imitate the movement, the leader opens and closes his or her hand. Finally, both hands are in the act. By starting slowly and matching the pace of the group, more activity is gradually elicited from the patients. Soon a member agrees to lead a simple movement while the others follow.

The major part of the group session is spent in activities especially selected for each day. These may include a series of games, each lasting a few minutes, or one long activity. For example, a regular feature of the Directive Group is the decoration of a large monthly calendar, used as a tool to help members stay oriented to the day of the week and the month. Depending on the needs and interests of the group, the sequence of events roughly proceeds from movement activities to interaction with objects to interaction with people (Robinson, 1977); the level of complexity increases from imitation to a few instructions to simple problem solving. Graded opportunities are available for leadership, decision making, expression of interests, helping others, and verbal interaction.

The last 10 minutes are spent in a verbal review of the activities and processes of the session. The leader lists on the board the patients' recall of the sequence of events, such as orientation of the board, name ball games, physical exercises, sitdown soccer, hangman, and the wrap-up. Then patients are asked to name the skills they used to perform these activities. With verbal structure, these patients are able to identify skills such as concentration, coordination, conversation, and having fun.

The wrap-up serves to attach meaning to the events of the group and provide feedback about each member's preferences and contributions. Because of the high patient turnover, group members must be helped to adjust to new members and say goodbye to old members during each session. A useful wrap-up activity is "Guess Who?" The patients answer questions like "Who was the first person in the group?" or "Who is wearing a red sweater?" or "Who laughed when we played sitdown soccer?" Such questions engage the patients' short-term memories, extend their attention, and create a supportive interactive focus.

The Coleaders' Role

The group is co-led by an occupational therapist and a psychiatrist. The leaders provide ongoing training experiences for other staff members and student coleaders.

Coleadership assures continuity of the group and consistency of meeting times. It provides security when a patient requires individual attention or assistance to leave the room in the event of out-of-control behavior. The severity of illness necessitates the presence of at least one other leader to counteract the patients' powerful pull toward extreme passivity, disruptiveness, and disorganization. Coleaders also provide support for each other when the daily demands of the group for creative, patient, and individualized approaches become overwhelming.

Coleaders plan activities, facilitate the assumption of group roles, and modify the structure of the group to meet the changing needs of the patients. Coleaders must be flexible and able to adapt activities on the spot. For instance, based on the group's level of attention, energy and interaction on the previous day, the leaders plan a game of modified bowling. But the group shows no interest and does not respond to other alternatives offered. The leaders than engage the group in yelling "yes" and "no." Breaking the action with humor gives patients a face-saving and empathic way to get involved.

As the main providers of feedback to the patients about the effects of their actions, the coleaders encourage, cajole, limit, refocus, and challenge the group members. The main message is acceptance. There is a strong expectation that each member, when ready, will be successful and will be supported in all attempts to participate. Patients are offered choices whenever possible to enhance their sense of control and to encourage their expression of interests. The choices can be graded to offer progressively more control. For instance, patients can decide if they would rather play bean bag toss sitting or standing up; if they want to have relay races in a circle or by teams; if they would prefer one activity over another, like geography or the card game Uno; if they want to suggest an altogether different activity based on their own experiences.

Physical Environment

Space is used to emphasize the expectations of participation. The room is fairly large and has tables and chairs that can be used as needed. There is a blackboard, storage cabinets, and a sink. Attendance is made clear by a daily list, which patients check off when they enter. The environment provides cues for role behavior, orientation in time, and performance.

Materials are used to engage patients' interests and inclination toward activity. Care must be taken to select activities that are appropriate for the current low functional level of the patients but do not demean their self-esteem as adults.

Often word games allow patients to associate with the memory of more pleasant times and elicit responses that surprise everyone. For example, one day a group was playing an alphabet game in which each letter is matched with the name of a country with the corresponding first letter. When no one responded to the letter "N", an elderly woman who was very depressed suddenly spoke up and said "Nepal." Her accurate response was applauded by all.

By listening to the patient's preferences during the wrap-up sessions and by observing patient responses throughout the sessions, leaders can develop a vast array of suitable resources. Other activities that have been used successfully include simple crafts (such as making, a memo pad or small terrarium), parachute activities, basic food preparation, coloring adult designs, adapted common games (like balloon volleyball, or wastebasket basketball), structured communication exercises, and memory games.

Individualized Goals

The most effective way to ensure the effective use of activities and interactions within the Directive Group is to individualize each member's pattern of participation. Explicit and reasonable short-term goals are important for the patients as well as for the family members who may feel overwhelmed by the patients' level of impairment. Confusion, anxiety, and concrete thinking make it difficult for these patients to conceptualize realistic goals for themselves. The coleaders develop and review individual goals each week in staff meetings.

The Directive Group leaders identified a series of individual short-term goals that address the behaviors patients frequently exhibit in the group. The four main goals for the patients are (a) to participate in the activities of each session, (b) to interact verbally with others around the common tasks, (c) to attend the group on time and for the full 45 minutes, and (d) to initiate relevant ideas for group activities.

Specific steps have been delineated to help patients achieve these goals. For example, a withdrawn patient who has difficulty interacting verbally may first be given the goal to respond once to a question asked within the group. During the session the leader would be sure to provide the patient with an opportunity to answer a neutral question. The patient's success in engaging may again be supported by other group members during the wrap-up by identifying patients who met their goal.

Patients who are paranoid or extremely disorganized may not even tolerate attending the group. For those patients, staying in the group for 5 minutes may be a reasonable first goal. If patients have to leave, they are given support for the length of time they did stay and told they are welcome to rejoin the group as soon as they can.

A different kind of goal may be developed for an adolescent who has adequate skills to participate in group activities on a regular basis but complains about every activity, thus discouraging people from interacting with him or her. For example, a young man's negativity is first accepted and then turned into a constructive contribution by giving him the goal to name at least one thing he did not like about the group during the wrap-up. It is likely that after a few days with such a paradoxical instruction (Watzlawick, 1978), the young man will ask to mention something he liked, too. At this point he has taken some initiative. The next step would be to ask him to help lead an activity or make a suggestion to the group.

Patients generally like having personal goals. Often they are written down for them on their own cards, which they show to their nurses or post on the doors to their rooms. The leaders consider the development and presentation of goals in the same way they analyze the use of games and other activities.

The positive feedback started in the Directive Group continues in other groups on the unit and in the community. Patients who meet the four main goals of the group are given a graduation certificate and are referred to other groups in the program. Some patients do not complete the program. These are patients who initially made substantial gains, but then failed to make further progress. They are given a certificate of participation and can be assessed for readmission to the group at a later date.

Documentation and Outcome

To monitor daily functioning, the patient's performance in the Directive Group is assessed after every session using an ordinal rating scale, which corresponds to the four main goals of the group (see Table 12-2). A patient's longest consecutive level of attention is rated from does not attend (1) to attentive throughout the entire session (5). The extent to which a patient participates in group activities and in verbal interaction is rated separately based on the amount of structure and support the patient requires. For most patients, initiation is the hardest response. Therefore, even slight indications in this area receive a high rating.

Unit staff members are taught how to use the scale through participation in the group. By understanding the meaning of the scores, they can monitor their patients' progress and compare the individual participation of the patients in the group. In this way, small increments of change, not otherwise appreciated, can be noted. Additional information, such as monitoring effects from changes in medications or electroshock therapy, or indications of organicity based on a patient's response within the group, is reported during team meetings and documented in the problem-oriented format in the patient's chart.

Using the rating scale, outcome measures for a 6-month period indicated that out of 146 patients, 129 (88%) improved their ratings on at least one of the four measures by 1 or 2 points. Over one half of the patients improved on at least two or three of the goals. About a quarter of the patients remained in the Directive Group until they were discharged from the hospital. These were generally the patients who required additional follow-up care in a nursing home or a day treatment program. Only a few patients (4%) appeared not to benefit from the group.

The behavior changes noted by the rating scale cannot be attributed only to the group because it is difficult to isolate the combined effects of medication, structure, and relationships. However, our clinical observation repeatedly revealed a marked difference between patient behavior in the group and elsewhere on the ward. The group is effective because it elicits and helps maintain more organized behavior.

DISCUSSION

The comprehensive group program presented here can be the starting point for occupational therapists to analyze and reconceptualize other inpatient group programs. The systems approach integrates the special and unique contributions of each group and therefore has the potential for decreasing the professional rivalry that is typical of many inpatient group programs.

The group program gives patients an opportunity to reflect on and restructure their lives. Some patients increase their level of functioning to a new level, some return to their previous level of functioning, and some acquire enough basic skills to function in a transitional setting, such as a day treatment program, halfway house, or brief stays in the community.

A limitation of the Directive Group is that no follow-up has been done to determine, as the research suggests (Mattes, Rosen, & Klein, 1977), that patients who attended the Directive Group are more likely to attend other groups because of their successful group experience. In our program, although no control group has been systematically studied, the Directive Group appears to enable patients functioning at minimal level to reorganize their lives faster than they could in other basic groups or with the help of medication only.

Conducting the group requires consistent, dedicated leaders and good cooperation with other staff members to help patients get ready for the group or to help them structure the remainder of their day. Interdisciplinary coleadership is recommended. Where this is not feasible, the alternative would be to have one identified leader and several rotating staff members or students. Based on our experiences, certain personality characteristics seem desirable in a leader. Patients respond best to leaders who are warm, enjoy being active and playful, and are not afraid of psychotic behavior. The leaders must be able to set limits in a supportive manner and be creative in developing goals and activities. It helps if at least one of the leaders is knowledgeable in group dynamics and psy-

Table 12-2

Directive Group: Key Model Variables and Clinical Characteristics

Model Variables	Patient Problems	Referral Criteria	Group Goals/ Individualized Goals*	Rating Scale
Performance Subsystem: Problems and Motor Skills	Passive Confused Distractible	Unable to find room or meal tray Unable to focus on a simple task for 5 min. Hyperactive or slowed activity level	Participation in Activities (showing active involvement) (focusing on activities) (following instructions)	5. Cooperates activity in all group activities without assistance 4. Needs minimal assistance to cooperate actively in group activities 3. Needs consistent support and structure to assure involvement in activities (or demonstrates hyperactive involvement) 2. Participates minimally 1. Uncooperative or resistive toward involvement in group activities
Performance Subsystem: Communication/ Interaction Skills	Isolated Aggressive Withdrawn Competitive	Speaks infrequently Monopolizes despite repeated feedback Makes inappropriate responses	Verbal Interaction (responding to question) (listening to others) (making one comment on his or her own)	5. Gives spontaneous and appropriate verbal responses to remarks and comments 4. Responds verbally and appropriately to direct questioning 3. Responds moderately to direct questioning (or monopolizes) 2. Responds minimally or offers inappropriate responses to direct questioning 1. Does not respond verbally
Habituation Subsystem: Habits	Dependent Disoriented Disorganized	Unable to stay in group for 5 min. Has difficulty performing basic self-care	Attending Group (on time) (dressed in street clothes) (for full 45 min.)	5. Attentive throughout entire session (45 min.) 4. Attends for 15 to 30 min. 3. Attends for 5 to 15 min. 2. Attends for 5 min. or less 1. Does not attend, highly distractible
Volitional Subsystem: Goals Interests Personal Causation	Unmotivated Resistant Fearful	Has difficulty identifying interests Lacks goal-directed behavior	Initiating Group Activities (helping lead activity) (explaining an instruction) (suggesting new idea)	5. Suggests, explains, or demonstrates at least one group activity (spontaneous initiation) 4. Makes suggestions (which may be inappropriate) 3. Elaborates on activity ideas with direct assistance 2. Can choose between two alternatives 1. Unable to volunteer activities on his or her own

chopathology so that the meaning behind psychotic behavior is understood and appropriate interventions are made. The leaders have to guard against taking over and against being punitive, rigid, interpretive, or passive with patients to avoid the problems associated with countertransference.

During the author's 6 years of developing this group, certain principles emerged, which are recommended in starting a Directive Group. They are as follows:

- provide a predictable routine for patients through the organization of the group and sequence of events
- develop realistic and individualized short-term goals for each patient
- offer leadership and role models to patients for action, support, and collaborative interaction
- create a playful arena which legitimizes the activities and interactions of the group and allows patients to develop skills and confidence
- modify the physical environment and materials to foster patient participation and encourage spontaneity
- establish a baseline of patient group behavior, monitor daily progress, and document achievement of individual goals

Within a supportive program, the Directive Group could be adapted to different patient settings. For instance, in a long-term facility with chronically ill patients, the group would probably need a set duration of attendance before graduation so that the many patients at the same level could eventually attend. The Directive Group has been used successfully by other occupational therapists to help patients with head injuries, stroke, mental retardation and chronic psychiatric problems, as well as for disoriented elderly patients in nursing homes. As part of a total treatment program, the Directive Group provides a first step toward self-direction.

ACKNOWLEDGEMENTS

The author thanks Marc Hertzman and Gary Kielhofner for their roles in the clinical and conceptual development of the Directive Group and Sandra Cohen and Colburn Cherney for their help in the preparation of the manuscript.

REFERENCES

Barris, R., Kielhofner, G., Levine, R., & Neville, A. (1985). Occupation as interaction with the environment. In G. Kielhofner (Ed.). *A model of human occupation* (pp. 42-62). Baltimore, MD: Williams & Wilkins.

Bednar, R., & Lawlis, G. (1971). Empirical research in group psychotherapy. In A. E. Bergen & S. L Garfield (Eds.). *Handbook of psychotherapy and behavior change* (pp. 812-838). New York, NY: John Wiley.

Bertelanffy, L. von. (1966). General system theory and psychiatry. In S. Aries (Ed.), *American handbook of psychiatry* (pp. 705-721). New York, NY: Basic Books.

Boulding, K. (1956). General systems theory—The skeleton of science. *Management Science, 2,* 197-208.

Cubie, S., & Kaplan, K. (1982). A case analysis method for the model of human occupation. *American Journal of Occupational Therapy, 36,* 645-656.

Decker, J. (1972). Crisis intervention and prevention of psychiatry disability: A follow-up study. *American Journal of Psychiatry, 129,* 2529.

Duncombe, L (1985). Group work in occupational therapy: A survey of practice. *American Journal of Occupational Therapy, 39,* 163-170.

Herz, M., Endicott, J., & Spitzer, R. (1977). Brief hospitalization: A two year follow-up. *American Journal of Psychiatry,* 34, 502-507.

Keith, S. (1982). Drugs: Not the only treatment. *Hospital and Community Psychiatry, 33,* 793.

Kielhofner, G. (1978). General systems theory: Implications for theory and action in occupational therapy. *American Journal of Occupational Therapy, 32,* 637-645.

Kielhofner, G. (1985). The human being as an open system. In G. Kielhofner (Ed.), *A model of human occupation* (pp. 211). Baltimore, MD: Williams & Wilkins.

Kielhofner, G. (1985). Occupational function and dysfunction. In G. Kielhofner (Ed.). *A model of human occupation* (pp. 63-75). Baltimore, MD: Williams & Wilkins.

Linn, M., Caffey, E., Klett, C., Hogarty, G., & Lamb, H. (1976). Day treatment and psychotropic drugs in the aftercare of schizophrenic patients. *Archives of General Psychiatry, 36,*1055-1066.

Mattes, J., Rosen, B., & Klein, D. (1977). Comparison of the clinical effectiveness of "short" versus "long" stay psychiatric patients. *Journal of Nervous Mental Disease, 165,* 395-402.

May, P. (1976). When, what, and why? Psychopharmacology and other treatments in schizophrenia. *Comprehensive Psychiatry, 17,* 683-693.

Meltzoff, J., & Kornreich, M. (1970). *Research in psychotherapy.* New York, NY: Atherton.

Moriarity, J. (1976). Combining activities and group psychotherapy in the treatment of chronic schizophrenics. *Hospital and Community Psychiatry, 27,* 574-576.

Mosher, L., & Keith, S. (1979). Research on the psychosocial treatment of schizophrenia: A summary report. *American Journal of Psychiatry, 136,* 623-631.

Parloff, M., & Dies, R. (1977). Group psychotherapy outcome research. *International Journal of Group Psychotherapy, 27,* 281-319.

Reilly, M. (1974). An explanation of play. In M. Reilly (Ed.). *Play as exploratory learning: Studies of curiosity behavior* (pp. 117-155). Beverly Hills, CA: Sage Publications.

CHAPTER THIRTEEN

A Living Skills Program in an Acute Psychiatric Setting

Kristin Ogren

This chapter was previously published in Mental Health Special Interest Section Newsletter, *6(4), 12. Copyright © 1983, The American Occupational Therapy Association, Inc.*

Training in community living skills has become recognized as one of the essential components in preventing the hospital readmission of chronic psychiatric patients by increasing their ability to cope with tasks of daily living. Traditionally, living skills programs have been a part of long-term treatment—either in preparation for reentry to the community from state hospitals or in after-care treatment in the community. While the area of living skills deserves attention in the acute care setting as well, time limitations imposed by a short stay and the high priority given discharge planning necessitate a different approach. This chapter describes a living skills program designed to meet the needs of an acute care setting.

SETTING

Located in a large metropolitan area, Overlake Hospital is a general hospital with a 30-bed inpatient psychiatric unit. The hospital contracts with the state to provide treatment to individuals committed by the courts, which results in a diverse patient population of both private and state patients. A wide range of levels of functioning and varied diagnoses are represented. The average stay is… days and planning for disposition is usually initiated as soon as the patient is admitted. In addition to discharge planning, inpatient treatment includes medications, milieu, and group therapy, and occupational and recreational therapies (OT/RT).

The OT/RT staff views the patient from the perspective of human occupation, or purposeful activity performed in everyday living. In the initial screening, the patient's work, leisure, and community living prior to hospitalization are considered. Based on this history and the patient's current functioning on the unit, assignment is made to appropriate groups for treatment.

LIVING SKILLS GROUP

Candidates for the Living Skills Group include individuals who have never lived independently or those with a history of poor adjustment in the community. Occasionally, patients who have functioned independently, but are currently clearing from acute psychosis, may be assigned to benefit from the structured, reality-based activities. Participation in the group requires that the patient be able to tolerate an hour of discussion and activity.

In response to the needs of the acute care setting, the goals of the Living Skills Group are: 1) to facilitate an appropriate and stable disposition through ongoing evaluation of the patient's living skills; 2) to promote the patient's participation in discharge planning by increasing awareness of community resources and agencies; 3) to increase independent functioning by providing information and practice of daily living skills.

The group of eight to ten patients meets daily Monday through Friday. Leadership is provided by an OTR assisted by a nursing staff member. The first three days of the week an educational format is used, with information presented through lecture, discussion, and printed handouts. Skills are practiced using paper and pencil tasks, role-playing and real-life situations. Five weekly units, each consisting of three related sessions, have been developed. Each week the unit that best meets the needs of the current patient group is selected for presentation. The units, in order of increasing complexity, are:

I. Self-Care: grooming, clothing, and nutrition
II. Health and Safety: safety, first aid, and health care
III. Community: public transportation, housing, and community resources
IV. Money Management: banking, budgeting, and shopping
V. Time Management: assessment, planning, and goal setting

Date:
Living situation prior to hospitalization:

Independent	Needs Help	
_____	_____	SELF-CARE (Reported by Nursing Staff)
_____	_____	Grooms self
_____	_____	Comes for medications by self
_____	_____	BASIC SKILLS
_____	_____	Follows written directions
_____	_____	Can use telephone book
_____	_____	HEALTH and SAFETY
_____	_____	Aware of household safety hazards
_____	_____	Knows emergency phone numbers
_____	_____	Gives proper response to emergency situations (grease fire, bleeding)
_____	_____	Knows where to obtain medical care
_____	_____	TRANSPORTATION
_____	_____	Identifies independent means of transportation method
_____	_____	Knows how to use metro transit
_____	_____	MEALS
_____	_____	Describes adequate diet
_____	_____	Able to locate and purchase food in grocery store
_____	_____	Carries out food preparation
_____	_____	MONEY MANAGEMENT
_____	_____	Identifies own source of income
_____	_____	Handles cash transactions (Counts money, makes change)
_____	_____	Budgets money for food and housing
_____	_____	Knows how to use bank accounts
_____	_____	USE OF TIME
_____	_____	Able to structure daily routine
_____	_____	Identifies leisure interests
_____	_____	Engages in work or is preparing to work

COMMENTS:

Figure 13-1. Living skills evaluation.

The group often serves to support the patient in discharge planning by providing information about local agencies and resources, i.e., the features of various halfway houses, the availability of vocational programs, etc. Patients practice decision-making and goal-setting, strengthening skills needed to develop and implement plans.

The last two days of the week the format changes to a cooperative group task. The patients plan a meal and shop for groceries one day and prepare lunch the next.

Instruction is informal as they experience planning a balanced meal within a budget, shopping from a list, handling money transactions and preparing a meal. As staff and patients cook and eat together, there is an opportunity to model and reinforce basic social skills.

Living Skills Evaluation – (Figure 13-1)

Knowledge of a patient's level of skills for community living can help assure an appropriate discharge placement. Informal assessment is done within the Living Skills Group, but in some cases there is need for a more formal evaluation. For this purpose a tool was developed that covers a broad range of skills but requires minimal time to administer. For the evaluation, information is gathered in three ways: 1) a report of the patient's functioning in selfcare is obtained from nursing staff; 2) in an individual session, the patient is given a series of tasks to perform in five areas (basic skills, health and safety, transportation, money management and use of time); and 3) the patient participates in the weekly grocery shopping and meal preparation. The shopping trip affords a unique opportunity to observe behavior in the community. Performance on each task is rated "independent" or "needs help." With these observations, the therapist then recommends a type of living situation that corresponds to the skill level of the patient. Most frequently indicated are independent living, halfway house, or nursing care facility.

Staff members from other disciplines, particularly those involved with placement, have responded favorably to the practical contribution of the Skills Program. A review of the discharge placements of patients whose living skills were evaluated over the past six months has shown that 91% of the actual dispositions were in accordance with the occupational therapy recommendation.

CHAPTER FOURTEEN

A Wellness Model for an Acute Psychiatric Setting

Peggy Swarbrick

This chapter was previously published as "Wellness Model for Clients" in the Mental Health Special Interest Section Quarterly, *20(1), 7-14. Copyright © 1997, American Occupational Therapy Association. Reprinted with permission.*

Proactive health promotion interventions are essential for persons with psychosocial problems to improve and maintain a level of wellness. Wellness is the process of adapting patterns of behavior to lead to improved physical, emotional, and spiritual health and heightened life satisfaction (Johnson, 1989). Wellness is a lifestyle that incorporates a good balance of health habits, such as adequate sleep and rest, productivity, exercise, supportive thought processes, and social resources. This balance influences social roles and associated activities.

Wellness includes physical, emotional, social, environmental, and spiritual dimensions (Dossey, Keegan, & Guzzetta, 1989). Self-management skills—the ability to manage stress and related factors, time management, and self-control—enable a person to maintain a self-defined level of balance among wellness dimensions (American Occupational Therapy Association, 1994). Life crises, stress, and psychosocial problems (mental illness) create an imbalance within wellness dimensions. Problems associated with a psychiatric diagnosis often require health promotion interventions to restore and maintain wellness.

The Wellness Model (see Figures 14-1 and 14-2) is a psychoeducational group program model that I developed that serves as the framework for groups, unit structure, and therapeutic approaches for an acute care psychiatric unit at a state psychiatric facility. The clients in this facility demonstrate symptoms and behaviors associated with life crisis that result in self-management skill deficits. These clients are admitted to an inpatient facility due to difficulty maintaining a level of wellness within their community environment.

It has been my experience that state psychiatric facilities do not foster wellness (see Table 14-1). The medical model approach and environment engenders dependence and lowers a person's sense of power and control (Leete, 1987/2000). Because the medical model does not explore health promotion choices, it is not congruent with adequately preparing persons with the skills and motivation needed to assume an active role in improving and maintaining wellness.

THE WELLNESS MODEL

The notion of wellness generates clients' internal motivation and active participation in treatment so that they can learn to manage problems and stress to prevent unnecessary inpatient hospitalizations. The treatment of diabetes is analogous to maintaining wellness. Management of diabetes, like mental illness, requires that the client designs, complies, and commits to a daily routine of medication, exercise, adequate nutrition, sleep and wake cycles, and rest. This regimen enables the client to maintain a level of physiological balance that affects his or her physical, social, spiritual, and emotional wellbeing. A focus on health, positive features (strengths), and personal responsibility rather than dependence and illness can engender optimism and a belief in the client's capacity to exert personal control in managing health needs, which can help prevent noncompliance with treatment.

The Wellness Model was developed through an interdisciplinary team approach. The client was identified as the most important active member. The strengths of clients and staff members were drawn on to coordinate treatment plans, environmental structure, and interventions. Specific attention was focused on developing and strengthening the person's self-management skills to strengthen a belief in that ability to manage their physical, social, emotional, and spiritual health needs. The daily routine and environment was designed to model the balance required to assume a wellness lifestyle. Balance included a regular routine of activity, exercise, group participation (psychoeducation group formats), and constructive community interactions.

The predictable routine offset the inner chaos many clients described and provided a pattern to help them regain

ABCs of the Wellness Model

Activity and Attitude

1. Foster a positive attitude toward assuming an active role in the pursuit of wellness.

2. Empower clients by fostering a positive attitude toward wellness and health.

3. Explore and engage in health promotion activities of daily living to promote an improved quality of life and satisfaction in achieving goals and interests.

Balance

1. Structure the unit routine to allow clients to experience the balance of productive activity, positive social support, emotional expression, and environmental interactions.

2. Promote a balanced approach (flexibility) in thinking, behaving, adapting, and coping.

Control and Choice

1. Explore and educate clients on healthy behaviors, activities, and coping skill strategies (choices and alternatives).

2. Educate clients on behaviors that they can choose to achieve a state of wellness.

3. Promote self-control and responsibility.

Figure 14-1. A simplistic overview of the Wellness Model's concepts for consumers.

control and order in their lives. Clients were provided opportunities to explore positive health choices while exerting control over events in the community and treatment. This strengthens belief in their ability to maintain greater control over their lives.

Wellness engenders a positive attitude rather than focusing on problems and illness. This seems to spark internal motivation and strengthen an optimistic attitude. Clients are empowered to manage life crises and stress and direct their attention to wellness lifestyle goals.

WELLNESS GROUP CONTENT

The content of all psychoeducational groups and environmental structure centered on wellness dimensions. The format of groups included a didactic component, experiential activities, audiovisual psychoeducation materials, and health promotion supplemental materials. The environment was analyzed, and specific attention was directed to promote positive community interactions and interdependence. Environmental stimuli such as noise level, content of music, and tel-

Physical

- Involve clients in medication education and psychoeducation groups on physical health needs (e.g., nutrition, AIDS education, smoking cessation, symptoms of stress, stress reductions).

- Involve clients in balanced daily exercises (e.g., walking, moderate levels of activity and productivity to promote health and counteract negative stress responses).

Spiritual

- Explore, respect, and incorporate personal values, beliefs, and life goals into treatment plan.

- Examine spiritual beliefs as a strength rather than negatively focusing on symptomatology.

- Respect spiritual beliefs as strengths and encourage healthy expression of spiritual beliefs and practices.

- Provide opportunities for self-reflection, meditation, and relaxation.

Emotional

- Promote healthy, constructive expression of needs, wishes, values, beliefs, and goals.

- Promote self-control, self-direction, and self-regulation.

- Foster self-esteem and self-control through successful activities that allow for expression of choice, self-control, and self-responsibility.

Social

- Structure community interactions to promote positive interdependence.

- Provide opportunities to work cooperatively to maintain the community environment.

- Explore social support networks and self-help groups.

Environmental

- Structure a pleasant, stimulating environment that supports physical, social, and emotional interactions.

- Provide music that promotes learning and relaxation.

- Structure balanced routines and procedures so that clients assume personal control and responsibility to maintain a clean, supportive, and cooperative environment.

Figure 14-2. Wellness dimensions.

evision were addressed. Often, there was a lot of noise and chaos due to sensory overload (i.e., radio and television going at once), which puts clients in conflict and crisis. The community voted on the type of music permitted favoring classical, jazz, and instrumental music rather than hard rock or heavy metal, which seemed to create noise pollution and provoke aggressive behaviors.

As occupational therapist, I played a major role in designing the activity component of the psychoeducational groups. I adapted health promotion educational media to address the clients' varied cognitive levels. Traditionally, much of the educational material was directed at clients of a higher cognitive level and higher socioeconomic and sociocultural

Table 14-1

Characteristics of the Traditional Psychiatric (Medical) Model Compared with a Wellness Model

Traditional	Wellness
Focuses on one aspect of the client. Fails to address the effect of dimensions on each other.	Focuses on all aspects of the client (physical, emotional, social, spiritual, and environmental) and the effects of each on the other.
Aspiritual. Spiritual issues are viewed as pathology.	Acknowledges a spiritual dimension.
Focuses on problems, what is wrong and is negative and pessimistic. Has less focus on promoting health.	Promotes strengths, health, what is right, and is positive and optimistic.
Treats symptoms and behaviors and dictates treatments.	Works with symptoms and behaviors.
Prefers the client to be externally controlled. Medications are administered in a controlled environment.	Fosters internal control and personal responsibility.
Dictates treatment; service is a parental role that engenders dependency. Has less focus on promoting health.	Promotes active participation in activities and treatment to achieve treatment goals. Occupational therapists, physicians, and nurses serve in roles of educators and coaches.
Quality of life is not a major focus.	Emphasizes quality of life.
Treatment dictated to client by physicians, occupational therapists, nurse and others.	Collaborative treatment team approach with the client as an active member of the team.
Uses fear as a motivator.	Uses good health and personal control as motivators.

background. However, many clients were of a lower socioeconomic status; therefore, psychoeducational materials were designed to address their unique needs. Often clients demonstrated various psychosocial sequelae along with secondary physical conditions such as AIDS, substance abuse, and life in socially and economically deprived environments, which do not support wellness lifestyles.

The tenets of the Wellness Model are health promotion and client responsiveness. An example of this was when a state-mandated "no smoking" policy was enacted. Clients and staff members cooperatively worked to develop strategies to make the unit smoke-free. Clients adapted to not being able to smoke and attended groups more often and with less resistance. This occurred after clients requested a smoke-ending group so they could learn to decrease smoking.

I adapted client education smoke cessation material to develop activity-based groups, which were used as a component of the physical health and self-management psychoeducational groups. Clients were instructed on the cost and health benefits of decreasing smoking (many were on limited budgets and realized how much money they could save). During group sessions, they explored leisure and productive activities they could engage in to occupy their time. Clients were educated on the physical health benefits of not smoking and engaged in exercise and relaxation techniques to replace smoking behaviors that many often used to decrease anxiety and stress. Alternative strategies to deal with stress and anxiety were explored through active participation in hobbies, crafts, group activities, and unit routines.

During the time management group, many clients said that they smoked because of boredom. Hobbies and activities were explored so clients could learn to productively occupy time and engage hands and minds in doing something other and possibly more meaningful than holding a cigarette.

OUTCOMES

A component of program evaluation includes soliciting feedback from clients. At the end of treatment, clients are asked to provide written feedback on a satisfaction questionnaire, a sampling of which is provided here.

Summary of Client Responses

- "Very glad I was given choices and the opportunity to state my opinion about my treatment instead of only being told what I should do."
- "Very educational. Felt like I was in health class in school where you can learn about good health."
- "Felt my opinion was respected."
- "Glad that I was given choices and could learn new ways to deal with my anger."
- "I really liked the positive focus. I want to be well and just the word wellness gives me hope."
- "I need to learn how to occupy my time because I have a lot of free time which gets me into trouble. I learned some things to do to keep out of trouble."

- "My depression makes me not feel well. I think I can stop feeling so depressed by thinking that I can be well."
- "Just the word wellness makes me feel better. I learned some ways to get rid of the negative tapes in my mind that make me feel depressed and replace them with positive tapes like talking about wellness."
- Negative responses included: too many people in some groups, want more groups, want more specific groups such as crafts and activities, want to go outside of the unit more.

Staff Member Responses

- "Unit is more controlled and cleaner."
- "Clients were more active in cleaning the unit and seem more willing to participate in their treatment."
- "There were less outbursts and conflicts between staff and less conflicts and fights between consumers."

Administrative Responses

- The director of the unit was very supportive of programming structure and securing supplies, materials needed for programming.
- Quality improvement measures and risk management report reflected fewer incident reports.
- Fewer consumers placed in quiet and seclusion rooms.
- Less staff on sick leave injury.
- Improved staff morale. Staff appeared more willing to do their jobs because they were given choices in the tasks and groups they conducted.

No specific data was collected to describe functional outcomes after discharge, at the time of this program. Future recommendations are to develop mechanisms to track functional outcomes and to implement closer follow-up by the state facility.

OUTGROWTHS

This program model has also been implemented for other services. Currently, the Wellness Model is being conducted on a crisis intervention program, and I provided consultation for wellness program development.

CONCLUSIONS

Occupational therapists can play an important role in empowering clients and the community by using a health promotion and wellness approach. Persons with psychosocial problems possess strengths, values, goals, and needs that should be addressed through optimistic and collaborative treatment team initiates. It is vital that occupational therapists work to collaborate with clients and other health care professionals to shift from a medically modeled paternalistic mode of treatment to a mode of treatment that addresses the total wellness dimensions of the clients they serve. Occupational therapists can play a pivotal role in the design of innovative, optimistic wellness approaches to empower persons with psychosocial problems to achieve goals and dreams and to maintain a personally defined level of wellness.

APPENDIX

Resource List

Fetzer Institute
9292 West Kl Avenue
Kalamazoo, MI 49002

Krippalu Center
PO Box 793
Lenox, MA 01240

New York Open Center
83 Spring Street
New York, NY 10012

REFERENCES

American Occupational Therapy Association. (1994). Uniform terminology for occupational therapy—Third edition. *American Journal of Occupational Therapy, 48,* 1047-1054. (Reprinted in Cottrall, R. P. (Ed.) Perspectives on purposeful activity: Foundations and future of occupational therapy (pp. 651-665). Bethesda, MD: AOTA.)

Dossey, B., Keegan, L., & Guzzetta, C (1989). *Holistic health promotion. A guide for practitioners.* Gaithersburg, MD: Aspen.

Johnson, I. (1989). *Wellness: A context for living.* Thorofare, NJ: SLACK Incorporated.

Leete, E. (l987). The treatment of schizophrenia: A patient's perspective. *Hospital and Community Psychology, 38,* 486-491. (See Chapter 9 in this text.)

RECOMMENDED READING

Goleman, D. & Gurin, J. (Eds.) (1993). *Mind-body medicine.* New York, NY: Consumer Reports Book.

Romas, J. & Sharma, M. (1995). *Practical stress management: A comprehensive workbook for managing change and promoting health.* Boston, MA: Allyn & Bacon.

Szasz, T. (1974). *The myth of mental illness: Foundations of a theory of personal conduct.* New York, NY: Harper & Row.

White, V. K. (1986). Guest editorial—Promoting health and wellness: A theme for the eighties. *American Journal of Occupational Therapy, 40,* 743-748.

CHAPTER FIFTEEN

Psychiatric Consultation-Liaison: Role of the Occupational Therapist

Dale Y. Watanabe and Linda J. Watson

This chapter was previously published in Mental Health Special Interest Section Newsletter, *pp. 1, 6, 7. Copyright © 1987, The American Occupational Therapy Association, Inc.*

Occupational therapy has a long and rich history in psychiatry. While contributing to the multidisciplinary treatment of psychiatric patients, occupational therapy uses functionally based activity groups within the context of the therapeutic community. Our own role as psychiatric occupational therapists is nontraditional in that we work with medically or surgically ill patients who experience psychological or emotional problems secondary to their illness. In fact, only about 2% of our patients have a diagnosed psychiatric disorder. This chapter will describe our involvement as psychiatric occupational therapists within the psychiatric consultation-liaison service of a large teaching hospital.

Rush-Presbyterian-St. Luke's Medical Center is a 1100-bed, private, tertiary care hospital. The Psychiatric Consultation-Liaison Service, a specialty within the Department of Psychiatry, has been in existence for approximately 12 years. Psychiatric occupational therapy has been involved in some capacity with this service for 7 years. Our involvement has grown from occasional referrals to a patient caseload requiring the services of two full-time occupational therapists. The therapists are an integral part of a multidisciplinary team consisting of six psychiatrists and two psychiatric nurses. Each discipline has the capacity to generate its own referrals or to cross-refer. Biweekly rounds are held to review the patient's treatment as provided by any one or a combination of team members. Occupational therapy receives approximately 65% of our referrals from nonpsychiatric physicians; consequently, we welcome these opportunities for clinical supervision and support.

OCCUPATIONAL THERAPY SERVICES

Psychiatric occupational therapists serve patients who are diagnosed with problems involving cardiology, nephrology, organ transplant, high-risk obstetrics, neurology, orthology, infectious disease, pulmonary (ventilator-dependent) and oncology (in particular bone marrow transplantation and gynecologic oncology). Patients who are appropriate for referral are those exhibiting any one or more of the following:

- disturbances in interpersonal relationships—anger, withdrawal; behaviors that are demanding, attention-seeking, complaining, and/or manipulative.
- disturbances in cognition-memory, orientation, concentration, perception, and/or judgment impairment.
- disturbances in affect and attitude—agitation, anxiety, lability, mood swings, anhedonia, uncooperativeness, and/or lethargy.

While all patients may demonstrate these characteristics at some time during their hospitalization, therapy is indicated when these disturbances are severe, pervasive, and/or interfere with treatment (Pasnau, 1982). Given the acuity of the patient's medical condition and/ or refusal to participate in treatment, therapy is done at bedside. A physician's referral initiates therapy.

LIAISON ROLE

As liaisons, our role is one of troubleshooting. The primary purpose is to facilitate early detection of problem situations and help staff to develop intervention strategies. We do this informally in response to staff, patient, or family requests and formally through participation in patient staffings. It is important to assess each request for timeliness, clarity of problem, and emotional tone (Hengeveld, Rooymans, & Hermans, 1987). The milieu of the unit is evaluated with regard to its flexibility, attitudes, norms, and values (Strain & Grossman, 1975). Some questions to be considered include: How does the staff discuss patients who are medically or psychologically unresponsive? Are there underlying conflicts with this particular patient from previous admissions? How sophisticated is the staff's understanding of psychological problems and interventions? How does the staff deal with terminally ill patients when the physician chooses not to discuss a change in status with the patient or family? How open is the unit to support and intervention from an outsider (non-nurse, non-unit staff)? Are there other causes of stress, such as staffing changes or unexpected patient deaths on the unit, and how have they been dealt with?

Formal meetings and informal contacts also serve to educate and support staff. Education is an important aspect of the consultation-liaison role. Describing psychological issues in common, understandable terms and reframing the patient's behaviors as a response to stress rather than vindictiveness or malicious intent can renew and foster empathy among staff. Assisting staff in the identification of their own behaviors and attitudes that may be contributing to the problem situation and developing a workable plan from the staff perspective are significant features of the liaison role (Strain, 1981). A supportive position with the staff is often necessary to manage conflicts, set limits, and deal with issues of death and dying.

Any staff consultation or patient referral is to be interpreted and respected as a plea for help. However, at times the request may seem hidden (Bustamente & Ford, 1981). For example, the referral may describe a patient as bored and needing something to do, but on observation, the patient appears severely withdrawn, disinterested, and lethargic and [demonstrates] self-deprecating signs indicating a possible depression. Staff members may not be able to articulate the need for therapy instead of volunteer services. Yet when questioned, they may be able to provide more specific clinical indicators of the patient's failing coping skills (Cohen-Cole & Friedman, 1983). Staff may feel protective of a patient (e.g., they prefer to see a favorite patient as bored rather than depressed) or may be responding to bias and prejudice within the milieu toward psychiatric problems (Perl & Shelp, 1982). Patients with personality disorders can split staff, and depressed patients can evoke a sense of anger and helplessness among staff. These issues may be difficult for non-psychiatric staff to recognize (Strain, 1978).

THEORETICAL ORIENTATION

The psychodynamic frame of reference and the model of human occupation provide the basis from which we assess and plan intervention strategies. Assessment begins with an understanding of the patient's fears, worries, and anxieties (Blumenfield, 1983). Illness or disability often represents a loss of dreams, hopes, and fantasies about the future. Treatment issues are primarily in the areas of control, self-esteem, independence, separation, and death and dying. Conflicts may occur regarding attitudes, values, ideals, and goals as a result of illness or disability. Problems may reflect a response to current stresses and/or unresolved conflicts from earlier periods in the patient's life (Mailick, 1985). The therapist examines the patient's use of defense mechanisms to manage stress, considering both adaptive and dysfunctional features. Patient regression is understood as an inadequate

coping response to a perceived threat. Poor coping results in impaired functions in one or more of the following areas:

- ability to restrain or delay tension discharge
- frustration tolerance
- problem-solving abilities
- judgment
- anticipation of consequences
- ability to regulate energy
- self-constancy
- interpersonal relationships
- use of language to communicate needs
- reality testing
- perception
- affect
- motor control

PERSONALITY

Personality is composed of a life-long style of relating, coping, behaving, thinking, and feeling and is adaptive and flexible within a variety of situations. However, illness and hospitalization may create stress that interferes with normal patterns of coping. Personality characteristics may become more rigid, exaggerated, and/or maladaptive. Stress may be caused by perceptions of illness, constraints of hospitalization, and heightened fears. Only a very small percentage of the patients we see meet the DSMIII, Axis II criteria for the diagnosed personality disorders.

The amplification of specific personality characteristics may cause the patient's behavior to become inappropriate and disruptive. The orderly and controlled patient may rely on knowing as much about his or her situation as possible in order to maintain control and handle anxieties. The dependent and thus over-demanding patient may become abusive in requests for nursing care and additional attention (Kahana & Bibring, 1964). The patient may over-use the call light, request special treatment, and refuse to be satisfied with the level of care given. These behaviors are often viewed by the unit staff as manipulative (Groves, 1978).

For some patients, familiar methods used to cope with stress may not be acceptable within the hospital setting. When confronted with the stress of hospitalization, coping methods become extreme. For example, the older man who normally manages his anxiety by yelling at his family will become loud and demanding when requesting care from nursing staff. Comfortable, familiar methods are employed in spite of their unacceptable nature within the hospital environment (Silverberg, 1985). In other situations, strange and uncomfortable behavior may be considered justifiable by patient and staff, given the traumatic situation and stress (Millon, 1981). This is demonstrated by a 37-year-old white male who received the sudden diagnosis of testicular cancer, resulting in the surgical removal of part of his genitals. Following recovery, the patient chose to lie in his bed in a double room totally exposed. Staff, roommates, and visitors complained to one another but not directly to the patient.

When questioned, the patient initially denied that it was a problem and reported he was following what the doctor wanted. In further discussion he reported feeling ashamed, embarrassed, and emasculated and said he worried about his return to work.

DEPRESSION

Depression is quite common among the medically ill; Cavanaugh (1984) reports that one-quarter to a third of all hospitalized medically ill patients experience feelings of depression. Behaviors and cognitions associated with the depressed mood hinder the patient's ability to participate in medical care.

The degree of depression ranges from mild and transient, usually representing an adjustment disorder as a result of illness and hospitalization, to severe and incapacitating with suicidal ideation (Cavanaugh, 1986). As with all clinical states, the intensity, duration, and pervasiveness of symptomatology and the interference with normal functioning become decisive features in a diagnosis. In the medically ill, patients may refuse treatment or not comply and subsequently jeopardize their medical condition.

In a psychiatric setting, disturbances in sleep, motor activity, and appetite are significant vegetative criteria for differential diagnoses of depression. However, in a general hospital setting these criteria may be less applicable due to the requirements of the hospital regimen (e.g., special diets for specific medical conditions and testing procedures that periodically awaken the patient). Robinson (1984) provides a description of how the hospital environment influences body integration, control separation, and somatic preoccupation. Saltz and Magruder-Habib (1985) describe feelings of hopelessness, helplessness, and [a] sense of sadness or loss as key manifestations of depression in the medically ill. Often the loss may not be concrete, but may be related more to a diminished sense of self as a result of an illness. The patient may describe himself as a failure or worthless. Former roles and habits may no longer be attainable. The patient may struggle with his perception of self-worth and efficacy (Kielhofner, et al., 1985).

Loss of interest or pleasure in usual activities is a significant indicator of depression (Cavanaugh, Clark, & Gibbons, 1983). The patient may be uninterested in his hygiene, meals, and course of treatment. Loss of interest in family characterizes deepening depression. Such [was] the case with Mr. W., a 66-year-old man who was referred because of his lack of motivation. The therapist found the patient lying in bed staring at the ceiling. As the therapist entered the room, he quickly closed his eyes and appeared to be sleeping. He refused to open his eyes but would answer by shaking his head to short, superficial questions. His only comment with eyes still closed was, "What's the use? No one cares, no one understands," in response to the therapist's explanation of services and need for treatment. In the most severe cases, the patient wishes to be dead and minimally participates in rehabilitation or maintenance efforts.

ASSESSMENT

Assessment with this population is an ongoing process from initial evaluation to discharge. It not only provides a baseline of information for patient treatment but also contributes to the formulation of a differential diagnosis. A semi-structured interview format is used to gain information about premorbid functioning in the areas of work, leisure, and activities of daily living. Therapists evaluate coping skills based on current life circumstances, medical condition, social surroundings, and effectual state. Some assessments we use include the Allen Cognitive Levels Test, Oakley's Role Checklist, Johns Hopkins' Mini Mental Status, and Lewinsohn's Pleasant Events Scale. Formal assessments and task evaluations are useful but are secondary to establishing a therapeutic rapport and meeting the patients on their own level (Watson, 1986).

CASE ASSESSMENT EXAMPLE

Mike is a 14-year-old, obese, black male hospitalized for the third time in a year for non-compliance with his diabetic diet and insulin adjustment. The referral to psychiatric occupational therapy followed an incident where the patient had persuaded his mother to sneak food to him from home. He said he ate because there was "nothing else to do around here."

On initial contact the patient reported that everything was fine. He explained that the food incident was an accident and had only happened once. He appeared defiant and questioned why staff was making "such a big deal about one little thing." Mike said he was tired and asked if the therapist would leave so he could get some rest. The therapist then asked if he'd rather do something other than talk and his response was "like what?" with a softened affect. He was offered an assortment of projects and was asked to complete some homework that included an adapted version of Black's Adolescent Role Assessment and Holland's Self-Directed Search (HSDS). The therapist returned the next morning to find Mike's woodworking magazine rack near completion. His work was of high quality. He had carefully followed directions on his own. When complimented, Mike stated he liked woodworking and had missed "doing stuff like that" because he had been skipping school a lot. We reviewed his evaluation and ascertained that since being diagnosed as diabetic, he had received "special treatment" at home. He was excluded from any household responsibilities, and illness had become an acceptable excuse for missing school. "I sit around and eat a lot, watch T.V." He reported having fun with the test (HSDS). "Thinking about the future.... I hadn't done that for a while. I never gave it much thought and since I've been sick no one seems to care much about (my future) anymore." When asked about his understanding of his medical problems, he reported "At first I was scared to death.... I guess I could die, you know.... I forgot the rest.... Now I just don't think about it. I don't think about much really."

TREATMENT

Treatment centers around conflicts in self-esteem, loss of control and independence, separation, and death and dying. These conflicts may be addressed directly and/or indirectly. Often activity serves as a vehicle. A major component of treatment is the therapeutic use of self. Counseling is done in conjunction with activity involvement or can be the primary mode of treatment. Appropriate treatment activities can act as precursors to the discussion of role changes, body image, personal worth, and self-management. Applied activities must be meaningful, pleasurable, and appropriate to the patient's physical and emotional tolerance.

A SHIFT IN ROLE

As a member of a psychiatric consultation-liaison service, the occupational therapist must feel comfortable in a role that requires a high degree of autonomy with little of the customary "team approach." Strong clinical and interpersonal skills are necessary for the therapist. Many times the therapist is the only psychiatric professional working with a particular patient. Thus the therapist must be able to articulate psychological and rehabilitative concepts fluently at a variety of levels. Ideas and recommendations prescribed to unit staff may be new and/or unpopular and may not be readily welcomed.

Working with acute medically ill patients requires a period of adjustment to the signs, symptoms, and physical treatment of illness, such as the Hickman catheters, ileostomies, suctioning, and dialysis. Having an active interest in medical conditions is essential to developing a working hypothesis about symptomatology. For example, how incapacitating is the patient's pain, nausea, or fever in relation to his or her current medical status, and are these symptoms symbolic of a deteriorating psychological condition?

In this capacity the occupational therapist feels the primary nature of each relationship and the subsequent responsibility. Helping a patient to deal with issues regarding the quality of life and death and dying is often painful and complex (Purtilo, 1983). In each relationship, the emotional availability of the therapist is important for listening and deeply understanding the meaning of each person's experience. Supporting the patient to clarify and progress with these issues is another important aspect of this work. The occupational therapist must have basic skills in assessing the family's coping methods in relation to the illness of the patient. Interventions with patients and their families may

tangibly reduce symptoms or complaints (Shapiro, 1986). Helping someone to live a more satisfactory, if brief, life is its own reward.

REFERENCES

Blumenfield, M. (1983). Patients' fantasies about physical illness. *Psychotherapy & Psychosomatics, 39,* 171-179.

Bustamente, J. P., & Ford, C. V. (1981). Characteristics of general hospital patients referred for psychiatric consultation. *Journal of Clinical Psychiatry, 42*(9), 338-341.

Cavanaugh, S. (1984). The diagnosis and treatment of depression in the medically ill. In F. G. Guggenheim, & M. F. Weiner (Eds.). *Manual of psychiatric consultation and emergency care* (pp. 211 222). New York, NY: Jason Aronson, Inc.

Cavanaugh, S. (1986). Depression in the hospitalized inpatient with various medical illnesses. *Psychotherapy & Psychosomatics, 45,* 97-104.

Cavanaugh, S., Clark, D. C., & Gibbons, R. D. (1983). Diagnosing depression in the hospitalized medically ill. *Psychosomatics, 24*(9), 809-815.

Cohen-Cole, S. A., & Friedman, C. P. (1983). The language problem: Integration of psychosocial variables in medical care. *Psychosomatics, 24*(1), 54-60.

Groves, J. E. (1978). Taking care of the hateful patient. *The New England Journal of Medicine, 298*(16), 883-887.

Hengeveld, M. W., Rooymans, H. G., & Hermans, J. (1987). Assessment of patient-staff and intra-staff problems in psychiatric consultations. *General Hospital Psychiatry, 9,* 25-30.

Kahana, R. J., & Bibring, G. L. (1964). Personality types in medical management. In N. E. Zinberg (Ed.). *Psychiatry and medical practice in a general hospital* (pp.108-123). New York, NY: International University Press.

Kielhofner, G., Shepherd, J., Stabenow, C. A., Bledsoe, N., Furst, G., Green, J., Harlin, B. H., McLellan, C. L., & Owens, J. (1985). Physical disabilities. In G. Kielhofner (Ed.). *A model of human occupation: Theory and application* (pp. 170-247). Baltimore, MD: Williams & Wilkins.

Mailick, M. D. (1985). The short-term treatment of depression of physically ill hospital patients. *Social Work in Health Care, 9*(3), 51-61.

Millon, T. (1981). *Disorders of personality DSMII: Axis II.* New York, NY: Wiley Interscience.

Pasnau, R. (1982). *Consultation-liaison psychiatry.* Kalamazoo, MI: Upjohn.

Perl, M., & Shelp, E. E. (1982). Psychiatric consultation masking moral dilemmas in medicine. *The New England Journal of Medicine, 307,* 618-621.

Purtilo, R. B. (1983). Ethical issues in cancer. *Journal of Psychosocial Oncology, 1*(1), 3-15.

Robinson, L. (1984). *Psychological aspects of the care of hospitalized patients.* Philadelphia, PA: F. A. Davis.

Saltz, C. C., & Magruder-Habib, K. (1985). Recognizing depression in patients receiving medical care. *Health and Social Work, 10,* 1522.

Shapiro, J. (1986). Assessment of family coping with illness. *Psychosomatics, 27*(4), 262-271.

Silverberg, R. A. (1985). Men confronting death: Management versus self-determination. *Clinical Social Work Journal, 13*(2), 157-169.

Strain, J. J. (1981). *Psychological interventions in medical practice.* New York, NY: Appleton-Century-Crofts.

Strain, J. J., & Grossman, S. (1975). *Psychological care of the medically ill: A primer in liaison psychiatry.* New York, NY: Appleton.

Watson, L. J. (1986). Psychiatric consultation-liaison services in the acute physical disabilities setting. *American Journal of Occupational Therapy, 40*(5), 338-342.

CHAPTER SIXTEEN

The Remediation of Role Disorders Through Focused Group Work

Hilda P. Versluys

This chapter was previously published in the American Journal of Occupational Therapy, 34, *609-614. Copyright* © 1980, The American Occupational Therapy Association, Inc.

Despite advances in medicine and rehabilitation, a high percentage of patients are discharged from the hospital unprepared to meet the demands of daily living and are not motivated to reach and maintain projected functional levels of performance. Their return to the community may be followed by social withdrawal, depression, regression, and multiple readmissions.

Harby and Smith define disability as the inability to perform the usual role activities as a result of a physical or mental impairment of long-term duration.[1] The idea central to this (chapter) is that loss of or change in valued personal roles can result in role disorders. Role disorders may produce social, psychological, and behavioral problems more profound than the disabling condition[2,3] and signal the need for occupational therapy intervention.

ROLE THEORY

The therapist committed to restoring a patient's physical function should also consider the patient's need to continue to meet role responsibilities. An understanding of the developmental aspects of role acquisition and the tasks and social skills that support adult roles is indispensable both in the evaluation of role loss and disorder and in the design of treatment programming.[4,5]

Berger states that Man directs considerable energy and commitment to the development of a variety of role functions resulting in the formation of personal identity and a unique lifestyle.[6] This process is a continual life task and might be thought of as part of Man's career.

Reilly and Moorehead have described the hierarchical development of a role through play, chores, and activities. This development is conceived of as a fluid process continuing through the life span and requiring continual adaptations and acquisitions of new skills and habits.[7,8]

Sociologists agree that the genesis of the adult role occurs in childhood through play, exploration, and relationships developed within the family and community. The child tests out or practices the role tasks and social interaction skills that allow adult roles to be successfully performed. These early maturational experiences of the child may be viewed as a learning laboratory or clinic where role models can be observed and role possibilities experienced, thus providing an indispensable process leading to adult role taking.[6]

The resulting adult roles—such as sexual, occupational, family, avocational, and social—allow an individual to participate in his or her culture and to satisfy human needs. The mature, well adjusted person integrates all his or her roles into a balanced life style.[7,9]

ROLE DISORDERS

Physical illness and disability may adversely affect personal role functions on a continuum from minor changes to complete obliteration of all major roles. A hospitalized and disabled patient struggling to maintain role responsibilities may experience a reduction or fragmentation in functional role skills that undermines confidence and may lead to depression, formation of a poor self image, and lack of motivation for the rehabilitation task. Functional role skills include maintenance tasks such as shopping and cooking, and work, occupational tasks such as driving, using the telephone, and caring for children. Patients may also temporarily have to shelve role tasks such as meeting financial obligations, maintaining personal standards, and meeting social commitments.[10,11]

Role disorders are often compounded by the patients' fears that their customary lifestyles will change irrevocably. Patients may deal with these anxieties by resorting to maladaptive behaviors such as dependence, denial, and regression.[12,13] For example, a cardiac event may precipitate fear, anxiety, and depression, which may result in unnecessary retirement, the termination of many adult roles, and entrenchment in a sick role.[14]

The residual effects of disability may prevent the performance of those "physical" skills that make the execution of major roles possible and thereby result in the exacerbation of role disorders.[3] For example, the loss of the physical skills that allow driving cancels the patient's ability to drive a car. Driving can be a vocational necessity and also influence participation in recreation and social activities. The loss of these physical skills severely limits the patient's ability to meet his or her human needs and prevents a balanced and rewarding lifestyle.

Avocational experiences fill needs for creativity and physical action. The loss of physical functions required to dance or ski may not only lead to the termination of pleasurable recreation, but also affect the release of tension through activity. The inability to perform these physical skills means that the role or role tasks must be changed and human and occupational needs must be met in a different manner.[15]

Patients vary in their ability to deal with role loss and to accept role substitutes. The loss of a valued role may present a barrier to role substitution for those patients who had invested time and effort in roles that increase status and self-esteem.

The time required for medical treatment, the stress of rehabilitation, the lack of mobility, and concern with changing personal appearance may precipitate a number of crises for the patient. The patient's response to this stressful or traumatic situation may be the development of avoidance behaviors that protect him or her from fear of rejection and contribute to social isolation. A family role such as father and provider carries certain expectations and responsibilities. Discontinuation of these roles, even for a short time, may result in crisis for both the patient and the family.[10,13]

Although dedicated to rehabilitation, the hospital system has its own overt and covert rules for patients' conduct and behaviors that may contribute to role dysfunction. Patients are no longer in charge of their own destiny and may find that they are unable to exert control over the use of their own time (i.e., when to eat, when to go to bed, and when to leave the hospital to visit their family). The patient is expected to adhere to decisions made by others, often without his or her knowledge or input. The patient's special skills prized in the community or at work are not useful in the hospital nor are they recognized by the hospital staff as significant. Personal initiative and problem solving are discouraged.[10]

Goals of rehabilitation should include the preservation and maintenance of adult roles or the development of strategies to compensate for the loss of social, task, and performance skills that make major role performances possible.

stand the hospital system, and thus be in a better psychological position to benefit from rehabilitation. The second strategy is to assist the patient in maintaining role responsibilities during the period of treatment. However, if the prognosis indicates permanent dysfunction, including the patient's inability to fill previous life roles, the goals of treatment are to rehabilitate by the transformation and reassignment of roles.

Based upon the premise that adult roles with their resulting identities are socially bestowed and sustained, it follows that role transformation or the reassignment of roles is a social, interactive process. Perhaps the most important influence in role maintenance and transformation is the contribution of the family. The attitudes the family maintains toward the patient's roles, their willingness to reestablish or contribute to role maintenance, and their identification and assignment of roles useful to the family and within the patient's capabilities are essential in reaching rehabilitation goals.[5,10,16]

Human roles influenced by cultural definition may be limited in the options for role change and reassignment.[6] Patients and their families may assume that there is only one way to be a successful man or woman, or a worker, or to fill family membership roles. The considerations of alternative life styles and concomitant adult roles may be difficult for the patient and resisted by the family.

The patient may accept the need to try a few work options, devise a new lifestyle, and work to experience and develop different leisure time interests. However, these choices must also be supported by family and reflect the reality of the patient's background experiences, interests, and real skills, both physical and intellectual. Failure to achieve in new endeavors may discourage the patient's progress in rehabilitation and his or her wish to become a viable part of the community upon discharge.

Role loss and lack of role acquisition should be assessed developmentally and chronologically before a problem list for treatment programming is identified. The occupational therapist should be aware that the patient's major life roles vary in priority at different times in the life cycle. Treatment goals should consider the patient's present and future role needs. After the degree of physical and role dysfunctions have been determined, treatment emphasis is placed upon guiding the patient in reexperiencing early developmental tasks through role-focused group experiences. Conditions for change within such groups include interpersonal transactions within a human group, opportunities for exploration and play, and the choosing and use of activities.[6,7,17] The patient involved in such a treatment program must also identify the need and purpose for maintaining and/or acquiring new skills.[18]

FACTORS INFLUENCING ROLE TRANSFORMATION

Occupational therapy intervention into role disorders is first aimed at assisting the patient to adjust to and under-

FOCUSED GROUP WORK

Occupational therapy believes that change occurs through action and involvement that reinforce the learned tasks or new skills. The patient, after the traumatic event or as a result of long illness and hospitalization, may not have the ego, strength, and energy to handle formal discussions concerning disability, role skills and psychosocial needs. Didactic or vicarious teaching, independent of an experiential component, is not successful in increasing self-esteem or in helping the patient to explore new role possibilities.[10]

Focused Group

A focused group experience provides a training ground where patients test their ability to deal with problems of living, decision making, and risk taking involved in the change process.

Patients are encouraged to continue responsibility for role tasks in the hospital, family, and community. The patient can be assisted in identifying and maintaining major role responsibilities through a problem-solving process. Graded social roles can be designed for and assigned to the patient for practice in the hospital and in the community.[10,19]

Cohesive Group

A cohesive group sustains patients while they experiment and master the skills necessary for physical and psychological survival in the community.[16,21] These necessary role skills are called "Weapons of Life," by Kutner.[15] To maintain viable adult roles and personal independence, patients need an arsenal of social and interpersonal skills, the ability to deal with everyday problems of living, and to take social responsibility.

Yalom states that, in the intrinsic act of giving, patients receive a boost to their self-esteem and find that they can be altruistic and important to others.[20] The physically disabled patient who encourages, responds, and become actively involved in supporting and sharing with the group members, including family, feels immediately more confident and useful, more in control, and more positive about his/her ability to handle change.

Role-Focused Group

A role-focused group assists in the ventilation of feelings concerning the permanence of disability, allows the patient to see that others have struggled and succeeded, amplifies the motivation for change, and encourages the patient to feel more socially acceptable and to plan more realistically toward transition into the community.

Through group interaction patients are exposed to a variety of social roles. Through activities and involvement in encouraging, planning, organizing, helping, and sharing, patients discover they are capable of being productive within their physical and medical limitations.[17,21,22]

Also important in treatment for the atrophy or loss of adult roles and underlying role skills is the kind of stress inherent in society. The removal of all stress in therapy groups will impoverish role expectations and thus limit the available number and complexity of roles the patient can play.[23] It becomes the responsibility of the therapist to esti-

mate when the patient can handle stress and to program experiences to meet individual learning needs.

The design of role-focused groups includes the following six factors: a group of patients that have the potential to become cohesive; role-building experiences that allows the patients to explore and test new behaviors[5]; the freedom to seek out and use activities to please the self and others and to feel competent[17]; clear communication system of supportive and realistic feedback that encourages adaptation and reinforces learning[24]; social recognition of group members and their role functions; and opportunities for role experience that are compatible with the patients' values, culture, and preferred lifestyles.[5,7]

Role Disorders

Certain responsibilities are specifically the therapist's task. The first is evaluation of role disorders. Guidelines include: 1.) a diagnostic projection to identify the degree of permanent functional limitation; 2) patient and family interviews to identify the importance to the patient of each adult role and those role areas central to preservation of the patient's self-esteem and identity; 3) an analysis of the elements of each role most prized by the patient to determine whether these needs can be met through substitute role activities, or compensated for by adaptive equipment or acquisition of new task skills; 4) evaluation of the family commitment level and the skills available in the family to achieve role requirements; 5) recognition of cultural and religious influences; and 6) determination of the patient's interests, values, background, experience, and preferred life style.

In addition to evaluating the patient, the occupational therapist should also: 1) facilitate insight concerning coming changes in adult roles and role skills; 2) design strategies to circumvent those role tasks the patient can no longer perform; 3) develop and encourage realistic treatment goals with the patient; 4) counsel and investigate alternative ways of filling role requirements; 5) prevent role saturation by insisting that role acquisition proceed cautiously and progressively so that new role tasks and behaviors become well-integrated within one major role; 6) stimulate development of follow-up programming within the community to strengthen and internalize new roles.

The patient's performance must be facilitated and monitored skillfully. Tasks need to be assigned, and dialogue and feedback that reinforce the direction and pace of new learning must be provided.[5,24]

Rehabilitation staff may feel that role disorders will remedy themselves when patients return to the community, or that the social and emotional needs of patients are not part of the total rehabilitation goals. Such concepts must be rejected since role disorders cannot be treated quickly, at the last minute, or post-discharge. The timing of treatment is important and should occur concurrently with physical rehabilitation, beginning at the time a patient is admitted to the hospital. The inclusion of experienced role models as group leaders or group members provides evidence to patients that others have been successful in building satisfying lives.

ROLE-FOCUSED GROUP MODELS

Homemakers' Group

In this group, members consider alternative ways of home management with emphasis on such specialty areas as child care, cooking, architectural and interior design, and social entertaining. They also deal with feelings about change in living style and the loss incurred in relinquishing familiar ways of meeting personal and family needs at home. Techniques the therapist might use include education, problem solving for individual situations, role playing, direct experience at home, and role models as teachers and consultants. Families are invited to participate.[15]

Role Maintenance Group

This group would assist the patient in maintaining role responsibilities while hospitalized. Emphasis is on identification and realistic appraisal of those role tasks that can be maintained during rehabilitation and separation from work and family. The occupational therapist and group members are responsible for facilitation of negotiations with community and family in problem solving as well as in continual feedback and monitoring of the maintenance process. For example, the salesman who can handle some of his accounts at the hospital through meetings with clients who visit him requires cooperation of the hospital administration and the employer. The group helps him negotiate with these authorities. Also, a mother is encouraged to give input to child care [sic], children's activities, and home management via the telephone and family visits. Meeting the family at the hospital to establish role responsibilities may be helpful. A patient's social obligations and committee tasks can be handled via the telephone. Community, work, and family responsibilities can be redesigned to allow patients continued participation. Family, friends, and business associates are encouraged to attend some of these group sessions.

Social Skill Development

In this group, the emphasis is on maintaining social and communication skills by providing structured learning experiences within a patient group. Mature social skills may have atrophied because of isolation and lack of opportunity to practice, or may be developmentally delayed. Treatment is focused on the development of age-appropriate social and communication skills through interactive exercises, social club activities, end expressive media—for example, poetry and literature. The end goals of community participation are stressed. For example, to illustrate this role-focused group, a patient may learn new social games within his or her physical capacities and then join a community group—for example, chess, bowling, musical club.

Sensitivity Training

This group is designed to assist patient's in coping with feelings about community reentry, being visible in the community, and dealing with rejection. Techniques include sequenced social experiences, planned tasks within the community such as shopping, luncheon, or parties, and dialogue with role models.[17,19] There is an emphasis on group design of experimental community assignments. The patients assigned to community tasks report back to the group on their personal experiences and feelings. The group provides feedback and support, and assists in solving problems encountered in mobility, access to public buildings, and poise in public or social situations.

Family Task-Oriented Groups

These are inter-hospital groups formed to strengthen and maintain family relationships and encourage the maintenance of the patient's roles within the family constellation. Patients and family are involved in dialogue concerning the adjustments to disability, the treatment process, [and] planning for discharge, and in social and recreational activities. Emphasis is on programming that provides opportunities for families to interact with the member.[16,25] Participation in task-oriented activity groups helps to reduce the tension a family feels toward relating to the patient who is physically ill or disabled. Activities include dinners prepared by patients and families, trips, game nights, parties, and expressive media experiences. Role models allow the family to observe the potential for good functioning after rehabilitation. Activities involving the patient and family allow the family to observe how the staff relates to the patient and what independent behavior is possible; for example, the patient's ability to eat independently, [to] organize activities, or to research and present information used for group planning.

Transitional Group

This group offers transitional or bridging activities designed to provide linkage between the hospital and the community. The patients consider ways to participate in family activities and work/social relationships. They prepare to meet their future social and emotional needs by participation in community groups while still hospitalized, and practice the social role skills necessary upon discharge. Group techniques include dialogue and activities with family, friends, community volunteers, and anticipatory guidance by consultants. Group design of transitional or bridging activities includes both interhospital and community activities, such as patient organization. For example, patients make and carry out plans to go to church, arrange job interviews or preliminary visits to the old work area, participate in volunteer experiences to teach skills to hospital staff or community groups, and find ways to maintain old friendships and to make new ones.[5,21,22]

SUMMARY

Patients with a physical illness or disability may find that their usual adult roles must be modified or permanently changed. Role disorders occur when patients are no longer able to meet their usual role responsibilities. The resulting social and psychological disturbances may be a permanent response to the physical trauma and more profound than the residual limitation warrants.

Treatment goals for such patients should include not only the mastery of physical and compensatory skills required for activities of daily living and mobility, but also parallel programming to treat the psychological and social effects of role disorders, hospitalization, and isolation from the family and community.

Remediation of role disorders can occur through an involvement in experience-based activity groups focused on maintaining and/or transforming major adult role functions. Group goals include remastery of social and communication skills, role building, the development of new and satisfying role experiences, and the enhancement of family cohesiveness.

Within the transitional programming between the hospital and community, the patient learns that intergroup roles are also relevant to family, work, and the social community.

Role-focused groups are specialized, flexible, and designed to meet the individual and changing needs of a patient population with role disorders secondary to physical disability.

ACKNOWLEDGMENT

This (chapter) is based on a program developed in the occupational therapy department at Highland View Hospital, Cleveland, Ohio, and on a presentation at the AOTA Annual Conference, Detroit, April 26, 1979. The author also appreciates the assistance of Phillip Shannon and Willem Versluys in editing and organization.

REFERENCES

1. Kutner, B. (1971). The social psychology of disability. In W. Neff (Ed.). *Rehabilitation psychology*. Washington, DC: American Psychological Association.

2. Wright, B. A. (1960). *Physical disability—A psychological approach*. New York, NY: Harper and Row.

3. Kutner, B., Rosenberg, P. P., & Berger R. (1970). In A. S. Abramson. *A therapeutic community in rehabilitation medicine*. New York, NY: Albert Einstein College of Medicine of Yeshiva University.

4. Thomas, E. J. (1966). Problems of disability from the perspective of role theory. *J Health Hum Behav, 7,* 2-14.

5. Kutner, B. (1968). Milieu therapy. *J Rehab, 34,* 14-17.

6. Berger, P. L. (1963). *Invitation to sociology.* New York, NY: WW Nortin Co.

7. Kielhofner, G. (1973). *The evolution of knowledge in occupational therapy—Understanding adaptation of the chronically disabled.* Unpublished masters thesis. University of Southern California, Los Angeles.

8. Moorhead, L. (1969). The occupational history. *Am J Occup Ther, 23,* 329-334.

9. Duncombe, L. & Versluys, H. (1979). *Occupational therapy theory in psychiatry.* Unpublished Course Manual. Occupational Therapy Department, Sargent College of Allied Health Professions, Boston University (2nd Edition).

10. Kutner, B. (1967). Role disorders in extended hospitalization. *Hosp Admin, 12,* 52-59.

11. Carmechail, H. T., Gruber, H. W., & Sletten, C. O. (1963). *Meeting the social needs of long-term patients.* Chicago, IL: American Hospital Association.

12. Oulgley, J. L. (1976). Understanding depression—helping with grief. *Rehabil Gazette, 19,* 2-6.

13. Siller, A. (1969). Psychological situation of the disabled with spinal cord injury. *Rehabil Lit, 30,* 290-296.

14. Naughton, J. (1979). Coronary head disease. J. F. Garrett, & E. S. Levine. (Eds.). In *Rehabilitation practices with the physically Disabled. Coronary heart disease.* New York, NY: Columbia University Press.

15. Safilios-Rothschild, C. (1970). *The sociology and social psychiatry of disability and rehabilitation.* New York, NY: Random House.

16. Versluys, H. P. (1977). In C. A. Trombly, & A. D. Ott Sr. *Occupational therapy for physical dysfunction. Psychological adjustment to physical disability.* Baltimore, MD: Williams & Wilkins Co.

17. Gels, J. (1972). The problem of personal worth in the physically disabled patient. *Rehabil Lit, 33,* 19-37.

18. Taylor, D. P. (1974). Treatment goals for quadriplegic and paraplegic patients. *Am J Occup Ther, 28,* 22-29.

19. Cogswell, B. E. (1968). Self socialization: Readjustment of paraplegics in the community. *J Rehabil, 34,* 11-35.

20. Yalom, I. D. (1970). *The theory and practice of group psychotherapy.* New York, NY: Bask Books.

21. Romano, M. D. (1976). Social skills training with the newly handicapped. *Arch Phys Med Rehabil, 57,* 302-303.

22. Gordon, E. W. (1971). Race, ethnicity, social disadvantagement and rehabilitation. In W. Neff (Ed.). *Rehabilitation psychology.* Washington, DC: American Psychological Association.

23. Bennett, O. H. (1975). Rethinking rehabilitation: No bedlam in Bethlehem. *Innovations, 2,* 13-14.

24. McDaniel, J. W. (1976). *Physical disability and human behavior,* New York, NY: Pergamon Press.

25. D'Afflitti, J. G., & Weitz, G. W. (1977). Rehabilitating the stroke parent through patient and family groups. In R. H. Moss (Ed.). *Coping with physical illness.* New York, NY: Plenum Medical Book.

CHAPTER SEVENTEEN

Options for Community Practice: The Springfield Hospital Model

Sharon Baxley

This chapter was previously published in the Mental Health Special Interest Section Newsletter, *17(1), 3-5. Copyright © 1994, The American Occupational Therapy Association, Inc.*

For persons with severe mental illness, the transition from inpatient psychiatric services to community placements is a challenge for both the clients and health care professional. Persons with chronic mental illness experience a variety of problems that interfere with their ability to succeed in a community setting. Difficulties that I have witnessed include an inability to adapt to a new environment, limited independent living skills, and weak social support systems.

The Occupational Therapy Department at Springfield Hospital Center in Sykesville, Maryland, recognized those problems approximately 10 years ago. The occupational therapists believed that they could make a vital contribution to the transitioning problem by lessening the gap between inpatient and outpatient services and allowing clients to experience the least restricted environment possible. Several corrective steps were instituted, the first of which was within the hospital

The hospital began to offer predischarge groups, co-led by occupational therapists and social workers, during which clients were introduced to the concepts of community rehabilitation programs (CRPs) and various options upon leaving the hospital. CRPs are day programs that offer training in various vocational components and operate on a day-to-day basis.

These readiness groups allow clients to voice their concerns about leaving a hospital setting, availability of outpatient programs, and expectations of programs in the community. In the groups, staff members encourage the exploration of concerns, feelings, and questions about community living. They provide facts about various programs, including the referral process, scheduling, expectations, and prevocational components.

This first phase allows persons who are not yet ready to leave the hospital to slowly gain exposure to concepts of community living and discuss their experiences and concerns with others. Often, participants remain in this phase for an extended period of time, because merely discussing leaving the hospital can cause increased anxiety and exacerbation of symptoms.

The next step established to assist with continuity of treatment services was that of staff sharing agreements. Visitation contracts were made between staff members at CRP agencies and occupational therapists at Springfield Hospital Center and implemented with nine different programs over the years. Occupational therapy staff members, in essence, became liaisons between the CRPs and the hospital.

Contracts specified that clients, accompanied by occupational therapy staff members, would make regular visitations to a specific community program. This arrangement allowed clients to experience a community program and CRP staff members to become familiar with visiting members. Occupational therapists have been scheduled one or two times per week to provide consistent exposure. A sample contract explains responsibilities of both parties (See Figure 1). Other state facilities have established similar visiting programs to aid in transition of their populations.

CONSULTATION MODELS

Occupational therapists at Springfield Hospital Center have assisted in successfully placing persons ranging from 25 to 76 years of age from a variety of cultural, ethnic, and socioeconomic backgrounds. Their diagnoses have included schizophrenia (chronic and paranoid types), depression, affective disorders, atypical pyschosis, substance abuse, and personality disorders. Despite a slow and careful transition, some clients ultimately find community living overwhelming. These persons may need to return to the hospital but often the duration of stays are shorter and they are able to gain some confidence to attempt discharge again. The ability to sustain oneself in the community for a few months can be seen as success, especially for someone who has been hospitalized for many years. Occupational therapists at Springfield

This letter of understanding is written to clarify the methods by which Hospital and Community Rehabilitation programs shall coordinate to provide a more complete continuum of care on behalf of citizens with long-term mental illnesses. This coordinated effort is to continue unless or until either party recommends modification or termination.

Methods of Cooperation

A. Hospital agrees to assign an occupational therapist a minimum of _____ days per week to:

1. Maintain active, regular communication regarding discharge planning and patient disposition for all clients referred to Community Rehabilitation Program.

2. Transport clients to and from Hospital and the Community Rehabilitation Program during their predischarge planning within the Community Rehabilitation Program. Transportation shall be with appropriate staff members.

3. Provide simultaneous referrals, with client's written consent to the Community Mental Health Clinic for those clients referred to Community Rehabilitation Programs.

B. The Community Rehabilitation Program agrees to:

1. Develop an individual rehabilitation plan for each person accepted into their program.

2. Maintain active communication with client's hospital treating staff to provide ongoing information as necessary for client's diagnosis and treatment.

3. Maintain active communication with Mental Health Clinic in regard to discharge planning of clients from the Hospital.

C. Mutual Responsibilities

Both the Hospital and the Community Rehabilitation Programs recognize that while the person is a client at the Hospital, the Hospital is responsible for the client's care and treatment. However, while the client is on leave from the Hospital at the Community Rehabilitation Program, before the client's actual discharge from the Hospital, the Community Rehabilitation Program is responsible for the client's care and treatment.

Figure 5-1. Letter of Understanding Between a Hospital and Community Rehabilitation Program. Copyright ©1992 by Springfield Hospital and Rehabilitation Center. Reprinted with permission.

Hospital Center believe that this success is more likely to occur with careful transitioning and consultation between hospital and community personnel.

CLIENT-CENTERED CASE CONSULTATION

Caplan (1970) described four types of consultation, based on function and target of services. The first type is client-centered case consultation, in which the health care professional maintains repeated contact with the client, assists with evaluation and screening, focuses on needs of the client, and evaluates the process by changes in the client (Dutton, 1986).

At the Springfield Hospital Center, this process begins with the occupational therapist, with referrals from various treatment teams to the CRP. Readiness of the client to attend the program is assessed through interviews, input from other rehabilitation staff members regarding involvement in treatment, and examination of the client's identified needs and anxieties. Reactions and behaviors of the client continue to be evaluated by the occupational therapist through the aforementioned predischarge groups and ongoing visitations.

The occupational therapist provides support, reassurance, and assistance during the client's initial visits to the community so the experience will be less stressful. This first exposure is designed to establish attitude and acceptance of the program. The occupational therapist becomes an advocate and ally during this phase of transition and remains a support as the client begins to connect with the community program.

Occupational therapists assist visiting clients to gain acceptance from staff members and members who are already living in the community with gradual introductions and increased interactions. The visiting client is encouraged to interact with CRP staff members, which is a subtle way to shift the support to community-based staff members. Also of importance in assisting clients is successfully engaging the client in existing CRP programs. The individual person's needs are explored and matched with units available at the center. Basic units include maintenance, clerical, or food service, but may also include specialty groups such as units for geriatric members or transitional members. Hands-on assistance may be necessary whereby the occupational therapist actually joins the unit with the visitor. Staff members can intervene to reduce anxiety, assist with tasks, and interact with others. Gradually, as the confidence of the visiting client increases, this contact can be decreased.

The roles of staff members take on a different meaning with less supervision and monitoring of behaviors. Mutual goal setting and consistent feedback both ways are crucial to allow modifying behavior and, at times, unlearn certain behaviors. In one instance, a special transitional unit was developed at a CRP to specifically address coping skills, educate on becoming a consumer, increase social networks, and promote personal growth through support and collaboration in regard to goals. Problems encountered on weekly visits can be addressed as they arise, and occupational therapists can focus and clarify goals for clients in their new environment. Clients often have difficulties moving from a more dependent type of environment such as the hospital. Effective problem-solving and decision-making skills may be lacking as a result of long-term hospitalization. Generally, due to restrictions necessary in a hospital, clients have limited opportunity to schedule and manage their own time, and make decisions (e.g. food selection, money management). Lack of responsibility for behaviors also poses a problem when the client enters the community, because consequences for undesirable actions may be quite different than for those in a hospital setting.

Consultee-Centered Case Consultation. The next type of consultation identified by Caplan is consultee-centered case consultation, which focuses on problems of CRP staff members, such as lack of knowledge or education, skill confidence, or professional objectivity (Dutton, 1986). Often the staff members' limited background or experience with persons with mental illness and their inability to plan programs for these persons make it difficult for clients to receive needed services. Typically, CRP staff members who lack knowledge of the needs of clients may begin to lose confidence in their ability to perform their job effectively.

Occupational therapists can dispense information, explain typical behaviors of clients, and address effective communication skills. Resource awareness is another area in which the occupational therapist can expand staff members' knowledge and competence. Developing skills in the areas of group dynamics and process, activity analysis, documentation, program planning, and time management can also be important.

Few disciplines are trained in the area of activity analysis and adaptation of tasks, which can become a problem because community units are task-oriented. Occupational therapists can offer assistance in individual units by breaking down the jobs into specific graded steps to allow facilitators to explain tasks more clearly to members. At the same time, the occupational therapist can show the staff member how to match clients' abilities to particular tasks.

Consultee-Centered Administrative Consultation. The third type of consultation, consultee-centered administrative consultation, focuses on CRP staff members' relationships with people and psychological characteristics of an organization (Dutton, 1986). Some occupational therapists have assisted with interviewing and hiring of staff members and reviewing skills that staff members can offer units and overall programs.

For existing staff members, morale is assessed during this consultation process, and formal inservice programs may be provided on burnout, stress management, and team functioning. Informal venting may also help staff members feel comfortable, dismissing perceived difficulties with the occupational therapist who is not part of the immediate staff. The occupational therapist should cultivate these relationships because consultation can only benefit those who do not feel threatened and see the occupational therapist as a helper. Recommendations have also been given as to placement of staff members in certain program positions that best use their potential.

Programs-Centered Consultation. Finally, a consultation method that is frequently used by occupational therapist liaisons is the programs-centered consultation, during which new programs are developed or present ones are improved (Dutton, 1986). I believe that occupational therapists' skill in program planning, organization, and implementation are valuable to community programs. CRP administrators often welcome suggestions, especially in the areas of staff utilization, space and environmental concerns, unit ideas, and future plans. I have found from experience, however, that community programs may not be in a position to make changes quickly or accept options fully.

I once entered into an agreement with a community program that was running at a minimum, barely managing to prepare lunches for clients and keep the building clean. Clients would sit and play cards during most of the day. Staff members were overwhelmed by the idea of implementing structured units for the clients and, when combined with the clients' difficulties in accepting this structure, most believed that the program would never change.

Today, this program offers eight units, each providing necessary components to meet needs of both the client and agency. Gradual evolution of a program is an exciting and rewarding experience, although the steps leading to it can seem small.

Because clients reentering the community have diverse needs and functional levels, it is crucial that community programs meet the needs of the individual consumer. Mutual goal setting and activities that promote success make consumer-based programming viable. CRPs need to meet the challenge of individualizing present programming, instead of expecting clients to adapt to existing programs.

Occupational therapists can become leaders in a consumer-oriented system that offers more choices. Clients will also continue to require assistance in learning new behaviors or adapting current behavior. Occupational therapists have been using skill-training techniques for years in inpatient treatment groups and, as I have outlined in this (chapter), have also implemented them successfully in transitional and community services. As health care systems strive to meet current challenges and issues, occupational therapists must continue to educate others about what they have to offer, assist with providing quality of care, and become advocates for clients and of their own profession.

REFERENCES

Caplan, G. (1970). *Theory and practice or mental health consultation.* New York: Basin.

Dutton, R. (1986). Procedures for designing an occupational therapy consultation contract. *American Journal of Occupational Therapy, 40,* 160-166.

Hays, C. (1992). Letter of understanding between a hospital and community rehabilitation program. Available from Springfield Hospital Center, 6655 Sykesville Road, Sykesville, MD, 22784.

CHAPTER EIGHTEEN

The Quarterway House: More Than an Alternative of Care

Deborah Wilberding

This chapter was previously published in Occupational Therapy in Mental Health, 11*(1)*, 65-91. Copyright © 1991, *Haworth Press. Reprinted by permission.*

Rehabilitation of the chronically mentally ill encompasses a wide range of psychiatric needs that are life-long. These needs are a result of severe psychiatric illnesses, such as schizophrenia, and thus involve a wide range of mental health services. For those individuals who receive their treatment in hospitals, aftercare becomes a crucial and life-saving issue for some patients and the main concern for their families and treatment providers. Aftercare means a continuation of the range of services started in a good hospital setting, but to the patient involved, aftercare can mean moving to a strange place, with totally different players and a totally different set of expectations. Adjusting to the community setting can be not only traumatic and fragmenting, but also a source of continual failure unless consideration is made as to what is needed to make the transition more comfortable and complete.

Residential rehabilitation is the logical and less costly next step after hospitalization for the severely and chronically mentally ill who show extensive lack of basic living skills. Myerson and Herman (1983) cited in a December 1980 report by the Department of Health and Human Services, that "the lack of adequate and stable housing opportunities linked with support services was perhaps the major unmet need of the chronically mentally ill," and noted "that increasingly large number of patients are living in board and care homes, single room occupancy residences and other settings that are generally run down and unsafe, and that offer few meaningful activities for residents" (p. 336). The report recommended transitional group homes and apartments that are rehabilitative, and homes that provided support and sustaining environments. That was 10 years ago (now 20).

The following (chapter) describes one private psychiatric hospital's attempt to help meet the residential aftercare needs of its chronically mentally ill (CMI) patients through the development of a quarterway house.

LITERATURE REVIEW

The following literature review explores the development of residential care for the CMI in this country; the forces that have influenced its development or lack of development; and finally, the concept of the quarterway house and its distinctiveness from other residential care homes. Three themes seem to stand out in regard to community-based residential programs for the CMI: (1) the relatively young age in this country of community-based residential programs and the forces that influenced their development; (2) a common assumption of replacing hospital or institutional care with community-based care as opposed to utilizing the hospital as part of the criteria, and policies distinguishing one type of residential program from another. The following explores these themes.

Historical Development of Residential Care

Arce and Vergare (1985) state that "a current pressing need to examine the role and utilization of community-based residential facilities for the mentally ill" exists and is the "result of significant changes in the mental health delivery system over the past three decades" (p. 423). They attribute these changes to "powerful medical, social, legal, and economic factors," and view the changes historically. They cite the 1950s as the period when social and psychopharmacological forces influenced the shift from hospital care to community care. This was the beginning of an "explosive increase in the types and number of residences for the mentally disabled" (pp. 423-424). According to the authors, when the federally funded community mental health centers began, transitional housing was one of the many services mandated to reduce the need for hospitalization. The number of such facilities had grown from 10 in 1960 to 128 in 1969. Subsequently, legal forces influenced change in the 1970s when, beginning with

Wyatt v. Stickney (1971), the courts "repeatedly affirmed a constitutional right to treatment, affirming protection from involuntary hospitalization, and care and treatment under the least restrictive conditions" (pp. 424-425). In the last decade, economic factors have impinged on hospital care even more forcefully, leaving the CMI with less hospitalization coverage, both in the private and public sectors and have forced the CMI into more vulnerable, often homeless situations.

As a result of all of these forces, Arce and Vergare maintain that "serious conceptual and operational deficiencies" characterize alternative programs, and the "lack of planning for alternative housing facilities at different levels of care to form a continuum for the patient population" is a prime example (p. 425). In addition, they claim that "local communities" and the "free enterprise system" influence the housing alternatives rather than the meeting of the needs of a "diverse patient population" (p. 425).

A Relationship to Hospital Care

Again as a result of social, economic, political, and medical forces, change has come about in the delivery of care systems. However, the patient's clinical needs and realities, based on the research and further understanding of the illness itself, are still left in question and are given last priority. According to Mechanic (1986), the community mental health movement was a blend of idealism, optimism, opportunism, and naiveté, and that "developing integrated systems of community care for chronic patients is limited less by inadequate knowledge than by organizational, political, economic, and professional barriers" (pp. 893-894).

Myerson and Herman (1983) maintain that what exists are "substantial barriers to the development of housing arrangements, such as community opposition, lack of funding for suitable and affordable facilities", and, an important one for this paper, "the lack of involvement of the private sector" (p. 337). Among their conclusions, justified by several studies made on the effect of community programs, was that the "effectiveness of the programs is enhanced by thorough integration with the original referring inpatient service" (p. 340). This leads into the second common theme or observation in this literature review, the assumption that community programs replace hospitalization.

As stated above, integration with the original referring inpatient service implies use of the hospital as the professional referral service and as part of the continuum of care as opposed to the "costly enemy" of effective treatment. Mechanic (1986) pointed out that the movement away from hospital care to the community was greatly influenced not only by cost benefits but by an ideology based on scientific research demonstrating secondary disabilities associated with custodial hospital care and inactivity. "No recognition was made for good hospital care nor possibly some patients benefiting from asylum" (p. 893). Hospital level care is needed, and must remain a part of the whole continuum of care. It is the logical resource for safe psychiatric treatment of the

CMI when warranted, but always in preparation for and toward the sustaining of a patient's illness management and skill learning beyond its walls in various levels of community care. According to Wilberding (1987), "the goal of inhospital treatment does not necessarily lead to complete independence but rather to an ability to successfully participate in outpatient programs and break the cycle of more costly rehospitalization" (p. 46). According to Hefmeister, Weller, and Scherson (1989), the private sector "has been reluctant to develop residential programs because of a lack of replicable models, limited outcome data, and uncertain third-party reimbursements" (p. 927).

Toward a Definition

The third theme found throughout the literature was the lack of definitional criteria, program standards, and policies for residential programming. Rarely mentioned was the concept of quarterway group homes. A definition of types of community residences is important to establish because it lends to their effectiveness and efficiency, and also serves to recognize and clarify the effect that facility characteristics play on the management of illness factors. According to Arce and Vergare (1985), the lack of "unifying policy, program standards, or precise definitional criteria" contributes to "confusing communication between professionals and across jurisdictions" (p. 426). Names, such as halfway house, transitional facility, board and care home, [and] quarterway house have become commonplace, but are used imprecisely—identical labels applied to dissimilar settings.

Arce and Vergare (1985) cited a 1982 task force of the American Psychiatric Association that surveyed existing residences of all 50 states and found them named under 100 different labels. They recommended a uniform typology consisting of seven types of possible residential settings for the CMI based on programmatic factors. These progressed from most restrictive and intensive to least restrictive and intensive and were as follows:

1. Nursing facility (both skilled and intermediate care)
2. Group home
3. Personal care home
4. Foster care
5. Natural family placement
6. Satellite housing (supervised apartments)
7. Independent living (p. 497)

This typology described the full range of residential facilities used as alternatives to hospitalization and again was based on a series of programmatic criteria. The group home category included a variety of program names, i.e., halfway houses, transitional living facilities, group care homes, hostels, [and] residential homes. (This category came the closest in definitive criteria to include the quarterway house concept, but it was not mentioned in this particular study.) The category was still broad in definition. The definitive criteria covered a wide range of populations, age groups, [and] lengths of stay, but was very focused in its criteria in regards to purpose, licensure, and staffing. The program goal in the group home category was psychosocial rehabilitation within a group of eight to 15 clients through use of a milieu, utilizing a 24-hour, full-time staff (professionals and paraprofessionals), and served mostly mildly to moderately disabled. The severely disabled were mentioned as being appropriate for the group home category, if appropriate staffing and support services were available. (This also would include the quarterway house concept because this type of program serves the severely disabled, as will be described later.) What broadened the definition of this category even further, was the described range of uses of group homes. They were as follows:

1. Alternative to acute hospitalization
2. Shorten inpatient length of stay
3. Transition from hospital to community
4. Permanent placement
5. Respite care (p. 432)

However broad and general in description, the group home category at least was a start toward a formal definition of residential group homes, including quarterway homes.

Assuming community integration is the goal, when further definition is made of the characteristics of the facility (and program), the community in which the facility is located, and the clients themselves, the differences between the various programs considered "group homes" becomes even more apparent. A study was done by Kruzich (1985) to identify not only client characteristics, but also facility and community characteristics. Their impact was shown to influence community integration of 87 former state hospital patients residing in residential facilities. Kruzich found that "as the number of daily living skills programmed in the facility increases, so too does the residents' level of participation in the larger community" (p. 557). Other characteristics cited as important were:

1. Level of personal, individualized care
2. City size and availability of community resources
3. Discharge planning in regards to matching client needs and environmental (program) demands
4. View of the clients themselves regarding suitability of facilities' environments
5. Staff attitudes and involvement

Kruzich emphasized the importance of management practices in determining residents' community integration through staff and administrators' explicit and implicit expectations (p. 562). Kruzich concludes, "These findings point to the importance of residential care administrators articulating a philosophy through their programming, physical environment, and emotional climate that supports clients' attempts to become part of the larger community" (p. 562).

The term "quarterway" used to describe a type of group home, was cited in only a few articles, and was usually a part of a continuum of residential care. Gudeman, Dickey, Rood, Hellman, and Grinspoon (1981) describe the Quarterway House of the Massachusetts Mental Health Center, founded in 1978. It is located in a refurbished unit of a public psychiatric hospital, and designed for "unplaceable" psychiatric patients with both behavioral problems and lack of basic living skills.

Mann (1976) describes a quarterway house set up in a building on the grounds of Harlem Valley Psychiatric Center in New York for both acute and chronic patients with psychiatric illnesses. This is the earliest recorded quarterway house found in the literature, but has dissolved after the center's inpatient census shrunk. A third quarterway house program was cited in an article by Purnell, Jackson, and Wallace (1982) for chronic patients in New Jersey. They described a three bedroom house on a state hospital grounds, with the program supported by the then federally funded CETA program (Comprehensive Employment Training Act). The program terminated when funds expired. A fourth quarterway house program is described by Ranz (1989). Located in a separate building on the campus of Rockland Psychiatric Center, the 16-bed facility is part of a well developed series of supervised residences on Rockland's state hospital campus, and is designed as the first step of their continuum of residential care. It is important to note that many articles were reviewed describing residential programs that have some elements of quarterway" level of programming. but were referred to as "halfway," "transitional," or "shelter care" homes. Again, the importance of a precise nomenclature is a focus of this (chapter), therefore these programs were not included here.

A Proposed Definition

To summarize, then, a quarterway house can be defined as a group home, transitional in nature and the first step after hospitalization in preparation for community placement. The quarterway house serves the most disabled and chronic psychiatric patients, whose only alternative is long-term institutional care. Its focus is psychiatric rehabilitation, specifically designed to teach and to promote the learning of basic living skills in the areas of work, self-care, and leisure through a daily, structured program within a home environment. Its location is usually on or near a hospital setting, which serves as both a referral source and clinical support when necessary. Its thrust, however, is to promote its residents toward integration in the larger community by utilizing a wide variety of community resources. A quarterway house provides a high staff to patient ratio, 24-hour coverage, and is comprised of both professionals and paraprofessionals trained in the philosophy, purpose, and methods of the program.

Its methods are well defined and behavioral in orientation. It provides clear, reasonable expectations, rules, and standards of behavior that are both socially acceptable and promote stabilization, and, finally, a quarterway house promotes illness management, through the use of medications and formal education.

The following is a description of the Mt. Airy House, a quarterway house program that was designed to meet the needs of moderately to severely disabled patients, based on the psychiatric reality of a lifelong illness and thus lifelong dependence on some level.

THE PROGRAM COMPONENTS

The Mt. Airy House is a freestanding, two-story, Tudor-style home, on the campus of The Sheppard and Enoch Pratt Hospital (SEPH) in Baltimore, Maryland. Licensed by the state of Maryland as a group home for 16 mentally ill adults, Mt. Airy is part of the range of outpatient services in the Ambulatory Division of the hospital. The facility, from its inception, was specifically designed to rehabilitate the CMI.

The Resident

Patients with severe mental disorders often share common characteristics. The Mt. Airy House was designed for certain diagnoses within the CMI population, i.e., schizophrenia, schizoaffective disorder, major affective disorder, and mild organic brain syndrome.

These diagnoses were selected due to [the] homogeneity of their characteristics, and this selection provided for a certain amount of specialization in assessment and treatment. Those characteristics are as follows:

1. Ongoing psychotic symptoms not likely to remit.
2. Cognitive deficits apart from psychotic symptoms.
3. High vulnerability to stress.
4. Extreme dependency.
5. Difficulty sustaining activities.
6. Difficulty in establishing interpersonal relationships.

Admission criteria were developed based on these characteristics to help assess appropriateness of placement. Some of the criteria also describe the patient's behavioral problems and strengths. They are as follows:

1. Be between the ages of 18-65 years old.
2. Seek voluntary admission.
3. Have the ability to comprehend rules of the home and be willing to sign a contract agreeing to comply with house rules.
4. Have been previously hospitalized for a psychiatric disorder such as schizophrenia, major affective disorder or organic brain syndrome. Sociopathic, borderline disorders, severe brain damage, or a diagnosis of mental retardation without psychotic features are not appropriate.
5. Have demonstrated the absence of alcohol/drug abuse for 90 days prior to admission. Not have a primary diagnosis of alcoholism or drug abuse.
6. Have minimal physical disabilities.
7. Be stable on a medication regime and be willing to take medications under supervision.
8. Not be actively suicidal, homicidal, or destructive of property, and not exhibit current violent or seriously disruptive behavior (hitting others, throwing things, verbal threats, loud yelling, stealing consumable items, dangerous smoking, fire setting, elopements) for a period of at least 30 days.
9. Be able to tolerate the presence of others, follow simple instructions, observe basic hygiene principles, and have a minimum of regressed behaviors such as vomiting or incontinence.
10. Be able to take appropriate action for self-preservation under emergency conditions.
11. Be able to take care of own possessions and laundry with minimum supervision.
12. Furnish proof of freedom from or control of communicable disease, such as tuberculosis.
13. Be able to remain in the program for a minimum of 6 months.

Another descriptive source of the residents' characteristics is in the behavioral assessment used at Mt. Airy. Behavioral problems, as a result of the disease process and maladaption to the environment, can be a serious impediment to a patient after discharging from the hospital, and some maladaptive behaviors are described in the criteria just mentioned. Once a resident is accepted into the program, a careful assessment of his/her behaviors is made. These behaviors are considered either behavioral deficits (absence of adaptive behaviors); excesses (acting out, bizarre, or odd behaviors); or behaviors present or absent in functional skill areas.

Two sources used for assessing these behaviors are the formal assessment (Figure 18-1), which is done after a resident is in the house for two weeks; and an assessment based on the "excessive behavior list" (Figure 18-2), which is also used to determine readiness for progressing in the tier system of the program. The list of excessive behaviors was developed by the residents themselves during a formal group meeting after the first year of operation. Once a resident is assessed by these tools, a clearer description of his/her behavior and individual characteristics is attained. Often, recognition of these behaviors by the residents themselves is the first positive step toward managing them.

The Community

The Mt. Airy House is on the 110-acre campus of SEPH located in a suburb of Baltimore, Maryland. The integration into the community from a psychiatric hospital campus is a challenge for both the staff and residents of Mt. Airy, and is done in a variety of ways.

The dependency that usually develops between the patient and the hospital, both practically and emotionally is discussed with the new resident. It is made clear that after discharge these ties will change and most of the resident's needs will be met in the community. This is usually stated periodically, and then experienced immediately and routinely through the weekly schedule of activities. Medications are purchased at the local pharmacy; medical and dental needs are met through local doctor and dental offices; groceries are purchased at the local grocery; a passbook savings account is set up at the local bank where the resident is welcomed and introduced to the bank's services by the manager; a library card is applied for at the local library; a mall trip or movie or bowling trip is planned in the afternoons or evenings; and the Sunday trip to some event in the city is organized.

Mt. Airy House
RESIDENT ASSESSMENT

Resident's Name: Date:
Person Filling Out Form:

SCALE: 1. Good Functioning or Not a Behavior Problem
              2. Mildly Impaired Functioning or Mild/Infrequent Behavior Problem
              3. Moderately Impaired Functioning or Moderate Behavior Problem
              4. Seriously Impaired Functioning or Serious/Frequent Behavior Problem
              Content areas below contain both functional behaviors and problem behaviors.

	1	2	3	4
I. EATING				
1. Eats and drinks neatly				
2. Chooses a well-balanced diet				
3. Eats or drinks too much				
4. Eats or drinks too fast				
5. Refuses regular meals				
6. Takes food or drink that has been discarded or that belongs to another				
II. HYGIENE				
7. Bathes or showers using soap daily				
8. Brushes or combs hair daily				
9. For males, shaves as needed or keeps beard neat				
10. Takes care of nails				
11. Brushes teeth at least once a day				
12. Changes clothes daily				
13. Wears appropriate clothing				
14. Has noticeable body odor				
15. For females, wears excessive or bizarre makeup				
16. Changes clothes excessively				
17. Disrobes publicly or exposes self				
III. PERSONAL DOMESTIC ACTIVITIES				
18. Gets up in a.m. on time				
19. Makes bed daily				
20. Keeps room neat and clean				
21. Changes bed linens as needed				
22. Stores soiled clothing for washing				
23. Does personal laundry				
24. Puts clean clothes away				
25. Prepares lunch and snack food for self safely				
26. Uses smoking materials safely and smokes only in designated areas				
27. Sleeps excessively				
28. Bedroom has noticeable odor				
29. Is incontinent				
IV. HOUSEHOLD DOMESTIC ACTIVITIES AND JOB READINESS				
30. Follows requests and directions				
31. Follows through on tasks started				
32. Starts and completes tasks promptly, neither too fast nor too slow				
33. Able to work independently				
34. Cooperative with others in completing tasks				
35. Consistent in work performance				
36. Has adequate duration of attention and ability to focus on tasks				
37. Maintains own schedule throughout day without being reminded				
38. Participates in shopping for, and stocking, house supplies				

Figure 18-1. Formal assessment.

	1	2	3	4	
39. Performs household clearing tasks					
40. Prepares meals adequately and safely for house					
41. Cleans up after house meals					
42. Performs other household chores as assigned or needed					
V. INTERPERSONAL SKILLS					
43. Speaks up in community meetings appropriately					
44. Initiates conversations with others					
45. Establishes relationship with resident advisor					
46. Maintains relationship with family/significant others					
47. Able to express positive feelings					
48. Able to express negative feelings					
49. Able to respond constructively to anger and/or criticism					
50. Goes on staff-accompanied group outings					
51. Uses telephone appropriately					
52. Threatens others					
53. Makes hostile, vulgar, rude comments					
54. Shouts or yells					
55. Talks too much					
56. Intrudes on others					
57. Talks to self					
58. Engages in inappropriate sexual behavior					
59. Is uncommunicative or withdrawn					
60. Hits others or throws things					
61. Steals or takes things from others					
VI. HEALTH					
62. Able to identify psychiatric problems/symptoms					
63. Understands nature of psychiatric illness and need for treatment					
64. Reports physical problems appropriately to house staff and/or doctor					
65. Follows through on advice from doctor or nurse					
66. Treats own minor physical problems appropriately					
67. Cooperates with person who dispenses medication					
68. Can reliably self-administer medication					
VII. MONEY MANAGEMENT					
69. Buys own clothes					
70. Purchases own personal items					
71. Budgets money for the week					
72. Makes deposits/withdrawals at bank as needed					
73. Counts change in store					
74. Behaves inappropriately at store					
VIII. TRANSPORTATION					
75. Cooperative on van trips					
76. Walks to places on grounds and in Towson					
77. Follows pedestrian rules					
IX. LEISURE					
78. Works regularly on a hobby					
79. Takes walks outside					
80. Works in the garden or yard					
81. Listens to the radio or watches TV appropriately					
82. Goes to the movies or sporting events					
83. Plays sports or table games					
84. Reads the newspaper, books, or magazines					

X. COMMENTS:

Figure 18-1 continued. Formal assessment.

This is what we mean by "excessive behaviors":

1. Impulsivity

   a. money
   b. massive consumption of anything
   c. splitting (running away)
   d. shoplifting
   e. substance abuse
   f. self-destruction
   g. threatening others
   h. destruction of property

2. Poor Boundaries

   a. asking for things beyond what is reasonable
   b. acting in an intrusive manner toward others
   c. wandering off

3. *Socially Inappropriate Behavior

   a. vulgar and rude comments to others
   b. talking and/or laughing to yourself while out and about
   c. dressing in bizarre ways
   d. poor hygiene
   e. inappropriate sexual behavior

*This means behaving in ways that would embarrass someone else, make someone else nervous, or make people look at you funny.

4. Angry outbursts

5. Dangerous smoking

6. Inability or unwillingness to respond to limits or requests

Figure 18-2. Excessive behavior list.

After the initial month, usually the new resident has established him or herself in to both the house program and the community by participation on a supervised group level. A more independent and individualized level comes about much later depending on behaviors and skills.

The community resources used (grocery, pharmacy, bank, library, etc.) have been exceptional in providing the attention, acceptance, and care for the residents' situation. It was, however, important to recognize that both incentives and information were needed and given to the grocery, pharmacy, and bank to establish the relationships. Initially, they were formally asked if they would be willing to participate in the Mt. Airy experiment. Social responsibility appeared to be as important as increased business to the managers. All were somewhat familiar with severe mental illness at some level, and were clinically curious, asking good questions to make themselves more informed. Were these exceptional people or is the public becoming more informed? This is hard to assess, but trust has been established both through the reputable name of the hospital, and the fact that the Mt. Airy staff have been clear to the managers and personnel that they would

provide supervision and behavioral limits for the residents. After a year in operation, the grocery manager commented on how well residents behaved. This was after a year not free of incidents, but was a year of incidents properly handled.

The second source of community integration is through community programs. A psychosocial program, funded by both the state and SEPH, is well utilized and has a very active recreational and vocational component that uses a wide variety of community resources. The Adult Day Hospital of SEPH is also used, as well as an outpatient vocational service supported by both SEPH and the State Department of Vocation Rehabilitation.

The Facility

Architecture and the decor were very important in the design of Mt. Airy. For example, the organization of the kitchen was designed to provide space as well as ease of use; comfortable but durable and non-reclining furniture was bought; the color scheme and decor was chosen not only to look coordinated and pleasing to the eye, but also to create a soothing, less stressful environment; ample space was provided for self-care and storage of personal belongings.

The house supports 16 residents with ample space and substantial supplies and equipment to allow for resident participation in all the cooking and cleaning chores, as well as recreational and formal learning activities. Of most importance is the home-like atmosphere and the first impression the facility makes on the incoming new resident—an impression of self-worth.

Program Components

The Mt. Airy House is a 16-bed residential rehabilitation program, with an aim toward providing chronically hospitalized patients with the next step in transition between hospital and community placement. The goal is to enable each resident to become a community participant rather than a community dependent.

The philosophy of the Mt. Airy House is based on the belief that successful adjustment to community life requires understanding the specific and unique problems of each resident. This understanding, coupled with the value of a meaningful, less isolated, and more rewarding life, is the cornerstone of the Mt. Airy House. In order for the resident to learn new and more adaptive skills and behaviors, the program model is based on behavioral rehabilitation principles.

The program objectives are to:

1. Provide an atmosphere for the learning and maintenance of the highest attainable levels of functioning.
2. Focus on building social skills, daily living skills for community participation.
3. Reduce loneliness, isolation, and lack of meaningful activity.
4. Provide emotional and practical support.
5. Set expectations at levels within which the resident is able to function.

6. Assist in arranging placement for residents at time of discharge from the program.

These objectives are reflected in the focused areas of rehabilitation, the rehabilitation characteristics and strategies, and the rehabilitation goals. The nine components of rehabilitation constitute the assessment areas: eating, hygiene, personal domestic activities, household domestic activities/job readiness, interpersonal skills, health, money management, transportation, and leisure (see Figure 18-1). The program is based on the self-care work/leisure model, adapted from the work-play-rest model proposed by Reilly (1966), rest being considered part of self-care. Rehabilitation strategies are characterized by the structure and routine provided, the kind of support given by the staff, the contained emotional environment maintained, behavioral contingencies, and use of community resources.

The daily schedule begins with the morning wakeup call, encouraging the resident to use an alarm clock when ready. The morning routine, i.e., completing hygiene, room care, breakfast, and obtaining morning medications, is expected to be completed by the time of the Planning Meeting. The Planning Meeting is used to give the schedule for the day on both a collective and individual basis; at this time, residents obtain their credits for the previous day's work accomplishments. Each resident possesses a folder containing their credit card and Budget Sheet that they are responsible for bringing to the meeting. Some residents have personalized their folders, reminding the staff of how much like a school it becomes, which also is a good sign of self-identity forming. The weekly schedule includes activities in all the nine focused areas mentioned, and is followed both routinely and repetitively (Figure 18-3). It is also balanced and scheduled so as not to overwhelm the residents.

Staff are trained in providing both emotional support, task assistance, and active involvement of a process quoted from Fidler (Wilberding, 1987) of "learning by doing." Techniques used are in the forms of behavioral reinforcements (verbal praise and encouragement, credits/money earned, privileges earned) and are constantly being individualized. Problem behaviors are contained within the expectations and limits well known by both staff and residents through the house rules. The staff are very firm, and try to remain neutral in their approach. Written Behavioral Contracts are used to formalize and make clear the steps toward eventual gain of behavioral control. Skills are learned through active participation and are taught by the use of demonstration, redirection, written instruction and check lists developed by task analysis. Independence from staff is gained by eventual use of only the written instructions and checklists (see Figures 18-4 and 18-5).

The overall treatment goals of the Mt. Airy Program are in four areas: maintaining the management of the illness itself (taking meds, keeping therapists' appointments, symptom control); the learning and maintenance of daily living skills; the acquisition of a place to work; and the acquisition of a place to live. Discharge planning is based on these four areas. In order to reach these goals, the program is designed for a

MT. Airy House **Weekday Schedule for Residents**	
7:30 a.m.	WAKE-UP CALL
	BREAKFAST PREPARATION (DUTY ROTATES)
8:00 a.m.	BREAKFAST SERVED
8:30 a.m.	BREAKFAST CLEANUP (DUTY ROTATES)
	MORNING MEDS
9:00 a.m.	DAILY PLANNING MEETING
9:30 a.m.	DAILY EXERCISE GROUP (REQUIRED)
10:00-11:30 a.m.	MORNING ACTIVITIES
	Monday—menu planning, inventory, grocery list, healthy eating group
	Tuesday—communications group, gardening
	Wednesday—house cleaning, budgeting
	Thursday—personal shopping, banking
	Friday—health workshop, community outing
12:00 p.m.	LUNCH
1:00 p.m.	LUNCH CLEANUP (DUTY ROTATES)
1:30 - 3:00 p.m.	AFTERNOON ACTIVITIES
	Monday—grocery shopping
	Tuesday—recreation (structured)
	Wednesday—beachball (volleyball)
	Thursday—leisure planning, video
	Friday—gardening, recreation
3:00 - 4:00 p.m.	AFTERNOON BREAK
4:00 p.m.	DINNER PREPARATION (DUTY ROTATES)
	Monday- pharmacy
6:00 p.m.	DINNER
6:30 p.m.	DINNER CLEANUP (DUTY ROTATES)
7:30 p.m.	EVENING ACTIVITIES
	Monday- library
	Tuesday - double trouble group, games
	Wednesday – communications/movie, budgeting
	Thursday—personal & grocery shopping
	Friday—mall night
8:30 p.m.	EVENING MEDS

Figure 18-3. Mt. Airy weekly schedule.

minimum of 6 months to a maximum of 4-year stay. Within this time, a resident can learn the skills needed to meet expectations, but is set within a three-tier system (see Figure 18-6). Movement from one tier to another is based on meeting expectations, and attaining behavioral control of any excessive behaviors (see Figure 18-2).

Dinner and Clean-Up Crew Responsibilities

Cook 1

Start at 4:00 p.m.
Main dish
Vegetable
Side dish

Cook 2

Start at 4:00 p.m.
Salad—if none, then vegetable.
Set the table, including condiments and 2 jugs of milk and 2 pitchers of ice water. Wash prep dishes, including any leftover dishes from the day. Make coffee.

Clean-Up 1

Start immediately after dinner.

Clear the table.

Put food away.

Wipe off and put away placemats.

Vacuum the dining room if needed.

Take out trash, replace bag.

Clean-Up 2

Start immediately after dinner.

Put away clean prep dishes. (in drainer & dishwasher).

Scrape and rinse dishes.

Wipe off all counters.

Empty and clean the coffee pot.

Clean-Up 3

Start immediately after dinner

Scrape, then wash pots, pans, utensils (in sink by window).

Sweep the floor.

Put dishes away by 7:30 p.m.

Straighten utensil drawers to insure neatness.

Snack Person

Start at 8:00 p.m.

Take out snack and place in activity room.

Fill blue cooler with ice.

Fill bowl 1/2 way with ice

Place jug of milk inside and take to act. room. Place cups in activity room.

Snack Clean-Up

Start at 9:00 p.m.

Put away milk and snack.

Wipe counters, tables, and ashtrays. Empty trash and replace bag. Load all dishes into dishwasher. Sweep the floor.

Figure 18-4. House chore written instruction based on task analysis.

The Staff

The characteristics of the resident population described at Mt. Airy House warrant a high staff/resident ratio for several reasons: lack of motivation coupled with problem behaviors; the complex and often stressful level of individual needs; and the coordination and execution of the wide variety of daily tasks involved in maintaining the program and facility. The House opened in September 1988 with a skeletal program. The staff developed and refined most of the structure, the related forms, protocols, and organization of the program,

	Date:	
Dinner Prep 1:	Dinner Prep 2:	
	You check when done	Staff check

Clean-Up Person #1 Checklist

1. Table cleared
2. Cond., milk, and water put away
3. Placemats wiped off and put away
4. Table wiped off
5. Dining room vacuumed
6. Trash taken out, new bag put in

Clean-Up Person #2 Checklist

1. Prep dishes put away
2. Dishes scraped and rinsed
3. Dishes washed
4. Counters wiped off—including pantry
5. Empty and clean coffee pot
6. All clean dishes put away

Clean-Up Person #3 Checklist

1. Pots, pans, and utensils washed—2nd sink
2. Sweep the floor
3. Put clean pots, pans, and utensils away
4. Straighten utensil drawer to insure neatness

Snack Person Checklist

1. Take out snack and place in activity room
2. Fill blue cooler with ice
3. Fill bowl 1/2 way with ice—place milk in bowl, take to activity room
4. Place cups in activity room

Snack Clean-Up Checklist

1. Put milk and all food away
2. Wipe all counters, tables, and ashtrays
3. Empty all trash and replace bag
4. Load all activity room dishes into dishwasher
5. Sweep the activity room floor

Figure 18-5. House chore checklist.

and thus have become dedicated and invested in seeing that it runs according to the guiding philosophy and principles.

The staff consists of the following: the Director (a master's level occupational therapist); The Psychologist Consultant; the Program Nurse (master's level); six full-time Rehabilitation Workers; two part time Rehabilitation Workers; and five 16-hour per week Rehabilitation Workers for weekends. The staffing pattern provides for both the Director and the Program Nurse to be available for day shifts and some evening shifts. Team Meetings are held daily during shift change to include the total staff. Day staff consists of two Rehabilitation Workers, whereas evening staff consists of three full-time plus one part-time Rehabilitation Workers. Weekends are separately staffed with the 16-hour Rehabilitation Workers. These are ideal positions for students in psychology or related fields. The majority of rehabilitation workers, even though considered paraprofessionals, come to the program with various levels of experience, and expertise, and some with degrees in a related field.

The Program Nurse serves not only as part of the day shift, assisting in all the daily tasks of the program for the residents, but also serves as the primary liaison to all of the doctors involved. Each resident has his or her own private psychiatrist. The Nurse oversees all medications which are prescribed by physicians. The medical needs of the residents are extensive, partly due to somatic complications and complaints that are part of the illness. The Nurse provides management of these needs, conducts a health workshop for residents, and also is a good resource for overseeing the menu and daily diet of the residents and providing state of the art education for both residents and staff in healthier ways of eating. The Program Nurse is in charge in the absence of the Director.

The Psychologist Consultant not only serves as a primary consultant to the program, but also is the Assistant Service Chief of the Chronic Schizophrenic Research Unit, and is the primary liaison between the House and Inpatient Division. The Psychologist Consultant, with the Director, screens all applicants as well as mediates when problems arise, consults in treatment, and educates staff.

The Director is in charge of the overall administration of the program, providing staff supervision, direction and consultation to overall policies, procedures, licensure, and program development and is on 24-hour call. The Director is also the primary liaison between the program and third party reimbursement case managers. Currently 70% of the residents are funded by private insurance.

Each staff member has two residents for whom he/she is responsible, as both a case manager and a resident advisor. The role of a case manager at Mt. Airy is to:

1. Provide all necessary documentation.
2. Conduct team meetings for establishing the residents' Rehabilitation Plans and monthly reviews.
3. Serve as a liaison to families, therapists, and community programs regarding residents' status.
4. Assure information regarding entitlements is procured.

The role and function of a resident advisor at Mt. Airy is to:

1. Serve as the primary advocate for his/her resident.
2. Give both practical and emotional support.

TIER I

1. Participate in the daily House program.
2. Earn *at least* 70% of your credits on a regular basis.
3. Follow the Basic House Rule.
4. Comply with any contracts that have been designed for you.
5. Take your meds consistently.

On Tier I you can earn a maximum of $30.00 per week so that:

90 - 100% = $30.00

80 - 90% = $25.00

70 - 80% = $20.00

To move to Tier II you must "present your case" and the reasons why you should be able to move with your resident advisor to the rest of the staff.

TIER II TRANSITIONAL

1. Earn 90-100% of your credits consistently (3 out of 4 weeks).
2. Consistently do your hygiene (showering, laundry) without being reminded.
3. Take your meds without being reminded.
4. Attend your regularly scheduled appointments without being reminded after planning meeting (i.e., therapy).
5. Use cabs, the bus or walk to where you need to go.
6. Own and use an alarm clock to get up—you may have one wakeup call after the alarm.
7. Can responsibly budget $40 per week.
8. Participate in movie and/or mall trips.

To move to Tier III you must "present your case" and the reasons why you should move with your resident advisor to the rest of the staff.

TIER III

1. Can maintain a weekly schedule (instead of a daily schedule) that you work out with your resident advisor. This includes getting yourself up.
2. Can get yourself wherever you need to go—i.e., find and use your own means of transportation.
3. Can make and keep all of your own appointments—i.e., doctor, dentist, therapist.
4. Can take your meds and take care of your prescriptions on your own.
5. Have an overall absence of "excessive behaviors."
6. Can budget on your own and keep up without being on the credit system.

Figure 18-6. The Tier System (I, II, III).

3. Meet weekly with the resident for budgeting and planning.
4. Assist the resident in establishing goals in response to problem areas.
5. Assist the resident in [his or her] formal presentation to staff for Tier promotion.
6. Draft behavioral contracts in response to problem behaviors and promote cooperation.

SUMMARY

The Mt. Airy House is a model based on a formal definition of a quarterway house. This definition was drawn from years of experimentation and research in the mental health field toward meeting the residential after care needs of the CMI. It represents one step within a needed spectrum of housing particularly suited for the CMI, and fully acknowledges the need for a network of support services in conjunction with housing.

According to Fine (1983), "Both rehabilitation and traditional treatment models have been guilty of addressing their efforts to the healthiest sectors of the patient population. Successful outcome with a chronic population should not be measured by the same yard stick used for the acutely ill and less disabled" (p. 12). She adds that important determinants of outcome in all rehabilitation efforts are repetition and frequency of practice in skill learning, appropriate performance expectations, supportive staff attitudes, movement into more normative settings with social supports, and appropriate length of time allotted to such an effort. Based on this premise, Mt. Airy House represents a good model and first step in a crucial continuum.

Mt. Airy House is approaching its third year of operation. To date, the program is operating to capacity, of which nine out of the 16 residents are approaching their second and third years in the program. The future of these residents depends on continuing to explore and creatively provide even more normative housing arrangements in the effort toward better community integration. For some residents, there is evidence that a supervised apartment would be suitable as the next step after Mt. Airy, if given enough social supports. For others, there is beginning evidence that a permanent group home setting is warranted. What is clear, however, is the need for a system that is available and open to the fluctuating needs of the CMI, and according to Crowel (1988), "enable patients to view housing changes as routine and normal, and not a sign of failure" (p. 66).

REFERENCES

Arce, A. & Vergare, M. (1985). An overview of community residences as alternatives to hospitalization. *Psychiatric Clinics of North America, 8,* 423-436.

Crowel, R. L (1988). The integrated clinically managed housing network. *New Directions for Mental Health Services, 40,* 59-64.

Fine, S. B. (1983). Psychiatric treatment and rehabilitation: What's in a name? *NAPPH Journal, 11*(5) 8-13.

Gudeman, J. E., Dickey, B., Rood, L., Hellman, S., & Grinspoon, L. (1981). Alternatives to the back ward: A quarterway house. *Hospital and Community Psychiatry, 32,* 359-363.

Hcfmeister, J. F., Weller, V. E., & Ackerson, L. M. (1989). Treatment outcome in a private-sector residential care program. *Hospital and Community Psychiatry, 40,* 927-932.

Kruzich, Jean M. (1985). Community integration of the mentally ill in residential facilities. *American Journal of Community Psychology, 13,* 553-564.

Mann, W. C. (1976). A quarterway house for adult pychiatric patients. *American Journal of Occupational Therapy, 30,* 646 - 647.

Mechanic, Ph. D. (1986). The challenge of chronic mental illness: A retrospective and prospective view. *Hospital and Community Psychiatry, 37,* 891-896.

Myerson, A T. & Herman, G. S. (1983). What's new in aftercare? A review of recent literature. *Hospital and Community Psychiatry, 34,* 333-342.

Purnell, T. L., Jackson, S. M., & Wallace, E. C. (1982). A quarterway house program for hospitalized chronic patients. *Hospital and Community Psychiatry, 33,* 941-942.

Ranz, J. M. (1989). Home II: Preparing chronic mental patients for on-campus living. *Hospital and Community Psychiatry, 40,* 1190-1191.

Wilberding, D. (1987). Rehabilitation through activities for the chronic schizophrenic patient. *The Chronically Mentally III: Issues in O.T. Intervention, Proceedings,* AOTA, Inc., pp. 37-47.

CHAPTER NINETEEN

Community Living Skills: A Psychoeducational Community-Based Program

Patricia Hickerson Crist

This chapter was updated by the author in September 1999, and originally published in Occupational Therapy in Mental Health, *6(2), 51-64. Copyright © 1986, Haworth Press. Reprinted by permission.*

AUTHOR'S REFLECTION—RE-VISITING COMMUNITY LIVING SKILLS: 14 YEARS LATER

I am pleased that this 1986 manuscript is being selected for reprint in *Proactive Approaches in Psychosocial Occupational Therapy* due to its clinical relevance for today's practice in occupational therapy. "Be careful not to throw the baby out with the bath water," and "everything old is new again," are two phrases that encapsulate the reason for including this older work now. Psychoeducation provides a relevant practice approach to mental health problems as an alternative to the biomedical model. Certainly, it is client-centered and empowering, both which address contemporary service delivery concerns. Psychoeducation is congruent with teaching-learning principles used in occupational therapy practice.

In lieu of doing extensive revisions within the text itself, the editor and I have agreed to update parts of this text through this mechanism to keep the entire concept intact but also respectfully place the content within today's practice environment. The literature review can easier be updated by doing a library search primarily of non-occupational therapy sources beginning with the words "psychosocial rehabilitation" or "psychiatric rehabilitation".

"Be careful not to throw the baby out with the bath water." The psychoeducational approach is a classic approach whose use waxes and wanes historically. These changes have been reflective of emerging approaches to mental health problems as well as funding for services.

A Historical Perspective: For occupational therapy, the last major practice thrust in community-based psychoeducation occurred in the late 60s and 70s in response to the 1963 Community Mental Health Act signed by President Kennedy. The act provided federal funds to create community mental health centers to serve a wide array issues including outpatient, inpatient (short-term stay), crisis intervention, day treatment or partial care and even prevention through community education. The goal was that over a seven- to eight-year funding cycle, the proportion of federal fends supporting a given center would decrease and be replaced by state funds.

Consequently, a large number of occupational therapists, including myself, found stimulating jobs that supported our occupational therapy philosophy in community mental health programs. With the advent of this act the primary role of the occupational therapy practitioner was being a team member serving individuals with chronic, long-term or chronic mental health conditions following de-institutionalization. Many community-based occupational therapists also provided services for long-term adjustment to physical disabilities and chronic illness such as stroke, multiple sclerosis, head injury, and Parkinson's disease. Many had exhausted traditional physical rehabilitation funding but were depressed or stressed emotionally by the continual adaptation to their condition. Occupational therapists were and still are uniquely and many times "the best qualified" in mental health settings to provide services for psychosocial adaptation to physical disabilities and chronic illnesses. Many of these individuals benefited then as well now from psychoeducational programming also. The goal was to maintain or rehabilitate these individuals to live safely and as independently as possible in the least restrictive community living environment.

Unfortunately, the states did not deliver the matching funds and consequently, community mental health centers had to generate revenue to continue. Rapidly, day care and partial care programs closed as these were not self-supporting through fees for service. While occupational therapists moved to "greener pastures," many also left mental health practice due to the continual lack of funding for services. Worse, insufficient funds were not available to address the critical health and quality of life needs of individuals who had been deinstitutionalized or have since been diagnosed with severe, persistent, mental health problems.

NAMI (1999) states that mental illness is more common than cancer, diabetes or heart disease with one in every five families affected in their lifetime by a severe mental illness. Besides the over 300,000 individuals with severe mental illness who are homeless or incarcerated, 21% of our hospital beds are filled by people with mental illness. Following a five year study of schizophrenia alone, more than 1/2 of the two million individuals with schizophrenia were receiving substandard care proven to reduce symptoms and improve recovery. Psychological treatments, family interventions, vocation rehabilitation and assertive community treatment were among the seven treatment recommendations included in outcomes of this extensive study. Occupational therapy could address these recommendations.

Abandonment and Continuation: As occupational therapists left community mental health for survival or for some "greener pastures", we, too, left the use of psychoeducation practice within the client's lived context. Psychoeducation continued as a viable approach to service. However, these services were allocated to mental health caseworkers or volunteers to sustain programming; yet, neither group had the fund of information held by occupational therapists to enhance these services. A walk into most community-based mental health settings reveals some type of psychoeducation programming being undertaken such as cooking, money management, pre-vocational planning, leisure groups, etc. Services are delivered in groups as they are cost-effective and generate cross learning between participants. Even some professions, such as education, social work, and psychology are beginning to cite in their literature the importance of "doing" and activity in the therapeutic process to stimulate more reliable change.

The time is now to reconsider what was begun in occupational therapy nearly 30 years ago and integrate our new resources into this model to re-engage in delivering community living skills in the form of psychoeducation. Our pioneers, our sage practitioners can be mobilized to help with this effort.

"Everything old is new again": Today you can walk into safe houses, clubhouses, outreach programs, homeless shelters and community day centers and see a form of psychoeducation being directed by paraprofessionals and volunteers. The concept presented in this manuscript lives but in a simplified form. Certainly, basic community living skills are teachable by nearly anyone. However, to make it comprehensible and meaningful to an individual with mental health problems, an occupational therapist must be involved with the program to adapt the program to individual learning styles and therapeutic goals. Certainly, incorporating home visits to understand the client's living environment is essential in order to match psychoeducation and the needs of the individual.

Second, all intervention programs are accountable to document individual change as well as global program outcomes. Now, more than ever, the occupational therapy practitioner can make a significant contribution to measuring the efficacy and effectiveness of psychoeducation programming. With the advent of such evaluation tools such as the *Canadian Occupational Performance Measure* (COPM), the *Assessment of Motor and Processing Skills* (AMPS), and the *Occupational Case Analysis Interview and Rating Scale* (OCAIRS), to identify, measure and assess change in community living skills, occupational therapists can make a significant addition. For instance, a recent visit to a community day treatment program revealed psychoeducation programs in place. Discussion with non-occupational therapy staff who delivered these programs expressed frustration that individuals could not apply the information to their own setting, limited ability to create individual goals and most importantly, inability to measure change related to psychoeducation.

Further, we can demonstrate through clinical studies comparative value of having an occupational therapy practitioner as an integral member of the treatment team in today's mental health settings. I believe that the overall outcome of psychoeducation intensifies when our skills are present.

Combined with a client-centered approach, our recipients can be empowered to attain a personal quality of life through the teaching-learning mode as a student, a less stigmatizing approach than the therapeutic one. Thus, they may be more likely to return to psychoeducation versus therapeutic programs for support and even additional learning.

INTRODUCTION

Persons with chronic mental health problems are frequently found residing in the community, participating in various support systems and living at varying quality of life levels. This variety is related to the development of community resources, the accessibility of services and the needs of persons being served. Most communities have developed crisis, acute and long-term partial care facilities in response to the Community Mental Health Act of 1963 (Pub. L. No. 88-164) and its revisions.

However, insufficient funds have been allocated for many of these programs and deinstitutionalization has increased demands for community-based programs; therefore, significant service gaps exist in most communities.

Though rehabilitation programs are suitable for patients with acute or initial exacerbations of mental health pathology, these programs alone are necessary but not sufficient to meet the long-term needs of the chronic person.

Long-term reliance on biomedically-based rehabilitation produces dependence on the system and maintains reliance on the "sick role". A major problem among persons with chronic mental health problems results from the ambivalence created between being dependent on a biomedical rehabilitation service delivery system versus independence in community life; the latter having greater social value. To close the gap between dependence-inducing models and client desires for independence with minimal labeling, psychoeducation emerges as a potential alternative.

Occupational therapists have indirectly been led in this direction for several years. Lorna Jean King (1978) provided a salient example when she stated that "Mental health is achieved through the learning of new adaptive behaviors and/or the unlearning of old maladaptive patterns".

One way to learn new adaptive behaviors is through the teaching-learning process where the student (person with a chronic mental health problem) is taught new information and given [the] opportunity to explore and practice new living skills. Psychoeducation can be supportive of one of occupational therapy's central philosophical tenets—to learn by doing. (Lillie & Armstrong, 1982). By using an educational model, new living skills which have been acquired can result in an increased independence among persons with chronic mental health problems which in turn should enhance their quality of life.

MENTAL HEALTH SERVICE DELIVERY

In 1975, 50 million Americans were considered to be peripherally or socially marginal due to chronic mental health problems (Spiegler & Agigian, 1977). This was attributed to skill deficits, maladaptive behavior or stresses and deficiencies in one's social environment. Neither the environment nor personal interactions alone can account for the variations or dysfunctions in human performance but a person-environment, interaction-based, service delivery model could offer solutions to this complex problem (Short & Pagliaro, 1981).

Skill training programs that teach new methods of effective interpersonal interaction through appropriate object use and adaptive task performance are likely to be effective (Lillie & Armstrong, 1982). The authors further states that if mental disorders are reclassified as problematic behaviors in community living, then the replacement of skill deficiencies through skill training experiences is the primary focus, not symptom alleviation. In the past, this training has been couched in the current service delivery system or environment and consequently, the processes and outcomes of skill training have reflected the central philosophies or beliefs of the selected service delivery model which are not always matched to the essential needs of the clients.

Early mental health paradigms promoted dependency among service recipients (Lillie & Armstrong, 1982). The primary stimuli for the dependency was three-fold: reliance on the medical model which gave authority to the medical personnel and reinforced submission by the recipient, labeling and pharmacologic intervention (Berkell, 1982; Lamb, 1976). In a system where authority is prescribed to select individuals, usually a physician, due to education and/or power, dependency of the recipient on the authoritarian figure is expected and reinforced. With skills training, the recipient must wait for the prescription and then follow the treatment regimen as deemed by others to be appropriate. Labeling has also generated dependency in that it reinforces that the recipient is sick, ill or stereotypically unable to care for [him or herself]. Further, due to diagnostic labeling, persons with mental health problems are not expected to be responsible for their activities. A case in point is the legal system and its allowance for the plea of "not guilty by reason of insanity", which indicates social belief that a person who is mentally ill is not accountable or responsible for [his or her] actions. Skill training is hampered by these lowered expectations for responsible performance associated with mental health problems. At one point pharmacology was perceived as the panacea or answer. Pharmacology must not be underestimated, as it permits clients previously too disturbed to benefit from therapy or the opportunity to participate in skill training. Pharmacologic intervention only alleviated symptoms and skill dependency remained, creating problems for community adjustment.

Milieu and social learning therapies were alternatives to programs which reinforced dependency issues. Milieu or therapeutic communities created environments where group pressure and confrontation were used to promote responsible behavior. The underlying assumption for most of these programs was that the clients possessed the requisite social behavior in their current repertoire, which was seldom the case (Berkell, 1982). Token economies created a similar atmosphere. Social learning therapies eliminated the problems of token and milieu therapies by providing modeling, positive expectancy and reinforced rehearsal to learn new skills (Hersen & Bellack, 1976; Falloon, Lindley, McDonald & Marks, 1977; Lillie & Armstrong, 1982). The problem with these therapies is that the usual focus was on interpersonal communication and not task development in functional living skills. Occupational therapists' major contribution to mental health services, besides understanding the implications of physical disabilities on mental health, has been to provide services not simply based on "talking" but on "doing". This active process is central to occupational therapy, and chronic mental health problems and other therapies, such as psychology, counseling and nursing, are increasingly reporting in their literature this core concept of occupational therapy as important to individual and overall program gains.

At the same time that these two models were popular in addressing the problems of the chronically mentally ill, several socio-political events were occurring which changed the mental health environment: (1) deinstitionalization became a central focus but frequently occurred without adequate development of community living resources for the special population released; (2) the biomedical model became less desirable and efficient as mental health care values changed and the perceived pressure of deinstitutionalization was felt; (3) community mental health services were proposed and federally funded; and, (4) quality of life issues became prime movers in health care service delivery. Dissatisfaction with the medical approach to mental health problems and its reductionistic dependence on disease, symptoms, and diagnosis was emerging. Trends toward enhanced moral or humanistic treatment in community settings were promoted. Holism coupled with self-responsibility were values for recipients of healthcare in the future. A comprehensive review of this movement is provided by Schulberg and Killilea (1982) in their edited book on community mental health.

Unfortunately, the promise of this movement has not been realized and mental health consumers and advocates continue to fight for resources to implement critical changes within the healthcare delivery system.

PSYCHOEDUCATION

With the advent of community mental health in the '60s and '70s, when mental disorders were defined in more functional modes, occupational therapy philosophy was closely allied with the new system. Mental disorders were seen as problematic behaviors which resulted in skill deficiencies. The interaction of the environment and human performance abilities was central in analyzing skilled performance or action. The pressure to assume self-responsibility for one's action was advocated. Fidler (1984) stated basic goals for occupational therapy in mental health: (1) to create a performance skill learning and practice environment so that skills become habitual patterns of behavior; (2) to provide acting-doing experiences that enable clients to acquire a repertoire of self-care, work, and leisure skills in order to achieve maximum independence, develop appropriate socio-cultural role expectations, and experience self satisfaction and self-worth; (3) to alter the role orientation from passive recipient to self agent in order to develop a sense of being able to influence and have some control over daily life; and, (4) to reduce dependency on external motivational forces and increase self-initiating behavior. All four goals can be facilitated through occupational therapy as part of a community-based psychoeducational program while addressing limitations of the other service delivery models as noted earlier.

Psychoeducation is a mental health service delivery model which is closely allied to community mental health but yet sufficiently different in practice. Both psychoeducation and community mental health have major differences with the biomedical model, which can be seen in Table 19-1. Psychoeducation advocates for the learning process through an educational system, which is different than the biomedical service delivery system. The therapist becomes teacher; patient or client becomes student and the clinic becomes a classroom. The treatment plan is replaced by the course syllabus and treatment takes the form of educational courses. Medical diagnosis is not the admission ticket to service but voluntary motivation to acquire new living skills. Reviews of several psychoeducational programs are available (Bakker & Armstrong, 1976; Berkell, 1982; Hewett, 1967; Lamb, 1976; Lillie & Armstrong, 1982; Short & Pagliaro, 1981; Speigler & Agigian; 1977; and Stern &

Minkoff, 1979). These reviews explore programs offered for students with chronic mental health problems who have problems with living skills. Training living skills is a high priority among the domains of concern for occupational therapy. In an educational model, occupational therapists can contribute their skills in analyzing and teaching the basic, non-academic skills of independent learning when coupled with mental health problems. This is essential considering, as stated earlier, that many of the problems seen among persons with chronic mental health problems begin with the basic skills of living or survival. Though seldom mentioned, it is apparent the relevance of occupational therapy to these programs is self-evident.

The philosophy and values of occupational therapy can be implemented in a psychoeducationally-oriented setting as it seeks to create a learning environment to foster learner independence and provide maximal control over one's life (Bakker & Armstrong, 1976). Educationally, the goal is to teach the student to set attainable goals for personal change and to develop skills required for reaching them. The occupational therapist will introduce positive expectancy in a more normalized environment such as a classroom, community center or vocational/trade school which enhances the students' self esteem and self-confidence as [the therapist] mobilizes to meet the needs of persons with chronic mental health problems (Lamb, 1976). Through the voluntary practice of new skills in a safe environment, community survival and enhancement skills are learned and practiced. Since the students elect which courses to enroll in, the expectation is that motivation for new learning will be great as content will be student-specific, desired by the student and, thus, habitually practiced outside the classroom. The last major component is time orientation as these programs are time-limited. This may increase the student's sense of urgency to acquire the new skills.

Many chronic mental health clients who live in the community desire normalization through acquisition of socially appropriate skills and behaviors. A model based on educational premises teaches new skills while decreasing the dependence on the day-care programs so frequently used in community mental health as management or maintenance programs. The dependence on and reinforcement of the diagnostically-related "sick role" will be replaced by the student's participation in the study and practice of life-related tasks in self-care, work and leisure Though not unique to occupational therapy, as these tasks are frequently addressed, the educational way in which they are delivered provides an alternate model which encourages student responsibility for skill acquisition. The vital link will be the application of learned material to the natural environment (Bakker & Armstrong, 1976). As Lamb (1976) so eloquently stated, the chronic mental health client will assimilate that basic skills are learned and not magically bestowed talents or abilities that some have and others do not. Consequently, much of the mystique about "making it" in the world is taken away.

Table 19-1
Occupational Therapy In Mental Health

	Biomedical Model	*Community Mental Health Model*	*Psychoeducational Model*
Central focus:	Medicine	Long-term care	Education
Environment:	Institutions; clinics	Community; some institutions	Educational settings
Therapeutic role:	Clinician	Clinician or case manager	Educator
Recipient's role:	Dependency	Semi-dependency	Independent/interdependent
Recipient's expectation:	Get well	Maintain or improve	"Learn"
Recipient's name:	Patient	Client	Student
Responsibility:	Therapist responsible for client	Dependent on CMH's philosophy	Client responsible for self
Control:	Therapist directs treatment	Mutual responsibility	Student selects learning opportunities
Referral to service:	Can be coercive/involuntary	Mixture	Non-coercive/voluntary
Service base:	Treatment plan	Treatment plan	Course syllabi

DEVELOPING A PSYCHO-EDUCATIONAL PROGRAM

In developing a psychoeducational program for persons with chronic mental illness, several suggestions concerning the setting, curriculum and students are necessary. The school-like setting should be characterized as a learning environment preferably outside the typical mental health service environment, which encourages dependency and identification with the "sick role"; and in which the students are further integrated into the community, such as an adult education program or continuing education unit in a local college or university. By locating the program in an educational setting, the role is one of a student engaged in learning new skills versus a patient hoping someone will be able to rid him or her of the symptoms. The teachers may be multidisciplinary professionals such as occupational therapists, vocational rehabilitation counselors or adult educators, volunteers from the community, program graduates or students in health or education careers who have [the] skills to be educators and tutors. Though a school nurse may be present, planned intervention with severe symptomatology is non-existent except during medical emergencies. Students are expected to have symptomatology controlled sufficiently in order to benefit from the educational program. Thus, it is desirable to be in contact with the community mental health center and inpatient psychiatric unit should services be needed during a student's medical leave of absence from the educational program. Tuition for the program can be charged and, if a nominal amount is paid by the student, is considered to enhance student motivation. Most programs run in similar duration to other educational units using the semester or quarter format which enhances the student's ability to

respond to schedules, facilitates goal-directed behavior and allows testing of behavior generalization at semester or quarter breaks (Spiegler, 1977).

The curriculum is planned by developing educational goals and objectives into logically coherent didactic and experiential learning opportunities with assigned homework for practice in the naturalistic setting, such as the student's current residence. Persons currently teaching in academic environments could serve as excellent resources in preparation of classroom activities and materials. Topics could include: money management, leisure time, job hunting, self-care, communication, sex education, nutrition, meal preparation, household safety, transportation, assertiveness training, and stress management, to name a few of the limitless options (Fidler, 1984; Lillie & Armstrong, 1982; Arbesman, Armacost, Hays, Rauschi and Swindle, 1984). Use of videotaping, films, field trips and guest speakers with expertise for the classroom topic would be advantageous. For example, contacting the local dental hygienists group can result in a presentation on dental care or, by contacting the local dairy council, charts on the nutritional value of various foods along with workbooks on nutrition can be obtained. With computers, information on a wide array of daily living topics is available which also gives students experience with a socially-valued and current technology. Most educational software programs are listed through software directories and educational software distributors. Use of software should supplement, not replace, classroom learning activities. All educational opportunities should provide training in new skills and develop problem-solving strategies for independent living based on the individual needs of the student.

The person with chronic mental illness must be ready to voluntarily identify himself as a learner and not a patient. Key elements to this process include student participation in planning the curriculum, assessment of skill ability and learning need in relation to student goals and attitude of educator, in order to reinforce learner responsibilities instead of the expectations associated with patient-therapist relationships. The student role must be encouraged and begins with an assessment of learning needs in a skill area by a student advisor who provides information concerning appropriate coursework for the student to reach his or her goals. Evaluations which may serve as useful tools include the Kohlman Evaluation of Living Skills (McGourty, 1979); Task Check List (Lillie & Armstrong, 1982); Phillip's Social Skills Criteria Scale (Phillips, 1978); Solving Community Obstacles and Restoring Employment (Kramer, 1984); Basic Living Skills Battery (Skolaski and Broekema, 1975); and Scorable Self Care Evaluation (Clark and Peters, 1984), as each evaluation gives specific but different composites of living skills. Two other sources include general educational tests over specific content domains and the development of community/life skills questionnaires which reflect course objectives or content and community skill needs. To individualize course content, a portion of the assessment should solicit student goals which can be used to develop open topics in each class as well as plan the student's course of study. This cooperative planning process sets a tone of reciprocity between student and teacher, each with his or her own prescribed responsibilities. Students should be encouraged to take notes, do homework, collect related handouts and meet timelines while instructors prepare coursework, give feedback to the students concerning their performance and provide student evaluation of overall course success.

Two psychoeducationally-related programs for persons with chronic mental illness will be briefly exemplified:

CASE STUDY #1

In a local community mental health setting, persons seen in a partial-care program were invited to participate in a basic living skills program designed to assist with problems in living. Each potential student was informed about the educational format of the program and assessed using the Basic Living Skills Battery (Skolaski & Broekema, 1975), which was adapted to reflect the community in which the students resided. An interview identified their goals and interest in participation. The program was developed and instructed by two community mental health occupational therapists. The majority of students were not coerced into participation.

Clients selected the content groups they desired based on the skills they wished to acquire and were informed that they must attend and participate in each session. Participation included: listening, practicing skills while in the group, completing homework based on the new information learned and sharing (the following week), their success in completing their homework.

Based on the initial group's cumulative assessment, the occupational therapists began initially with three separate programs on interpersonal communication, self-care, and nutritional meal preparation. Eventually, the programs were expanded to topics on leisure planning, vocational readiness skills, financial management and communication. Program entrance was voluntary.

Example: Though all members had some degree of problem with cleanliness, one particular female will be discussed. During the assessment, she indicated that she washed her hair, took a bath and brushed her teeth once a month. During the interview, she indicated that the day on which all this happened was a very busy one for her. Later, one of the sessions was allotted to dental care. A local hygienist was invited to instruct the course. She demonstrated proper dental brushing and flossing as well as explored healthy snack foods. A highlight of the demonstration was the red-dye tablets each member chewed to demonstrate brushing deficiencies. In addition, each member was given a free toothbrush. The previously mentioned female student agreed to brush her teeth daily and a chart was developed for her to keep track of her homework assignment. At each consecutive session, she reported progress on her contract. A generally successful change was noted by the end of the class sessions which was maintained after the class terminated. In fact, more than this behavior changed due to the cumulative impact of contracts added at the end of each session.

The program was viewed by agency administrators and accreditors as beneficial to not simply maintaining clients in the community but also improving their quality of community life. A major hindrance to this program was that the clients were still seen in the mental health environment (day care program) and it would have been interesting to see their performance in a strictly educational setting.

(Due to funding reimbursement constraints, psychoeducational programs are often offered at clinical practice settings rather than school settings; although therapists can refer individuals to appropriate course offerings at community colleges and continuing education programs to acquire skills in natural contexts.).

This program is related to usual day care programs but is different due to the expectations for student acquisition of new skills and the teacher-student relationship in contrast to the usual therapist-client one.

CASE STUDY #2

Through contacts with the local community mental health center, the vocational rehabilitation division, and support groups for families of the chronically mentally ill, it is becoming apparent that a vital community service-link is missing. Several persons with chronic mental health problems wanted to be "normalized" within the community and no longer identified with mental health services. It is known that these persons are employable, but hiring is easy compared to retention on the job due to maladaptive secondary behaviors which prevent job survival. Families of the chronically mentally ill desire increased options for their family members which go beyond recreational diversions only.

Simultaneously, the free-standing sheltered workshop for persons with chronic mental health problems was moved to the same enclosure as one for the developmentally disabled amidst concerns for economics and promises for new, unique job training which has not been forthcoming over the past two years. This has created frustration among staff and consumers in the community.

In response, three occupational therapists are in the initial stages of developing a psychoeducational program to be housed at the university. Instructed by community persons/professionals on given topics, with tutors made available through students completing occupational therapy practicums. Initial evaluation of persons with chronic mental illness interested in the curriculum format will decide which course content to develop first. The overall outcome of the program will be job evaluation and placement by providing skill courses in core readiness behaviors. Though an eventual training grant will be applied to support the complete development of the program, the initial pilot studies are being conducted through the resources of the university (primarily the occupational therapy department and the division of continuing education), the local community mental health center, and, hopefully, the division of vocational education. By housing the program within the university environment, an educational atmosphere will be promoted. The initial challenge at this time is to continue to maintain an educator's viewpoint and avoid slipping into a therapeutic model. Collaboration between the three occupational therapists is helping to keep this in check.

Currently, occupational therapy students in a research methods class are performing a needs assessment of the community to identify services needed by the chronically mentally ill. It is anticipated that this initial evaluation will give direction to the curriculum as well as identify potential registrants. Further, it will provide evaluation objectives for the future to assess outcomes of the program.

Future program expansions include developing learning materials for any student regardless of their physical, psychological or social disability as long as they desire to develop new living skills to increase their productive community involvement. Research efforts are planned to document the impact of the program on participants' quality of community living. Both of these programs, one underway and the other evolving, support potential benefits of the psychoeducational model for service delivery to persons with chronic mental health problems. They offer a community-based alternative, which from initial entry into the curriculum, anticipates student self-responsibility and investment in learning. The student is seen as the responsible change agent and the instructor a guide to resources and skill development. Of course, the success of this program is directly related to students entering who are motivated to learn and the provision of appropriate coursework to meet their objectives. If the two are present, relevance or meaningfulness to the student will become the prime motivator.

CONCLUSION

The intent of this (chapter) was to review the potential benefits of a psychoeducational program to meet the needs of the chronically mentally ill. Psychoeducation and its relevance was described and exemplified via two brief case studies.

This model has broader benefits since there are numerous individuals who are beyond the capacities of usual rehabilitation programs, particularly if they are coping with a long-term, irreversible disability, such as spinal cord or head injury. Programs such as the ones described above focus on problems in living, not diagnosis. Thus, if the instructor is able to adapt his or her teaching strategies, many persons who have peripheral social status due to their disability could benefit from a psychoeducational program. Occupational therapists are professionally suited to provide services in such a holistic manner.

In a psychoeducational model, [those] with chronic mental illness will benefit as they will be participating in a self-development program whose central organization focuses on normalization and self-direction. Occupational therapists will be able to utilize their teaching expertise in naturalistic settings which support underlying philosophies. The community will benefit from more socially independent and productive members who are less dependent on costly mental health services. Additionally, as noted in the second case study, occupational therapy curricula could offer relevant fieldwork experiences to their students. In these days of cost effectiveness and managed care for mental health services, the advantages of psychoeducation cannot be understated as a community-based alternative in the health care delivery system and the potential contributions of the occupational therapist in providing leadership to these community living skills programs are exemplified.

REFERENCES

Arbesman, F., Armacost, P., Hays, C., Rauchi, M., & Swindle, S. (1984). *Occupational therapy protocols in mental health*. Baltimore, MD: Betty Cox Associates.

Bakker, C. B. & Armstrong, H. E. (1976). The adult development program: An educational approach to the delivery of mental health services. *Hospital & Community Psychiatry, 27,* 330-334.

Berkell, D. E. (1982). Psychoeducational and task-analysis models. *Educational Technology, 22,* 2-29.

Clark, E. N., & Peters, M. (1984). *Scoreable self-care evaluation.* Thorofare, NJ: SLACK Incorporated.

Falloon, I. R. H., Lindley, P., McDonald, R., & Marks, I. M. (1977). Social skills training of outpatient groups: A controlled study of rehearsal and homework. *British Journal of Psychiatry, 131,* 599-609.

Fidler, G. S. (1984). *Design of rehabilitation services in psychiatric hospital settings.* Laurel, MD: Ramsco.

Hersen, M., & Bellack, A. S. (1976). Social skills training for chronic psychiatric patients: Rationale, research findings, and future directions. *Comprehensive Psychiatry, 17,* 559-580.

Hewett, F. M. (1967). Educational engineering with emotionally disturbed children. *Exceptional Children, 33,* 459-467.

King, L. J. (1978). Occupational therapy research in psychiatry. *American Journal of Occupational Therapy, 32,* 15-18.

Kramer, L W. (1984). Solving community obstacles and restoring employment. *Occupational Therapy in Mental Health, 4,* 1-135.

Lamb, H. R. (1976). An educational model for teaching skills to long-term patients. *Hospital & Community Psychiatry, 27,* 875-877.

Lillie, M. D., & Armstrong, H. E. (1982). Contributions to the development of psychoeducational approaches to mental health service. *American Journal of Occupational Therapy, 36,* 438-443.

McGourty, L K. (1979). *Kohlman evaluation of living skills.* Seattle, WA: KELS Research Box 33201.

National Alliance for the Mentally Ill. (1999). Arlington, VA. (www.nami.org)

Philips, E. L (1978). *The social skills bases of psychopathology.* New York, NY: Grune & Stratton.

Schulberg, H. C., & Killilea, M. (Eds.) (1982). *The modern practice of community mental health.* San Francisco, CA: Jossey-Bass.

Short, R. H., & Pagliaro, L. A. (1981). A psychoeducational model of counseling. *International Journal for the Advancement of Counseling, 4,* 111-118.

Skolaski, T., & Broekema, M. C. (1975). *The basic living skills.* Madison, WI: Dane Mental Health Center.

Spiegler, M. D., & Agigian, H. (1977). *The community training center.* New York, NY: Brunnar-Mazel.

Spiegler, M. D., & Agigian, H. (in press). *Schools for living.* New York, NY: Brunner-Mazel.

Stem, R., & Minkoff, K. (1979). Paradoxes in programming for chronic patients in a community clinic. *Hospital and Community Psychiatry, 30,* 613-617.

CHAPTER TWENTY

Ramsey County Day Treatment Services: Day Treatment to Extended Day Treatment Centers to Focus Groups

Ronna Linroth, Suzanne Zander, Sunja Forde, Mary Hanley, and Jeanne Lins

This chapter was previously published in Occupational Therapy in Health Care, 10*(2), 89-103. Copyright © 1996, Haworth Press. Reprinted by permission.*

INTRODUCTION

Partial hospitalization, which has been a major treatment modality since the late 1940s, covers a broad, sometimes poorly differentiated, range of patient care. Controlled studies have shown partial hospitalization to be a flexible and cost-effective alternative to inpatient hospitalization and its proponents believe that it is used far less than treatment outcomes justify (Rosie, I987; Fink, 1982). In the Mental Health Centers Construction Act of 1963, partial hospitalization was designated as a mandated service for community mental health centers in the United States. The American Association for Partial Hospitalization recommends classifying partial hospitalization programs according to their function (Casarino, Willer, & Maxey, 1982). Rosie (1987) suggests from his review that the terms "day hospitals," "day treatment programs," and "day care centers" adequately describe the three broad catagories. Anthony, Cohen, and Farkas (1982) have articulated a number of basic partial care principles or "ingredients" that are necessary to support a client's skills necessary to live, learn, and work in their chosen environment at the most appropriate level of functioning and with the least amount of support from the mental health system. These ingredients include functional assessment, individualized treatment plans, skill teaching, and client involvement.

Partial hospitalization has enjoyed acceptance by third-party payers. Managed care looks favorably on the mode. Equitable coverage can now routinely be pursued through established case management procedures. In 1987 services rendered in hospital-based partial hospitalization programs became reimbursable under Medicare, and in 1991 Medicare coverage was extended to community mental health centers. In a report from the conference on managed care in mental health, *Psychiatric News* summarized a presentation from one of the leaders of the managed care industry (Herrington, 1990): "In the future, Feldman envisions the rapid development of alternatives to inpatient care, a new environment in which funds are available to pay for partial hospitalization, structured outpatient programs, and more. Focus will be on measuring whether a service has improved a patient's functioning both at work or at home."

The efficacy of an intensive day treatment program for patients who manifest significant difficulties associated with affective and personality disorders was evaluated by Piper et al. (1993). Treated patients showed significantly better outcome than control patients for seven of the outcome variables: social dysfunction, family dysfunction, interpersonal behavior, mood level, life satisfaction, self-esteem, and severity of disturbance associated with individual goals of treatment. Hoge et al. (1992) stress that the critical question regarding partial hospitalization is no longer its comparative effectiveness to inpatient treatment, but rather its comparative effectiveness to intensive outpatient approaches that may enhance continuity of care while providing care in more normalizing environments.

Partial care programs tend to provide extended care to persons with severe psychiatric disability. Client data collected in a study by Fishbein (1988) revealed that the mean length of time clients were enrolled in partial care programs was 11 months.

Dr. Mary Langley (1992) says that the perception of need for inpatient setting is often unduly influenced by a woeful lack of alternatives. Developing alternatives is exactly what many professionals interested in the concept of deinstitutionalization are trying to do. The following presentation of the day treatment services offered through Ramsey County is intended to be an encouragement to those professionals who wish to develop programs.

Ramsey County Extended Day Treatment is an eclectic model that uses cognitive behavioral therapy (CBT) and skill development to treat persons with serious and persistent mental illness in community-based settings. Day Treatment provides a structure for the individual's day, where they can learn a holistic approach for stabilizing and maintaining mental health. The program is an alternative to hospitalization. Clients attend several days per week and participate in verbal group therapy, mental health education, occupational therapy, recreational and movement therapy, independent living skills, sexuality, socialization, stress management, and weekly goal-setting groups. Involvement averages 6-18 months depending on individual needs. Clients may self-refer or be referred by health care professional. Clients may be recently discharged from the hospital, be seeing a counselor for one-to-one visits, or be in the community with or without support services. New clients call an intake screener who gathers information about their current situation as well as their history. Case management services for clients with a diagnosis of major mental illness are addressed as needed.

INTAKE AND REFERRAL GROUP

Clients attend an intake and referral group for three hours one time a week for 2 to 6 weeks. The group consists of large and small verbal groups and an occupational therapy session. The referral group is facilitated by staff representing all the extended day treatment groups. This gives clients an opportunity to experience the basic structure of a day treatment program and gives staff an opportunity to observe how a client interacts with others.

Staff observe the quality and amount of contact with people a client can tolerate. Observations specific to occupational therapy are how a client takes instructions, follows through, initiates and responds to interactions, and the level of cognitive skill exhibited. The amount of structure or support a client needs will determine their placement in a group. Staff are also able to consider how a client will fit in with the members currently attending the groups. For example, they can avoid placement of a male with predatory behaviors into a group with young vulnerable females with histories of victimization.

Placement will be recommended for one of the six Day Treatment Programs described below. Programs are listed from most intensive to least intensive.

Day Treatment Central

A four-day per week cognitive-behavioral therapy program. Clients deal with depression, anxiety or behavioral problems related to personality disorders. Individuals selected for this group have major dysfunction in most spheres of their lives, poor vocational histories, problems with relationships, and self-concept. Other problems include a history of abuse and impulse control problems. They may have an Axis I personality disorder but typically do not have a chronic and persistent diagnosis. These clients may be on antide-

pressants or anti-anxiety medications. They are likely to have lived independently of the mental health and/or welfare systems for a period of time. Axis I depressive symptoms are lessened by developing coping skills. Goals are to alleviate depression and anxiety, to control impulses and self-defeating behaviors, to gain employment. When these individuals leave the program, they are expected to be actively involved in school, work, or a volunteer position; to resume "normal" functioning. The average stay is three to five months. They meet in the basement clinic at the county's mental health office building, Monday, Tuesday, Thursday, and Friday from 9:00 a.m. to 2:30 p.m. See Appendix A for Central's schedule of therapeutic activities. Absenteeism is discouraged by an emphasis on personal responsibility and accountability. Upon completion of this program, clients are given a graduation party.

Day Treatment East 4

This is a four, half-day per week program using supportive cognitive behavioral therapy to alleviate depression, anxiety and to improve social skills. Clients in this program may have chemical dependency issues, have a borderline personality, and often need to work on victimization issues. Individuals referred to this group may have had a psychotic episode and may be living independently. They may require up to a year to make behavioral changes and become generally functional. East 4 has the same graduation expectations as Central. They meet in a school building Monday, Tuesday, and Thursday from 9:00 a.m. to noon and Friday from 10:00 a.m. to 2:30 p.m.

Day Treatment Fort Road 4

This is a four-day per week supportive therapy program for adults who have disabling conditions such as bipolar affective disorder or schizophrenia; with or without chemical dependency issues. Less intensive confrontation and more supportive groups place an emphasis an practical problem-solving and social skills building. Clients may have had an extensive mental health history. Clients stay 6 to 12 months. They meet in a storefront building, Monday, Tuesday, and Thursday from 9:00 a.m. to noon and Friday from 10:00 a.m. to 2:30 p.m.

Day Treatment West 3

Day Treatment West 3 is a three-day per week supportive therapy program for adults who have serious and persistent mental illness. Individuals referred to this group will have had more severe psychosis, be more dependent, and utilize more vocational support programs as well as supportive work programs. They may be involved in supported educational, volunteer, or social programs. In this group, struggle with day-to-day living seems more apparent. Although some live independently, many live in supported apartment living programs and others live in structured supportive living environments such as a Board and Care facility. This program focuses on awareness, support, developing problem solving, stress management, coping skills, and planning goals. Clients stay six to twelve months. They meet in a church building, Tuesday, Thursday, and Friday from 9:00 a.m. to noon.

Day Treatment East 2 and Fort Road 2

This is a two-afternoon per week supportive therapy program for adults who have serious and persistent mental illness. The program focuses on structured activities and socialization. Goals are set weekly around socialization, structure, and hygiene. There is a high degree of acceptance and caring for one another. The majority of individuals in this group require supervised living settings or are in supported apartment living programs. The length of stay in the program is open-ended but averages 12-18 months. East 2 meets in a school building and Fort Road 2 in a storefront building, Tuesday and Thursday from 1:00 p.m. to 4:00 p.m.

OCCUPATIONAL THERAPY IN DAY TREATMENT

Occupational therapy varies depending on the population served. At Day Treatment Central, occupational therapy is designed to:
1. Provide balance to the more intense parts of the program.
2. Help clients "compartmentalize" problems. They need to learn how not to work on problems as well as how to work on them.
3. Challenge old beliefs; support fledgling, more productive ideas about self, the world, and the future.
4. Provide a laboratory to practice interpersonal skills.
5. Help with action-oriented goal setting.
6. Help counter the anhedonia of depression.
7. Help develop the "lightening-up" strategies need to accomplish many clients' goal of not taking oneself so seriously.
8. Lighten up and have fun right now!

The therapists choose activities that are interactive and build group cohesiveness. Tasks promote self-awareness and insight and encourage experimenting with new behaviors and ways of perceiving a situation. Activities are supportive of cognitive behavioral underpinning and a client's work.

The occupational therapy structured task groups in the 4 and 2 day programs are also intended to improve skills in areas of self-awareness, awareness of others, social skills, coping skills, and stress rearrangement. At East 4, craft activities have a prevocational focus. Clients are expected to do day-to-day problem-solving. Occupational therapy uses group community art projects to develop interaction and collaboration skills. West 3 and programs of lower intensity use craft modalities that are less involved, foster success and problem-solving, skill development and may be leisure oriented. Utilization of community resources is encouraged. Craft activities at the two day programs are designed to improve structuring the use of time, following directions, decreasing impulsivity, and increasing organizational skills. Building interpersonal skills along with decision-making, planning and problem-solving are also benefits of the purposeful craft activities.

All programs use occupational therapy structured groups focusing on issues related to group participation. These range from warm-up and group building activities, and from self awareness to awareness of others. They include problem solving, assertiveness, coping skill development, time management, and task groups.

APPLYING TREATMENT TOOLS AND THEORY

New clients to Day Treatment are given a folder that contains information on the program such as a weekly schedule (Appendix A), rules that clearly delineate the expected conduct and respect for confidentiality, guidelines for writing a contract, and a glossary of terms.

Cognitive Behavioral Theory (CBT) was developed by Beck and Steer (1987). All parts of all day treatment programs use a cognitive behavioral approach or some modification of it, as is evident in the recurrent monitoring question, "What were you thinking when you said/did that?" Dysfunctional thought is challenged. Staff encourages clients to use the following questions when questioning thoughts and beliefs: What is the evidence for or against this belief? Is there another way of looking at this? What are the implications if this does happen? What good will it do to dwell on this? Will it be helpful or counterproductive?

Staff teach four rules that have been developed from Claire Weekes' Anxiety Management Inventory (Weekes, 1972):
1. Body Awareness—Identifying muscle tension, breathing pattern, heart rate, and restlessness.
2. Label— "This is anxiety."
3. Reassure— "Anxiety won't kill me."
4. Do nothing to stop the anxiety—Do something to get it in the here and now.

Day Treatment clients are expected to submit a *Day Treatment Contract* (Appendix B) to the group after two weeks of attendance. The contract states a client's problems, goals, the work to be done to achieve their goals, and the strengths available to apply to the problem resolution. The contract must be negotiated with the group and therapists, and must be signed by everyone. After agreement, the contract is posted for continued reference. A Contract Review is requested when a client has reached a plateau or is thinking about setting a graduation date. In preparation for leaving a day treatment program, the client must design and present a Relapse Plan (Appendix C). The Plan identifies likely trouble spots, red flags, and an action plan to prevent falling back into old behavior patterns.

The Day Programs address a wide range of mental health consumers over all the programs. They have found CBT to be the best approach for persons with Axis I Depression and Anxiety but less successful with individuals with Borderline Personality Disorder who tend to be more responsive to behavioral modification approaches. The staff have also found that clients with abuse issues benefit from dealing with the crisis first, then family of origin, work, and then back to CBT.

Single Issue Focus Groups

Compared with the general population, persons with serious and persistent mental illness are disproportionately unemployed or underemployed (Jacobs et al., 1992). According to the Mental Health Group Issues Transition Briefing for the Clinton Administration, 85% of people with psychiatric disabilities are unemployed (1992). The C4 Program: Creative Careers and Community Contributions was designed for people with serious mental illness that has kept them from finding productive career or community niches where they can use their abilities to aid themselves and society. The program examines a variety of possible approaches to develop work skills.

The target population for the 15 three-hour weekly sessions is people who have long-term, chronic mental illness, but have also have talent, intelligence, previous training or skills. Such people are encouraged to move forward along a course that recognizes their disabilities as important factors but not automatic disqualifiers for interesting lives. The C4 Program is intended to: utilize a client's high potential; help them make contributions to society that are somewhat in accord with their high capabilities; confront the prejudices of society about people with serious disabilities, especially psychological; and aid self-expression and self-esteem.

The definition of career used in this program is not just paid full-time work, but a dynamic path toward personal fulfillment and accomplishment meaningful to the individual over a long-term effort. A "career path" may involve a delay in earning money while receiving training or making vocational contacts. Training can be academic, apprentice-based, or a practical internship fieldwork experience. Many careers, in this sense, may be hobbies, collecting things, sports, or other applications undertaken while not working, or working in a less interesting or low-paying job used to finance the person's key interest.

Peer Relationships and Sensuality Group is for those clients who have had trouble with personal relationships both romantic and otherwise. Sex education is part of the curriculum. To build skills, assigned homework tasks may include making a social contact during the week, making phone calls, making plans for an outing to a zoo, a movie, a museum, etc.

Self-Trust/Self-Control and Anger Management Group is for people who may have had domestic problems or behaviors that have led to arrests. Clients learn how to modulate acting on their feelings by learning strategies. Self-esteem is also addressed in this group. Clients are challenged to express negative feelings without having to bully or pull a power move. Clients discuss how their dehumanizing of others leads to violence. The course is 10 weeks in length.

Wellness: Avoiding Relapse and Maximizing Health is a group that started out as medication management. It is now being expanded cover stress management and self-nurturing activities to promote a healthy lifestyle. The focus is on what the clients can do; what is positive for them, and what keeps them on an even keel. The group meets for two hours for 10 weeks. Group members include people newly diagnosed with mental illness and/or people having difficulty coming to terms with mental illness.

Coping Skills Training is a very basic social skills group that is in the planning stages. Clients will learn to make eye contact, express themselves tactfully, and be groomed and dressed appropriately. It will be taught as four five-week modules which address stress management, time management, social skills training, and cognitive restructuring.

Quantifying Outcomes

A Graduate Group is available for graduates of several of the day treatment programs. Clients return for an evening or late afternoon group that is available one time a week. Graduates come for a "tune-up" after a few months or a few years. Their return is usually issue-oriented and on a short-term basis.

The Day Treatment Staff are looking at using the Burns Depression Checklist (1993), the Burns Variety Inventory (1993), and a relationship satisfaction scale as pre- and post-measures. The self-rated check lists are simple and take approximately 10 minutes to administer. These copyrighted scales have been demonstrated to measure change over time in treatment.

Trends in Treatment

The staff of the Day Treatment Programs have been seeing an increase in dual diagnoses with mental illness and chemical dependency. Treatment is less compartmentalized where mental illness and chemical dependency are dealt with as two separate issues. The Day Treatment Staff have sought to eliminate the shuffle between mental health and chemical dependency programs by recognizing people who relapse are depressed. If clients can't maintain sobriety they can't work in therapy and are therefore referred for a chemical dependency evaluation. Chemical dependency treatment practitioners also seem to be more flexible about the use of antianxiety medications in these cases. Views about the use of medication appear to be changing as more is discovered about the effects of certain chemicals on brain function.

The clients are coming into the day treatment programs more dysfunctional and more often through the criminal justice system. Many are on provisional discharges from hospitals and on occasion may be on probationary status.

CONCLUSION

The fiscal issues of the current health care system make alternative service delivery in mental health care more attractive. The opportunity to maximize on third party payment can, at the same time, be beneficial to the clients in need of mental health treatment if practical and clinical concerns are addressed first. Ramsey County Day Treatment Service incorporate the "ingredients" necessary to support a client's ability to live, learn, and work in their chosen environment at the most appropriate level of functioning. Day treatment programming is a viable option as an alternative to hospitalization if it is well-designed and graded to meet the existing functional capabilities of clients with mental illness. Occupational therapy is an integral part of day treatment in the model presented because it is the laboratory in which clients try out and practice new behaviors. In day treatment programs this occurs in a more normalized setting with a greater chance for generalization of skill. The action-oriented, concrete tasks and opportunities to demonstrate new behaviors are evidence of the plans and goals of the verbal groups. Occupational therapy staff are valued, collaborative partners in each of these programs.

Clients are introduced to what day treatment can offer them with this summary from the Ramsey County Day Treatment brochure entitled, "Welcome to Day Treatment."

...the Day Treatment Program is designed to assist you through a planned program of group activities to learn more about yourself and what there is about your behavior that is self-defeating for you so that you may change. We make no guarantee you will always be comfortable during your stay here. Hopefully, you will learn a great deal about yourself and acquire some new skills that will make your future life more enjoyable and productive.

BIBLIOGRAPHY

Anthony, W.A., Cohen, M., Parkas, M. (1982). The psychiatric rehabilitation treatment program: Can I recognize one if I see one? *Community Mental Health Journal, 18* (2), 83-95.

Beck, A.T., Steer, R.A. (1987). *Beck Depression Inventory manual.* San Antonio: Psychological Corporation.

Bums, D. (1993). *Ten days to self-esteem.* New York: Willis Morrow and Company.

Casarino, J.P., Wilner, M., Maxey, I.T. (1982). American association for partial hospitalization standards and guidelines for partial hospitalization. *International Journal of Partial Hospitalization. 1,* 521.

Fink, E. (1982). Encouraging third party coverage of partial hospitalization. *Hospital Community Psychiatry, 33*(1), 3841.

Fishbein, S. M. (1988). Partial care as a vehicle for rehabilitation of individuals with severe psychiatric disability. *Rehabilitation Psychology, 3*(1), 57-64.

Herrington, B. S. (1990). Time is running out to protect mental health benefits. *Psychiatric News, October 19,* 12.

Hoge, M. A., Davidson, L., Hill, L. W., et al. (1992). The promise of partial hospitalization: A reassessment. *Hospital and Community Psychiatry, 43,* 345-354.

Jacobs, H. E., Wissusik, D., Collier, R. (1992). Correlations between psychiatric disabilities and vocational outcome. *Hospital and Community Psychiatry, 43,* 365-369.

Langley, M. E. (1992). Letters to the Editor. *Hospital and Community Psychiatry 43*(7), 743.

Mental Health Liaison Group Issues. (1992). *Transition Briefing for Clinton Administration. NASMHPD Report 1031.* Washington, D.C., National Association of State Mental Health Program Directors, December 16.

Piper, W. E., Rosie, J. S., Azim, H. F., Joyce, A.S. (1993). A randomized trial of psychiatric day treatment for patients with affective and personality disorders. *Hospital and Community Psychiatry, 44*(8), 757-763.

Rosie, J. S. (1987). Partial hospitalization: A review of recent literature. *Hospital and Community Psychiatry, 38*(12), 1291-1299.

Weekes, C. (1972). *Peace from nervous suffering.* New York: Hawthorne Incorporated.

Appendix A
Day Treatment Schedule

Monday	Tuesday	Wednesday	Thursday	Friday
9:00-10:30 Therapy Group	9:00-10:30 Therapy Group		9:00-10:30 Therapy Group	9:00-10:30 Therapy Group
10:30-10:45 Break	10:30-10:45 Break		10:30-10:45 Break	10:30-10:45 Break
10:45-12:00 Movement Therapy	10:45-12:00 Media Communications	Take Care of Business Day	10:45-12:00 Self Awareness	10:45-12:00 Stress Management Goals Group
12:00-1:00 Lunch	12:00-1:00 Lunch		12:00-1:00 Lunch	12:00-1:00 Staff & Group Lunch
1:00-2:30 Mental Health Mgt/ Recreational Therapy	1:00-2:30 Sexuality Group		1:00-2:30 Cognitive Behavioral Therapy	1:00-2:30 Volleyball

Appendix B
Day Treatment Contract

First name _____

Date _____

Problems	**Goals**	**Work**	**Strengths**
List 5 or fewer problems that bring you to Day Treatment. Be specific and concrete.	For each problem— how do I want to change?	Exactly how am I going to work on this goal in Day Treatment?	What personal quality do I have to apply to this problem— In myself or my environment?

How long will you be in Day Treatment?

Projected Graduation Date: _____

Appendix C
Relapse Plan

As you prepare to leave Day Treatment, take some time to think about and plan for how to handle a future relapse as well as for continued growth.

It is only realistic to expect that life will continue to present you with challenges, upsets and disappointments. On these occasions you will find yourself relapsing into old behavior thinking and feeling patterns that have been self-defeating for you in the past. Take some time to plan ways to handle these situations in the future.

STEP 1

Likely Trouble Spots	**Red Flags**	**Action Plan**
(List situations, thoughts, feelings, wants, or behaviors and how they are self defeating.)	Earliest point that I am aware of a trouble spot (a certain situation, thoughts, wants, feeling or behavior.)	When this happens, what is my plan?

STEP 2
What are the situations that help stabilize my life, help to avoid self-defeating behavior and keep me on an even keel? (Exercise, social contact, work, planning weekends, meds, having goals, support group, etc.)

STEP 3
What are the activities that I know will bring me enjoyment that I want to continue to cultivate after I leave?

STEP 4
Future plans for school, employment, volunteer work, and therapy, if needed. Don't forget to plan two months of Graduate Group, Wednesday 3:00 pm to 4:00 pm.

CHAPTER TWENTY-ONE

Day Activities Programming: Serving the Severely Impaired Chronic Client

Mira Coviensky and Victoria C. Buckley

This chapter was previously published in Occupational Therapy in Mental Health, *6(2), 21-30. Copyright ©1986, Haworth Press. Reprinted by permission.*

Every mental health system has a history of "treatment failures": those severely impaired chronic clients who have not responded to traditional forms of psychiatric treatment (Anthony, 1979; Sullivan, 1981; Liberman & Foy, 1983). Despite psychotherapy, family therapy, chemotherapy, partial hospitalization, intensive day treatment, electroconvulsive therapy, insight-oriented groups, task-oriented groups, vocational programs, and whatever else has been tried, these clients remain symptomatic and dysfunctional. They may have made gains, but still cannot function even within traditional sheltered mental health settings in the community.

These are clients whose paranoia may decrease but never disappears, who hear voices daily and can't ignore them to focus on reality, and whose internal world is so chaotic that the slightest change in their external world upsets whatever modicum of stability they may have achieved. These clients' cognitive-perceptual-motor problems make the simplest task into a major challenge, and seriously restrict their role functioning and performance of daily activities. For the most part, these clients are severely depressed and dissatisfied with their lives; their capacity for pleasure has diminished to the point of nonexistence (as noted also by Gruenberg, 1982). Typically, the problems have been of long-term duration, necessitating multiple, extensive psychiatric hospitalizations.

With deinstitutionalization and the creation of community residential programs and nursing home placements, these clients no longer need to spend their lives in hospitals. There is now an "uninstitutionalized generation" of chronic clients (Pepper, Ryglewicz, & Kirshner, 1982) who have spent little time in hospitals yet share similar psychiatric and functional limitations with the deinstitutionalized clients.

Without programming designed specifically for their needs, these clients are unable to use their time in a gratifying way. For them, deinstitutionalization without daily structure only increases their social isolation and emphasizes the impoverishment in their lives. Repeated exacerbations and rehospitalizations, known as the "revolving door syndrome" (Liberman & Foy, 1983), emerge as the pattern for their lives in the community.

For these reasons, in 1982, a long-term adult day activities program was designed to be a partner program to an already existing transitional intensive day treatment program. Program designs are not readily transferable from one setting to another due to culture-specific and internal idiosyncratic factors (Bachrach, 1980, 1982). Fully recognizing this, the program description offered below is intended to highlight certain essential principles generalized to the treatment of the severely impaired chronic client.

THE DAY ACTIVITIES PROGRAMS

Philosophy and Structure

The major goal of the day activities program is to give meaning to the lives of these clients in hopes of both increasing their satisfaction and decreasing the need for rehospitalization. The emphasis on quality of life inherent in this program reflects a model of health different from the traditional medical model, with the focus on occupation as opposed to cure.

The program provides an environment enabling clients to establish a health-enhancing work/play/rest balance (described by Reilly, 1966). Prior to enrollment in the program, the daily pattern of these clients was largely made up of rest and aimless wandering. Clients identified themselves as patients and as disabled. By changing the pattern of their daily activities, the program provides the opportunity for them to develop both new occupational identities, such as worker and hobbyist, and new social identities, such as friend and responsible adult. The program day has two major components: work and recreation, within a supportive milieu environment. The milieu is based on three tenets: consistency, concreteness, and normalization.

Consistency and predictability are crucial, given these clients' low tolerance for change. In addition, repetition is important for the clients to internalize norms and routines and to develop skills. Within this consistent, predictable framework is built-in flexibility and respect for individuals' needs. Clients exhibit a wide range of abilities and intellectual functioning, as well as mental status, and activities need to be adapted accordingly in order to meet clients on their own level.

The clients in the program have difficulty abstracting, and therefore have difficulty accepting the value of a process without a product. The activities and interventions are centered around tangible, concrete requirements. The clients' concreteness is also addressed by staff role modeling, allowing clients to learn new skills through direct practical observation.

Normalization is important throughout the program structure. The norms of the larger community are the norms of behavior at the program, and activities are always designed to reflect cultural relevance and the values of the larger community.

Considering the tenets of consistency, concreteness, and normalization, the balance between work, play, and rest must be actually experienced by the clients in a unified way. For this population, using isolated groups focusing on prevocational skills or leisure skills will only result in the learning of isolated skills rather than the generalization to the daily pattern of activities. The actual structure of the program must provide the concrete opportunity for clients to routinely experience the balance of work, play, and rest.

Work Component

Much of the clients' sense of failure is due to their repeated inability to succeed in one arena identified as the proper arena for adult activity: work. These are clients who have failed in prevocational programs, sheltered workshops, and transitional employment programs. They are keenly aware of the difference between meaningful productive work and "busywork." For this reason, the main criteria for the work activity is meaningfulness: the work must be considered worth doing in the values of the larger community. This sense of being truly productive may be more incentive than earning money.

There are two categories of work at the program. The first is volunteer work for other nonprofit agencies, such as the Red Cross, nursing homes, and the hospice. Typical tasks involve stuffing envelopes for mailing and making holiday decorations for nursing homes. The second is work necessary for the program itself. Examples of tasks include chores, preparing meals, gardening, and building furniture. Due to the wide range of task performance skills, the occupational therapist needs to adapt the tasks to each individual's cognitive, perceptual, motor, and psychosocial needs. Staff participate in the work itself for the purpose of role-modeling.

Due to their concreteness, it is difficult for clients to see the value of work that is not readily tangible. Details such as visibly stacking the stuffed envelopes as they are completed, or having clients involved in actually delivering the products to the nursing home, can add to clients' satisfaction with their productivity.

Since the normal pattern in society is to work first and then play, the work activities always take place in the morning. The consistency of this routine is important in addition to the aspect of following cultural norms.

Recreational Component

Chronic clients have an abundance of free time but cannot make use of the recreational resources in the community. This is due to a variety of reasons: poor task skills, unawareness of social norms, bizarre behaviors which set up rejection, paranoia, depression, inability to experience pleasure, agoraphobia, confusion, disorganization, and fear of failure. In general, the clients have little understanding of how to select or adapt recreational activities to their needs.

As for other adults, recreation should provide a balance to work. It is a chance to explore interests, establish different social contacts, and enjoy relaxed expectations of performance. As in the work component the main criteria for selecting the activities is meaningfullness. For clients to develop a sense of themselves as responsible adults, their recreations as well as their work must be consistent with normal adult values: cards, board games, trivia games, sports, walks, reading, outings, music. Several concurrent recreational activities are offered so that clients can learn to select those appropriate to their abilities and interests. Staff participate, respect individual interests, and adapt activities accordingly.

Recreation normally provides a chance to meet new people. To expand clients' social network, the recreational component of the program is open to drop-in clients from the rest of the mental health system three times a week. This serves the additional purpose of providing programming to clients unable to make a commitment to the full program. Staff again role-model so that clients can develop and practice appropriate verbal and non-verbal social skills in a nonthreatening situation.

Due to their need for concreteness and their pervasive inability to experience pleasure, it is difficult for clients to simply have a good time without a concrete task and a tangible product. It has been helpful to provide concreteness to nontangible events by such things as using prizes for games and having clients bake cakes and make decorations for parties.

Supportive Milieu Environment

As deviants in their society, these clients seldom feel a sense of belonging. Even in hospitals, they are often the ones unable to tolerate therapy groups and are only too clearly able to see the difference between themselves and the less functionally impaired patients. The milieu is therefore designed to foster a sense of belonging and security.

To encourage group cohesion, the day begins with a brief community meeting to focus on upcoming events and clients' evening or weekend plans. Lunch break provides an unstructured time for socialization in self-selected groups with staff remaining readily available to facilitate interactions.

To feel a sense of belonging, clients must have some control over their environment and choice over their participation. These choices must be respected. Clients are encouraged to be as active in decision-making and activity planning as they are comfortable with doing. Decision-making needs to be graded to not overwhelm the client, beginning with offering a clear choice between two alternatives within a consistent, predictable framework, and then gradually becoming less directive and more open-ended, making more choices available.

Throughout the program, expectations are structured in ways designed to minimize stress. These clients are hypersensitive to the demands of the environment, often misperceiving external demands due to feeling so much overwhelming internal pressure. What to staff is meant as gentle persuasion may be experienced by the client as a stressful expectation. Therefore, although every attempt is made to adapt activities to the individual, varying levels of participation are acceptable and advisable. For these clients, learning how to match the amount of stimulation and interaction to their own level of tolerance is a skill to encourage.

When clients do exceed their tolerance level and lose control, as does occasionally happen, they are given space, both in a physical and in an emotional sense. There is a lounge always kept free from groups to which clients retreat when overwhelmed. Staff interventions are supportive rather than interpretative. Depending on the situation and the needs of the particular client at that moment, one of several approaches is employed to minimize stress. These approaches include redirection, refocusing, distancing, involvement in activities, and, when appropriate, socialization. These interventions seem the most effective with this population and have the added advantage of being generalizable for clients to use in other settings and situations where trained staff are not available.

General behavior or dress inappropriate to the social norms of the larger community is dealt with as it comes up in context. The issue-oriented groups approach usually used with less severely impaired clients does not work due to the concreteness of this population. This population cannot generalize the skills learned in an isolated group, such as a grooming group, to the natural context. Therefore, a more concrete approach is needed. Bizarre behavior and dress have their natural consequences: rejection by storekeepers, stares on the street, avoidance from other clients. Behaviors are addressed by acknowledging these consequences as they occur and by offering specific concrete solutions to target problem behaviors. Self-care issues and task skills are addressed in the same way: in natural context as they arise.

The program encourages integration into the community to the extent that clients are comfortable. Lunch break is often a time during which clients shop. The location needs to be within walking distance from stores and restaurants for this to occur with minimal stress.

The site must be large enough for clients to find their own comfortable physical distance from each other and from staff. This is particularly important as clients begin to feel cohesion and closeness, an unfamiliar and initially unsettling feeling for most of them. Minimally, the program needs several large group rooms, a large kitchen, a client lounge kept free of groups, an area for gardening, and office space for staff. The setting and decor should be as nonclinical as possible to discourage clients from seeing themselves as patients.

Since the program is based on an occupational model, staff must represent disciplines which believe in the value of doing: occupational therapists, expressive therapists, rehabilitation counselors, and recreation therapists. Although volunteers are useful to augment the staff, a full-time core staff adequate for program need is crucial to provide the consistency and predictability which clients need. Currently, this program operates with a staff:client ratio of one:four.

Coordination of Treatment

These clients need a multitude of services, of which day activities programming is only one. Services provided outside the program include medication, monitoring, individual and family therapy, residential placement, case management, and crisis intervention. These additional services must take place at other sites for the day activities program to serve its purpose. Clients cannot develop identities as workers and adults in the same setting where they are treated as patients.

A well-coordinated system of communication along treatment providers is crucial, particularly to ensure smooth transitions and provide support for changes. Each client is assigned a case coordinator from among the program staff, whose role is to collaborate with the client on their treatment plans, to maintain documentation, and to coordinate with other treatment providers.

DISCUSSION

As has been previously stated, programs are not easily transplanted from one system to another. However, basic treatment principles are generalizable, and similar programs will likely encounter similar challenges.

The effectiveness of this type of programming is difficult to assess and to report to funding sources, although there is some evidence from this program and from others that day programs are in fact helpful in maintaining clients in the community (Polak & Kirby, 1976; Task Panel, 1978). Since it is neither the goal nor the expectation, the efficacy of the program cannot be judged by progressive movement out of the program. For many clients, it will take months for them to feel comfortable even within the program. Research has indicated that programs providing more occupational therapy and non-threatening milieu environments with lowered expectations are more successful with the chronic population than those expecting progressive movement (Linn, Caffey, Klett, Hogarty, & Lamb, 1979).

Changes seen in clients involve the quality of their lives and life satisfaction. The clients smile more frequently, are more socially appropriate and relaxed, and the more verbal clients can state that they feel happier.

Research needs to be done, however, to find ways to quantify such intangibles as life satisfaction with this population in order to see if day activities programming meets its stated goal of improving the quality of life. If so, the issue which can then be explored is whether there is any correlation between life satisfaction and the need for other services, particularly rehospitalization.

Although the program was established to be a long-term placement, this has been difficult for other treatment providers to accept. As clients have developed task skills and stability, there has been pressure to graduate them to a "higher level" program, despite repeated evidence from these clients' pasts that this will only lead to decompensation, and despite clients' strong desires to stay at the day activities program. Resistance to long-term placement seems related both to the values placed in society on achievement and upward mobility and the cure-oriented medical model of the mental health system.

Since long-term programs do not discharge clients, they can only expand. This is a problem both with the site capacity restrictions and with availability and adequacy of funding sources. It is also a problem for the clients. As has been noted, a major characteristic of this population is an inability to tolerate change. Each new admission has been viewed as a major disruption, and each new client has had a difficult period of entering a tightly knit group.

For staff, the clients' low tolerance for change can be frustrating. The consistency and predictability so necessary for these clients can become tedious for a creative, energetic staff.

IMPLICATIONS FOR OCCUPATIONAL THERAPY

Many of the program concepts are based on the theories of occupational behavior (Reilly, 1966, 1969; Black, 1976; Heard, 1977; Kielhofner, Burke, & Igi, 1980); however, within community mental health centers, program proposals are often judged by nonclinical administrators and members of consumer boards and need to be written in lay terms. The proposals for this particular program stressed the fact that occupational therapy was the one crucial discipline for staffing, while presenting program concepts in as non-technical language as possible. These proposals provided a unique opportunity to educate consumers and administrators about occupational therapy.

Due to their unique view of the health enhancing value of a work/play/rest balance and their ability to translate the theory into practice, occupational therapists are particularly suited to design and direct day activities programs for this population. Assertiveness is necessary to advertise this expertise and initiate programming. Occupational therapists must educate others that concentrating on psyche and symptoms can prove nonproductive and frustrating. For the severely impaired chronic client, the focus of treatment on occupation is both more meaningful and more fruitful.

REFERENCES

Anthony, W. A. (1979). The rehabilitative approach to diagnosis. In L. I. Stein (Ed.), *Community support for the long-term patient: New directions for mental health services, No. 2* (pp. 20-36). San Francisco: Jossey-Bass Inc.

Bachrach, L. L. (1980). Overview: Model programs for chronic mental patients. *American Journal of Psychiatry, 137,* 1023-1031.

Bachrach, L. L. (1982). Program planning for young adult chronic patients. In B. Pepper & H. Ryglewicz (Eds.). *The young adult chronic patient: New directions for mental health services, No.14* (pp. 99-109). San Francisco, CA: Jossey-Bass Inc.

Black, M. M. (1976). The occupational career. *American Journal of Occupational Therapy, 30,* 225-228.

Gruenberg, E. M. (1982). Social behavior in young adults: Keeping crises from becoming chronic. In B. Pepper & H. Ryglewicz (Eds.). *The young adult chronic patient: New Directions for mental health services, No. 14* (pp. 4350). San Francisco, CA: Jossey-Bass Inc.

Heard, C. (1977). Occupational role acquisition: A perspective on the chronically disabled. *American Journal of Occupational Therapy, 31,* 243-247.

Kielhofner, G., Burke, J. P., & Igi, C. H. (1980). A model of human occupation: Part 4, Assessment and intervention. *American Journal of Occupational Therapy, 34,* 777-788.

Liberman, R. P., & Foy, D. W. (1983). Psychiatric rehabilitation for chronic mental patients. *Psychiatry Annals, 13,* 539-545.

Linn, M. W., Caffey, E. M., Klett, J., Hogarty, G. E., & Lamb, H. R. (1979). Day treatment and psychotropic drugs in the aftercare of schizophrenic patients: A Veterans Administration cooperative study. *Archives of General Psychiatry, 36,* 1055-1066.

Pepper, B., Ryglewicz, H., & Kirshner, M. C. (1982). The uninstitutionalized generation: A new breed of psychiatric patient. In B. Pepper & H. Ryglewicz (Eds.), *The young adult chronic patient: New directions for mental health services, No. 14* (pp. 14). San Francisco, CA: Jossey-Bass Inc.

Polak, P. R., & Kirby, M. W. (1976). A model to replace psychiatric hospitals. *Journal of Nervous and Mental Disease, 62,* 13-22.

Reilly, M. (1966). A psychiatric occupational therapy program as a teaching model. *American Journal of Occupational Therapy, 20,* 61-67.

Reilly, M. (1969). The educational process. *American Journal of Occupational Therapy, 23,* 299-307.

Sullivan, J. P. (1981). Case management. In J. A. Talbot (Ed.), *The chronic mentally ill* (pp. 119-131). New York, NY: Human Sciences Press.

Task Panel reports submitted to the President's Commission on Mental Health: Vol. 11, Appendix. (1978). Washington, DC: US. Government Printing Office.

CHAPTER TWENTY-TWO

Changing Helplessness to Coping: An Exploratory Study of Social Skills Training with Individuals with Long-Term Mental Illness

Sisko Salo-Chydenius

This chapter was previously published in Occupational Therapy in Mental Health, *8(2), 21-30. Copyright © 1996, Haworth Press. Reprinted by permission.*

INTRODUCTION

The development of an occupational therapy program for social skills training in individuals with long-term mental illness was based on a cognitive-behavioral frame of reference. The key in helping a patient is to identify adaptive social skills through the use of goal-directed activities. The collaborative intervention process is a core of occupational therapy. Data were collected through the Group Interaction Skills Survey administered by occupational therapists and through patient self-assessment. Analysis of the results showed that social skills can be learned effectively in structured groups based on cognitive-behavioral methods.

What are Social Skills?

Social interaction is an essential part of human activity. This interaction can be described as social skills. These skills generally mean the ability to manage effectively the situations and problems of everyday life. Social skills include such everyday actions as greeting, explaining, asking, listening, discussing and interacting with others. Communication with others is both verbal through word and nonverbal through facial expressions, gestures, postures, eye contact, bodily movements and interpersonal distance. These include voice volume, fluency, pacing, affect, tone, latency to respond, and meshing of responses in a conversation and speaking. A part of nonverbal behavior may be consciously controlled, but there are other behaviors that are unconscious and involuntary (Liberman, DeRisi, & Mueser, 1989).

Social skills are a totality of behaviors that help us to communicate our emotions and needs accurately and allow us to achieve our interpersonal goals (Liberman, DeRisi, & Mueser, 1989). Social skills are influenced by cultures, rules, norms, habits and roles and a person's own conscious and unconscious needs and goals. Social skills can also be defined as purposeful ways of interaction (Salo-Chydenius, 1993).

According to Liberman, DeRisi, and Mueser (1989) communication can be broken down into a three-stage process that requires a unique set of skills.

1. *Receiving skills* are necessary to attend to and to perceive accurately the relevant social information in situations. For example, a person must recognize the environmental and interpersonal cues that will lead to communication.

2. *Processing skills* are the ability to generate response options, to assess the consequences of each alternative and choose the response that is most likely to be successful in achieving a goal. Processing skills are guided by cognitive planning ability which includes problem solving. We need to know what we want to achieve and how to achieve it. To solve the problem we need a list of possible solutions; we must evaluate the strategies and the consequences of each solution; we must select the best solution or a combination and decide how to put them into action.

3. *Sending skills* are both verbal and nonverbal actions for appropriate social responses. The style of communication is often as important as what one transmits, because it determines the effectiveness of our social

interaction. Nonverbal and paralinguistic components are the media that convey a large part of the meaning of communication, e.g., how we communicate, and what is communicated and understood by the individual receiving the message.

Deficits in Social Skills

People with long-term psychiatric disorders such as schizophrenia, depression and personality disorders usually experience deficits in social skills. This prevents these individuals from successfully engaging in everyday verbal and non-verbal communication such as initiating conversations, exchanging ideas with others, making friends, dating, negotiating or interacting with others. The deficits may prevent individuals from performing basic self-care activities, managing finances, and engaging in work and leisure pursuits. People who are unable to clearly communicate their feelings and desires to others can become lonely and vulnerable to physical or emotional problems. Being unable to express feelings and being incapable of understanding another's expressions and not having mutual satisfying relationships, is a human tragedy and an enormous, intolerable suffering (Salo-Chydenius, 1992).

There is evidence to suggest that people with serious mental illness are unable to adequately receive information and cues from the environment, as a result of attention and concentration impairments. Psychotic symptoms may also distort their interactions. Once information is received, there may be deficiencies in the way a person generates, evaluates and selects response options. (Liberman & Mueser, 1989; Franklin, 1990; Vaccaro & Roberts, 1992).

Gilbert (1992) has suggested that there is a basic need to present oneself as attractively as possible to others. We use non-verbal communication as social signals to strengthen our intentions. Mostly social signals are designed to elicit a positive interest and a sense of belonging to the other person, rather than exerting social control via threat or aggression. Ability to reach and control the attention of others in a positive way and taking the initiative in social interaction, is known as *social attention holding power* (SAHP) (Gilbert, 1992). The motivation to gain positive attention and a sense of belonging is an important part of social interaction. We try to live in the minds of others. There are various reasons for individuals who cannot direct positive social attention to themselves: lack of skills, shame, fear of rejection, lack of self-monitoring and a deficit in understanding social behavior. Individuals who do not take the initiative tend to get ignored and are experienced as indynamic. A person who shows himself or herself as not being interested, may activate feelings of resentment from others. Trust in one's own abilities and skills acts like a first opening to social interactions. A person's own estimation of his or her SAHP strongly influences, for example, taking an interest in others, showing appreciation of others, exploring another person's viewpoint and generally using a mutually valuing interactional style (Gilbert, 1992).

To understand SAHP we should focus on the social signals a person is sending and receiving. Second, we should also focus on the social signals a person would like to receive: How would you like others to behave towards you, and how do you behave toward them? We can ask ourselves: What kind of impression is a person trying to create in the minds of others? What is he or she trying to elicit from others? What kind of behavior raises (or lowers) his or her estimations of SAHP and self-worth? What is the image he or she has of himself or herself?

Why Practice Social Skills?

There are many social skills deficits which are common among individuals with long-term mental illness such as poor verbal and nonverbal communication skills, information processing difficulties and deficient problem solving abilities (Liberman & Mueser, 1989).

The aim of social skills training is to enable a patient to be more comfortable in social situations and to be more effective in communications. The focus of training is on developing coping skills, and practical and useful social skills. The desired outcome is to help a patient use these skills to become more socially competent in everyday encounters. The goals in social skills training include: teaching how to express oneself, listening to other people, problem solving, negotiating and working effectively with others. The therapy sessions are planned in advance; behavior simulation, drawing, sociodrama and role-playing are scheduled. In viva exercises and home assignments are emphasized to develop practical social skills. A supportive and positive therapeutic relationship is the core of social skills training.

Theoretical Assumptions Underlying Social Skills Training

Cognitive-behavioral theories provide important insights and operational procedures for social skills training. Controlled studies have demonstrated that structured social skills training can be effective both in enhancing the social competence of long-term patients and in reducing their vulnerability to psychiatric symptoms (Liberman & Mueser, 1989). There are many studies, that have documented the linkage of social skills to wellness. Interaction with other people is necessary for obtaining practical skills. Communication skills are intimately connected with the process of socialization; for example, learning to use, and to experience, various social roles. Several studies have found that social skills training significantly reduces symptoms and the risk for relapse in individuals with schizophrenia and depression. The patients report often that social skills training improves their quality of life. (Duncombe & Howe, 1995; Eklund, 1994; Howe & Schwartzberg, 1986; Liberman, DeRisi, & Mueser, 1989; Salo-Chydenius, 1994a.)

Social skills training has also been found to be useful when added to a holistic program including activities of daily living, independent living skills, community reintegration, vocational training, family therapy, psychotherapy, medication, housing and social support groups (Liberman, DeRisi, & Mueser, 1989).

The following premises are summarized from the findings from Falloon & Liberman (1983), Gunderson, Frank & Katz (1984), Hogarty, Anderson, & Reiss (1986), Wallace & Liberman (1985), Liberman & Mueser (1989), Liberman, DeRisi & Mueser (1989), Franklin (1990), Gilbert (1992), Ojanen (1992), Birchwood & Tarrier (1992).

1. A variety of practical skills and communication skills can be learned in structured social skills groups.

2. Moderate generalization of acquired social skills can be expected, but generalization is less with more complex social relationships. Generalization is enhanced when patients are encouraged and have demands made of them by their peers, relatives and caregivers to use their social skills in their natural environments.

3. Social skills are learned tediously or little at all by patients who are floridly symptomatic, aggressive and highly distractible. Patients who are not motivated, have little insight into their disabilities and harbour negative attitudes towards caregivers, may not benefit from the program.

4. Initially some patients report feeling anxious during the program in spite of receiving emotional and social support from the occupational therapist and other members of the group. After social skills training many patients report a decrease in their anxiety.

5. Incorporation of acquired social skills in everyday interactions depends upon duration of training and follow-up and booster sessions. Social skills training, when provided for three months to a year and integrated into a comprehensive psychiatric rehabilitation program including medication, emotional and social support, and work and leisure activities, reduces relapse and improves self-managing and social functioning of everyday life. However, many patients need continuous support to maintain their coping skills. Social skills training should be long-term, as its benefits do not become apparent before one year and are even greater after two years. As for psychiatric rehabilitation generally, social skills training is similarly optimized by continuous practical reinforcement.

RESEARCH METHOD

The goals of this study were to investigate the development of coping and social skills and to evaluate outcomes as part of a structured occupational therapy program for individuals with long-term mental illness. Changes in social skills were used as an outcome criteria. Evaluation was based on the patient's self-evaluations and it was measured through self-assessment and goal attainment forms. Occupational therapists evaluated group process systematically through the Group-Interaction Skills Survey designed by Salo-Chydenius (1994b).

An analysis of previous social skills studies (for summarized findings see above) compared with this occupational program. Social skills were evaluated through the Group Interaction Skills Survey (Salo-Chydenius, 1994b) before the group period, ongoing after every session and at the end of the occupational therapy group period by the occupational therapists leading the group. Structured and open-ended interviews with patients were used to evaluate the level of group interaction skills and social skills before the group. The assessment of group interaction skills was derived from Mosey (1986) and Gilbert (1992). Self-assessment and goal-attainment forms (Salo-Chydenius, 1994c, 1994d) were based on the work of Wallace and Liberman (1985), Liberman, DeRisi, and Mueser (1989) and Liberman (1992).

Data were collected from thirteen patients (three woman and ten men) in two groups. Each group gathered weekly, 12 times, for a 1 1/2 hour session. Two of the patients were outpatients living in a rehabilitation house, the others were inpatients. The age range was 20-55, the mean age being 30 years. All patients were diagnosed with severe psychosis and had a long history of long-term and serious mental illness. Staff were interviewed and cooperated throughout the program.

The social skills group used various methods, such as:

- self-assessment and goal-attainment forms (see Forms 2 and 3)
- drawing (e.g., descriptions of feelings, fears and hope, or through color)
- music (listening, singing, and moving)
- social skills tasks and games (e.g., small talk, greeting, thanking, congratulation, policing, 'how do you know your friend?')
- role-playing, simulation and drama (e.g., introducing oneself and introducing a fellow group member; travelling in underground trains; visiting the doctor and requesting changes in medication; getting together at a party; how to be assertive in conflict situations; how to start a discussion with another person)
- discussing feelings, hopes, fears and rules in a group.

Techniques of self-evaluation, how to set goals and problem solving were taught step by step. Charts were used to describe progress, for example:

1. eye contact
2. voice tone and volume
3. speak clearly-verbal content
4. listening to another
5. ask or answer in friendly manner.

The most important goals of the group were to facilitate communication and socialization in a small group. Group size (6-7 members plus 2 occupational therapists) was an important determinant of group processes and related not only to the goals of the group but also to the number of interactions between members (Howe & Schwartzberg, 1986). Video was a useful tool for self-evaluation, feedback and discussion.

Principles of social skills training were:

- teaching (suggestion and demonstration of the appropriate way of behavior)
- coaching (showing a model or giving practical tips to the patient when he or she is performing a task)
- giving feedback (positive and constructive feedback, both social and emotional support and feedback confronted through actions, encouraging a patient to make positive statements of himself or herself). Below is a case study example of one of the participants in the social skills training group.

CASE STUDY

Hans is a 38-year-old single man diagnosed with paranoid schizophrenia. Hans was initially hospitalized when he was 20 years old. He had symptoms of an acute psychosis (auditory hallucinations and a suicide attempt). Since this initial hospitalization, Hans has spent most of his life in a hospital. He has tried living in a halfway house, but has succeeded only for short periods. He also has problems with alcohol and is diagnosed as having polydipsia. Hans has qualified through a vocational school to become a baker, but he has not been able to acquire any work experience. His parents keep in contact with him and he regularly spends his weekend holidays at home with his parents.

Hans has received occupational therapy to increase his independence in activities of daily living. He was also referred to occupational therapy for social skills training. His main problems now were social, i.e. difficulty in expressing his own thoughts and desires, difficulty in relating to others and preoccupation with drinking alcohol.

Session 1. This was the interview. Hans answered questions mechanically without being spontaneous. He related that he was interested in joining the social skills group and he would like to initiate a friendship. His group interaction skills were at the parallel level. He smiled when the occupational therapist told him that he had been chosen to become a member of a social skills training group for six patients (Two women and four men). Two occupational therapists would be leading the group that would meet for 11 sessions.

Session 2. The goals and the methods used in the group were carefully explained to the six patients. Goals were: to express oneself, to listen to other people and to work cooperatively with others. Methods, rules and models of behavior were explained and repeated in the beginning of every session. The philosophy of the group was "learning by doing." Rules stated were:

- confidentiality
- the right to say 'no'
- respect for each other.

The occupational therapists structured the group with rules and method and ended each session with a music exercise. A self-evaluation form (Form 2) was introduced and the patients filled it out in every session. Hans needed support and help in formulating his goals, i.e.:

- I want to learn how to express myself.
- I want to learn to hold my own.
- I want to learn to compromise.

His evaluation of his social skills was realistic and he realized the need to practice his skills. Finally, when the session ended, Hans stated that 'this is hard work'.

Session 3. Problem-solving was discussed and demonstrated. One problem worked through by a patient was: How to say 'no' nicely but firmly when someone asks you to do something that you don't want to do. First, all of the alternatives were stated. The patients were encouraged to state their options, no matter how good, bad or funny they sounded. The advantages and disadvantages of each alternative were discussed in the group and the most suitable option was chosen. The situation was then role-played by two patients with the help of the occupational therapists. The occupational therapist asked Hans to role-play a person who refuses nicely, but Hans requested that he just wanted to watch.

Session 4. This was started as in previous sessions with warm-up activities. The warm-up activities (listening to music and moving to the rhythm) had become rituals at the beginning and end of each group session. The patients were instructed to 'paint all the colors in their names'. They were encouraged to be original and creative. Each patient explained his or her painting and other patients were asked to be supportive and to make positive comments.

Problem-solving and role-playing were repeated using the question raised by a patient: How do you start a discussion with another person? Videotaping was used during the role-playing and after the exercise all the other patients viewed the tape. The occupational therapists asked the patients to identify themselves in the tape and comment on their experiences. Hans told the group that he had always wanted to see himself on television.

Session 5. Videotape exercises were continued. First, everyone presented himself or herself. Second, in pairs, patients presented each other. Charting was done on: eye contact, voice tone and volume, clarity of speech, listening to others, and asking or responding in a friendly manner. These observations were used by the occupational therapists for coaching and support. Hans was worried about confidentiality and he came back after the session to see if the videotape was erased as promised.

Session 6. The theme "How to cope with hearing voices when traveling underground in a train" was presented by a patient. It was role played twice. Hans didn't want to take an active role but he participated as a silent traveler.

Session 7. This was started with coping skills exercises. Members were asked to write down as many activities as they could think of that make them feel good. They were encouraged to make suggestions to each other. Hans suggested, with a smile, that drinking beer would be nice activity that would make him feel better. Problem-solving was used to list the advantages and disadvantages of Han's behavior. The occupational therapists asked for suggestions on helping Hans to select other activities instead of drinking beer. Members suggested listening to music, calling a friend, going to the movies, watching TV. Hans realized that he shouldn't drink and he promised to alter his behavior when he had the urge to drink, for example, by calling up a group member to go for a walk.

Session 8. The theme for the role-play suggested by a patient was: "Visiting the doctor and asking to decrease medication". The theme was role-played three times changing doctor's and patient's roles. Hans was asked to play the doctor, but he refused. However, he wanted to see himself in the video and he requested he role-play the patient. Hans was coached to take a polite attitude and he managed the task very well. This was first time that he demonstrated good eye-contact with another person in the group.

Session 9. The theme "Organizing a party at home" was suggested by a patient. The patient mentioned that this is a real life problem for her and she would like to have a party with some friends but she doesn't know how to organize it. With the help of other members the simulation was done. The patient asked the group members if they had any good ideas for games or competitions. The patients suggested doing something that had been done in the group, such as free dancing. The occupational therapists suggested a 'chair-dance'. A chair-dance is started with one chair less than there are dancers. For a while the music stops and everyone tries to get a sitting place. Because there are not enough chairs somebody has to sit on someone's lap. As the dance progresses chairs are taken away one by one, and the dancers continue until there is only one chair left. Hans enjoyed this game and said that he hoped to play it again.

Session 10. Hans suggested the theme: "How to manage a conflict situation". He was asked to describe a real life situation in which there was a conflict. Hans described a problem with his father, who blames him for being lazy with housework chores. Hans wanted to role-play himself and he chose another member to role-play his father. In the conflict situation Hans shouted and argued with his "father". After discussing and watching the taped video, the situation was role-played again. Hans was coached to decrease his temper and the "father" was told the same. Hans was happy with the result, and he told his "father" that he "feels bad when his "father" blames him". The "father" was coached to respond to Hans by asking: "What can we can do together to get your room clean?" At the end of the session Hans said that he was exhausted but he appreciated the experience.

Session 11. The theme was discussion skills. As a warm-up exercise a collection of art picture cards was distributed to the members. They were asked to name as many feelings as they could that they associated with these cards. They shared their feelings in a discussion. The session ended with a discussion about group closure. Everyone was asked to collect their memories for the last session. Hans said that he would not like to end the group. He felt this would leave a vacuum in his life.

Session 12. The self-evaluation form (Form 2) for patients was completed. Hans evaluated his experience by stating, "I am working toward reaching my goals". His estimation of his own social skills had become more realistic ("I need to practice"). In response to the question about how he had been working, interacting and cooperating in the group he stated, "I have done my best, but I know that I need more practice to improve social skills". Hans related that his most important memories of the group were being engaged in various activities and the positive feedback from group members and the occupational therapists. There was a significant improvement in his group interaction skills in the evaluation by the occupational therapists. (See Figure 22-1).

RESULTS AND CONCLUSIONS

Accurate assessment of social skills is one of the most difficult areas of psychiatric rehabilitation. This study was based on the assumption that patients can give valid information in understanding their skills and abilities. Gilbert (1992), Eklund (1994), Liberman, DeRisi and Mueser (1989), and Ojanen (1992) consider patients' self-assessment and a sense of efficacy as the two most important factors in social skills development.

The results and conclusions of the study are summarized from data from two clinical groups that met for 12 sessions. The group members were selected in cooperation with the staff. There were group interviews for selecting the members. The interview gave a basic knowledge of the level of group interaction skills of the patients.

Three phases of development were clearly seen in the group. First there was the initial phase (Session 13) when the members got to know the rules and mores of the group, how to act in this group, and find out whether they could trust the occupational therapists leading the group. The atmosphere filled with expectations, and patients felt the excitement of anticipating the group. The second phase was the working period (Sessions 4-9), where new possibilities were examined and rules and norms were tested through role-playing conflictual situations, and problem solving. The atmosphere was unpredictable; sometimes members were anxious, sometimes happy and funny; while some members enjoyed activities others used more time for arguing. The third phase was the closure period (Sessions 1-12) where new information was integrated and new behavior tried out. The atmosphere was both relief and sadness, but at the same time some members started giving positive feedback and support to each other.

Form 2 was completed by the patients at the beginning of the group period. Goal-setting was taught, and patients who were not able to fill out a form were helped by the occupational therapists. The results were discussed together. Form 3 was treated in the same way at the end of the group period.

Patients reported that they experienced learning social skills training as demanding, challenging and meaningful. The following components were identified by the patients as helpful:

- being engaged in various activities
- learning new ways of dealing with problems
- peer interactions

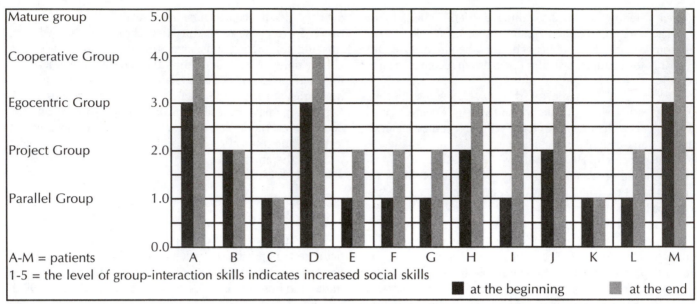

Figure 22-1. Comparing the level of group-interaction skills at the beginning and at the end of the group.

- gaining increased insight
- positive feedback from others
- empathy from the occupational therapists

The occupational therapists completed The Group Interaction Skills Survey (Form 1) after every session. The occupational therapist observed that the use of the Group Interaction Skills Survey gave them important new information. For example, in planning the next session:

- Who needs more encouragement, and who must be confronted?
- What subjects aroused interest in the group and need to be discussed?
- Which individuals demonstrated more improvement in the level of group-interaction skills than was expected?

The staff reported significant improvement in social functioning and in daily living skills.

Analysis of the results showed that social skills can be learned and improved in a structured group. There were significant positive changes in group-interaction skills. Figure 22-1 compares the level of group-interaction skills at the beginning and at the end of the group evaluated by the occupational therapists. The level 15 indicates increased social skills. A-M identify the scores for each patient.

Evaluation

The results to date are promising. However, further research is needed. Social skills are important for individuals interaction with other people and for obtaining other practical goals. There are many documented studies (Duncombe & Howe, 1995, Liberman; DeRisi & Mueser, 1989) which show the importance of social skills training as a part of a comprehensive psychiatric rehabilitation program. These studies of group occupational therapy demonstrated an increase in patient socialization and communication skills.

The role of the occupational therapist in leading the group and organizing activities is essential for the success of the group. The therapeutic relationship, supportive and positive feedback both verbal and directive, and the use of activity constitute the core of occupational therapy practice. A therapeutic relationship can be seen as a vehicle for positive change because it provides powerful social signals like compassion and empathy while appreciating another person's point of view. These signals, in turn, facilitate further communication and interaction (Liberman, 1992, Salo-Chydenius, 1992).

Enthusiasm in conducting social skills training is a key ingredient in successful outcome in addition to using goal-directed activities as a media. An understanding of activity evaluation and analysis are important tools for group leaders and will enable them to guide the group to achieve specific goals through purposeful activities. Teaching self-assessment and positive self-expectations (e.g., through drama and role-playing, self-assessment measures) encourages a patient to explore his or her thoughts, feelings and behavioral skills and to acquire new skills to develop more effective coping behaviors. Exploration and evaluation of activities together become a shared experience, which gradually increase the self-concept of a patient in becoming more active and a positive participator in social interactions. The active participation by a patient helps him or her to develop the social skills and communication tools to cope with problems in the future. Positive shared experiences increase mutual understanding and help a patient to build up purposeful coping skills which allow him or her to function at a higher level of interpersonal relationships.

IMPLICATIONS FOR FURTHER RESEARCH

In this study the occupational therapist facilitated social skills training through varied group media and used patient self-assessment. Results were encouraging. However, questions remain:

- How can the effectiveness of social skills training be most usefully measured?
- What are the factors inherent and distinctive in occupational therapy that promote desired change?
- What is the meaning to the patient of the process of activity in this change? Are therapeutic factors in occupational therapy groups as effective (or more effective) in promoting change as in those groups using discussion only?

Self-assessment and evaluative research designs may prove to be better suited for evaluating the complex factors of effectiveness in occupational therapy. Clinical research can also help us to develop new instruments and strategies for occupational therapy.

REFERENCES

Birchwood, M., & Tarrier, N. (Eds) (1992). *Innovations in the psychological management of schizophrenia.* Chichester, UK: John Wiley.

Duncombe, L., & Howe, M. (1995). Group treatment: Goals, tasks, and economic implications. *The American Journal of Occupational Therapy, 49*(3): 199-205.

Eklund, M. (1994). *First report of a progress outcome study: An occupational therapy group treatment program in a psychiatric day care unit.* Sweden: Lund University.

Falloon, I., Liberman, R. P. (1983). Interactions between drug and psychosocial therapy in schizophrenia. *Schizophrenia Bulletin 9,* 40-45.

Franklin, L. (1990). Social skills training. In J. Creek (Ed), *Occupational therapy and mental health: Principles, skills, and practice.* Edinburgh, England: Churchill Livingstone. (pp 229-246.)

Gilbert, P. (1992). *Depression. The evolution of powerlessness.* Hove UK: Lawrence Erlbaum.

Gunderson, J., Frank, A., & Katz, H. M. (1984). Effects of psychotherapy in schizophrenia. *Schizophrenia Bulletin, 10,* 564-589.

Howe, M. D., Schwartzberg, S. (1986). *A functional approach to group work in occupational therapy.* Philadelphia, PA: JB Lippincott.

Hogarty, G. E., Anderson, C. M., & Reiss, D. J. (1986). Family psychoeducation, social skills training and maintenance chemotherapy. *Archives of General Psychiatry, 43,* 633-642.

Liberman, R. P., DeRisi, W. J., & Mueser, K. T. (1989). *Social skills training for psychiatric patients.* Washington, DC: Allow & Bacon.

Liberman, R. P., Mueser, R. T. (1989). *Psychosocial treatment of schizophrenia.* Baltimore, MD: William & Wilkins.

Liberman, R. P. (1992). *Social skills training and functional assessment.* Workshop, 22nd Congress of the European Association for Behavior Therapy, Coimbra, Portugal.

Mosey, A. C. (1986). *Psychosocial components of occupational therapy.* New York, NY: Raven Press.

Ojanen, M (1992) Psykososiaalinen kuntoutus. *Psykologia, 27*(2): 145-155.

Salo-Chydenius, S. (1992). *Toimintaterapia mielenterveystyossa.* Helsinki, Finland: VAPK-kustannus.

Salo-Chydenius, S. (1993) Jakamisen ilo sosiaalisten taitojen tutkiminen ja hankkiminen. *Toimintaterapeutti, 4,* 35.

Salo-Chydenius, S. (1994a). Application of occupational therapy in the treatment of depression. *Occupational Therapy International, 1*(2), 103-121.

Salo-Chydenius, S. (1994b). *The occupational therapist's evaluation for group-interaction skills. Form 1.*

Salo-Chydenius, S. (1994c). *The self-evaluation form for patient A. Form 2.*

Salo-Chydenius, S. (1994d). *The self-evaluation form for patient B. Form 3.*

Wallace, C. & Liberman, R. P. (1985). Social skills training for schizophrenics: A controlled clinical trial. *Psychiatry Research, 15,* 239-247.

Vaccaro, J. & Roberts, L. (1992). Teaching social and coping skills. In M. Birchwood, N. Tarrier (Eds), *Innovations in the psychological management of schizophrenia* (pp. 103-144). Chichester, UK: John Wiley.

APPENDIX

Form 1: The Occupational Therapist's Evaluation of Group-Interaction Skills
(Developed by Salo-Chydenius, 1994b)

The Group-Interaction Skills Survey (Adapted from Mosey, 1986, and Gilbert, 1992)

Name: Date:

1. Parallel group
- the ability to participate in presence of others (1/2-1 hour)
- the ability to concentrate and receive information and commands
- awareness of others in the group
- have verbal and non-verbal interactions with others

2. Project group
- the ability to involve oneself in short-term tasks requiring some shared interaction and cooperation
- seeks assistance from others when needed
- the ability to help another when confronted or requested
- tries to reach and maintain social attention holding power for a while (low SAHP)

3. Egocentric group
- the ability to involve relatively long-term tasks requiring some shared interaction and cooperation
- recognizes the goals and the norms of the group
- recognizes his or her rights and responsibilities
- values the other group members
- recognizes and uses himself or herself with positive social signals
- self-motivation to reach and maintain social interaction (medium SAHP)

4. Cooperative group
- participates as an equal and mutual member
- the ability to express both positive and negative feelings to others
- recognizes the feelings of others
- behaves in an appropriate assertive way
- helps others when approached
- seeks social support and receives help.
- the ability to share thoughts, control inappropriate behavior and evaluate one's own behavior and its consequences, (high SAHP)

5. Mature group
- the ability to involve oneself in long-term tasks requiring cooperation and interaction
- flexibility in taking a varied of purposeful roles
- the ability to take the leadership task when it is appropriate
- the ability to express and recognize various feelings
- the ability to maintain long-term social interaction (high SAHP)

Form 2: The Self-Evaluation Form for Patient A
(Developed by Salo-Chydenius, 1994c)

The aim of this form is to help you to evaluate your own social skills.

My goals are:

1.

2.

3.

My own evaluation of my social skills are (good / very good / I need to practice)

1. I am able to maintain appropriate eye contact
2. I express my feelings and desires clearly
3. I am able to discuss issues appropriately
4. I listen to what others say
5. I am interested in other people and what they say
6. I understand that other people don't always agree with me
7. I am able to negotiate conflict and compromise on issues
8. I keep agreements or promises
9. I am able to behave in an assertive way
10. I would like to learn: _____

(name the social skills e.g. to express myself, to listen to others, to discuss, to accept others, to behave in an assertive way, to make compromises, to cooperate, or something else)

Form 3: The Self-Evaluation Form for Patient B
(Developed by Salo-Chydenius, 1994d).

The aim of this form is to help you to evaluate your social skills and the way you learn the new skills.

At the beginning of the group state three goals of your own.

A. Please look again at Form 1. Have you reached these goals?

B. Choose the most descriptive statement from the following:

    1. I have reached all my three goals.

    2. I have reached some of my goals.

    3. I am working toward reaching my goals.

C. My estimation of my skills in this group (good / very good / need to practice)

    1. I am able to maintain appropriate eye contact

    2. I express my feelings and desires clearly

    3. I am able to discuss issues appropriately

    4. I listen to what other people say

    5. I am interested in other people and what they say

    6. I understand that other people don't always agree with me

    7. I am able to negotiate and compromise

    8. I keep agreements or promises

    9. I am able to behave in an assertive way

    10. I would like to learn-name the social skills _____

(for example, express myself, to listen to others, to discuss, to accept others, to behave in an assertive way, to make compromises, to cooperate or something else)

D. I have been working, interacting, and cooperating in this group (Please mark your own choice in the following list)

    1. I have participated in group activities and I have been interested in other people.

    2. I have listened to other people in this group, but I have not participated very much.

    3. I have done my best, but I know that I need more practice to improve my social skills.

CHAPTER TWENTY-THREE

Occupational Therapy in Geriatric Mental Health

Susan Trace and Timothy Howell

This chapter was previously published in the American Journal of Occupational Therapy, 45, *833-838. Copyright* © *1991, The American Occupational Therapy Association, Inc.*

Elderly persons with mental illnesses present a complex picture to geropsychiatry teams. Problems such as dementia, depression, and psychotic disorders are often compounded by nonpsychiatric problems. For example, health problems or physical disability, changing or stressed support systems, loss of major life roles, and impaired performance of activities of daily living all may exacerbate the impact of the psychiatric disorder on the older person's life. The occupational therapist, with an eye toward functional skills and limitations and an educational background in physical, psychosocial, and environmental factors, can provide important information and insight to the multidisciplinary team as it strives to provide optimal services for this population.

This (chapter) describes the specific contributions of the occupational therapist to the mental health of the aged. On the basis of our clinical experience, we have identified three important outcome areas of occupational therapy intervention: preserving autonomy, enhancing integrity, and increasing personal and community safety.

Older persons with psychiatric disorders are often at risk of losing their independence at many levels, ranging from being deemed unable to choose where to live to being restrained in a geriatric chair. The occupational therapist can assist these persons in maintaining independent living (or in instituting the least restrictive measures necessary) and maximal autonomy.

The engagement or integration of older people within their life context is vital to their well-being and integrity. Detachment and inactivity are often seen among this population. The occupational therapist can contribute to the support system that is often required to enhance the integrity and productivity of aging persons.

Concerns about unsafe behaviors associated with psychiatric impairment are often paramount in the treatment of elderly persons. Measures taken to ensure safety may at times oppose the older person's desire for autonomy. While the health care team sorts through the clinical and ethical questions surrounding these issues, the occupational therapist can help to support the older person's autonomy while improving his or her safety.

Barriers to the provision of occupational therapy services to this population include limited resources, inadequate alternatives, an insufficient number of occupational therapists, need for an improved knowledge base in occupational therapy, need for quality assurance methods, and the underutilization of mental health services by the elderly.

PRESERVING AUTONOMY

Difficulties in performing instrumental activities of daily living are often experienced by persons with dementia, depression, or other psychiatric problems. These limitations raise a question as to whether a supervised setting may be required for such persons to function adequately. These persons may be capable of living independently but may have one or two limitations in instrumental activities of daily living. A thorough evaluation of their ability to perform such instrumental activities as managing money, keeping house, preparing food, and managing medications along with an evaluation of external available resources (Williams et al., 1991) allows the occupational therapist to assemble information about their abilities and areas of difficulty as well as available informal supports needed.

Often, if a problem and its cause can be identified, a solution may be reached through adaptation or assistance that can postpone or eliminate the need for institutionalization. Once the nature of the problem is determined, various measures can be implemented. Examples of adaptations for the improvement of instrumental activities of daily living abilities are enlarged telephone buttons, compartmentalized daily medication boxes, and checkbooks printed in large type. Other physical adaptations may facilitate the client's mobility or compensate for physical or perceptual difficulties. When more than adaptation is necessary, the therapist can refer the client with limitations in instrumental activities of daily living to services designed to support independent living, such as chore services, meal delivery services, and visiting nurses. These services often deter a move from the home to a nursing home or group home. To ease the caregivers' stress, the therapist may refer the family to respite programs or adult daycare centers, which also may facilitate the person's remaining in the home longer.

If the client wishes to remain in the home and has the requisite skills or resources, the therapist may advocate the client's position to the family, the clinical team, or the legal system by proposing alternatives. In areas where services, living options, and other types of resources are limited or unavailable, the therapist can advocate for these persons by increasing public and government awareness of their problems and needs. Advocacy is a natural role for occupational therapy; our therapeutic tradition has been one of subscribing to the value of independence and respecting the individual's right to choose (see Harvey, 1984, for a description of this role).

Chemical and physical restraints are used more often with the elderly than with any other population (Robbins, Boyko, Lane, Cooper, Jahnigen, 1987). Restraints are used to control behaviors considered to be dangerous or disruptive (e.g., falls, agitation). Recent legislation limits this practice and challenges the interdisciplinary team to find alternatives to controlling these behaviors (Omnibus Budget Reconciliation Act of 1987 [Public Law 100203]). The engagement of a person in a meaningful task usually reduces his or her agitation, anxiety, and wandering by channeling energy in a positive direction, thus reducing the need for restraints. Selection and modification of an activity that will be both accepted by an agitated person and successful, however, can be difficult. Activity selection requires consideration of the client's motivation, task simplification, and potential for risk if agitation escalates (e.g., the use of sharp or heavy objects is not wise when working with agitated clients). Engagement in activity can provide not only therapeutic value but also information on the precipitants of agitation, aggressive behavior, or catastrophic reactions. The therapist can share this information with other health care professionals and with caregivers to develop strategies to prevent these behaviors from recurring.

When people are restrained to prevent falls secondary to unsteadiness, poor judgment, or both, they may become physically deconditioned and thus more unsteady. Often, there may be treatable but overlooked reasons for the unsteadiness (e.g., orthostatic hypotension, sedation from psychotropic medications). Because the occupational therapist focuses on maintaining or improving function, he or she may be able to recommend interventions other than restraints. The risk of falling must be weighed carefully against the psychological and physical risks involved in the use of restraints.

ENHANCING INTEGRITY

Purposeful activity is essential to one's integrity and well-being throughout the life span (Erikson, Erikson, & Kivinick, 1986; Smith, Kielhofner, & Watts, 1986). Withdrawal or disengagement of one's usual level of activity can be a major consequence of mental illness. Due to performance deficits associated with mental illness (e.g., changes in memory, perception, energy level, or coordination), persons may develop increased expectations of failure, avoid activities, and thus experience a decline in their skills. The occupational therapist can interrupt this cycle by ensuring success or partial success in activities. Clients can thus regain a sense of productivity or even mastery, which in turn increases the likelihood that they will participate in future activities.

The loss of life roles, common in the aged, contributes to the exacerbation of a psychiatric disorder. By interviewing the client or using a role-oriented assessment tool such as the one offered by Oakley (1982), the therapist can gain insight into the current status of valued roles and how role changes have affected the client. This information, together with an idea of the client's current abilities and limitations, allows the therapist to help the client reactivate roles, even through alternative means, if necessary (Levy, 1990/1996). For example, with the move to a sheltered living situation, one may expect to lose the roles of home maintainer, hobbyist (e.g., gardening), and religious participant. Although these roles have been strongly valued and central to a person's identity, they may no longer be assumed because the client believes that he or she can no longer participate in the activity. The therapist can help the client identify the importance of these roles and ways to continue practicing them. In the sheltered facility, the client may be able to do his or her own laundry, have a windowbox garden, or be escorted to religious services. With help in identifying the importance of valued life roles and support in continuing them, the client is less likely to lose those roles.

Anhedonia, or lack of pleasure in previously enjoyable activities, is a major symptom of depression and other psychiatric disorders and can disrupt activity patterns that are conducive to good health. Activities with successful outcomes are likely to improve the client's appraisal of his or her own abilities, facilitate a belief in his or her skills, and foster a renewed sense of pleasure from doing. A determination of the presence of anhedonia is diagnostically valuable in the identification of depression and in the differentiation of depression from dementia. Persons with depression may have the component skills needed to complete a task but may show little enjoyment initially. Conversely, persons with dementia will generally enjoy a task until their skills fail them and they are unable to continue. They then may provide a spurious excuse (i.e., "My hands are sore" or "I have other things to do") to avoid a sense of failure.

Group activities are efficacious in working with this population, not only because of the inherent therapeutic benefits of group process, but also because the therapist's use of time is maximized. Due to the clients' decreased initiation of and involvement in activities, the enlistment of their participation in a group activity becomes problematic without skilled and patient intervention. Persons with psychiatric impairments living in nonspecialized (e.g., nursing homes, retirement centers) or minimally staffed settings may never engage in the groups available. Group leaders, therefore, must understand the dynamics behind a person's reluctance or refusal to participate as well as provide the time and support necessary to help the person over the hurdle of first attempting to participate. This process can be time consuming, especially with clients with dementia. Zgola (1987) described the difficulty that patients with dementia have in initiating activities as well as ways in which to facilitate engagement. She interpreted a client's refusal as being a response to the stress resulting from an inability to conceptualize what is expected, a difficulty in initiating, and the fear of failure" (p. 70). Clear directions, concrete cues, and specific first-step instructions are some of the techniques that Zgola employed to get beyond a client's reluctance to engage in the group.

In selecting activities for clients with performance anxiety or deficits, the therapist may find it helpful to build on the clients' existing skills and special interests as well as to use familiar tasks rather than tasks requiring new learning. Compensating for mistakes rather than drawing attention to them is usually more therapeutically valuable in working with persons with depression or dementia. For example, by pointing out to a woman with dementia that she is redrying dishes that she has already dried, the therapist is augmenting the client's inability to remember. Conversely, by putting the dried dishes away, redirecting the client to the wet dishes, and acknowledging the client's contributions, the therapist will be more helpful in improving the client's feelings of self-worth and integrity.

In group activities, a playful and safe arena together with positive regard for the aged client provides an encouraging foundation for exploratory behavior and helps to minimize interpersonal failures. The therapist facilitates a therapeutic psychosocial environment by modeling playful behaviors, providing an atmosphere of acceptance, and minimizing the consequences of failure. We have found the Directive Group Therapy Model (Kaplan, 1988) to be most useful in maximizing performance and facilitating group process in lower-skill level groups.

INCREASING SAFETY

Elderly patients with cognitive impairment who no longer retain skills adequate to cope with the perils of everyday life may engage in a variety of unsafe behaviors (Howell & Watts, 1990). Risky behaviors, such as reckless or inattentive driving, unsafe use of heating devices, and careless smoking, may jeopardize both the client and the community as a whole. Other examples of risky behaviors include the mismanagement of medications, neglect of nutritional and health concerns, and consumption of spoiled food. Memory loss, inability to recognize or appreciate the consequences of actions, and lack of insight concerning physical or mental impairments may contribute to such behaviors. Restrictive decisions (e.g., selling the car, hospitalization) are often made by the family, medical team, or legal system and compromise the client's personal liberty. The risk of an activity and its consequences must be carefully weighed against other factors, such as whether the benefits of protection are worth the loss of autonomy (Watts, Cassel, & Howell, 1989). The discovery or development of measures that will improve safety with the use of the least restrictive means will yield workable solutions in such situations. The insights that the therapist lends to this search can help ensure that the goals of safety and autonomy are optimally balanced.

Functional assessment is of critical importance and is a key contribution of the occupational therapist in the assessment of safety issues. By using assessment tools and observing task performance, the therapist obtains information about the client's ability to maintain safe behavior and the likelihood of a risky situation recurring. For example, watching the client perform the simple task of making a cup of instant coffee allows the therapist to observe the client's judgment, memory, ability to understand the implications of abstract concepts (i.e., heat), coordination, and praxis. Does the client remember to attend to the pot without cues? Does he or she handle and pour hot materials safely? Does he or she turn off the stove when finished? Through observation, the reasons for an unsafe behavior like hazardous cooking can often be identified. For example, unsafe use of the stove may be due to problems with memory, awareness, judgment, or vision. Once the reason is ascertained, the therapist can recommend specific environmental adaptations or treatment to decrease the recurrence of the unsafe situation.

In the home or institutional setting, the occupational therapist can suggest critical environmental adaptations that may decrease the older person's risk of harm to self or others. For example, the therapist can mark stairs and remove or tape down throw rugs to compensate for the client's perceptual difficulties and to prevent falls, thus preserving mobility and saving costly medical bills. Adaptations to a stove unit also may improve safety. Marked dials for improved visibility or automatic shut-off features to compensate for forgetfulness are examples of such adaptations. Visible cues such as labels or pictures on doors or drawers may assist persons with memory or orientation deficits. The removal of items that could be misused by a person with cognitive impairment (e.g., poisons, sharp objects, weapons, heating devices) may also decrease the risk of harm. (See Skolaski-Pellitteri, 1983, 1984, for more information on this topic.)

Medication management can be important for the maintenance of safety and well-being. Elderly persons are prone to misuse both prescription and over-the-counter medications (Carruthers, 1986). They commonly have multiple medical conditions, each of which requires medication, thereby adding to the complexity of medication management. Additionally, because elderly persons are often more sensitive to medications than are younger people, there is less margin for error in the avoidance of side effects. The occupational therapist can assess the skills needed for the independent administration of medication, including the client's memory, orientation to time, fine motor dexterity, vision, and understanding of possible side effects. This assessment may indicate the need for a supervised trial of self-medication. Adaptations such as pillboxes holding premeasured amounts, easy-opening containers, large print, and color-coded labels may facilitate the client's independence in this task. Simplification (e.g., having the physician adjust times or dosages) may also improve the potential for correct medication use.

Another related role of the occupational therapist is to monitor functional performance as psychotropic medications are titrated (Allen, 1985). With the narrowed margin of effectiveness of such medications in the elderly, close monitoring can prevent improper medication or over-medication. Medication may have adverse effects on mobility, attentiveness, continence, communication, and cognition. These effects may be associated with akathisia, confusion, incontinence, sedation, and even delirium. The occupational therapy session provides a more natural environment in which to observe a person for a longer period than that usually provided in a brief visit with the physician.

BARRIERS TO OPTIMAL SERVICE PROVISION

One cannot discuss occupational therapy in geriatric mental health without also addressing barriers to optimal outcomes of intervention. In the health and social service systems, as well as within the profession, there is often a lack of sufficient resources to best meet the client's needs.

Although the range of care alternatives for the elderly client has grown considerably in recent years, for most clients options for services are inadequate in several ways. There continue to be, especially in rural areas, limited sheltered housing options, too few respite or specialty area within the profession. Higher visibility is of primary importance in continued efforts by the profession to recruit therapists in geriatric mental health.

The need for standardized, validated assessments for elderly persons with psychiatric problems will continue. Measures of abstract concepts (e.g., quality of life) are needed for quality assurance. Advocacy and education of the public and government to increase awareness of the growing needs of elderly persons with mental illness and their families will continue to be important issues for both the practicing therapist and the profession as a whole.

REFERENCES

Allen, C. (1985). *Occupational therapy for psychiatric diseases: Measurement and management of cognitive disabilities.* Boston, MA: Little, Brown.

Carruthers, S. G. (1986). Principles of drug treatment in the aged. In I. Rossman (Ed.), *Clinical geriatrics* (pp. 114-124). Philadelphia, PA: Lippincott.

Erikson, E. H., Erikson, J. M., & Kivinick, H. Q. (1986). *Vital involvement in old age.* New York, NY: Norton.

Ezenky, S., Havazelet, L., Scott, A. H., & Zettler, C. L. B. (1989). Specialty choice in occupational therapy. *American Journal of Occupational Therapy, 43,* 227-233.

Gibson, O. (1990). The challenge of adaptation: Shaping service delivery to meet changing needs. *Hospital and Community Psychiatry, 41*(23), 267-269. (Reprinted in Cottrell, R. P. (1993). *Psychosocial occupational therapy: Proactive approaches* (pp. 11-14). Bethesda, MD: AOTA.)

Harvey, L. (1984). Advocacy and the aged: A case for the therapist-advocate. *Physical and Occupational Therapy in Geriatrics, 3*(2), 515.

Hasselkus, B., & Dickie, V. (1990). Themes of meaning: Occupational therapists' perspectives on practice. *Occupational Therapy Journal of Research, 10,* 195-205.

Howell, T., & Watts, D. (1990). Behavioral complications of dementia: A clinical approach for the general Internist. *Journal of General Internal Medicine, 5,* 431-436.

Kale, R., Ouslander, J., & Abrass, L., (1984). Essentials of clinical geriatrics. New York, NY: McGraw-Hill.

Kaplan, K. (1988). *Directive group therapy: Innovative mental health treatment.* Thorofare, NJ: SLACK Incorporated

Levy, L. (1990). Activity, social role retention and the multiply disabled aged: Strategies for intervention. *Occupational Therapy in Mental Health, 10,* 1-30. (Reprinted in Cottrell, R. P. (1996). *Perspectives on purposeful activity: Foundation and future of occupational therapy* (pp. 423-435). Bethesda, MD: AOTA.)

Oakley, F. (1982). *The Model of human occupation in psychiatry.* Unpublished master's research project, Virginia Commonwealth University, Richmond.

Omnibus Budget Reconciliation Act of 1987 (Public Law 100-203). Title IV, Subtitle C, Nursing Home Reform.

Robbins, L. J., Boyko, E., Lane, J., Cooper, D., & Jahnigen D. W. (1987). Binding the elderly: A prospective study of the use of mechanical restraints in an acute care hospital. *Journal of the American Geriatric Society, 35,* 290-296.

Skolaski-Pellitteri, T. (1983). Environmental adaptations which compensate for dementia. *Physical and Occupational Therapy in Geriatrics, 3,* 25-32.

Skolaski-Pellitteri, T. (1984). Environmental intervention for the demented person. *Physical and Occupational Therapy in Geriatrics, 3,* 55-59.

Smith, N. R., Kielhofner, G., & Watts, J. H. (1986). The relationships between volition, activity patterns, and life satisfaction in the elderly. *American Journal of Occupational Therapy, 40,* 278-283. (Reprinted in Cottrell, R. P. (1996). *Perspectives on purposeful activity: Foundation and future of occupational therapy* (pp. 299-305). Bethesda, MD: AOTA.)

Watts, D., Cassel, C., & Howell, T. (1989). Dangerous behavior in a demented patient: Preserving autonomy in a patient with diminished competence. *Journal of the American Geriatric Society, 37,* 658-662.

Williams, J., Drinka, T., Greenberg, J., Farrell-Hoitan, J., Euhardy, R., & Schram, M. (1991). Development and testing of the Assessment of Living Skills and Resources (ALSAR) in elderly community-dwelling veterans. *Gerontologist, 31,* 84-91.

Zgola, J. (1987). *Doing things*. Baltimore, MD: Johns Hopkins University Press.

CHAPTER TWENTY-FOUR

An Expanded Community Role for Occupational Therapy: Preventing Depression

Alisa Ofsevit Eilenberg

This chapter was previously published in Physical and Occupational Therapy in Geriatrics, *5(1), 47-57. Copyright © 1986, Haworth Press. Reprinted by permission.*

Depression is a formidable illness currently threatening the well-being of countless community elderly. Their social isolation, the physical changes of aging and a societal focus on youth and the roles and skills of the young cause this group to be particularly vulnerable to depression. Therapeutic approaches employed by occupational therapists can be effectively applied to promote mental health and prevent depression in the community elderly.

After several years of working with institutionalized elderly psychiatric patients, many of whom had been admitted for depression, the author's focus turned to prevention stimulated by a course taken in the advanced Occupational Therapy Program at Columbia University. As part of a related practicum at a senior center, the author designed and implemented a time-limited program to foster independence and prevent depression, as well as to observe the multidisciplinary efforts being made toward this end on an experimental basis. This preparation helped in the planning of the theoretical and practical aspects of the "Wellness Program" now carried out at the Mamaroneck Senior Center in Westchester.

FRAMES OF REFERENCE

The wellness program is based on several frames of reference that form a comprehensive approach to preventing depression and promoting the health of the community elderly. The first frame of reference is developmental. Erikson, as cited in Belkin, described the chief challenge of old age as a struggle of "ego identity versus despair." Successful resolution of this life stage involves a sense of peace and acceptance of life's accomplishments and failures, an overall sense that one's life has been worthwhile. He suggests that depression results if this perspective is not attained (1980). Peck, as cited in Weiner, elaborates on Erikson's view by listing more specific tasks of old age, including adaptation to work and family role changes by the establishment of varied, valued activities. He stresses the importance of transcending physical and cognitive limitations and discomforts while enjoying social interaction. A further task is the focusing on making some contribution to the welfare of future generations rather than the preoccupation with death that so often accompanies depression (1978). The Wellness Program seeks to help members attain these goals and overcome the limitations of aging as each individual finds him or herself at a different point of development.

A sensory-integrative frame of reference focuses on the human need for adequate, varied and meaningful stimulation. Ideally, this input is then processed by the brain and permits daily adaptive behavior. Sensory integration is typically compromised in the elderly. Sensory systems such as sight, hearing, taste and smell are commonly diminished. The sense of joint movement and position in space may be impaired because of arthritic changes and reduced nerve conduction. The consequences of these changes are frequently slowed and cautious movement and decreased overall activity.

Socialization, a most important type of sensory and mental stimulation, is also compromised in the aged. This is due to death and relocation of friends [and] relatives (particularly spouses), and the scarcity of extended family systems in this society.

The author's previous research into the sensory integrative needs of the elderly indicates that disuse of existing sensory-motor abilities only accelerates the deterioration of these systems. The inactivity and withdrawal that can accompany these losses puts the elderly at great risk of depression.

Numerous studies of sensory deprivation demonstrate that inadequate stimulation and/or processing of information have devastating physical, cognitive and emotional effects, including vulnerability to disease, confusion, decreased motor skills, irritability and general withdrawal (Ofsevit, 1980).

Given the importance of sensory-integrative function, it is crucial that these needs be addressed in any program designed to prevent depression in the elderly. In the Wellness Program, a dance and movement part of each session is an important tool in meeting sensory integrative needs of members.

A learning model is another useful frame of reference in the design of the Wellness Program. There is an assumption that given the motivation, new skills can be learned and changes made in a lifestyle late in life. Mosey (1971) states that learning takes place as a consequence of positive reinforcement. In the Wellness Group, the reinforcement includes peer and leadership support for constructive changes, as well as the innate satisfaction that comes from mastery of one's environment. The forming of individualized goals, which, when met, increase members' sense of their autonomy, is a valuable approach to preventing the sense of helplessness that so often accompanies depression. The group problem-solving approach is a useful means to this end.

An additional frame of reference is the systems approach. This approach is useful in understanding the structure of any organization: staffing patterns, membership composition, goals, mandates, and constraints of the institution. It was helpful in initially determining how occupational therapy skills could be applied toward furthering the existing goals of the senior center through the implementation of a new program and in maintaining open lines of communication for the ongoing success of the program.

Program Setting

The Mamaroneck Senior Center has a membership of approximately two hundred from the Westchester area. It provides hot lunches Monday through Friday, daily activities, special events, and referrals for members in need of community services. Mamaroneck Human Resources is particularly involved in this regard. Staffing includes a chief administrator, site manager, a secretary, assistants, kitchen workers, as well as volunteers and consultants who conduct activity programs. The senior center is supported by federal funds which are scheduled to be gradually phased out, as well as by the town of Mamaroneck. Local community organizations frequently contribute toward special needs or events at the center.

The senior center aims to meet the social and recreational needs of its membership. There is also an awareness of the increasing frailty of members and the difficulties faced by them in terms of remaining well and independent in the community. The administrators were thus receptive to the idea of a Wellness Program which would have the aim of promoting health in this group at risk for physical deterioration, social isolation, and depression.

In introducing the Wellness Program at the center the author described the role of occupational therapists in different settings and with varied age groups. Life tasks change with the aging process. Older adults have tremendous adjustments to make to role changes, as children leave home, retirement arrives, and a spouse dies. The many physical changes that occur with aging often begin to interfere with the performance of daily activities. The purpose of the Wellness Program was to help older people make the fullest possible use of their abilities and to stay well and able to live in the community as long as possible.

An open discussion and written survey were provided to determine the unique health concerns of this population. Large and small group meetings were held as well as two consecutive sessions with individuals. Physical concerns expressed included arthritis, managing household tasks, improving posture, coping with pain, and getting adequate exercise. Psychosocial subjects of concern included living alone, using time more fully, and meeting new friends.

Following the written survey, members were invited to sign up for the Wellness Group. Potential participants were encouraged to give the group a try. The group was to be conducted in time-limited phases, after which members were free to continue or to leave. Individuals were pleased to know that the program would be geared to their needs, [and] that no one would be pressured to participate beyond what was comfortable for them. Staff was helpful in identifying individuals who could benefit from the program. The response was enthusiastic. So many members signed up that a waiting list had to be started.

Methodology

The Wellness Group's objectives were influenced by the expressed needs of the population. This approach fostered the objectives of helping participants to discover and make use of their strengths, express their health needs and thus to realize the impact they can have on shaping their lives and environment. Another objective is for group members to form a supportive network of friendships at the senior center. A further objective is for members to gain and share knowledge about preserving physical abilities and compensating for deficits as these relate to activities of daily living. Yet another objective is for participants to understand a balanced, fulfilling use of time for them personally.

The group has a maximum enrollment of 15 members per 8-week phase; each phase covers a specific topic. Every group begins with a 1-hour discussion, using a group problem-solving approach. A half hour of movement follows, including posture, breathing, and warm-up exercises along with selected ballroom, folk, and free-style expressive dance. The author meets with individuals during the final half hour. At the end of each 8-week phase, members are asked to assess the program via discussion and written survey.

The senior center's site manager helps publicize the group through the monthly calendar, weekly announcements, and an attitude of enthusiastic support. Senior center staff set up the group's meeting area in advance. Periodic meetings are held with the site manager and the chief administrator to discuss the outcome of the group, and any difficulties or questions that arise.

The Wellness Group meets in the one long, large, often crowded room that comprises the temporary accommodations for the senior center during its renovation. A corner of the room is set up with a record player and a circle of chairs. Tables are pushed away to allow for needed space. The membership is asked to assist the group by keeping their voices lower than usual, since a high noise level interferes with discussion.

SAMPLE SESSIONS

Physical discomforts and increasing dependency that stem from arthritic conditions so common in the elderly can produce feelings of depression. The first series of sessions was devoted to arthritis and learning joint protection concepts, since this was the main priority indicated in the initial survey. Topics covered included resources for relieving and coping with pain, safety and management issues around the home, posture and body mechanics, and resources for coping with arthritis.

The theme of one particular session was finding a balance between rest and activity. The group was asked how they determined whether a household or other task was too much for them to handle. One woman described the enormous task of cleaning her fish tank. She had made it more manageable by emptying it out cup by cup. It was still exhausting and she felt that the only solution was to give up having the fish. Although this solution would be acceptable if the fish were no longer important to her, it was suggested that an alternative might be found if an effort were made to creatively solve the problem. That led to the topic of when, whom, and how to ask for help. Possible resources, such as family and friends, were mentioned. The group discussed the advantages of calling upon them, the "price paid" for doing so or for not doing so. The importance of the timing of a request was discussed, along with consideration of the resource person's mood and obligations

The tone of voice and attitude of the person making the request were explored. Participants pointed out that a demanding or hurried tone could make others less willing to help. It was also noted that firm self-advocacy was at times needed in case of hazards, such as when one member's window would not close during a harsh winter.

Mamaroneck Human Resources was mentioned as an additional resource. Members had heard that high school students and retirees were available for assistance with heavy tasks such as household repairs and that senior center staff might know more about specifics.

The group concluded with posture, breathing, and warm-up exercises. There was dancing in pairs and as a group to old-time jazz. All were encouraged to take part within their individual limitations and capacities. The mood of the group was light-hearted and cheerful. There was much enthusiastic participation.

The second phase of the Wellness Program dealt with developmental social concerns that can be handled constructively or make the elderly more vulnerable to depression. In this sample session, the group discussed the benefits and drawbacks of living alone. One member said that she thought it was fine for younger people to live alone, but that she would not want to do so at this time of life. Another woman had managed to live alone with no difficulty for many years. After her marriage late in life, however, when her husband was hospitalized, she found it a shock and nerve-wracking to suddenly be alone again.

One participant is usually withdrawn, in pain and has memory problems. He complained that it was terrible to live alone. When the group suggested he consider taking in a "boarder," he was emphatic that such a step would impinge on his freedom and independence. He didn't want to answer to anyone or be dictated by their needs. The group laughed in response to his description of some of the benefits of living alone.

A member whose husband lives in an institutional setting expressed her contentment with the flexibility of living alone. No one tells her when to go to sleep or get up, and she feels able to find all the company she needs outside of her home. Her one concern was security. She had worked to improve the building's security by fighting to get a front entrance lock, and so was no longer afraid of break-ins.

The group discussed security problems and measures to be taken, including getting a free security appraisal by the police.

Another member of the group had never married. Living alone was never a problem until recently, when she began to feel the need to have "someone around." We discussed the fact that needs often change over time. The group discussed housing alternatives and the fact that many older people are trying group living situations and taking in roommates.

The movement session following the discussion included warm-ups, dancing in pairs to square dance music, and free-style expressive dance.

Other topics covered in this phase were members' work and family backgrounds, current living situations, relocating, and making friends later in life.

Additional Group Topics

The extensive leisure time that older people are often faced with after retirement can be a source of new enjoyment or it can be a source of burdensome loneliness. A fulfilling use of time is quite important in preventing depression. It is vital in meeting sensory-integrative needs for variety and meaningful stimulation. A 12-week phase of the program was devoted to the developmental task of exploring options to enhance or improve the use of time.

This particular session focused on adult education. The group was asked whether it was harder to learn earlier or later in life. One woman said she was concerned that she would not retain as much information now as she could when she was younger. Others had the same concern. We talked about ways to compensate for slight memory losses that affect many older people. One method mentioned was to have the instructor review material to reinforce learning. Other approaches discussed were practicing skills at home, reviewing with a classmate, and taking notes. It was pointed out that some types of courses such as film or music appreciation do not rely heavily on memory. It was noted that another aspect of successful learning later in life is one's attitude. If older students take a realistic and tolerant view of their abilities, they may enjoy the experience of learning without constantly comparing themselves to other learners.

Transportation as an issue that can help or interfere with taking classes was discussed. Accessibility and cost of transportation were considered. We discussed car pools, taxi pools, buses, and the possibility of exploring town funding to help older people attend classes.

The group concluded with exercise and dance to international folk music. Increased participation of members who had been reluctant to take part earlier was noted.

Additional topics covered during this phase were volunteer and work options, museums, theater and concert attendance, and other recreational options.

OBSTACLES ENCOUNTERED

Several factors have interfered with the group. One has been the physical setting of the Wellness Program. Leading a small group within a single, large and busy room has caused frequent distractions and interruptions. It poses a particular challenge to participants who are hearing impaired or distractible. This difficulty should be resolved with the completed renovation of the original senior center which will include small meeting rooms.

Another problem has been the varied demands on participants' schedules. In the community, events such as holiday preparation or even clothing sales can reduce attendance. Weather and illness inevitably interfere as well. Although flexibility is needed, participants should be reminded that attendance is a commitment and that each member is an important and valuable part of the group. The site manager has been most helpful in reinforcing the importance of attendance and in locating members who fail to attend.

Funding has severely limited the time that can be devoted to the Wellness Program. A more extensive program could reach more people, allow for more teaching and reinforcement of the kinds of adaptive skills mentioned earlier, and permit leadership in time consuming projects that would benefit a large portion of the senior center membership.

ASSESSMENT OF THE PROGRAM

After the first eight-week phase of the group, a written survey was provided to assess the effectiveness of the group.

Eleven of the thirteen regular members completed the survey. The following quotations are some representative responses to the questions, "How did the group benefit you, if at all?" and "Has the group influenced your lifestyle in any way?"

"I realized not to feel bad when I can't do ordinary things but to accept it and work around it. There always is a way." "I exercise more often."

"It helped to talk about the problem and bring it out in the open." "I realized I've got to get a little more exercise."

"It was a time to participate in the different exercises and to get to know the other people." "Made more friends, made me aware of how to help myself in many tasks, and to know where to look for help should I ever need it."

When asked how the group might be improved, participants who responded in the earlier survey expressed complete contentment with the structure of the group, praising the leadership as being motivating and enthusiastic. Only in the most recent survey were members at all critical. There were requests for a larger group, for craft instruction, and for more time to be devoted to movement. This suggests that over time, group members have become more secure and autonomous in terms of voicing their needs.

The group and leader have made various observations about members during the course of the sessions. The group spontaneously told one member who had been initially lethargic that she looked more awake and happy. Another participant reported feeling much more energetic after practicing some of the exercises at home. In time, this same group member took on greater responsibility within the senior center and demonstrated considerable creative abilities in that setting for the first time. Another participant who had always considered herself "just a listener" found that to her satisfaction, she was eventually able to express her own opinions. Two members began volunteer jobs in the course of the sessions, and one decided to take driving lessons in order to take fuller advantage of leisure options.

These changes occurred over weeks and months. The size and supportive nature of the group, as well as the structure, which is carefully tailored to address the needs of a specific group of older adults, has greatly helped members to make the most of their abilities and promote their health on many levels. Those who entered the group withdrawn and isolated clearly benefited from the program at least for short periods of time. Members who came with greater personal strengths have made fuller use of their resources and inspired their peers in the process.

IMPLICATIONS FOR OCCUPATIONAL THERAPY PRACTICE

There is a vast and increasing population of community elderly in need of preventive services. Some are obviously depressed, while many experience low levels of depression which are not dramatic, but nevertheless take a heavy toll in terms of socialization, disuse of existing living skills and physical abilities. Their potential contribution to their own welfare, to their families and communities is being lost.

Occupational therapists have the potential skill for organizing preventive programs. Our holistic training provides a perspective on the developmental needs of each age group. Our schooling in the basic sciences gives us a grasp of the physical changes and sensory-integrative needs of old age. We are creative teachers equipped to assess individual needs, teach living skills, and motivate clients in the face of many obstacles.

Occupational therapy educational programs need to focus more on prevention and the burgeoning needs of the elderly. Training must include an understanding of and practical experience in community organizations to help therapists feel secure in noninstitutional settings.

At the highest levels of the professional association, occupational therapists must take an active role in paving the way for community practice. Most community organizations that serve the elderly either are unfamiliar with occupational therapy or associate any kind of therapy with hospitals and the ill. The scarcity of funds for new programs within community organizations makes it equally difficult if not impossible for occupational therapists to support themselves doing preventive work in the community.

As a professional body, occupational therapists need to lobby government officials and endeavor to educate the public about the at-risk community elderly and how our services might be used to keep older people independent and well in the community as long as possible.

Occupational therapy can and should assume a substantial role in preventive services for the elderly. Prevention programs address a relatively neglected area: keeping older people healthy. The possibility of preventing unnecessary use of more costly care needs to be carefully explored through research. The author's experience indicates that much of the isolation, despair, boredom, and physical deterioration that face the community elderly can be reduced and to some extent reversed by preventive occupational therapy programs.

REFERENCES

Belkin, G. S. (1980). *An introduction to counseling* (pp. 262-263, 270, 280-281). Dubuque, IO: Wm. C. Brown.

Mosey, A. C. (1971). *Three frames of reference for mental health* (p. 109) (3rd edition). Thorofare, NJ: SLACK Incorporated.

Ofsevit, A. (1980). *The effect of a sensory integration movement group on life satisfaction for the frail elderly* (unpublished Occupational Therapy Masters Thesis) Columbia University.

Weiner, M. B., Brok, A. J., & Snadowsky, A. M. (1978). *Working with the aged—Practical approaches in the institution and community* (pp. 27-29). Englewood Cliffs, NJ: Prentice Hall.

BIBLIOGRAPHY

Burnside, I. (1984). *Working with the elderly group process and techniques* (2nd edition). Monterey, CA: Wadsworth.

Butler, R., & Lewis, M. (1977). *Aging in mental health: Positive psychosocial approaches* (3rd edition). St. Louis, MO: Mosby.

Caplow-Lindner, E., Harpaz, L., & Samberg, S. (1979). *Therapeutic dance movement—Expressive activities for older adults*. New York, NY: Human Sciences Press.

CHAPTER TWENTY-FIVE

Occupational Therapy for Independent-Living Older Adults: A Randomized Controlled Trial

Florence Clark, Stanley P. Azen, Ruth Zemke, Jeanne Jackson, Mike Carlson, Deborah Mandel, Joel Hay, Karen Josephson, Barbara Cherry, Colin Hessel, Joycelynne Palmer, and Loren Lipson

This chapter was previously published in the Journal of the American Medical Association, 278, *1321-1326.* Copyright © 1997. Reprinted with permission.

The number of Americans aged 65 years or older has risen dramatically from 3.1 million persons (4% of the US population) in the early 1900s to over 33 million persons (nearly 13% of the population) in 1995.[1] It is projected that over 17% of the American population will be elderly by the year 2020, that 42% of this group will be older than 75 years, and that the "oldest group" (aged 85 years or older) will more than double in size by 2030 and will nearly double again by 2050.[2] If present trends persist, it can be expected that longer life spans will be marked by poorer health-related quality of life.[3,4]

Health-related quality of life is generally thought of as "those aspects of self-perceived well-being that are related to or affected by the presence of disease or treatment",[5,p.1348] encompassing such dimensions as physical and social functioning, bodily pain, and vitality.[5,6] While aging, per se, may account for certain losses its role has generally been overstated.[4,7] For example, chronic disease has become the most severe health problem among older adults and often leads to chronic disability. Older adults are also presented with unique psychological stressors (e.g., financial hardship, death of a spouse, retirement) that can contribute to psychiatric disorders such as depression, paranoia, or anxiety that leads to substance abuse.[7,10-12] In addition, older individuals are confronted with social stressors (e.g., changes in roles, difficulty interacting with the surrounding environment, and logistical problems performing daily activities) that may lead them to discontinue lifelong pursuits and experience a decrease in life satisfaction.[12,13]

Studies of what is now referred to as "successful aging" reveal that considerations extrinsic to aging or disease such as diet, lifestyle and daily routine, degree of social support, amount of exercise, and sense of autonomy and control play a strong positive role in enabling older individuals to maintain their health and independence.[9,14-16] Research has shown that remaining active and productive is a key component of successful aging. Such findings offer hope for the potential to design effective activity-based interventions capable of enhancing the lives of elderly individuals. However, given the diversity of challenges faced by older adults, the complexity of interlocking physical, psychological, economic, and social factors must be taken into account.

In response to this need, we conducted between 1994 and 1996 a randomized controlled trial, the Well Elderly Study, to evaluate the effectiveness of preventive occupational therapy specifically targeted for urban, multi-ethnic, independent-living older adults. Typically, occupational therapy is provided to older individuals to facilitate independence after catastrophic illness or accidents when significant functional impairment or disability is present.[9,17-19] However, we reasoned that many of the principles of occupational therapy intervention, given their focus on fostering productive and meaningful activity (occupation), maximizing independence, and enhancing function, constituted a potentially effective approach to preventing illness and disability and promoting the health in this vulnerable population. We hypothesized that mere participation in a social activity program does not affect the physical health, daily functioning, or psychosocial well-being of well elderly individuals; and compared with participation in a social activity or an absence of any treatment, preventive occupational therapy positively affects the physical health, daily functioning, and psychological well-being of well elderly individuals (1-sided alternative).

METHODS

Study Subjects

The planned study population was independent-living, culturally diverse men and women, aged 60 years or older, who had the capacity to benefit in multiple outcome areas from involvement with occupational therapy. Subjects were excluded if they were unable to live independently or if they exhibited marked dementia. In response to the need to accrue study subjects and to assess the effectiveness of occupational therapy among a non-English-speaking population, the study population was augmented to include Mandarin-speaking subjects. Inclusion of Mandarin speaking subjects required the cultural adaptation and translation of the research protocol and testing instruments into Mandarin and use of Mandarin-speaking occupational therapists and social activity control group leaders during all phases of the study.

Subjects were recruited from residents of Angelus Plaza (a large government subsidized apartment complex for independent-living seniors in Los Angeles, Calif), from residents in private homes or other facilities in the surrounding areas who used the Angelus Plaza Senior Citizen facilities, or from residents of Pilgrim Tower (a government subsidized apartment complex in Pasadena, Calif). To maximize the resources at the Angelus Plaza and Pilgrim Tower facilities (the evaluation and treatment sites), to reduce the effects of seasonal changes on the study, and to minimize the effects on subject interaction, subjects were recruited at different times in 2 cohorts, with the second cohort completing each study phase approximately 11 months after the first cohort. Methods of recruitment included staffed recruitment tables placed in facility lobbies and at onsite functions such as dances and coffee houses, flyers, articles in the residence newsletter, presentations at regular meetings such as the Senior Citizens Club, and letters placed under residents' doors. All study volunteers sign an institutionally approved informed consent form prior to study enrollment.

A questionnaire was used to collect information on subjects' sex, age, ethnicity, medical conditions, number of current medications, disabilities, marital status, education level, number of children, languages spoken, and length of residence at Angelus Plaza or Pilgrim Tower (where applicable). An occupational therapist administered the Tinetti balance examination to each subject. A physician trained in geriatric medicine conducted a medical history, performed a physical examination, and evaluated the health status of each subject using standardized instruments including the Modified MiniMental State Examination (MMSE),[22] the (self-reported) Geriatric Depression Scale,[23] and the LaRue Global Assesment.[24]

Randomization and Treatment

Using a completely randomized design with computer generated random numbers and a blocking factor of 6, we assigned eligible subjects to one of three treatment groups within strata defined by language of testing: an occupational therapy group, a generalized group activity ("social") control group, or a non-treatment control group. Subjects in the occupational therapy group were encouraged to attend all treatment sessions and to refrain from discussing their treatment experience with other subjects. Subjects in the social control group were encouraged to participate in all activity sessions and to refrain from discussing their activities with subjects from other groups. The period of treatment was 9 months.

The central theme of the occupational therapy program was health through occupation, with occupation defined not in the conventional sense of type of employment, but more broadly as regularly performed activities such as grooming, exercising, and shopping. Findings from two previous studies,[25,26] principles extracted from the occupational science literature,[27-31] and approaches conventionally used in occupational therapy[18-20] were drawn on to design the occupational therapy protocol. The key intent of the treatment was to help the participants better appreciate the importance of meaningful activity in their lives, as well as to impart specific knowledge about how to select or perform activities so as to achieve a healthy and satisfying lifestyle.[32] The therapeutic approach entailed exposing the subjects to both didactic teaching and direct experience with a broad range of activities. Concurrent with this exposure, each subject was asked to analyze the role of each activity in affecting health and well-being in his or her personal life. Modular programmatic units centered on such topics as home and community safety, transportation utilization, joint protection, adaptive equipment, energy conservation, exercise, and nutrition. (Details of the occupational therapy protocol are available from the authors.)

Subjects randomized to the occupational therapy group received 2 hours per week of group occupational therapy and a total of 9 hours of individual occupational therapy during the 9-month treatment period. Up to 10 seniors were assigned to each group. Group sessions were individually administered by registered occupational therapists trained in working with elderly populations. Four therapists (two per cohort) were involved in administering treatments, each therapist received a minimum of 10 hours of instruction on the specific study intervention and was blind to the study hypotheses.

The social control program focused on activities designed to encourage social interaction among members of the group. During the generalized activity sessions, subjects went on community outings, worked on craft projects, viewed films, played games, and attended dances. The subject matter covered in these sessions was tailored to the interests of the participants. Subjects randomized to the social control group following a meeting schedule similar to that of the occupational therapy group. Up to 10 seniors were assigned to each group session. Group sessions were administered by non-professionals who were blind to the study hypotheses. Because individual sessions were not held for the subjects in the social control group, the weekly group sessions were extended to 2.25 hours to ensure that the total number of treatment hours experienced per subject in the social control and occupational therapy groups were similar.

No intervention was applied to subjects assigned to the non-treatment control group.

Primary Outcome Measures

To evaluate the effectiveness of the treatments, testing was performed both at baseline and at the end of the 9-month treatment period. Subjects were tested using self-administered questionnaires designed to measure physical and social function, self-rated health, life satisfaction, and depressive symptoms. Testing was overseen by paid research assistants, blind to group assignment and study hypotheses. Subjects were instructed not to interact with each other during testing. Large print versions of the forms were used, and subjects were assisted if they were unable to complete the forms independently.

The primary outcome variables assessed in the study were derived from the following battery of five questionnaires:

1. Functional Status Questionnaire. The Functional Status Questionnaire assesses potential functional disabilities or disruptions of daily activities in physical and social domains.[33] Physical function was measured using two subscales: basic activities of daily living (BADL) and instrumental activities of daily living (IADL), which assess such activities as walking and preparing meals. Social function was measured using two subscales: social activity and quality of interaction, which assess the subjects' social role performance and affective quality of interactions with others. All subscales were converted into a percentage scale ranging from 0 to 100, with a score of 100 indicating no functional disability.

2. Life Satisfaction Index-Z. The Life Satisfaction Index-Z is a 13-item questionnaire designed to measure life satisfaction in older populations[34] and has been used as an indicator of health-related quality of life.[35] Participants rated items such as "I am just as happy now as when I was younger" on a scale from 0 to 2. Summary scores range from 0 (low satisfaction) to 26 (high satisfaction).

3. Center for Epidemiologic Studies (CES) Depression Scale. The CES Depression Scale consists of 20 questions designed to determine the frequency with which participants experienced depressive symptoms within the previous week. Questions addressed symptoms such as depressed mood, loss of appetite, and feelings of hopelessness. Summary scores range from 0 (no depressive symptoms) to 60 (many symptoms).

4. Medical Outcomes Study (MOS) Short Form General Health Survey. The MOS Health Perception scale administered in this study is a subset of the MOS Short Form General Health Survey.[33] This scale consists of five questions that assess subjects' perceptions of their own general health. Subjects rated questions such as "My health is excellent" on a 5-point scale. Final scores reflect a percentage scale from 0 (poor) to 100 (good).

5. RAND 36-Item Health Status Survey, Short Form-36 (RAND SF-36). The RAND SF-36 measures a range of physical and mental health-related dimensions.[39-40] It specifically addresses eight health domains: bodily pain, physical functioning, role limitations attributable to health problems, general health, vitality (energy and fatigue), social functioning, role limitations attributable to emotional problems, and general mental health. One final item asks participants to rate how much their general health has changed in the past year. All subscales are scored on a 0 (low) to 100 (high) percentage scale. This instrument was administered only to the second cohort of subjects as part of a decision to broaden the study.

Statistical Analysis

Summary scores for each of the instruments were calculated by adding the scores for all answered questions on the particular instrument and converting to a percentage scale where appropriate. Items missing a response were either assigned a value computed by published algorithms based on the responses to the subject's completed questions or assigned the average value of the questions answered by the subject if such algorithms were unavailable. For each study variable, including demographic and control variables, x^2 analyses and analyses of variance were performed to test for differences at baseline across the 3 treatment groups.

For each outcome variable, treatment effects were examined by calculating signed change scores (post-treatment score minus pre-treatment score). Analyses of variance were performed to determine demographic factors related to the change scores independent of treatment groups. Factors found to be significant were used as covariance in subsequent analyses. Analyses of covariance were then conducted using the change scores for each variable to test for equivalency between the social and non-treatment control groups, and to test for differences between the occupational therapy group and an overall control group consisting of the combination of the social and non-treatment groups. Statistical testing as carried out at the .05 level, used detailed assessments to test for equivalency between the social and non-treatment control groups and detailed assessments to examine whether the occupational therapy group produced more positive mean change outcomes. In the later case, the direction of difference was specified on an a priority basis before the outset of the trial.

Assuming a 20% attrition of subjects over 9 months and conducting testing of hypotheses at the .05 level (1-tailed), a projected sample size of 360 (with a 2:1 allocation ratio) permitted a degree of power equal to 80% in detecting a moderate population effect size (greater than or equal to 0.3) attributable to the occupational therapy treatment.[41] For the RAND SF-36, which was administered to the second cohort, a projected sample size of 220 permitted 80% power in detecting a population effect size of 0.4 or greater.[41]

RESULTS

Baseline Characteristics

A total of 373 volunteers were eligible for the study. Of these, 12 withdrew prior to randomization for personal reasons (unwilling to make the time commitment). Of the 361 volunteers (97%) who were randomized (143 in cohort 1 and 218 in cohort 2), 216 (60%) were residents of Angelus Plaza, 74 (20%) used the Angelus Plaza Senior Citizen facilities but resided in private homes or other facilities in the surrounding areas, and 71 (20%) were residents of Pilgrim Tower. Randomization resulted in the assignment of 122 subjects to the occupational therapy group, 120 subjects to the social control group, and 119 subjects to the non-treatment control group (Figure 25-1).

No significant differences in demographic characteristics were found across treatment groups (Table 25-1). The mean (SD) age was 74.4 (7.4) years, and 65% of the subjects were female. Ethnic group representations were Asian (47%), white (23%), African American (17%), and Hispanic (11%). In the Asian group, 66% were tested in Mandarin. The majority (73%) of subjects lived alone, and 27% of the subjects reported at least one disability.

No significant differences were found across treatment groups in baseline medical history and physical examination results (Table 25-2). Overall, 77% of the subjects had good or excellent balance on the Tinetti, 89% of the subjects scored normal on the MMSE, 75% of the subjects were regarded as normal according to the Geriatric Depression Scale, and 80% of the subjects had fair or better health according to the LaRue Global Assessment. The median number of medications taken was three per day.

In general there were no treatment group differences in pre-test means on any of the questionnaire based outcome variables (data not shown in tables). However, the non-treatment control group had a lower average RAND SF-36 vitality score than did either the social control group or the OT group, both P values less than or equal to .05.

Follow-Up and Compliance

Of the 361 subjects, 306 (85%) were evaluable at 9 months: 102 (84%) in the occupational therapy group, 100 (83%) in the social control group, and 104 (87%) in the nontreatment control group (P=.62) (see Figure 29-1). For the 55 unevaluable subjects, the reasons for discontinuation were the following: 8 died, 3 became ill, 13 relocated, 11 active participants were unavailable for post-testing for personal reasons, and 20 were lost to follow-up. Except for quality of interaction on the Functional Status Questionnaire, there were no significant differences at base line between evaluable and unevaluable subjects on either the demographic or the primary response measures. Compared with unevaluable subjects, evaluable subjects had a significantly greater mean quality of interaction score at baseline (82.7 vs 77.7, P=.02). Sixty-five percent of the subjects randomized to the occupational therapy group attended at least half of the sessions (average percentage of sessions attended by subjects in the occupational therapy group=60%). Sixty-two percent of the subjects randomized to the social activity control group attended at least half of the sessions (average percentage of sessions attended by subjects in the social control group, 61%).

Baseline Factors Related to Outcome

Analyses of variance were performed to determine baseline factors related to outcome variable change scores independent of treatment groups. Demographic factors found to be significantly related to one or more change score variables were sex, age group, disability status, and living status (all P values

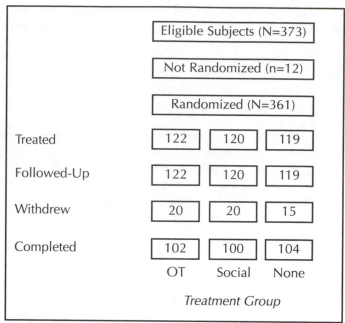

Figure 25-1. Profile for the Well Elderly Study. OT indicates occupational therapy group; Social, social control group; and None, nontreatment control group. Unwillingness to make the time commitment was the primary reason subjects were not randomized. Primary reasons for withdrawal were death (8), illness (3), relocation (13), personal matters (11), and loss to follow-up (20).

<.05). In addition, for each outcome measure, the baseline scores were significantly negatively related to the corresponding change scores (all P values <.001). Based on these results, all subsequent covariance analyses adjusted for these factors.

Equivalency of Control Groups

Analyses of covariance were conducted to compare outcomes between the two control groups (social vs. nontreatment). Except for the RAND SF-36 vitality scale, in which case the social control group fared worse than the nontreatment control group (social control mean change=6.3 vs nontreatment control mean change=4.1 P=.007; P=.04 after adjusting for baseline differences) no significant differences were found. Because of these findings the 2 control groups were combined for subsequent analyses.

Intent-to-Treat Analysis

Table 29-3 summarizes the results of the intent-to-treat analysis for subjects who completed the study. Shown are the mean pre-test and post-test scores for each outcome variable along with the unadjusted and adjusted mean change scores. Analyses of covariance revealed a significant benefit attributable to occupational therapy treatment for Functional Status

Table 25-1

Self-reported Demographic Characteristics by Treatment Condition*

Characteristics	Control			P Value
	Nontreatment (n=119)	Social (n=120)	OT (n=122)	
Sex				
Male	43 (36)	39 (33)	44 (36)	.80
Female	76 (64)	81 (67)	78 (64)	
Age group, y				
<70	28 (23)	39 (33)	29 (24)	
70-79	59 (50)	57 (47)	59 (48)	.38
≥80	32 (27)	24 (20)	34 (28)	
Ethnicity				
African American	22 (18)	20 (17)	19 (16)	
White	24 (20)	30 (25)	29 (24)	
Hispanic	15 (13)	15 (13)	9 (7)	.60
Asian (English speaking)	17 (14)	14 (12)	27 (22)	
Asian (Mandarin only speaking)	38 (32)	37 (31)	36 (30)	
Other	3 (3)	4 (3)	2 (2)	
Living alone	88 (74)	85 (71)	90 (74)	.83
Disabled	30 (25)	35 (30)	34 (28)	.78
No. of disabilities, mean (range)	0.4 (0-7)	0.4 (0-4)	0.4 (0-4)	.74

Values are frequency (column percent). OT indicates occupational therapy.

Questionnaire: quality of interaction (P=.03), Life Satisfaction Index-Z (P=.03), and MOS Health Perception (P=.05), and for 7 of 8 measures on the RAND SF-36: bodily pain (P=.03), physical functioning (P=.008), role limitations attributable to health problems (P=.02), vitality (P=.004), social functioning (P=.05), role limitations attributable to emotional problems (P=.05), and general mental health (P=.02). General health was marginally significant (P=.06). Benefit attributable to occupational therapy treatment was maintained on the RAND SF-36 after adjusting for vitality the single domain found to be significantly different at baseline across treatment groups. Analyses of outcomes within the occupational therapy group revealed that compared with other ethnic groups Asians (non-Mandarin-speaking) showed greater improvement as measured by the Life Satisfaction Index X-Z (P=.01), CES Depression scale (P=.03), and the MOS Health Perception Index (P=.04). Finally, compared with other ethnic groups, Hispanics showed greater improvement attributable to occupational therapy treatment on the RAND SF-36: general health (P=.01).

COMMENT

The Well Elderly Study provides the most comprehensive test to date of the effectiveness of occupational therapy. Although a limited number of prior investigations have examined the effects of occupational therapy on older adults the Well Elderly Study goes beyond previous studies in that it included a much larger sample size, incorporated a wider range of outcome domains, and included a greater degree of experimental control.

Significant benefits for the occupational therapy treatment were found across various health, function, and quality-of-life domains. In cases where a significant finding was present, the control groups tended to decline over the study, whereas the occupational therapy group either improved or exhibited a relative reduction in the extent of decline. Further, in a statistical analysis across all 3 treatment groups of all 11 significant outcome variables in Table 25-3, we found that the direction of effect favored the occupational therapy group in all 11 comparisons with the social control group and in 10 of the 11 comparisons with the non-treatment control group. Results of the present study therefore suggest that preventive occupational therapy programs may mitigate against the health risks of older adulthood.

Ory and Cox[4] suggest that health professionals have been reluctant to target older adults in preventive programs, assuming that this population would fail to benefit significantly from such efforts; however, results of the present study demonstrate that preventive programs designed for older adults can be effective. Moreover, a recent study by Ware et al[42] reported that older adults show more health-related decline in managed care programs than both other clientele within the same programs and adults comparable in age and socioeconomic status who used fee-for-service systems. Again, the current findings suggest that preventive occupational therapy programs could be used in conjunction with other services to proactively manage health care and either generate health improvements or at least slow decline.

The finding that only 5 of the 15 outcome measures that were studied failed to demonstrate a significant gain for the occupational therapy group relative to controls provides solid evidence of the comprehensive positive effects of the occupa-

Table 25-2
History and Physical Examination Results by Treatment Condition*

Nontreatment Characteristics	Control Social (n=119)	OT (n=120)	(n=122)	P Value
Tinetti Balance Examination (1-18)				
≤16 (Fair)	30 (26)	25 (21)	26 (22)	
17 (Good)	16 (14)	21 (18)	15 (12)	.70
18 (Excellent)	71 (60)	73 (61)	80 (66)	
Mini-Mental State Examination (0-30)				
≤23 (Impaired)	17 (14)	13 (11)	9 (8)	
>23 (Unimpaired)	101 (86)	106 (89)	111 (92)	.23
Geriatric Depression Scale (0-15)				
≤ (Normal)	90 (76)	87 (73)	93 (76)	
>5 (Depressed)	28 (24)	33 (27)	29 (24)	.74
LaRue Global Assessment of Overall Health (1-4)				
1 (Poor)	30 (25)	22 (19)	20 (16)	
2 (Fair)	54 (46)	58 (49)	63 (52)	
3 (Good)	21 (18)	23 (20)	24 (20)	.77
4 (Excellent)	13 (11)	15 (12)	15 (12)	
No. of medications, median (range)	3 (0-9)	3 (0-9)	3 (0-9)	.79

* Values are frequency (column percent). OT indicates occupational therapy.

Table 25-3
Outcome at 9 Months*

Response	Condition	Pretest Mean (SD)	Posttest Mean (SD)	Change Mean (SEM)	Adjusted Change (SEM)	P Value+ (1-Talled)
		Functional Status, Life Satisfaction, Depression, Health Perception				
B-ADL	OT (n=101)	94.2 (12.2)	90.1 (19.6)	-4.1 (1.8)	-2.3 (1.6)	.31
	Controls (n=202)	90.6 (18.6)	90.1 (16.9)	-0.5 (1.3)	-1.3 (1.1)	
I-ADL	OT (n=102)	78.7 (25.9)	79.1 (26.5)	0.4 (2.0)	0.9 (1.8)	.28
	Controls (n=202)	77.8 (25.1)	77.6 (22.8)	-0.2 (1.5)	-0.4 (1.3)	
Social activities	OT (n=100)	87.9 (24.7)	84.7 (28.2)	-3.2 (2.9)	-1.0 (2.4)	.38
	Controls (n=203)	83.6 (28.3)	82.8 (27.1)	-0.8 (2.0)	-1.9 (1.7)	
Quality of interaction	OT (n=102)	83.8 (12.1)	85.4 (12.2)	1.6 (1.3)	2.1 (1.1)	.03
	Controls (n=203)	82.2 (14.9)	81.9 (13.3)	-0.3 (1.0)	-0.6 (0.8)	
Life Satisfaction Index-Z	OT (n=102)	17.5 (5.9)	18.8 (5.3)	1.3 (0.4)	1.6 (0.4)	
	Controls (n=203)	16.4 (6.1)	17.3 (5.9)	0.9 (0.3)	0.7 (0.3)	.03
CES-Depression	OT (n=101)	10.9 (8.9)	10.8 (8.2)	-0.1 (0.7)	-0.8 (0.8)	
	Controls (n=203)	13.8 (9.8)	13.6 (9.8)	-0.2 (0.7)	0.2 (0.5)	.16
MOS Health Perception	OT (n=102)	60.6 (22.8)	62.2 (23.5)	1.6 (1.9)	2.4 (1.9)	
	Controls (n=204)	57.5 (23.7)	56.4 (25.5)	-1.1 (1.5)	-1.5 (1.4)	.05
		RAND SF-36				
Bodily pain	OT (n=49)	74.7 (19.1)	70.8 (20.1)	-3.9 (3.1)	-0.9 (2.7)	
	Controls (n=111)	65.8 (23.6)	60.2 (22.2)	-5.6 (2.1)	-6.9 (1.7)	.03

Table 25-3 continued
Outcome at 9 months (continued)

Response	Condition	Pretest Mean (SD)	Posttest Mean (SD)	Change Mean (SEM)	Adjusted Change (SEM)	P Value+ (1-Talled)
Physical functioning	OT (n=48)	77.0 (25.4)	72.9 (27.9)	-4.1 (2.9)	-3.2 (2.8)	
	Controls (n=110)	72.8 (23.3)	61.7 (25.7)	-11.1 (2.0)	-11.5 (1.9)	.008
Role functioning‡	OT (n=49)	75.5 (34.8)	71.9 (39.4)	-3.6 (6.0)	0.6 (5.4)	
	Controls (n=110)	62.5 (39.2)	51.8 (43.2)	-10.7 (4.0)	-12.5 (3.6)	.02
General health	OT (n=49)	73.3 (19.7)	72.8 (19.6)	-0.5 (2.1)	1.1 (2.3)	
	Controls (n=110)	64.6 (22.7)	62.0 (23.2)	-2.6 (1.7)	-3.3 (1.5)	.06
Vitality	OT (n=48)	66.0 (18.4)	70.1 (20.3)	4.1 (2.2)	6.2 (2.4)	
	Controls (n=111)	59.2 (23.0)	58.4 (20.9)	-0.8 (1.9)	-1.7 (1.6)	.004
Social functioning	OT (n=49)	86.0 (20.7)	85.5 (18.8)	-0.5 (3.2)	0.6 (2.7)	
	Controls (n=111)	81.3 (23.2)	77.1 (22.7)	-4.2 (2.1)	-4.7 (1.8)	.05
Role emotional§	OT (n=49)	83.0 (31.3)	77.6 (35.0)	-5.4 (6.0)	-3.6 (5.2)	
	Controls (n=111)	77.2 (37.9)	64.3 (39.6)	-12.9 (4.2)	-13.7 (3.4)	.05
General mental health	OT (n=48)	84.4 (15.5)	83.5 (12.7)	-0.9 (2.5)	1.1 (2.1)	
	Controls (n=111)	78.3 (20.7)	74.7 (18.4)	-3.6 (1.7)	-4.5 (1.4)	.02

* B-ADL indicates basic activities of daily living: OT, occupational therapy; I-ADL, instrumental activities of daily living: CES, Center for Epidemiologic Studies; MOS, Medical Outcomes Study; and RAND SF-36, RAND 36-Item Health Status Survey, Short Form-36.

† Analysis of variance performed with baseline, sex, age group, disability status, and living status as covariates. P values are given for adjusted change scores.

‡ Role functioning refers to role limitations attributable to health problems.

§ Role emotional refers to role limitations attributable to emotional problems.

tional therapy intervention. Examination of the structure of the CESD and the IADL, BADL, and social activity subscales of the Functional Status Questionnaire (ie, the variables that were not at least marginally significant) suggests that, because they have low ceilings, these tools are relatively insensitive to detect changes among the well elderly. In contrast, the RAND SF-36 subscales, which in general proved to be the most sensitive to treatment effects, had high ceilings and were therefore capable of detecting upward changes among well individuals. The design of this study provided a rigorous test of the relative effectiveness of a nonprofessionally led activity group (the social control group) and a professionally designed program based on occupational therapy principles. Because both programs involved subjects with activity, our findings call into question the cliche that "keeping busy keeps you healthy." Conversely, it appears that simply being regularly engaged in activity through the social control program was no more effective in promoting health than receiving no treatment.

How then might one account for the superior outcomes of the occupational therapy intervention? First, activities were chosen based on principles from the occupational therapy field that pertain to the relationship of occupation to health. Through the systematic application of such principles, the occupational therapy program enabled subjects to construct daily routines that were health-promoting and meaningful given the context of their lives. Fuhrer[13] has suggested that people experience elevated health and subjec-

tive well-being when they are engaged in activities that they view as health-promoting.

Second, in contrast to the social control intervention, the occupational therapy program was highly individualized, even though it occurred in a group context. As part of the treatment plan, participants were asked to apply the content to their own everyday experiences. This requirement is likely to have made the treatment activity sessions personally meaningful and effective within the participants' daily lives.

Third, the occupational therapy program included specific instruction on how to overcome barriers to successful daily living, an important consideration given that the participants had limited incomes and resources. For example, emphasis was placed on activities that required no financial outlay, and time was spent assisting subjects in learning to master public transportation systems. Through this approach, subjects were provided with the supports they needed to confront obstacles, take risks, and experience self-efficacy and personal control while participating in daily activity. Research outcomes have demonstrated the crucial role that such factors play in giving one a sense of forward progression rather than stasis.[9,12,14-16,43]

It is important to stress that the social control group was included in the study to rule out mere participation in group based activities as an alternate explanation for the effects of occupational therapy, and not to simulate any type of professional intervention. Consequently, no attempt should be made to equate the social control condition with alternate treatment approaches, such as recreation therapy, that use involvement in activity as a treatment focus, but that require trained personnel to administer.

Programs such as the currently studied occupational therapy intervention that focus on everyday practices of people are sometimes viewed as neither requiring the expertise of a professional to administer nor being sufficiently effective to warrant large-scale studies of their effectiveness. However, our study results demonstrate that superior outcomes can be expected when an activity-centered intervention is administered by professional therapists as opposed to being conducted by nonprofessionals. Further, our results suggest the need to perform more studies of this kind that may uncover additional positive effects of occupation-based treatment approaches. We believe that future research must also be directed toward uncovering the factors associated with activity, in general, that promote health and well-being. Finally, data on programmatic and medical costs obtained from questionnaires and telephone interviews with study subjects have been collected. A complete cost benefit analysis is the subject of the next facet of the study.

Limitations of the current research are that results may not generalize to older adults in different living situations (eg, single-family dwellers, nursing home residents) or of different socioeconomic status. On the other hand, a significant strength of the current research is that the outcomes can be extended to older adults of varying ethnicities. Future research is needed to replicate the positive effects of this preventive occupational therapy intervention for older adults in different living situations as well as to understand the mechanisms that underlie the positive effects found in the present study.

This study was supported by grant RO1 AG11810 from the National Institute on Aging, the National Center for Medical Rehabilitation Research, the Agency for Health Care Policy and Research; the American Occupational Therapy Foundation Center at the University of Southern California for the Study of Occupation and Its Relation to Adaptation; the RCK Foundation; Lumex, Inc. and Smith, Inc, & Nephew Rolyan.

REFERENCES

1. Statistical Abstract of the US. (1996). US Bureau of the Census. Washington, DC: US Government Printing Office.

2. Current Population Report: Special Studies: Sixty-five Plus in America. (1992). US Bureau of the Census. Washington, DC: US Government Printing Office. Publication P23-178.

3. Crimmins, E. M., Hayward, M. D., & Saito, Y. (1994). Changing mortality and morbidity rates and the health status and life expectancy of the older population. *Demography, 31,* 159-175.

4. Ory, M. G. & Cox, D. M. (1994). Forging ahead: linking health and behavior to improve quality of life in older people. *Soc Indicators Res, 33,* 89-120.

5. Ebrahim, S. (1995). Clinical and public health perspectives and applications of health related quality of life measurement. *Soc Sci Med, 41,* 1383-1394.

6. McHorney, C. A., Ware, J. E., & Raczek, A. E. (1993). The MOS 36 Item Short Form Survey (SF3G), II: Psychometric and clinical test of validity in measuring physical and mental health constructs. *Med Care, 31,* 247-263.

7. Rowe, J. W., & Cahn, R. L. (1987). Human aging: usual and successful. *Science, 237,* 143-149.

8. Bachelder, J. M. & Hilton, C. L. (1993). Implications of the Americans With Disabilities Act of 1990 for elderly persons. *Am J Occup Ther, 48,* 73-81.

9. Verbrugge, L. M. & Jette, A. M. (1993). The disablement process. *Soc Sci Med, 38,* 1-14.

10. Murrell, S. A. & Himmelfarb, S. (1989). Effects of attachment bereavement and pre-event conditions on subsequent depressive symptoms in older adults. *Psychol Aging, 4,* 166-172.

11. Gatz, M. (1995). Introduction. In M. Gatz (Ed.), *Emerging issues in mental health and aging* (pp. xv-xx). Washington, DC: American Psychological Association.

12. Pearlin, L. I. & Skaff, M. M. (1995). Stressors and adaptation in later life. In Gatz M., ed. *Emerging issues in mental health and aging (pp. 97-123).* Washington, DC: APA.

13. Krause, N. (1994). Stressors in salient social roles and well-being in later life. *J Geroutul Psychol Sci, 49,* 137-148.

14. Berkman, L. F., Seeman, T. E., Albert, M., et al. (1993). High, unusual and impaired functioning in community dwelling older men and women. *J Clin Epidenriol, 46,* 1129-1140.

15. Fisher, B. J. (1995). Successful aging, life satisfaction and generativity in later life. *Int. J Aging Hum. Devel, 41,* 239-250.

16. Seeman, T. E., Berkman, L. F., Charpentier, P. A., Blazer, D. G., Albert, M. S., & Tinetti, M. E. (1995). Behavior and psychosocial predictors of physical performance. *J Gerontol, 50A,* M177-M183.

17. Carlson, M., Fanchiang, S., Zemke, R., & Clark, F. (1996). A meta-analysis of the effectiveness of occupational therapy for older persons. *Am J Occup Ther, 50,* 89-98

18. Larson, K. O., Stevens-Ratchford, R. G., Pedretti, L. W., & Crabtree, J. L. (1996). *ROTE: The role of occupational therapy with the elderly.* Bethesda, MD: AOTA.

19. Levine, R. E. & Gitlin, L. N. (1992). A model to promote activity competence in elders *Am J Occup Ther, 47,* 147-153. (Reprinted in Cotrell, R. P. (Ed.). (1996). Perspectives on purposeful activity: Foundations and future of occupational therapy (pp. 557-564). Bethesda, MD: AOTA.)

20. Hopkins, H. L., & Smith, H. D. (Eds.). (1993). *Willard and Spackman's Occupational Therap* (8th ed.). Philadelphia, PA: JP Lippincott.

21. Tinetti, M. E. (1986). Performance oriented assessment of mobility problems in elderly patients. *J Am Geriatr Soc, 34,* 119-126.

22. Teng, E. & Chui, H. (1987). The Modified Mini Mental State (3MS) Examination. *J Clin Psychiatry, 48,* 314-317.

23. Yesavage, J. A., Brink, T. L., Rose, T. L., et al. (1983). Development and validation of a geriatric depression screening scale. *J Psychiatry Res, 17,* 37-49.

24. LaRue, A., Bank, L., Jarvik, L., & Hetland, M. (1979). Health in old age: how do physicians' ratings and self-ratings compare? *J Gerontol, 34,* 687-691.

25. Clark, F., Carlson, M., Zemke, R., et al. (1996). Life domains and adaptive strategies of a group of low income well older adults. *Am J Occup Ther, 50,* 99-108

26. Jackson, J. (1996). Living a meaningful existence in old age. In: Zemke R. Clark F, (Eds.), *Occupational science: The evolving discipline.* Philadelphia, PA: FA Davis.

27. Clark, F., Parham, D., Carlson, M. E., et al. (1991). Occupational science: Academic innovation in the service of occupational therapy's future. *Am J Occup Ther, 45,* 300-310.

28. Clark, F., & Larson, E. A. Developing an academic discipline: The science of occupation. In H. L. Hopkins & H. D. Smith (Eds.), *Willard and Spackman's Occupational therapy* (8th ed.) (pp. 44-57). Philadelelphia, PA: JB Lippincott.

29. Zemke, R. & Clark, F. (1996). *Occupational science: The evolving discipline.* Philadelphia, PA: FA Davis.

30. Clark, F. (1993). Occupation embedded in a real life: Interweaving occupational science and occupational therapy: 1993 Eleanor Clarke Slagle Lecture. *Am J Occup Ther,* 1067-1078.

31. Yerxa, E. J., Clirk, F., Frank, G., et al. (1989). An introduction to occupational science. *Occup Ther Health Care, 6,* 117.

32. Townsend, E. (1996). Institutional ethnography: A method for showing how the context shapes practice. *Occup Ther J Res, 16,* 179-199.

33. Jette, A. M. (1987). Clearly PD. Functional Disability assessment. *Phys Ther, 67,* 1854-1859.

34. Wood, V., Wylie, M. L., & Sheafor, B. (1969). An analysis of a short selfreported measure of life satisfaction. *J Gerontol, 24,* 465-469.

35. Burkhardt, C. S. (1985). The impact of arthritis on quality of life. *Nurs Res, 34,* 11-16.

36. Burkhardt, C. S., Woods, S. L., Schultz, A. A., & Zicbarth, D. S. (1989). Quality of life of adults with chronic illness: A psychometric study. *Res Nurs Health, 12,* 347-354.

37. Radloff, L. (1977). The CES-D Scale: A self-report depression scale for research in the general population. *Appl Psychol Means, 1,* 385-401.

38. Stewart, A. L., Hays, R. D., & Ware, J. E. (1988). The MOS Short Form Health Survey. (SF-36). *Med Care, 26,* 724-735.

39. Hays, R. D., Sherbourne, C. D., & Mazel, R. M. (1993). The RAND 36-Item Health Survey 1.0. *Health Econ, 2,* 217-227.

40. Ware, J. E., & Sherbourne, C. D. (1992). The MOS 36-Item Short-Form Health Survey (SF36), *Med Care, 30,* 473-481.

41. Cohen J. (1987). *Statistical power analysis for the behavioral sciences (Rev ed.).* Hillsdale, NJ: Erlbaum.

42. Ware, J. E., Bayliss, M. S., Rogers, W. H., Kosinski, M. L., & Tarlov, A. R. (1996). Differences in 4-year health outcomes for elderly and poor chronically ill patients treated in HMO and fee-for-services systems: Results from the Medical Outcomes Study. *JAMA, 276,* 1039-1047.

43. Fuhrer, M. J. (1994). Subjective well-being. Implications for medical rehabilitation outcomes and models of disablement. *Am J Phys Rehab, 73,* 358-364.

Adult Day Care: A Model for Changing Times

Laurie Ellen Neustadt

This chapter was previously published in Physical and Occupational Therapy in Geriatrics, *4(1), 53-66. Copyright © 1985, Haworth Press.*

Day health care for older adults is an exciting and innovative alternative to institutionalization. As will be illustrated below, it is extremely well suited to the skills and interests of many health professionals who assist individuals to attain their maximum levels of independence. This (chapter) discusses the need for adult day care, describes one center's program and offers some ideas for health professionals who are establishing their own programs.

HISTORY OF ADULT DAY CARE

Adult day care was first developed in Europe in the early 1940s. In l947, the Menninger Clinic became the first United States adult day care center, followed by the Yale Psychiatric Clinic in 1949. Both were established for psychogeriatric care (Rathbone-McCuan & Elliot, 1976-77). By 1969, there were still only twelve adult day care programs, whereas an estimated 800 centers existed by 1984.

Historically, families provided care for their own relatives. Aging was accepted as a part of the life cycle and not as a sickness. Family units were closer and more interdependent, with one or more family members at home to care for those who needed them. With the societal changes occurring over the past 25 years, the caregiver function of the family has changed.

Society responded to this change in family-provided care by increasing the availability of institutional care. Nursing homes became the alternative to care given at home by the family. Institutionalizing the elderly increased the general perception that aging is an illness, and unfortunately, promoted premature institutionalization for those lacking the family or community support needed to remain independent (Burris, 1981).

While nursing home placement became more widespread, it only provided services for a small segment of the elderly population. The majority were still living in the community and having a great many needs unmet (Kiernat, 1976). With the increased expense of institutionalization, and subsequent burden on families in particular and society as a whole, alternative options for geriatric care have become essential.

The traditional senior center recreational and nutritional programs met some of the community support needs of more self-sufficient older people. However, these programs were not geared to meet the needs of infirm, confused, or disabled adults, lacking the facilities or staff to provide nursing care or therapy.

Adult day centers were developed to provide a supervised, protective environment for participants. Services include nursing, social services, occupational and physical therapy, speech/language pathology, activity programming, transportation, and nutritional meals. Three models of these day care centers evolved—the medical model, the health maintenance model, and the social model—although some overlap exists among the three.

The medical model stresses nursing services, therapy, and rehabilitation while still providing recreational programming. The social model emphasizes socialization and recreation, but can also provide some nursing care and therapy. The health maintenance model is a blend of the two, but does not stress rehabilitation. Most day care centers enable elderly participants to receive coordinated health care at one site. Participants can utilize the program for ongoing health maintenance to avoid institutionalization, or as a temporary setting for rehabilitation after surgery, accident, or illness. The centers provide group involvement and promote wellness and independence which in turn increases the individual's quality of life, contentment, mental functioning, and activity level.

The adult day center also provides needed respite for family members engaged in the caregiver role, and increases the options for those who choose not to place a family member in a nursing home. This assistance often allows the family to continue providing direct care and often improves family relationships by alleviating the stress so common to family caregiver situations.

The following objectives, as established by the Levindale Adult Treatment Center in 1968 (Rathbone-McCuan and Elliot, 1976-77), summarize the overall role of adult day care: "(a) to provide socialization experience to physically and emotionally disabled older people; (b) to help maintain disabled older people in their own homes and communities; (c) to provide an integrated professional service to disabled people living in the community; (d) to preclude the institutionalization of disabled people by providing services through a day care center; and (e) to provide support and relieve the burden of families who care for their older disabled relative" (Rathbone-McCuan and Elliot, 1976-77, p. 159).

The adult day center creates a link in the continuity of care for the elderly between nursing home placement and home care, thus providing a choice for individuals and their families. Maintaining independence in the community, promoting wellness, and offering the option of continued family care, the day center becomes a welcome alternative to institutionalization

St. Mary's Day Health Center for Older Adults

St. Mary's Hospital Medical Center in Madison, Wisconsin, hired the Gerontological Planning Associates of Santa Monica, California, in February 1981 as consultants to help clarify the need for services to the elderly in its community. A committee made up of area professionals in aging explored a wide range of possible services and determined there was a need for a medical model adult day care program in the Madison area. The committee found one-third of the total St. Mary's Hospital Medical Center population was 65 years old and over, and discovered that among those elderly patients, the ones suffering from multiple chronic diseases or impairments needed a longer recovery time.

It was determined that the Day Health Center would allow elderly patients to be discharged sooner from the hospital. They would be able to obtain the coordinated therapies, health care, nutritional, and social needs they require, and still benefit from their home environment during recovery. As noted in the Certificate of Need Application, the Day Health Center would alleviate the problem of patients being admitted to nursing homes only because all family members held jobs, and the elderly person could not be left alone for eight hours.

St. Mary's Day Health Center for Older Adults opened its doors on July 19, 1982. The Center is open Monday through Friday from 8:00 a.m. to 5:30 p.m. and accommodates up to 20 clients per day.

Program and Staff

St. Mary's Day Health Center is a medical model day center established with the following objectives:

1. To promote or maintain independence.
2. To rehabilitate the participant to the maximum extent possible.
3. To maintain the participant in the community as long as it is medically, socially, and economically feasible.
4. To prevent inappropriate or premature institutionalization.
5. To provide daytime respite and educational support for families.

The general philosophy of the Center is to increase the independence of the clients physically, psychologically, and socially, and to assist them in maintaining the highest level of independence possible. Clients are encouraged to involve themselves not only in individual activities, but in the life of the Center itself. This approach has developed a sense of community and caring among the clients and the staff.

For each participant, a multidisciplinary team develops an individualized plan of care. Nursing services, social services, occupational and physical therapies, speech/language pathology, activity programming, pastoral care and religious services, transportation services, and a nutritional meal are provided at the Center. The staff includes one full-time Registered Nurse (RN) who is the coordinator of the program; one full-time Licensed Practical Nurse (LPN); one full-time Certified Occupational Therapy Assistant (COTA), who is the volunteer and activity coordinator of the program; one part-time Social Worker; one part-time aide; two part-time van drivers; and one part-time secretary.

Occupational and physical therapy and speech-language pathology are contracted through St. Mary's Hospital Medical Center on an outpatient basis. Clients who are referred to therapy by their physicians are seen by a hospital therapist at the Day Health Center. A parallel bar, full-view mirror, overhead pulley and weights, treatment tables, hydroculator, exercise bike, and a variety of occupational therapy equipment are on hand for use by the clients.

Nursing services. Nursing services are a vital part of this medical model day center. The RN and LPN administer medication and supervise and perform health assessment, counseling, and health education. They monitor specific illnesses such as congestive heart failure, diabetes, pulmonary diseases and hypertension. They provide specific treatments such as dressing changes, catheter care, and monitoring vital signs and weights. Nursing staff also assist with activities of daily living including feeding, toileting, ambulating, bathing, hair care, nail care, teeth or denture care, and shaving. Because of the long-term participation of clients of the Center and low staff turnover, the care given is consistent and personal. All Center participants must have a referral form filled out by their personal physician upon entering the program. The Nurse Coordinator then maintains close communication with the physician to assure the continuity of care given.

Pastoral care. Pastoral care is available, as requested by clients or family, through the Pastoral Care Department of the hospital. Catholic Mass is celebrated on Friday mornings, and most Christian and Jewish holidays are celebrated with the clients.

Social services. Social services at the Center are multidimensional and provide the necessary link between the day center program and the community. The social worker screens prospective clients and conducts initial intake interviews. Once a client has been accepted to the program, the social worker briefs staff members, makes sure the client has a physician, and sets up transportation, bathing and medication schedules. The social worker also provides informational services to clients and community agencies. She acts as a liaison between community services, clients, and their families to assure continuity of goals among services. Individual counseling to clients and families is provided, especially crisis counseling as problems arise. Group counseling is provided regularly on an informal basis through weekly membership meetings between clients and the social worker. An educational program for family caregivers is offered twice a year.

Support staff. The part-time Center aide assists with the activities, shops for supplies, assists clients with activities of daily living and helps with routine housekeeping at the Center. The secretary acts as receptionist and unit clerk, handles all billing and accounting, keeps Center statistics, and does all the secretarial duties required.

Transportation can be provided for those who need this service by the Center's wheelchair accessible van. The van accommodates seven individuals and makes two morning and two afternoon runs. The two part-time drivers have developed a particular rapport with the clients and their families and provide essential information on the home environment to the rest of the staff. Other clients are brought to the Center by community transportation services or by their families.

A nutritious noon meal is served daily at the Center, catered by a local business, and served by the staff and volunteers. Specific meals are ordered for those on special diets including diabetic, low salt, vegetarian, and kosher restrictions (Neustadt, 1982). Two snacks are served, one in the morning and one in the afternoon, planned and prepared by the licensed practical nurse.

Basic lab work such as urinalysis and blood work are available. Samples are drawn by the nurse coordinator and processed by the lab at Shared Laboratory Services of Madison.

Volunteers are an essential element of the Day Health Center. They act as an extension of the staff, allowing for a higher level of quality care and diminishing staff burnout. Volunteers assist with activities, visit with clients on an individual basis, help serve and clean up meals and snacks, and assist clients to and from activities and to and from the Center van. The certified occupational therapy assistant recruits volunteers from the community, universities, and churches, and supervises their activities.

The Center's entire staff meets once a month. The RN, LPN, COTA, and social worker meet once a week to be briefed on new clients and discuss plans of care and treatment approaches. The Center uses medical model documentation procedures and SOAP note charting techniques.

The Activities Program

The activities program is central to the success of the Day Health Center program. Through an organized activities program, clients can develop their self-esteem and self-worth, establish support systems, engage in socialization, and become involved with purposeful activity. Activities programming is a medium for creating community among the clients and a means of replacing the occupational and social involvements no longer existent in the client's lives.

The St. Mary's Activity Program is run by a certified occupational therapy assistant. In Adult Day Care Activities·one must work with and meet the needs of an extremely varied population with problems ranging from multiple physical handicaps to acute psychological disorders. The COTA is trained to work with varying degrees of minimal to multiple handicaps and in acute to chronic stages of disorder, both physical and psychological, and is competent in adapting activities for the problems encountered. The educational training program for COTAs—a strong focus on a variety of activities, the skill of needs assessment, and activities adaptation—make the COTA a logical candidate for Adult Day Care Activity Programmer.

The occupational behavior frame of reference, with performance components and occupational performance areas, is woven into the fiber of the activity program. Within the performance component areas, the physical component is addressed in the daily group exercise program, the "Willing Walkers Club," and a daily informal exercise group. Clients currently receiving treatment from the registered occupational therapist (OTR) do supportive exercises during this informal group with the COTA.

Sensory integration is directly addressed through the exercise program. Sensory stimulating props compensate for perceptual and cognitive deficits and assist clients unable to follow verbal cues. All the senses—taste, touch, smell, hearing, and visual stimuli—are incorporated in many of the planned activities. Perceptual deficits are also addressed in the informal exercise group with the COTA using input from the occupational therapist. Cards and table games, brain teasers, reminiscing groups, discussion groups, story reading, educational programs, and guest lecturers involve the cognitive component. Psychological and social components are touched upon in weekly membership group meetings. Specific issues that have come up with individuals or the group are discussed. These components are also addressed in other group discussions, programs, and in the daily interpersonal relationships that are an ongoing part of the Center.

The activities also include the occupational performance areas of self-care, work, homemaking, and play/leisure. Most of the clients' self-care needs are addressed by the nursing and occupational therapy staff on an individual basis. Clients are involved in homemaking activities through cooking, sewing, and gardening groups.

Some clients also assist in the homemaking chores of the Center such as watering plants, clearing the table, and help-

Table 26-1
Sample Weekly Activity Calendar

	Monday	Tuesday	Wednesday	Thursday	Friday
8 9	Individual Activity time with snacks, coffee, and juice served. Clients work on individual craft projects [and] occupational therapy exercises, read the newspaper, and participate in the Willing Walkers Club.				
10	Membership Group with the Social Worker	Poetry Group or Health Group	Reminiscing Group	Reading Group or Pet Visit	Current Events
11	Exercise Group to Music	Exercise Group to Music	Exercise Group to Music	Exercise Group to Music	Exercise Group to Music
12	Lunch Willing Walkers Club	Lunch Willing Walkers Club	Lunch Willing Walkers Club	Lunch Willing Walkers Club	Lunch Church Service
1	Cooking Group with L.P.N.	Feature Film Presentation of the Week	Volunteer Work Group	Cooking Group with L.P.N.	Brain Teasers
2	Bingo or Bowling	Feature Film Presentation of the Week	Storyteller from the Community	Drama Group	Stained Glass Workshop
3	Reading Group	Cards and Table Games	Brain Teasers	Crafts	Reading Group
4	Individual Activity time including reading, watching television or listening to music, individual exercise routines and craft projects, individuals visiting time with staff and volunteers.				

ing with dishes. Clients have expressed a need to remain involved in work-oriented projects. Volunteer projects such as preparing mailings, sewing projects, and sorting stamps are brought in from community agencies like the American Red Cross and Retired Senior Volunteer Program. The clients also planned and ran their own Christmas craft bazaar. The group voted to purchase a video recorder with the money it raised. Some clients also needed counseling and assistance in structuring their leisure time both at the Center and at home.

Often, activity programs remain structured and unchanged for many months, if not years. It is important to blend planned, stable events with spontaneity. A structured calendar of activities should exist, but it must allow for daily changes according to the mood, energy level, needs, and interests of the clients present that day. Spontaneity allows for those subtle changes which present themselves day to day, and also allows for those creative moments that cannot be planned. A large store of resources—cognitive games, craft ideas and samples and supplies, group projects, party ideas, and work tasks—make spontaneous activities possible. Offering a wide variety of activities will assist in reaching the varied interests of the participants. There are five group activities a day at the Center with approximately 15 different types of activities per week. (See Table 26-1 for a sample activity program.)

Philosophy, Approaches, and Ideas of an Activity Program

Developing an activity program which truly meets the needs of the clientele is always a challenge. Frequently the program represents what staff assume are the needs of the clients, or what might be good for them. It is a constant challenge to balance the staff's knowledge, skills, and talents with programs based on the actual needs and interests of clients.

"The challenge of activities programming in extended care and long-term care facilities is to provide opportunities for truly meaningful activity. Meaningful is a word that must be individually defined by the (clients) themselves, not by a staff which seeks to involve (clients) in activities which the staff perceives as meaningful. Later maturity is one of several developmental stages in the life continuum and has associated with it specific developmental stages and human needs. Consequently, activities which are defined as meaningful by a thirty-year-old staff member may not be similarly defined by an eighty-year-old (client). Careful assessment of (client) problems and needs by perceptive and empathetic professionals who have a thorough knowledge of the developmental tasks of later maturity is essential to gain an understanding of how elderly individuals define meaningful activity" (Curley, 1980).

Clients are approached individually about their specific activity interests. They are encouraged to follow through on individual activities and participate in group activities as they choose. There is a fine line between encouraging clients to attend group activities to increase socialization and diminish isolation and depression, and allowing them the freedom to be and do what they want. Staff members need to be aware of the strong need for elderly individuals to reminisce and to be listened to. One of the most important activities for some clients may be talking, and one of the most important activities for the staff may be listening.

Establishing trust is a critical element when working with people in any capacity, and becomes particularly important when working with confused elderly. Consistent approach assures a greater comfort level for the client. Verbal and physical affection help establish closer, more rewarding relationships for clients and staff.

Intergenerational programming creates a sense of normalcy which precludes the age separatism so prevalent in institutions. St. Mary's Day Health Center is located in a school building that also houses four preschools, two music schools, a gymnastics program, and a grade school. The preschool children join the Center's exercise group once a week and occasionally perform musical programs. The grade school children have conducted taped oral history interviews with clients, practiced storytelling, and performed class plays for the Center. A neighborhood Brownie troop adopted the Center and held their monthly meetings together with the clients. Parties, crafts, and service projects led up to the Brownies "flying up" ceremony at the Center, with clients escorting the girls across the symbolic bridge to Girl Scouts. The Girl Scouts voted to continue visiting the Center the following year, with some of the girls establishing one-to-one relationships with special clients. Young children seem to bring out expressions of love and affection from even the most confused and withdrawn of the clients. Between the visiting school children, volunteers, staff, and clients, five generations are integrated into the Center's community.

Most adult day centers are located in churches and school buildings, making it easier to involve resources from the community at large. Helping to keep individuals involved and aware of happenings within their own communities is important when working with the elderly. It is easy to become isolated and uninformed when involvements from the past—jobs, church affiliations, and clubs—are discontinued. The Day Center and its staff become an important link back into the community; inviting speakers, entertainers and artists to come to the Center is one approach toward reestablishing that link.

The local Humane Society "Love a Pet" program brings Red Cross volunteers with puppies and kittens to visit twice a month. Community artists have become the Center's resident artists, leading sculpture and stained glass workshops. Often, artists and musicians with City Arts Grants develop programs with this specific purpose in mind. Storytellers, musicians, dancers and choirs have all visited the Center. Speakers from the local Police Department, Save Our Security Organization, Brain Injury Association, the State Historical Society, and area health professionals, have presented their expertise. This outside involvement increases program quality and the level of interaction between the clients and the community.

Developing an internal sense of community is equally important to all the participants in the Day Center program. Clients spend the whole day together and are able to get to know each other and develop a sense of caring and interdependence. By involving clients in the planning and decision-making process, they feel a sense of ownership in the Center. Most staff members lead at least one formal activity, and all are involved in direct care. The continual interaction throughout the day among clients and staff adds considerable depth and vitality to the sense of internal community.

Description of the Population

St. Mary's Day Health Center can accommodate 20 clients a day. The Center accepts adults who need continuous individualized medical treatment and rehabilitation. Persons with walkers or wheelchairs, those who require supervision and help with medications, and those who are incontinent are accepted into the program. Clients are referred to the Center by hospitals, clinics, private physicians, health and social service agencies, their families, or by self-referral. Eighty-four total clients have been served at the Center since its opening. (See Table 26-2.)

In order to be eligible for admission into the Center, potential participants should meet one or more of the following: (1) have a primary physical diagnosis which includes a disability or chronic illness; (2) require continuing medical evaluation, treatment, and follow-up care as well as skilled nursing supervision and care, but not to the extent that institutionalization is required; (3) require rehabilitative services to improve or maintain level of independence; (4) require specific training in the taking of prescribed drugs, special diets, special diet preparation, catheter management, and care of the feet because of peripheral vascular disease; (5) the family of the disabled or chronically ill elderly person requires the education and respite support that a day health center offers in order to continue caring for the person at home.

Eligible participants must: (1) be older adults (exceptions are made for younger clients if they need day care and are at least 18 years of age); (2) not be bedridden, totally disoriented, harmful, or disruptive; (3) be able to tolerate four to eight hours in a day care situation and transportation to and from the Center; (4) have a physician referral; (5) live within metropolitan Madison or provide their own transportation.

Diagnoses submitted by client physicians include: (1) heart and vascular diseases; (2) brain disorders such as tumors, CVAs, Organic Brain Syndrome, and Alzheimer's Disease; (3) bone diseases and fractures; (4) cancer; (5) kidney and bladder disease; (6) vision and hearing impairments; (7) lung disease; (8) depression; and (9) alcohol abuse.

The majority of the Center's clients live either with their

spouse or one of their children. A few clients live with a hired live-in aide or live by themselves. The majority of the clients attend the Center for two or four days a week, with some attending one day a week and some five days a week. Clients arrive between 8:00 and 10:30 in the morning and leave between 3:00 and 5:30 in the evening.

The following case studies illustrate client types served by St. Mary's Day Health Center.

Case study Mrs. "R." Mrs. R came to the Center after suffering a right-sided CVA with left hemiplegia. She attends the Center five days a week and receives both physical and occupational therapy. She has shown great improvement with her perceptual exercises and is now walking with assistance. Mrs. R actively participates in most of the Center's activities and has developed many friendships with clients, staff, and volunteers at the Center. The improvement Mrs. R has made while attending the Center has made it feasible for her family to care for her at home.

Case study Mr. "K." This client is a 71-year-old male with congestive heart failure who attends the Center Monday, Wednesday, and Friday. Mr. K needs his lungs checked, and his weight, blood pressure and diet monitored by the nursing staff to maintain his delicate physical condition. His wife works during the day and he drives himself from home to the program. He is very alert and social and has many friends both among the clients and staff of the Day Center and among the many children attending preschool in the same building. This client had been physically unstable and frequently required hospitalization before attending the Day Health Center. During his 18-month involvement in the Center, constant monitoring and treatment have prevented further hospitalization.

Case study Mrs. "C." This client is a 77-year-old female with severe dementia. She attends the Center Monday through Friday. This client has difficulty communicating her needs and desires and attending to a task. She tends to wander and often requires individual attention for her own safety. Mrs. C participates in some Center activities, especially those involving small children, pets, and music. A number of the clients look out for her well-being and visit with her. Mrs. C lives with her daughter who works full-time. Due to the level of care she requires and the expense of in-home care, the Day Health Center provides the only alternative to institutionalization.

Future Program Goals

Future goals of the Day Center staff include: 1) spending more individual time with clients; (2) having more time for staff meetings and inservices; (3) developing regular family conferences and involving families more in the treatment process; (4) developing a formal evaluation for clients and their families to give feedback to the Center; (5) refining and utilizing the assessment tool the staff is now working on to classify levels of client care; (6) developing a system of intake according to levels of care, percentages of clients in each level

Table 26-2
Statistics Collected from July 1982 to January 1984

Total Clients Served: 84

Total Male: 35   Total Female: 49

Age Range of Clients Served: 29 to 97 years old

Age	Number of Clients
20 to 29	I
30 to 39	I
40 to 49	II
50 to 59	IIIII IIII
60 to 69	IIIII IIIII I
70 to 79	IIIII IIIII IIIII IIII
80 to 89	IIIII IIIII IIIII IIIII IIIII II
90 to 99	IIIII IIIII IIII

of care, and ability of the staff to care for the client accordingly; and (7) developing a work skills program.

St. Mary's Day Health Center for Older Adults is a successful medical model day center because of the consistent quality care given by its staff and the enthusiasm of the Madison community. It is a rewarding experience to be involved in an innovative program that may prolong people's independence while helping to relieve the stress experienced in family caregiving situations.

REFERENCES

Burris, K. (1981). Recommending adult day care center. *Nursing and Health Care,* 437-441.

Curley, J. (1980). *Methodist Health Center Activities Department Statement of Philosophy,* unpublished.

Kiernat, J. M. (1976). Geriatric day hospitals: A golden opportunity for therapists. *American Journal of Occupational Therapy, 30,* 280-289.

Levy, M. (1981). *Certificate of need application.* St. Mary's Hospital Medical Center, unpublished.

Neustadt, L. (1982). Developing a program for Jewish residents in non-Jewish nursing homes. *Occupational & Physical Therapy In Geriatrics, 2,* 13-23.

Rathbone-McCuan, E. & Elliot, M. (1976). Geriatric day care: In theory and practice. *Social Work in Health Care, 2,* 13-23.

Robins, E. *Keynote Presentation. Adult day programs for the elderly proceedings.* Publications and Advertising Office, Utica College and Syracuse University, 5-11.

CHAPTER TWENTY-SEVEN

Program Planning in Geriatric Psychiatry: A Model for Psychosocial Rehabilitation

Danielle N. Butin and Colleen Heaney

This chapter was previously published in Physical and Occupational Therapy in Geriatrics, 9(3-4), 153-170. Copyright ©1990, Haworth Press. Reprinted by permission.

Psychosocial rehabilitation in geriatric psychiatry is based on the premise that success in self-care, leisure and work is crucial to mental well-being. The objective of program planning is to comprehensively assess function and to promote optimal performance in areas of cognition, interpersonal skills, self-care, leisure, work, and utilization of community resources. Maintaining levels of activity involvement with adaptability and flexibility is an essential component of late life satisfaction. The geriatric activity program at the New York Hospital is a comprehensive rehabilitation model that positively impacts on patients' well-being.

The Westchester Division of the New York Hospital Cornell Medical Center is a university based nonprofit voluntary psychiatric facility. The 322-bed in-patient clinical service has a separate division of geriatric services, with three units totaling 66 beds.

Separate departments of medicine, nursing, social work, psychology, and therapeutic activities comprise the multidisciplinary team. Three of the five therapeutic activity professionals who treat geriatric patients are represented on each unit, and serve as case managers for their patients. The arbitrary age for admission to the geriatric service is 55, with potential range from 55-98 years old. The average length of stay is five weeks. Though a wide variety of neurological and psychiatric disorders are represented, the majority of patients are admitted for diagnosis and treatment of an affective disorder or an organic mood disturbance. Diagnosis, prognosis, chronological age and expected discharge environment often do not influence placement on any particular unit because bed availability is an overriding concern. Those persons with affective disorders, dementia, or long term chronic psychiatric illness may live on the same unit.

The wide variation in developmental and chronological age for this heterogeneous group, and the brief length of stay presented a significant challenge to activity program planning and treatment. Equally challenging for activity rehabilitation is that a medical model of treatment prevails, and in the past, psychosocial rehabilitation had been minimized or disregarded. Elderly patients, family members and many professional staff readily abdicated all clinical decisions to professionals, and symptom relief was seen as the ultimate answer. Prior to aggressive efforts to restructure activity rehabilitation, geriatric patients were treated biologically, received individual and family therapy, and participated in a largely diversional activity program. The patients generally were discharged free of major psychiatric symptomatology and were given a suggested aftercare plan. However, maladaptive behavior patterns and skill dysfunction that can accompany mental illness or result from loss of esteem and confidence was manifest throughout the hospitalization and evident at discharge. Patients were often at risk for noncompliance in following discharge recommendations, were unsuccessful in adapting to their discharge environment, and were risks for recidivism.

Over the past five years, the authors have worked extensively to develop a program that would more definitively address psychosocial aspects of rehabilitation and challenge patients, families and staff to acknowledge the importance of it. The complexion of professional staff in the Geriatrics Therapeutic Activity Division include a gerontological counselor, an occupational therapist, two recreational therapists, and a creative arts therapist. A liaison vocational counselor is also available for those persons who have work as a priority goal. Through collaborative efforts of these professionals, a framework for treatment has been established that uses counseling techniques to promote purposeful involvement in activity. Activity rehabilitation has gradually, but consistently become integrated into treatment in the geriatric division, and is currently recognized as tantamount to recovering from mental illness.

FRAME OF REFERENCE

Although the disengagement theory suggests that older people naturally become more self-involved and less interested in others or external events, clinical observations and scientific studies dispute this view of universal disengagement (Neugarten, 1965, Havighurst, 1968). Disengagement theorists claim that this reaction is a response to inner needs and not a response to sociocultural pressure (Cumming, 1961). A universal disengagement process is an over-generalization, and lacks the consideration and integration of an individual's lifestyle as a predictor of successful aging (Neugarten, 1965). In fact, social involvements and commitments are the factors most strongly associated with well-being during the natural adjustment to old age. Greater life satisfaction has been found among seniors who are active in both community activities and family roles. Since life satisfaction is more closely related to levels of activity than inactivity, older adults who maintain greater amounts of activity report high levels of gratification and contentment (Havighurst, 1961). Activity theory stresses the need for older adults to maintain active involvement and to augment and replace activities to assure continued satisfaction and mental well-being (Pikunas, 1969). Older adults age favorably if they remain active, cope with major life losses, and find meaningful replacement activities for those relinquished. Generally, older adults have the same psychosocial needs as middle-aged adults, with the exception of biological and health related changes (Havighurst, 1961).

As older people age, however, activity levels may decrease with restrictive opportunities for interpersonal pursuits. Life satisfaction tends to be greater when physical and mental health states are sound (Maddox, 1965). People limited in activities of daily living, access to community services and vocational opportunities are least likely to report feeling satisfied and fulfilled (Smith, 1972). Psychogeriatric patients are frequently faced with the dual burden of coping with a major psychiatric disorder, while attempting to adapt to physical changes and limitations. Skills in carrying out activities of daily living, working, or volunteering at a relatively satisfying job, enjoying avocational and creative pursuits, and relating interpersonally are frequently impaired among psychiatric patients (Mosey, 1970).

The overall goal of psychiatric rehabilitation is to promote patient satisfaction and provide learning opportunities for the skills necessary to accomplish tasks of everyday living (Fidler, 1984). The necessary components for a meaningful activity program for older adults with psychiatric illness are sensory stimulation and reality orientation for the cognitively impaired or severely regressed; remotivation for patients who are socially withdrawn and alienated from their surroundings but capable of coherent interactions and able to perform graded simple tasks; complex and challenging activities for those whose social and functional skills are relatively intact; and transitional activities or volunteer work to meet the needs of those returning home with community responsibilities (Weiner, 1978).

Following initial assessments of their needs, capabilities, and wishes for rehabilitation, patients are referred for individual or group treatment. This process encourages skill development and incremental progress toward attainment of individualized activity goals that are vital to the well-being of the elderly patient.

ASSESSMENTS

Comprehensive assessments are the cornerstone of psychosocial treatment in the geriatric division. These assessments help determine assets and liabilities in cognition, interpersonal skills, task performance, physical ability, leisure and social involvement and utilization of community resources. The assessments guide treatment, maximize individualized interventions and promote programming that is responsive to the expressed interests of each patient.

The rehabilitation process is initiated (within a few days of admission), when the Therapeutic Activities Representative meets with the patient and engages him/her in a planning dialogue. The Rehabilitation Activity Assessment helps determine the patient's overall goals in self-care, work, and leisure and elicits participation in identifying and prioritizing skills and behaviors needed to attain their goals. Patients who have the cognitive skills to participate meaningfully in this process value this tool as it promotes participation in a rehabilitation plan that is self-generated. This model gives patients the opportunity to identify goals, determine needed skills, select methods for skill acquisition and augment or modify their goals in relationship to their ongoing performance.

Sometimes the patients are seriously cognitively impaired, or too psychiatrically ill to realistically determine their goals and needs. In these cases, the Therapeutic Activity Representative provides assistance in referring to groups and recommending discharge plans that are consistent with their needs for support.

Consistent application of this initial dialogue with geriatric patients has generated some common rehabilitation goals and skills needed to achieve the goals. Individual and group treatment that reflects the patient's priority needs in self-care, work or leisure and focuses on their level of functioning have been conceptualized with regard to the patient's expressed interest for rehabilitation.

Self-care treatment generally focuses on skills needed for the patient to manage in his or her living environment following discharge. Treatment in the leisure category addresses the skills needed for the patient to spend free time qualitatively. Treatment in the work category focuses on skills needed to resume paid employment or acquire a volunteer job. Some common examples of overall rehabilitation goals and required skills in these areas are as follows.

SELF-CARE REHABILITATION GOALS

1. I will go to a nursing home when I am discharged from the hospital.
2. I want to move to my daughter's house when I leave the hospital.
3. I want to return home to my apartment when I am discharged from the hospital.

Skills:
- identifying self-care strengths and weaknesses
- improving attention to hygiene
- following schedule
- improving nutritional awareness
- managing money
- accepting help from a home health aide
- managing transportation
- cooking and meal planning
- expressing opinions
- tolerating others
- improving confidence
- expressing satisfaction
- following routine
- researching residences

LEISURE REHABILITATION GOALS

1. I want to participate in the activity program at the nursing home when I am discharged.
2. I want to find people to play bridge with in my location when I leave the hospital.
3. I want to join a senior center when I leave the hospital.

Skills:
- clarifying current and past leisure interests
- enriching or renewing leisure interests
- improving skill in a leisure activity
- finding community leisure options
- increasing confidence and independence in using community resources
- initiating leisure involvements
- initiating contacts with peers

WORK REHABILITATION GOALS

1. I want to be productive in my nursing home environment.
2. I want to find a volunteer job in the community when I leave the hospital.
3. I want to find paid employment in the community when I leave the hospital.

Skills:
- clarifying work/volunteer history and aspirations
- identifying concerns regarding retirement
- improving awareness of post-retirement options
- accepting supervision in the work setting
- increasing willingness to accept challenge and responsibility in work setting
- working cooperatively with others
- organizing tasks
- increasing productivity in tasks
- exploring community services
- interviewing for job
- identifying work related skills

The described assessment and planning dialogue almost always signals a need for additional assessments to supplement, validate or help patients measure the congruence between their goals, assets and liabilities.

The SHORTCARE (Comprehensive Assessment and Referral Evaluation) (Gurland, 1984) is often used to gather additional functional information. The SHORTCARE discourages reliance on typical symptoms only for resolution of psychiatric illness. It encourages a probing look at the etiology of specific areas of psychosocial dysfunction. This standardized, multidimensional semi-structured interview provides clinicians with scales for depression, dementia, and disability. The SHORTCARE assists therapists in becoming more cognizant of each patient's individual needs for rehabilitation and aftercare.

Patients are also assessed with the Activities Health Assessment. This tool provides both therapists and patients with information about time management, involvement in meaningful activities, and discharge planning.

Finally, patients are constantly assessed and observed while participating in functional activities. They have opportunities to critique their own performance while receiving feedback about the specific skills needed to attain their overall rehabilitation goal.

PROGRAM DESCRIPTION

The primary objective of activity rehabilitation in geriatrics is to help each patient identify his or her specific goals and needed skills in self-care, leisure and work. Because the therapeutic activity professionals recognize the broad range of dysfunction, there is commitment to meeting individual needs. The program and the therapists are highly flexible while maintaining a core structure that provides stability. This is accomplished by offering groups that closely parallel the expected plans for the individual's discharge environment. It is also accomplished by expecting the therapist to individualize treatment within the context of the group. For example, in a verbal group, one patient may be working on expressing opinions, while another patient might be working on the acquisition of listening skills because they are dominant interrupters. A moderately demented patient might cook in a group with patients preparing for discharge because they have maintained a skill in that one area.

Groups are generally organized with regard for the patient's functional status and need for different amounts of support.

Table 27-1
Leisure Planning Protocol

Days: MWF   Time: 1:30 to 2:45 pm

Problems

1. Patient unable to identify leisure interests.

2. Patient unable to independently plan or participate in meaningful activities.

3. Patient is unaware of leisure resources or how to access these services in the community.

Short-Term Goals

1. Patient will identify one or two interests within the group.

2. Patient will cooperatively plan and participate in one community activity per week with peers on the unit.

3. Patient will call two or three community resources per week to heighten awareness of available programs.

Long-Term Goals

1. Patient will commit to two-three community based activities based on identified interests.

2. Patient will initiate suggestions and plans for weekly community outing.

3. Patient will develop a resource file of meaningful activities in the community prior to discharge.

Interventions

1. *Identifying Leisure Interests*
Leader provides leisure interest finders and value surveys to encourage identification and exploration of interests.

2. *Planning*
Leader encourages group to cooperatively identify and plan one community activity. Patients utilize resource file to make arrangements and calls.

3. *Implementation*
Leader accompanies group on the community trip. Patients secure names on mailing lists and independently seek out information for their involvement.

This assures successful involvements while challenging the patient to continually use skills that have been neglected.

After assessments are completed, findings are collected and analyzed. The patients are then referred to groups that can provide them with skill acquisition that they, or the therapist, have determined as essential for success in their discharge environment. Patients are given large print schedules with a detailed description of groups. The schedules have a space for the therapist and patient to list the specific skills requiring attention within the context of each group. Since each group has a clearly defined protocol, therapists are aware of the specific guidelines and objectives for that group. As an example, the Leisure Planning Protocol is described in Table 1.

Each program cluster (self-care, work and leisure) has groups that respond to the requirement for maximum, moderate or minimum levels of support. As patients improve or plateau they are encouraged to participate in increasingly challenging activities. Examples of the program are provided to illustrate how assessment findings are applied to the level of support needed in group treatment.

GROUP STRUCTURE OFFERING MAXIMUM SUPPORT

Patient Population

This population is quite regressed due to depression, chronic schizophrenia, or dementia, and is moderately to severely cognitively impaired. They are alert, but frequently disoriented. If their level of function remains the same throughout hospitalization, these patients are usually discharged to an institutional facility, or return home with significant home care, and a structured day program.

Self-Care

Assistance and encouragement is needed in all activities of daily living, and patients are unable to follow simple 12-step directions. Decisions do not show good judgement and supervision is required to maintain safety. These are patients who have a limited investment in how they look, how they spend their time, and often deny, minimize or overlook difficulties.

Self-Care Skills:
- Following simple directions while grooming
- Eating independently
- Dressing with minimal cueing and encouragement
- Finding room on the unit
- Using notes to compensate for memory problems

Leisure

Activity participation is limited. They cannot generate interests or skills, and require constant encouragement and stimulation to remain engaged in purposeful activity. They minimally communicate with each other, and are withdrawn and isolative.

Leisure Skills:
- Attempting an adapted version of an activity from the past
- Tolerating the presence of others
- Initiating and completing a task within one group setting

Work

Patients are unable to work productively in organizing tasks to completion. They are easily frustrated and have no tolerance for stress. Difficulties sequencing logical steps in an organized manner are noted.

Work Skills:
- Asking for clarification or assistance
- Maintaining participation in task activities for 15 minute periods
- Sequencing simple steps in a logical order
- Following simple directions

Activity groups organized for this population illustrate ways to engage the seriously regressed geriatric population. The severely regressed begin each day with sensory stimulation and exercise. Old familiar show tunes lead even the most regressed patient through pleasurable movements. Balloon volleyball ends this daily session with increased alertness and heightened sensitivity to the environment.

Simple repetitive tasks are provided to encourage basic responsibility for one's immediate environment. Examples of volunteer jobs on the unit include folding laundry, ringing meal bell, dusting tables, and changing tablecloths. Jobs are listed weekly on the unit bulletin board, with the patient's name, and cueing is provided consistently by the interdisciplinary team.

Many strategies of an adaptive function model are incorporated in the remotivation group. Modalities utilized to increase socialization, and sensitivity to the immediate environment are memory games, elder trivia, reminiscent slide shows, pet therapy, nature outings, murals, improvisation, and simple baking.

For the more regressed, individual work includes sensory stimulation, and in some cases holding stuffed animals has been therapeutic.

GROUP STRUCTURE OFFERING MODERATE SUPPORT

Patient Population

This population represents those older adults with partial symptom resolution following biological, milieu, activity and counseling therapies. As patients improve, they need new challenges. Although they are alert and oriented, they may be mildly cognitively impaired, and still depressed. If their condition remains stable, they are usually discharged to a senior residence, or home with senior day treatment. Moderate support is required because the therapist must organize components of their projects, while encouraging greater self-reliance among group members. The leader encourages interaction, and promotes opportunities for group feedback, but must continue to be the facilitator.

Self-Care

Although needing help with problem solving, most can perform activities of daily living with minimal assistance. They are able to recognize areas of difficulty and may begin to ask for help and feedback.

Self-Care Skills:
- Following activity schedule independently
- Participating in meal planning and preparation
- Making bed
- Cleaning bedroom
- Organizing datebook with telephone numbers and appointments

Leisure

Interest and motivation for leisure involvements is inconsistent. They initiate activities within structured settings, but not outside of group opportunities. These are people who have difficulty asking peers to join them for a casual activity or conversation. They are dependent on a group leader for initiating interaction, and rarely generate involvement independently.

Leisure Skills:
- Setting up supplies needed for a group activity
- Attending all scheduled activities
- Identifying interests to pursue upon discharge

Work

Patients derive genuine pleasure from involvement in work-related projects, or commitments that improve the lives of others. They continue to rely on the group leader for directions and instructions to follow through on tasks appropriately.

Work Skills:
- Identifying ways to remain committed to meaningful work-related activity
- Improving investment in quality of work
- Increasing confidence in familiar tasks

Patients in this phase of treatment are expected to be familiar with unit and activity routines. They often begin their day with discussion of current events, and are encouraged to bring at least one or more topics of interest to the group. This intervention provides them with a nonthreatening way to participate in discussions.

Often patients demonstrate increased independence by participating in a cooking group. By making snacks for their unit, and initiating luncheons for peers, family members, staff or guests, they begin to regain confidence in a wide range of skills. A leisure skills group provides an opportunity to get acquainted with peers who share similar interests. Group leaders facilitate opportunities for patients who value bridge, shuffleboard, etc. to know one another and make commitments. This is important for those who will return to a center, because they will be expected to initiate and join social activities.

Finally, exposure to volunteer activity is popular at this phase of treatment. Community service projects help patients move outside themselves and offer something to others. This group has frequently made and contributed toys to homeless children, participated in clerical tasks needed for fundraising events, maintained bulletin, boards, designed advertisement flyers and contributed information to the patients' newsletter. The leader usually needs to provide tasks, direction and encouragement.

GROUP STRUCTURE OFFERING MINIMUM SUPPORT

Patient Population

This group is approaching discharge and has resolved a major depressive disorder. After a major depression has been treated with medication, maladaptive behaviors are often apparent. Patients continue to struggle with dependency; helplessness; anger over losses; and poor coping mecha-

nisms. They can use insight-oriented experiences to understand maladaptive patterns and initiate and practice alternate coping mechanisms. This population generally returns home with a clearly defined plan to pursue for community involvement. The therapist encourages increased leadership and opportunities for problem solving by operationalizing decisions made within the group, and helping members to see the carryover process. Although they are cognitively intact and usually physically healthy, they frequently have lifelong difficulties with adaptation, making and keeping friends, and interacting meaningfully in the community. They need careful individualized programs to help compensate for lifelong problems reaching out for help.

Self-Care

Any limitations in activities of daily living are minimized because of fears of dependency. They struggle with issues of interdependence, and lack the ability to comfortably ask for help. Familiar tasks, like cooking or balancing a checkbook, are resisted because of anxiety or lack of familiarity with the task (following the death of a spouse). Some self-care tasks may be difficult due to dependency and anxiety.

Self-Care Skills:
- Planning and ordering food for meals
- Arranging transportation for passes
- Practicing asking for help
- Identifying strengths in self-care

Leisure

Although motivated and interested in meaningful activities, they need encouragement and support to participate in new or challenging activities. They are quite anxious about engaging in community outings and returning home.

Leisure Skills:
- Identifying activities to pursue upon discharge
- Participating in a few community outings per week
- Planning and arranging details for community-based activities
- Asking peers to participate in unstructured activities
- Initiating meaningful activities during unstructured time

Work

They are motivated to translate interests into community service or employment. These skills are practiced while hospitalized and only assistance with major decisions is needed.

Work Skills:
- Identifying specific volunteer/paid employment interests
- Practicing skills needed for expected job
- Exploring community options for work
- Arranging details and interviews
- Identifying strengths and deficits

This population is approaching discharge to the community following treatment for a major depression. Generally, they have reacquired essential concrete skills, but maladaptive behaviors may resurface or continue to be apparent as the patient faces discharge without the intense support he or she had during hospitalization. Struggles with dependency, anger over losses, fears of incompetence and interpersonal problems are highlighted as expectations for more challenging functioning are indicated. Essential in this phase of treatment are opportunities to verbally express concerns and get support, but shift emphasis away from the activity therapist and toward themselves and others. Counseling groups that focus on increased autonomy, choice, and responsibility are introduced along with more challenging activities. These interventions help patients to identify concerns, explore coping strategies and practice activities designed to rekindle feelings of competence and worthwhileness.

The Leisure Planning Group is a three-part group that helps older adults identify interests, community events, and plan a weekly community outing. An extensive file of community resources is available. Group participants are expected to make appropriate calls and arrangements.

Goals Group uses activity and cognitive therapy models to empower and assist in regaining some control and mastery of life tasks. The action-oriented verbal-task group stresses exploration of coping and problem-solving skills, emphasizes collaborative involvement and encourages goal-directed activity that alters the person's role from that of subordinate to peer group member responsible to themselves and others. Homework is given and participants are encouraged to practice specific strategies to optimize their independence in preparation for discharge.

To practice better communicating strategies with their grandchildren, an intergenerational meal group was established in collaboration with hospitalized adolescents. An older adult patient was matched with an adolescent to foster and learn appropriate interactive strategies to carryover at home. The dyads interchanged responsibilities for meal planning, and each dyad assumed responsibility for the preparation of specific components of the meal. Older patients used past meal planning skills, while practicing appropriate interactive styles necessary for healthy relationships at home.

For those patients who have work as a priority goal, Vocational Services provides them with opportunities for volunteer jobs throughout the hospital. The placement is viewed as a vital reality testing tool. Examples of volunteer jobs used by hospitalized older adults have included a plant operations director volunteering in the hospital maintenance department, a retired secretary volunteering as a research librarian, and a knitting teacher volunteering as an instructor with older and younger long-term patients.

CONCLUSION

The geriatric psychosocial rehabilitation program has become well regarded and integrated into the fabric of comprehensive, multidisciplinary treatment.

Initial and ongoing assessment assure that the patient is continually being evaluated so that his or her treatment is specific and relevant to changing needs. Well-designed groups and flexible group leaders guarantee a structure that is perceived as stable, while being responsive to the unique needs of each patient.

The Geriatric Therapeutic Activities staff's distinct contribution in clinical rounds has impacted upon all disciplines planning for treatment, family therapy and discharge. The patients report valuing the program because it gives them the varied opportunities and support they need to meet the challenges of growing older with dignity and purpose.

REFERENCES

Cumming, E., Henry, W. (1961). *Growing old: The process of disengagement.* New York, NY: Basic Books.

Fidler, G. S. (1984). *Design of rehabilitation services in psychiatric hospital settings.* Laurel, MD: Ramsco.

Gurland, B., Golden, R. G., Teresi, J. A., & Chatlop, J. (1984). The SHORTCARE: An efficient instrument for the assessment of depression, dementia and disability. *Journal of Gerontology, 39,* (2), 166-169.

Havighurst, R. J. (1961). Successful aging. *Gerontologist, 1,* 8-13.

Havighurst, R. J., Neugarten, B. L., & Tobin, S. S. (1968). Disengagement and patterns of aging. In B. L. Neugarten. (Ed.) *Middle age and aging* (pp. 161-172). Chicago, IL: University of Chicago Press.

Maddox, G. L. (1965). Fact and artifact: evidence bearing on the disengagement theory from the Duke Geriatrics Project. *Human Development. 8,* 117-130.

Mosey, A C. (1970). *Three frames of reference for mental health.* Thorofare, NJ: SLACK Incorporated

Pikunas, J. (1969). *Human development: an emergent science.* New York: McGraw-Hill.

Smith, J. J., & Lipman, A. (1972). Constraint and life satisfaction. *Journal of Gerontology,* 77-82.

Weiner, M. B., Brok, A. J., & Snadowsky, A. M. (1978). *Working with the aged.* New Jersey: Prentice-Hall.

CHAPTER TWENTY-EIGHT

Health Promotion Through Employee Assistance Programs: A Role for Occupational Therapists

Marianne Maynard

In the 1970s, a series of articles in the *American Journal of Occupational Therapy* urged therapists to broaden their perspectives and practice to include community health promotion and disease prevention. During this period, health policy agencies also began to place more emphasis on keeping people well through health promotion programs. Occupational therapists, along with other allied health professionals, were encouraged to share their expertise in advocating a healthy life style through the prevention of disease and disabilities and the maintenance of wellness.

Wiemer and West (1970) found support for the role of the occupational therapist in health promotion and disability prevention in the American Occupational Therapy Association's (AOTA's) definition of occupational therapy as the art and science of directing a person's response to selected activity to promote and maintain health, to prevent disability, to evaluate behavior and to treat or train patients with physical or psychosocial dysfunction. The authors observed that our practice model was expanding from a hospital-based and treatment-oriented setting to a community-based and health-oriented setting. Walker suggested in 1971 that the emerging model of occupational therapy is concerned with the well community and the maintenance of health and prevention of deficits, disease, and disabilities. She identified areas of practice in home health, maternal and child health, community guidance, and chronic disease care. Wiemer proposed in 1972 that the role of the occupational therapist in preventive and community health should be that of a health advocate and counselor and that, by joining with other health professionals, occupational therapists can promote their special knowledge of the relationship between health and occupation. In the wellness community, therapists can function in all types of settings such as homes, schools, labor union halls, industrial plants, businesses, hospitals, and town halls.

Finn (1972), in her Eleanor Clarke Slagle lecture, traced changes in our professional role in the delivery of health services in the 1960s. She affirmed that, unless we begin to refocus our attention on keeping people well, we will never be able to stem the tide of human suffering in our country. She also urged us to move beyond the role of therapists and become health agents, to progress along the continuum from hospital and clinical services to community and health programs. Occupational therapists can make unique contributions to preventive health care and community programming because they understand the importance of activities in wellness. Grossman (1977) advised us to "be skilled in the techniques of primary prevention: consultation, education, and collaborative efforts to develop community resources, to establish natural support systems, and to use natural caretakers" (p. 351).

The official AOTA position paper on the role of the occupational therapist in the promotion of health and prevention of disabilities (AOTA, 1979) identified a framework to promote health and prevent disease and injury through primary, secondary, and tertiary programs:

> The provision of services for primary prevention most often focuses upon health promotion activities that are designed to help individuals clarify their values about health, to understand the linkages between lifestyle and health and to acquire the knowledge, habits and attitudes needed to promote both physical and mental health.... Secondary prevention services that help to prevent or retard the progression of a disorder to a more serious or chronic condition normally include early diagnosis, appropriate referral, prompt and effective treatment, as well as health screening, consultation, crisis intervention, and home health care.... Tertiary prevention programs encompass the provision of rehabilitative services to assist disabled individuals in attaining their maximum potential for productivity and full participation in community life (p. 50-51).

Occupational therapists are generally active in all three prevention levels and with most of the risk factors listed. However, their role has only recently become visible. New areas for occupational therapy services in health promotion and wellness activities will continue to emerge. One specific area that is expanding rapidly in business and industry is the employee assistance program (EAP). EAPs address both primary and secondary prevention health issues of employees, and many also incorporate health promotion activities. Occupational therapists can contribute to EAPs by identifying and providing services for workers who are at risk for occupational dysfunction or who have early signs of maladaptive occupational behavior.

EMPLOYEE ASSISTANCE PROGRAMS

For some time now companies and institutions as well as local, state, and federal agencies have been using employee assistance programs to handle their employees' personal and job-related problems. The earliest EAP may have been an alcohol rehabilitation program for employees instituted by Macy's department store in 1917. DuPont established the first corporate EAP in the 1940s because of alcoholism among its workers. After World War II, with the increase in drug and alcohol misuse and mental health problems at the workplace, more companies established EAPs. These programs have expanded or have grown from an estimated 50 in 1950 to over 5,000 in 1981 (Sakell, 1985). For example, General Motors' EAP provides services to 44,000 employees at over 130 sites (Galvin, 1983). The list of major corporations, private firms, state agencies, and universities with EAPs continues to grow, with many EAPs expanding their services into areas of health promotion, stress management, and fitness and recreation programs for employees and their families. In general, companies have found it more cost-effective to rehabilitate good workers with problems than to fire them and train new workers (Pelletier, 1984)

Staffing Patterns and Procedures

Depending on the organizational structure and the size of the facility, EAPs may be free-standing units reporting directly to top management or units within employee health or human resource departments. Employee assistance services are usually included as part of the company benefit package. For example, mental and physical health problems may be covered by employees' group health insurance plans.

The staffing pattern also varies in companies, depending on the location in the organizational structure and on the services provided. Most EAPs are staffed by counselors and human services professionals, including mental health and rehabilitation counselors, social workers, and perhaps industrial health nurses and related health personnel. As EAPs expand into health promotion and disease and disability prevention activities, there is a substantial role for occupational therapists to perform as members of the EAP team.

General Operational Procedures

The general purpose of an EAP in industry is to identify, confront, diagnose, treat, and follow up on employees' health problems:

The eight elements for program support identified by people who work in stress prevention are (a) a policy statement or performance contract; (b) union support; (c) clearly-defined work performance standards; (d) recognition that performance problems have a variety of causes; (e) a diagnostic and referral agent; (f) comprehensive treatment resources; (g) insurance coverage that is compatible with the EAP philosophy; and (h) an evaluation program (Gam, Sauser, Evans, & Lair, 1983, p. 62).

Most EAPs' procedures include the following steps: (a) referral of an employee either by supervisor, colleague, family member, or a voluntary referral; (b) screening process, including information gathering; (c) personal interview, assessment of problem/situation; (d) diagnosis of concern, problem, and situation; (e) intervention process, which may include employees, family members, or coworkers; (f) intervention in the form of counseling sessions, group support sessions, information and skill building classes, and seminars; (g) continuing follow-up and evaluation of services provided (Sakell, 1985).

If after the initial screening or diagnosis of a problem situation the EAP administrators are unable to handle the employee's problem within their unit, the employee is referred for follow-up to an appropriate community service agency. An important part of most EAPs is the training sessions, which teach supervisors how to identify and refer troubled employees to EAP services. In many cases, the supervisor provides the early guidance and referral that is so important in primary prevention.

The Richmond Employee Assistance Program (REAP), for instance, provides services to 10,000 employees in 16 organizations. Based on request or employees' needs, classes have been offered in assertiveness, communication skills, dealing with depression, financial planning, life planning skills, parenting skills, retirement planning, single parenting, stress management, substance abuse awareness, time management, and two-career family management. REAP also provides support groups for employees and their family members who are concerned about Alzheimer's disease and related disorders, battered women, aging parents, children with special needs, and separation and divorce (Krammer, 1984). Frequent services offered by EAPs are in the areas of retirement planning, stress management, family concerns, financial and legal concerns, and health and fitness. In addition to counseling employees, identifying problems, and finding solutions, the larger EAPs spend a large amount of time organizing and conducting support groups and special seminars and classes for their employees in occupational performance areas where occupational therapists have expertise, such as daily living management and encouraging a balanced work-leisure life style.

EAPs and Health Promotion

Some corporations include health promotion activities under the EAP, either providing in-house facilities for their activities or cooperating with a local YMCA or YWCA, Heart and Lung Association, or Red Cross to provide their activities. Some corporations provide incentives for employees to stay well, such as memberships in recreational and fitness clubs or discounts on goods and services (Pelletier, 1984).

Most companies disseminate health education information as part of their overall employee health promotion program. The larger companies may focus on stress management and physical fitness programs. Most health promotion programs also provide some type of risk assessment and screening for early detection of coronary, hypertension, and other lifestyle risk factors.

Health hazard appraisals or health risk profiles are two methods used to determine an employee's probability of becoming ill or dying from a particular cause. The concept of risk implies that there are specific links between habits and disease, such as between smoking and lung cancer or overeating and heart disease. Risk for certain diseases is related to a person's group membership based on heredity, environment, personal history, age, sex, and race. There are three basic types of risk (a) those of potential importance on a probabilistic basis in an otherwise asymptomatic person; (b) those indicating the early manifestation of disease; and (c) those indicative of fully developed disease (Mavis, 1984).

Employees may volunteer to complete a health risk profile questionnaire or be interviewed for such information. Those employees that evidence a high-risk lifestyle are especially encouraged to complete a health risk profile. The information is then processed by comparing the person's health data with the national morbidity data base, examining deviation from the average risks for the various causes of death. This process is usually built into the scoring process and interpretation of data with commercially available forms of health risk profiles. The EAP or health promotion counselor will then meet with the employee and family members if this is necessary for interpreting the profile results. The consultation usually focuses on employee habits, helpful resources, and a discussion of a course of action for changing habit patterns. The employee may be encouraged to participate in health promotion classes, exercise programs, or stress management seminars. Periodic follow-ups are made to check progress and provide additional encouragement and resources. High-risk employees are urged to see their personal physicians for monitoring. Health risk assessments have been found to be helpful for promoting a healthy lifestyle in that they help employees understand the choices involved in risk-taking behaviors in relationship to their lifestyle. The feedback and interpretation of a profile seems to communicate to the employee a sense of urgency to change risk behavior for a more healthy lifestyle (Mavis, 1984).

THE OCCUPATIONAL THERAPIST ON THE EAP TEAM

Occupational therapists' knowledge and skills can be used in EAPs, especially in the areas where a recognized void in services exists. Major contributions would be providing employee services in the areas of analysis and enhancement of daily living skills for maintenance of productivity, leisure, and home/family management; assessment and recommendations on adapting the work and home environment to improve health and well-being; task analysis and instruction in work simplification to reduce stress and strain on body parts; and conservation of energy and time for improved job performance. Other areas for occupational therapist services would include the identification and elimination of architectural barriers; instruction in the use of adaptive devices; modification of the work unit for the worker injured or disabled on the job; promotion of a milieu supportive of occupational role performance through interpersonal skill development; and support group process and activities such as health and fitness promotion, stress reduction, and retirement and leisure planning programs.

As EAP team members, occupational therapists would contribute their evaluation skills in functional assessment, self-maintenance, and occupational role performance, as well as their knowledge of adaptive and maladaptive role behaviors. Occupational therapists' experience in program planning, implementation, and evaluation, as well as their experience in collaborating with medical, human services, and education personnel for the purposes of referral, information, and follow-up, could facilitate EAP team efforts in program development and networking.

The Therapist's Approach

Depending on the EAP and organizational structure, the occupational therapist's intervention may include the procedures illustrated in Table 28-1. These interventions are part of a repertoire of services that may improve the quality of life. Johnson and Kielhofner (1983) suggest that occupational therapy's major contribution to prevention or health maintenance is to enable people to modify their health-threatening lifestyles and restore healthy patterns of work and play. The general areas of services of the EAPs either implicitly or explicitly address the occupational behavior perspective as described by Rogers (1983).

First, there is an emphasis on the health of persons in terms of their productive participation in society. Second, health is seen as correlated with daily experience, which consists of work, play, rest, and sleep. Third, daily experiences take place in a complex physical, temporal, and social environment, which is a critical factor in shaping behavior. Fourth, occupational

Table 28-1

Sample Profile of Occupational Therapy EAP Intervention Plan

Intervention Goals	Principles of Behavioral/ Situational Change	Techniques Used for Behavioral/Situational Change	Criteria of Success
To obtain information on worker's support networks and significant others that may be helpful in intervention plan	Assess worker's dysfunction areas, identify occupations and resources beneficial in meeting worker's need	Additional exploration, information gathering, and identification of resources. Collaboration with significant other in worker's network	Reeducation in high-risk habits and behavior detrimental to health
To support optimal health and well-being of workers by promoting a healthy and safe workplace, supportive milieu, and balanced life-style of work, play and rest	Design an intervention plan to improve worker's deficits and/or environmental conditions Facilitate and promote worker's and significant others' involvement and commitment to intervention plan	Problem solving sessions Goal setting and action planning	Resumption of normal occupational roles and function in work, home, and community settings
To assess worker's behavior and performance in terms of occupational role components (work, leisure, and self-maintenance) and areas of developmental delays (sensory, motor, cognitive, and psychosocial)	Assess worker's occupational role performance, adaptive behaviors, and skills to determine areas of deficit needs and overall capabilities and strengths	Observation of work unit and situation Consultation with employee, supervisor, and significant others	Improved state of health and well-being based on worker's self-report and reports from significant others
To assess work environment and milieu as to compatibility with worker's needs, skills, job requirements, and work condition	Assess environmental conditions (home, work, and community) that may be supportive or nonsupportive of worker's performance	Interview and occupation history Assessment of worker's role, tasks, and performance	Acquisition of skills Improved occupational performance
To promote, improve, reestablish, or maintain worker's occupational role performance, adaptive behavioral, and skills	Validate and share findings, make recommendations, and follow up results	Group sessions, educational classes, seminars, skill development or remediation, development, prevention, maintenance	Engagement in health-promoting life-style behaviors

dysfunction that may be recognized by symptoms such as boredom, futility, indifference, lack of self-respect, immobility and disorientation, disrupts daily life. Fifth, daily life may be reorganized through engagement in occupations, such as work, play, crafts, and sports. Sixth, occupational therapists assist the process of organizing behavior by habit training and socialization of patients to the expectations of the culture (p. 97-98).

The human development through the occupation model as described by Clark (1979a; 1979b) could also serve as a guiding framework for a therapist working on an EAP team. It can help in identifying the worker's (consumer's) problems, setting goals, facilitating role performance, and enhancing behavioral functioning. Employers are finding not only that an increasing number of workers are developmentally delayed or impaired in basic skills and knowledge such as cognitive, motor, and social performance areas, but also that they are psychologically handicapped in their ability to handle stress and interpersonal relationships. This model

recognizes that developmental delays can have a major impact on occupational performance and provides some directions for the therapists to deal with this problem. The basic concepts found in both these models seem to be compatible with the EAP's holistic approach to intervention.

Practice Considerations

Today, consumers have two alternatives for selecting health services: the medically-oriented, doctor-centered, hospital-based treatment program or the community-centered health-promotion, disease-prevention, and consumer-involved program. Therapists also have choices in considering community practice. Although job opportunities in hospital acute-care programs are on the decline, more opportunities for practice exist in community programs, such as home health agencies, business and industry, public school systems, community mental health programs, day care programs for the elderly, private and group practices, and health maintenance organizations. However, to take advantage of these opportunities, therapists must be prepared to work not only with pathology but also with health concepts within the normal life continuum of health-wellness and illness-disease. They need an understanding of the impact of personal lifestyles, environmental and sociocultural influences, and economic resources on health. In community health programs, occupational therapists must be prepared to intervene anywhere along the health-illness continuum as the need arises, be it in the home, school, agency, or institution. Our focus will be on the maintenance of health and the prevention of disease through lifestyle management in primary and secondary prevention programs. We will also continue to be active at the illness-disease dysfunctional end of the continuum, providing treatment, reeducation, and skill development in tertiary programs.

Education Considerations

Grossman (1977) suggests the following:

Students must be introduced to career opportunities other than the clinical model. The concepts and skills of community programming can be an integral part of theory and practice courses. Field placement in the community should emphasize interdisciplinary training for outpatient and outreach services. These experiences are better integrated when assigned after hospital-based placements with clear role models. More importantly, students should be exposed to multiple systems (family, hospital, community) and develop varied interactional patterns (p. 354).

Academic courses should stress critical thinking and problem solving along with disease prevention, health promotion, and treatment concepts and skills. Programs used in the industrial and business community, such as EAPs, require that the therapists have skills in interviewing, counseling, and group process.

One option for education programs is to provide fieldwork experiences in a community-based program such as an EAP. If there is no occupational therapist to supervise the student, an occupational therapist faculty member, a consultant, or a private practice therapist in the community could work with a staff member at the agency and provide the on-site supervision. Such collaborative ventures would not only promote the profession of occupational therapy, but also open new employment opportunities for therapists in community practice. For example, a 2-month affiliation with an EAP program under the cooperative supervision of a school faculty member and an EAP counselor would enable the students to enhance their skills in program planning, assessment procedures, teaching, group process, job and task analysis, and skill development. My own exploration with EAP directors has convinced me that they would welcome such an arrangement. Those located near universities are already providing field experiences for social work, rehabilitation, and psychology students, and several EAP directors have expressed a willingness to provide training sites for graduate- level occupational therapy students.

Another way that occupational therapists can become involved in EAPs is to provide training sessions for employees on a contractual basis. Many EAPs contract with either individuals or other agencies to provide specific classes in areas of employees' needs. Occupational therapists have the knowledge and expertise to conduct such classes, especially those related to lifestyle management and occupational performance. Role delineation tends to be more flexible in EAPs than in the hospital care system. Each staff member works in an area of expertise in addition to sharing tasks that are germane to all human services workers. The social worker may be focusing on the worker's family situation, the rehabilitation counselor on the job climate, and the psychologist on the emotional well-being or psychosocial adjustment of the worker. The occupational therapist can complement these efforts by placing emphasis on the worker's occupational dysfunction in work, play, leisure, and rest, and on the maintenance of a balanced lifestyle in daily living activities.

SUMMARY

The rapid expansion of EAPs provides a natural area for occupational therapy programming in the well community. If occupational therapists apply their skills and knowledge in the corporate work site, they are able to intervene in the health care continuum earlier than at the acute care stage. Occupational dysfunction can be corrected while the person is still functioning on the job. This approach provides a saving in both time and money for employees, employers, and society.

Occupational therapists are encouraged to take advantage of the opportunities to work as team members in EAPs. Educators can encourage students to consider this job opportunity by promoting fieldwork experiences at EAP facilities and by collaborating with faculty and agency staff for on-site supervision. As EAP team members, occupational therapists have the opportunity to inform the public about their services, to promote and maintain health and well-being, to prevent disease and injury, and to correct and improve occupational performance. We provide primary, secondary, and tertiary programs for children with impairments in the public school system. Let us also provide primary and secondary programs for adults in their place of work by assuming a place on the EAP team.

REFERENCES

American Occupational Therapy Association. (1979). Role of the occupational therapist in the promotion of health and prevention of disabilities: Position paper. *American Journal of Occupational Therapy, 33*(1), 50-51.

Clark, P. N. (1979a). Human development through occupation: A philosophy and conceptual model for practice, Part 2. *American Journal of Occupational Therapy, 33*, 577-585.

Clark, P. N. (1979b). Human development through occupation: Theoretical frameworks in contemporary occupational therapy practice, Part 1. *American Journal of Occupational Therapy, 33,* 505-514.

Finn, G. L. (1972). The occupational therapist in prevention programs. *American Journal of Occupational Therapy, 26,* 59-66.

Galvin, D. (1983). Health promotion, disability management, and rehabilitation in the workplace. *The Interconnector, 6*(2), 1-6.

Gam, J., Sauser, W., Evans, K., & Lair, C. (1983). Implement an employee assistance program. *Journal of Employment Counseling, 20,* 61-69.

Grossman, J. (1977). Preventive health care and community programming. *American Journal of Occupational Therapy, 31,* 351-354.

Johnson, J., & Kielhofner, G. (1983). Occupational therapy in the health care systems of the future. In G. Kielhofner (Ed.), *Health through occupation: Theory and practice in occupational therapy* (pp. 179-195). Philadelphia, PA: F. A. Davis.

Krammer, T. (Ed.). (1984). REAP: The Richmond Employee Assistance Program. *REAP Reader, 1,* 14.

Pelletier, K. (1984). *Healthy people in unhealthy places: Stress and fitness at work.* New York: Delacorte Press/Seymour Lawrence.

Rogers, J. (1983). The study of human occupation. In G. Kielhofner (Ed.). *Health through occupation: Theory and practice in occupational therapy* (pp. 93-124). Philadelphia, PA: F. A. Davis.

Sakell, T. (1985). EAPs develop human assets: Programs help to alleviate costly personnel problems. *Guidepost, March 21,* 1,12.

Wader, L. (1971). Occupational therapy in the well community. *American Journal of Occupational Therapy, 26,* 1-9.

Wiemer, R. B., & West, W. (1970). Occupational therapy in community health care. *American Journal of Occupational Therapy, 24,* 1-6.

CHAPTER TWENTY-NINE

Employment for Individuals with Mental Disabilities: ADA Unlocked the Door But Who Has the Handle?

Patricia Scott

This chapter was previously published in Occupational Therapy in Health Care, 10(2), 49-64. Copyright © 1996, *Haworth Press. Reprinted by permission.*

INTRODUCTION

The Americans with Disabilities Act (ADA) of 1990 has been proclaimed as the Bill of Rights for the disabled. The ADA specifically addresses equal opportunity for access to a broad array of goods and services, for individuals with disabilities both mental and/or physical. The intent of the law is to prohibit barriers to full participation in all aspects of life. Title I includes the employment provisions. Included in these provisions is the process for accommodating individuals who are qualified to perform the essential functions of a job, but, due to disability-related limitations, need accommodation. Provisions for non-discrimination on the basis of a mental disability were included in the Rehabilitation Act of 1973 (Feldbaum, 1991), but the ADA expands and strengthens these provisions especially in the area of employment protection. When accommodations are requested, the ADA details the process to determine how specific accommodations would enable an individual to overcome disability-related limitations and perform the essential functions of a job. But, herein lies a potential pitfall; while the ADA has "unlocked the door," the "handle" that "opens the unlocked door" needs to be turned. The ADA requires that an individual initiates the request for an accommodation and collaborate in the process of determining potential accommodations. Benefit is achieved only when an individual with a disability can represent their needs and work with the employer to implement the process.

The ADA specifies a collaborative process to determine whether a qualified individual with a disability could perform the essential functions of a job with or without accommodation. The process depends on clear understanding of disability-related limitations and strategies to overcome these limitations. While any typical individual could be overwhelmed by the task of assessing job demands and defending the need for specific accommodations, unique challenges are faced by individuals with mental disabilities. How well can individuals with mental disabilities articulate the impact of their disability on performance of job-related tasks? How comfortable are these individuals in discussing their disability? How effective is the health care system in preparing the mentally ill to advocate for themselves? How accepting is a potential employer of an individual with a mental disability? How accepting are fellow employees? What are the privacy issues? These are only a few of the questions that need to be explored to better understand how individuals with mental disabilities can open the newly unlocked door.

The purpose of this (chapter) is to address the particularly difficult issues facing individuals with mental disabilities as they attempt to activate the rights and protections that they are provided through the ADA. A case example is used to illustrate the accommodation process. Specific attention is given to the problems this population faces in representing themselves, and asserting what type of accommodation they require to overcome disability-related limitations. Specific attention is given to the role of the occupational therapist in preparing individuals for self-advocacy. Discussion of the problems inherent in the traditional way that health care professionals approach individuals with mental disabilities and recommendations for change, specifically in the area of occupational therapy services, are offered. The term "mental disability" is used in this paper to maintain consistency with the language found in the ADA.

ADA TITLE I—EMPLOYMENT PROVISIONS

An individual with a disability is defined by ADA as a person who has a physical or mental impairment that substantially limits one or more major life activities; a record of such impairment; or is regarded as having such an impairment. A "mental impairment" is "any mental or psychological disorder such as mental retardation, organic brain syndrome, emotional or mental illness, and specific learning disabilities." There is no definitive list of qualifying disabilities; examples that are provided include schizophrenia, depression, and personality disorders.

Discussion on the specific language and scope of the ADA is covered in depth elsewhere (Barlowe & Hane, 1993; Williams 1992; Feldbaum, 1991; Gostin, 1991; LaPlante, 1991; Shaller, 1991; Mancuso, 1990; Parmet, 1990). The most definitive resource is the EEOC Technical Assistance Manual (U.S. EEOC, 1992). An additional, very detailed guide is a resource manual for employers (Zuckerman, Debenham, & Moore, 1993). The role of the occupational therapist working with individuals with mental disabilities is specifically addressed by Christ and Stoffel (1992/1996).

The process of decision-making about an accommodation, when one is requested, is very specific. The responsibility for initiation of the process lies with the individual with a disability, the employee. Once the accommodation has been requested the process becomes interactive between the employee and the employer, and the employer is then bound to follow through. The case of an individual with a schizotypical personality disorder is presented here to illustrate this process and the inherent difficulties that individuals with mental disabilities face.

Derrick: A Case Illustration

Derrick was hired as a prep cook at a restaurant in South Beach. At the time of the hire the manager noted frequency of job changes and gaps in his work history, yet Derrick was enthusiastic and the manager needed someone right away so the manager agreed to give Derrick a try.

As a prep cook, it was Derrick's responsibility to prepare vegetables and condiments for use by the chef. During the week of training Derrick worked alongside another prep cook. During the training he kept to himself and showed some oddities of behavior, appearing somewhat silly and aloof, yet he was able to follow directions and complete the tasks required of the position. Training was completed on a Tuesday; on

Wednesday and Thursday Derrick performed his duties without any difficulties.

Problems became evident on Friday night. Derrick performed his job without difficulty until the rush hour occurred. Many people came into the restaurant at once and the kitchen was in chaos. The chef ran low on several items and was yelling to Derrick to hurry and prepare them. In response to the demands of the chef and the chaos in the kitchen, Derrick stood immobile. The manager came in and saw that the dishwasher was backed up and yelled for Derrick, who was standing, appearing to be doing nothing to help the dishwasher.

Derrick started mumbling to himself that the tomatoes cannot be cut until after the onions, shaking his head as he paced back and forth. The manager again requested to him that he help the dishwasher and the chef yelled for him to chop some vegetables. Derrick stared at them blankly then continued to pace and mumble. The manager then told Derrick to leave. Derrick left.

Background: The reason for the gaps in Derrick's work history are that he has been hospitalized for several brief psychotic episodes. He has been diagnosed as having Schizotypical Personality Disorder. He has had many jobs, some of which he quit due to his discomfort and anxiety, others he was fired from due to eccentric and odd behavior. He has a strong desire to work and is self-conscious about his poor work history.

His disability: Schizotypical Personality Disorder appears by early adulthood. Deficits are seen in the ability to relate to others and in peculiarity of ideas and behavior. During periods of extreme stress, transient psychotic episodes may occur. Individuals with this disorder are extremely anxious in social situations involving unfamiliar people. Thinking is either overly abstract or overly concrete, and they lack the ability to engage in a give and take interpersonal interchange. (APA, 1995)

First, it is necessary to establish that Derrick is a qualified individual with a disability, and that the disability must be substantially limiting in one or more areas of functioning. He is qualified for this job as a prep cook by virtue of experience; in fact, he performed the essential job functions for two days after the completion of his training. He has also been hospitalized for transient psychotic episodes and meets the DSM IV criteria for Schizotypical Personality Disorder (APA, 1995). Derrick is substantially limited in his ability to work as evidenced by his history of frequent job changes and long periods of unemployment. In fact, he has been fired from any job in which he has to deal with ambiguity or change. The ADA does not require a prior disclosure of disability; Derrick can state that he has a disability and ask for accommodation at any time, before, during, or after employment (Technical Assistance Manual; EEOC 1992). The question here is, what most realistically will happen to Derrick? When the question was posed to a group of EEOC investigators, the overwhelming response was that Derrick will get fired. Unfortunately,

Derrick probably will get fired. Is he protected under the ADA? The answer is yes. What would Derrick have to do to keep his job? The answer to this question can best be understood by a discussion of the process of determining reasonable accommodation.

Steps in Determining Reasonable Accommodation

The process for determining reasonable accommodation is defined by the ADA and described in the ADA Technical Assistance Manual published by the EEOC (1992). The process includes the following steps:

- Analyze the job to determine purpose and essential function.
- Consult with the individual having a disability to ascertain the precise job-related limitations imposed by the disability and how these limitations could be overcome by reasonable accommodations.
- Identify potential accommodations and assess the effectiveness that each would have in enabling the person to perform the essential functions of the position.
- Consider the preference of the individual and select and implement the accommodation that is most appropriate for the employee and the employer.

1. Job Analysis

A good job analysis is the key to determine essential job functions and lays the groundwork for understanding how the position can be adapted. The ADA requires that essential job functions be specified prior to the initiation of the hiring process (Barlowe & Hanes, 1993; Feldblum, 1991; Mancuso, 1990). The job description should specify the amount of time spent in each of the required tasks. Tasks that are not essential to the position, and could be assumed by others without changing the nature of the job, should be indicated. The qualifications needed to perform the essential functions of the job need to be carefully delineated.

2. Consultation on How to Overcome Special Disability-Related Limitations

The second step in the process is consultation with the individual to determine the specific disability-related limitations and how these limitations could be overcome by reasonable accommodation. This process requires that the individual with a disability be able to understand the demands of a job and identify specific areas in which he or she may experience difficulty. He/she must also be able to express abilities and limitations. The employer must be willing to understand an employee's limitations and maintain an open mind about potential for success. It is at this point the employer must confront personal biases and stereotypes about mental disabilities. In our society we have a long history of discrimination against individuals with mental disabilities based on myths and fears (Feldbaum, 1991).

3. Identify Potential Accommodations

The third step is for the employer to identify possible accommodations and to assess the potential effectiveness of each. Identification of alternatives requires an open mind and a willingness to do things in a different way. The adequacy to which steps one and two were conducted will facilitate or impede the accommodation identification process. Success depends both upon a thorough knowledge and understanding of the limitations imposed by the disability, and objectivity about alternative ways to complete a task. Determining accommodations for disability-imposed limitations, the requirement for equal treatment and non-discrimination, remains the primary objective.

4. Select and Implement the Most Appropriate Accommodation

Once potential accommodations have been identified, the employer and the employee together agree on the most acceptable accommodation. Although the final decision lies with the employer, acceptability of an accommodation for the requesting individual is also required by the ADA. Privacy issues and the process of implementing the accommodation to insure that privacy is respected is important; further, the individual must not be treated "special," thus establishing a potential for ostracization by fellow employees.

The law requires that the employer implement a reasonable accommodation, but does not demand an assumption of undue hardship or a change in the nature of the way business is conducted. Undue hardship addresses economic concerns, and is treated in the law as a relative term, dependent on the specific size, budget, and nature of the organization. Chirikos (1991) and Shaller (1991) examine the economics of employment and cost issues related to accommodation.

Derrick and the Accommodation Process

Assume that when the restaurant manager told Derrick to get out of the kitchen, Derrick left and went home. The most likely subsequent scenario is that either Derrick never showed up again or he showed up for his next shift only to be handed a check for the days worked, and told, sorry, it did not work out.

Let's change the scenario. Let's assume that Derrick went back to the restaurant the following day to speak with the manager. He explained to the manager that he has a disability that causes him some problems in the workplace. If Derrick asked for an accommodation then, by law, the manager would be required to initiate the accommodation process. The restaurant manager can ask for proof that Derrick does indeed have an impairment that is substantially limiting. Once Derrick's eligibility for accommodation is established, the manager would need to examine the job description, ask Derrick what tasks he would have difficulty with, and explore possible accommodations.

Areas of Difficulty	Possible Accommodations
Cognitive and Perceptual Distortions	Speak directly to Derrick and take the time to be sure that Derrick understands instructions the way they are intended. Have him repeat as needed for clarification.
Social Anxiety	Limit the number of unfamiliar people with whom Derrick has to be in contact. Do not expect friendly or relaxed behavior.
Odd or Eccentric Behavior	Recognize that Derrick may talk or mumble to himself and that he may have unusual gestures and facial expressions.
Peculiar Ideas	Clarify tasks required to perform the essential functions of the job. Recognize need for sameness and put in writing (simple and concrete) performance expectations.
Poor Stress Response	Decrease Stress. Possibilities include scheduling at times when the "rush" does not typically occur. Set up check system for Derrick to monitor amounts of vegetables that are ready. Work with the chef to identity shortages early and establish a system of written communication when variations in routine are required. Sensitize staff to need for calm and unambiguous communication.

Figure 29-1. Possible accommodations for "Derrick", an individual with Schizotypical Personality Disorder seeking to perform the essential functions of a "prep cook".

Derrick would need to explain that these problems include problems with social contact, poor attention span, odd or eccentric behavior and ideas, and difficulty with stress and changes in routine (APA, 1994). Derrick and the restaurant manager would then work together to explore possible accommodations. Some possible accommodations include: scheduling Derrick for shifts where the restaurant is less busy, providing instructions one at a time, utilizing calm and unambiguous communication, installing a blackboard for noting changes, and giving clear information, preferably in writing, about the amounts of different chopped vegetables needed on hand (Figure 29-1). The manager would then assess the potential effectiveness of each accommodation, make a decision about which accommodations have a potential for working out, and then determine, with Derrick, acceptable strategies for implementation. Derrick and the manager would then work together make the necessary accommodations, evaluate the effectiveness, and make adjustments on an on-going basis.

Does this scenario sound ludicrous? For many who have worked with individuals such as Derrick, and others familiar with the business of running a restaurant, it is at best unlikely and more likely absurd. Why? Why does the process of accommodating an individual with disabilities such as Derrick, who is qualified to perform the essential functions of the job, seem so unlikely?

There are reasons on both sides of the accommodation process. Some of the barriers include the knowledge of the restaurant manager about mental disabilities, his attitudes, fears, and stereotypes. A frequent comment that you never know when the person will get mad, pull out a gun, and start shooting, reflects a biased view of the over-prediction of violence in individuals with mental illness. Another problem is the similarity of some of the disability-related limitations to attitude problems such as moodiness, laziness, and irritability. There needs to be a willingness to spend the time to explore accommodations, in Derrick's case, to accommodate a prep cook. The attitudes of the other kitchen staff, a staff that may be characterized by high turnover and potentially little understanding of mental disabilities must be considered. Concern for equal treatment of staff and desire to avoid resentment for what may be perceived as special treatment is necessary. Fear of possible lost productivity and the consequence for business if the essential functions of the job are not met, and the vegetables are not prepared when they are needed to fill customers orders.

Barriers that Derrick face include his understanding of the performance limitations caused by his disability, and his ability to articulate these limitations. Mental disabilities are poorly accepted in our society and denial of having mental problems is not uncommon. Some individuals have the ability to articulate limitations, others do not. The nature of mental disabilities is that the course is variable and that in acute stages limitations may be substantial enough to preclude working. LaPlante characterizes this problem in his statement "the world of disability is dynamic, it can differ from one day to the next and varies according to the person and the situation" (1991, p. 55). Flexible work schedules, arrangements for time off, job sharing, and working at home are all specified by the ADA as possible accommodations. Of course accommodations such as working at home are possible for some jobs and not for others; obviously a prep cook needs to perform his work at the restaurant.

An equal number of limitations face Derrick. These include accepting his disability and taking the initiative to discuss his disability with others. He must have insight into the effect that having a Schizotypical Personality Disorder has on his ability to work. Further, he must be able to explain this to others.

IMPLICATIONS FOR OCCUPATIONAL THERAPY TREATMENT

While acknowledging the restaurant manager or employer issues, the intent of this (chapter) is to address the implications for the occupational therapist working with an individual with a mental disability. The EEOC technical assistance manual names occupational therapists as professionally qualified to assist in the determination of accommodations. The role of the occupational therapist is, however, larger than determination of accommodation; it is to prepare the individual as much as possible for self-advocacy, starting with education about the law, then moving toward a plan for activating the protections when and if needed. Unless this larger role is assumed, then the potential benefits of the ADA may not for many become realities.

Education about the ADA needs to be a part of all patient/consumer education programs. The comprehensive treatment plan should address vocational status and identify whether an individual is expected to return to previous employment, seek new employment, is in need of vocational training or supported employment, or is not expected to participate in employment or training (retired, too disabled, etc.). For those individuals who are expected to resume or assume a vocational role, five areas of intervention are suggested as appropriate for the occupational therapist:

1. Prepare the individual to disclose that they have a disability, if and when it is appropriate to do so.
2. Identify the types of positions for which a particular individual is "qualified."
3. Focus treatment around identification of disability-related limitations.
4. Educate the client how to read job descriptions, identify potential problems, and suggest accommodations.
5. Awareness of community opportunities and advocacy on the part of individuals with mental disabilities.

Preparation for Disclosure

The ADA only covers individuals who state they have a disability and request accommodations. There are three issues with disclosure: when, if, and how. Disclosure can take place at any time before, during, or after the hiring process. On an independent job search, when there is competition for a position with non-disabled applicants, it is recommended that individuals do not disclose until after the offer has been made. Once the offer has been made, the individual needs to decide the extent to which their disability will affect their performance on the job and disclose right away, or wait until a specific problem is encountered, then initiate the process.

The decision to disclose is a difficult one. Without disclosure, an employer can only speculate that an individual may have a mental disability. Unlike the situation where the obvious use of a wheelchair leads logically to a discussion about limitations in mobility and access that may affect job performance, an observation of an odd affect, distractibility, or hyper-vigilance, do not lead to easy employer initiated discussion about disability.

Open discussion by the occupational therapist and mentally disabled individual of the non-verbal and verbal behaviors that are readily observable helps to make the decision to initiate the disclosure or not. An individual with an obvious affective difference may be ostracized and perhaps discriminated against in a work situation, where an open discussion of the reason may facilitate understanding and result in acceptance and accommodations, which make the work situation more positive.

There are situations that an individual believes their disability will not preclude their ability to perform the essential job functions and they may choose not to disclose until problems arise. Derrick, for example, has major limitations in social and interpersonal relationships; he believes that he can perform the essential functions of the job, in fact, he did until the stress of the situation resulted in brief decompensation. Given his response to the chaos of the kitchen, Derrick was forced into the situation where he either has to explain his response to the manager or he will lose his job. His limitations in social and interpersonal relationships complicates his ability to participate in the collaborative process. An individual like Derrick will need a plan and most probably outside intervention. In fact, with accommodation, he may very likely be successful in performing the essential tasks of this position.

How disclosure takes place is important. The occupational therapist should use role-playing as part of the individual's treatment program. This role-playing needs to address to whom the individual should disclose—the original employer, or the immediate supervisor; the time and place; and include practice in explaining any disability-related limitations. Individuals need to understand the privacy protections and that they do not have to provide specific information on the actual diagnosis or answer any personal questions related to history or prognosis. Role-playing with facility personnel department staff is very effective. Videotaping is helpful in giving feedback after the role-play.

Individuals unable or uncomfortable in disclosing and discussing disability-related limitations, for whatever reason, need to have an alternative plan. Direct involvement of the occupational therapist with the potential or current employer may be appropriate. Often a family member or other caregiver can assist with the process. The key is that the individual has a plan when support and/or assistance is needed.

Established "Qualifications"

Individuals need to understand the concept of "qualified individual able to perform the essential functions of the job." The ADA covers a "qualified" person with a disability. The definition of "qualified" is an individual who: satisfies the requisite skill, experience, education, and other job-related requirements of the employment position such individual holds or desires, and who, with or without reasonable accommodation, can perform the essential functions of the position. (EEOC, 1992 p. 1-3)

The occupational therapist needs to work with clients to analyze qualifications, with a focus on education, prior experience, and training. This process may be done as part of a pre-vocational skills program, or where appropriate, in consultation with a vocational counselor. Once qualifications have been determined, practice in identifying potential positions by a search of the classified advertisements and job bulletins can be conducted. Once jobs are identified, the occupational therapist should review with the client their perceptions of the education and experience requirements of the position. Then have them call and ask about the actual education and experience required for the position. This actual calling verifies the client's perceptions and serves to desensitize an individual uncomfortable or unaccustomed to initiating contact with a potential employer for future contacts.

Disability-Related Limitations

The nature of mental illness is that there is a variable course with changes in intensity of symptoms. Symptoms, as outlined in the APA Diagnostic and Statistical Manual, guide the assignment of diagnosis. As much as the use of diagnosis is discouraged to deter stigma and labeling, the criteria, as outlined in the manual, can serve as a basis to understand limitations.

Discussion of diagnosis demystifies the disability and cuts through the denial. Results of task-based assessments such as the Bay Area Functional Performance Evaluation (Williams & Bloomer, 1987), or the Routine Task Inventory (Allen et al., 1992) need to be openly discussed with the client. Comparison of results at different points in time, upon admission, after stabilization, and later upon follow-up will clarify the variations that occur at different cycles of the illness. Specific attention needs to be given to the problems that would affect performance on a job. Derrick, for example, experiences ideas of reference and magical thinking, therefore needing clear and unambiguous directions.

Additional information regarding disability-related limitations can be obtained from past or present employers, family or others closely associated with the individual and observations or direct care staff (in in-patient settings). Simulations of work settings, or engagement in a task need to be followed by discussion and feedback. Comparison of task performance over time is useful. The therapist needs to be very careful to not only point out limitations but also help the individual to develop awareness of abilities. All task performance information needs to be systematically recorded and variability noted and discussed.

Suggesting Accommodations

In order to suggest an accommodation, job requirements need to be clearly understood. Reading sample job descriptions and discussion of the specific activities that are required of certain positions will initiate the client's understanding of essential job functions. Sample descriptions can also be used to reinforce with a client activities that present difficulty. Success in this step requires the ability to abstract and have insight into oneself. Awareness of one's limitations may be the most difficult and may be impossible for many individuals with mental disabilities. It is unlikely that Derrick, given his tendency towards odd ideation and impairment in interpersonal and social skill, would be able to fully engage in the collaboration needed to achieve accommodation. Discussion of the way to access resources is therefore important. Once a job is obtained, the client could bring a copy of the job description to the occupational therapist for consultation, or have the therapist, or another qualified individual visit the job site to assist the employer in the determination of potential accommodations.

For the individual who has been working in an established position and has now become under the care of an occupational therapist, there needs to be discussion of if and how their job tasks need to be accommodated. Accommodations may be short- or long-term. For example, a secretary experiencing a major depressive illness may be able to return to work and perform typing, filing and other task-based functions, but may have difficulty maintaining the positive cheery attitude the company requires of employees dealing with the public. Reassignment of duties in the office to accommodate her limitations may be appropriate. Initiation of the accommodation upon return to work will promote successful adjustment rather than initiating the process after poor performance is noted by the supervisor.

Employment Opportunities: Awareness and Advocacy

Determination of the needed level of accommodation and support will help ensure success in the workplace. However, merely determining what accommodations are needed by a particular individual does not lead to success in obtaining and retaining a job any more than reading the Dictionary of Occupational Terms determines qualifications. In the case of Derrick the goal was success in a competitive employment situation. The intent of the ADA is to eliminate the differences in treatment of individuals with disabilities from those without disabilities. To the extent that an individual can perform the essential functions of a position with or without accommodation this objective is possible. Many individuals with mental disabilities however will not succeed in competitive employment. Models have also been developed for workplace adaptation. Hearne (1991) provides a description of four types of programs that could assist in effective integration of individuals with disabilities into the workplace, with the caveat that all would require collaboration between people in the public and the private sector and persons with disabilities individually and in groups. These types of programs include:

1. Programs to make local labor markets work more effectively both for employers and for persons with disabilities
2. Projects with industry
3. Supported employment
4. Centers for independent living (p. 121)

The occupational therapist must be informed about available programs and involved in advocacy for expansion of opportunities. Advocacy can be done both directly and indirectly. Direct advocacy, the focus of this (chapter), occurs when treatment focuses on teaching the individual to advocate for themselves, and by interfacing between the individual and a potential employer. Indirect advocacy is accomplished by encouraging individual and family involvement in organizations such as the National Alliance for the Mentally Ill (NAMI). NAMI has local chapters in most areas. Another way to facilitate the process is through the myriad of technical and personnel assistance networks, such as those listed in the ADA Technical Assistance Manual. The utilization of resources by individuals with physical disabilities is seen in the proliferation of computer bulletin boards and support groups. Is it possible to envision a world where individuals with mental disabilities sit in the day room of the hospital or community program and share ways in which they cope with their disability-related limitations? The reality is that these individuals often lack the capacity for self-advocacy and are unable to identify the door handle without outside assistance, much less open the door for themselves.

SUMMARY

Individuals with mental disabilities possess a wide range of abilities and limitations. Mental disabilities are numerous, vary from each other and are manifested differently in different individuals. Many people with mental disabilities experience a variable course of symptoms. The ADA is a landmark piece of legislation that unlocks the doors for individuals with mental disabilities, yet the ADA does not open the doors.

Individuals with mental disabilities will be able to advocate for themselves only to the degree that they are aware of the ADA protections, able to make decisions about disclosure, and have an understanding of their disability-related limitations. Education about the ADA should be a standard part of patient education programs in all treatment programs. Vocational status should be addressed on the initial treatment plan and strategies put in place to prepare the individual for self-advocacy. Specific attention to establishing insight into disability-related limitations should be a primary focus of the occupational therapy treatment program.

Some individuals with mental disabilities represent themselves and work with employers to implement accommodations that allow for successful completion of essential job tasks. Other individuals are less comfortable with their disability and do not have the insight to know and/or the ability to articulate their limitations and thus have reduced capacity for collaboration. It is for therapists who work with these individuals that the recommendations in this (chapter) are provided.

There are large groups of individuals with mental disabilities too severe to be able to function in a regular employment setting. These individuals have neither the qualifications nor possibilities of reasonable accommodations to the limitations imposed by their disability. Some of these individuals will need adapted settings such the collaborative models proposed by Hearne (1991).

No one approach, no one solution, exists to address all the issues related to this very complex topic. Misunderstanding, lack of knowledge, fear, and the stigma of mental illness, are all obstacles to opening the door for individuals with mental disabilities. Occupational therapists have a critical role to play in the assuring that the provisions of the ADA work as a Bill of Rights for the disabled, and not represent an unlocked but still closed door.

REFERENCES

Allen, C. K., Earhart, C. A., & Blue, T. (1992). *Occupational therapy treatment goals for the physically and cognitively disabled.* Rockville, MD: AOTA.

American Psychological Association. (1995). *Diagnostic and statistical manual of mental disorders* (4th edition). Washington, DC: Author.

Americans with Disabilities Act of 1990, Pub. L. No. 101-336. title 42, United States Code. Section 12101 (1990).

Barlowe, W. E., & Hane, E. Z. (1993). A practical guide to the Americans with Disabilities Act. *Clinical Laboratory Management Reviews,* pp. 9-19.

Chirikos, T. N. (1991). The economics of employment. *The Milbank Quarterly, 69*(suppl. 1, 2), 150-179.

Christ, P. A., & Stoffel, V. C. (1992). The Americans with Disabilities Act of 1990 and employees with mental impairments: Personal efficacy and the environment. *American Journal of Occupational Therapy 46*(5), 434-443. (Reprinted in Cottrell, R. P. (Ed.). (1996). *Perspectives on purposeful activity: Foundations and future of occupational therapy.* Bethesda, MD: AOTA.)

Feldbaum, C. R. (1991). Employment protections. *The Milbank Quarterly, 69*(suppl. 1, 2), 81-110.

Gostin, L. O. (1991). Public health powers: The imminence of radical change. *The Milbank Quarterly, 69*(suppl. 1, 2), 268-290.

Hearne, P. G. (1991). Employment strategies for people with disabilities: A prescription for change. *The Milbank Quarterly, 69*(suppl. 1, 2), 111-128.

LaPlante, M. P. (1991). The demographics of disability. *The Milbank Quarterly, 69*(suppl. 1, 2), 55-77.

Mainstream, Inc. (1985). *Putting disabled people in your place: Focus on individuals with of history of mental illness.* Washington, D.C.: Author.

Mancuso, L. L. (1990). Reasonable accommodation for workers with psychiatric disabilities. *Psychosocial Rehabilitation Journal, 14*(2) 3-19.

McNulty, E. (Ed.). (1992). Legal Q's & A's. *Discharge Planning Update, 12*(1), 12-14.

Parmet, W. E. (1990). Discrimination and disability: The challenges of the ADA. *Law, Medicine, & Health Care, 18*(4),331-344.

Schelly, C., Sample, P., & Spencer, K. (1992). The Americans with Disabilities Act of 1990 expands employment opportunities for persons with developmental disabilities. *American Journal of Occupational Therapy, 46*(5),457-460

Shaller, E. H. (1991). "Reasonable accommodation" under the Americans with Disabilities Act—what does it mean? *Employee Relations Law Journal, 16*(4), 431-451.

U.S. Equal Employment Opportunity Commission. (1992). *A technical assistance manual on the employment provisions Title I of the Americans with Disabilities Act.* Washington, D C.: Author.

West, J. (1991). The social act and policy context of the act. *The Milbank Quarterly, 69*(suppl 1, 2), 3-23.

Williams, J. (1992). What do you know? What do you need to know? *ASHA,* 54-61.

Williams, S. L., & Bloomer, I. (1987). *Bay Area Functional Performance Evaluation* (2nd edition). Palo Alto, CA: Consulting Psychologists Press.

Zuckerman, D., Debanham, K., & Moore, K. (1993). *The ADA and people with mental illness: A resource manual for employers.* Washington D.C.: National Bar Association & Alexandria VA: National Mental Health Association.

CHAPTER THIRTY

Vocational Treatment Model

Frances Palmer and Donna Gatti

This chapter was previously published in Occupational Therapy in Mental Health, *5(1), 41-58. Copyright ©1985, Haworth Press.*

A major component of psychiatric occupational therapy is the restoration of functioning: work, play and self-care. For the adult psychiatric patient working represents a significant life skill challenge. Vocational programs offered by the Rehabilitation Services Department at McLean Hospital are structured to assist patients to identify and evaluate work behaviors which either enhance or inhibit successful performance. This (chapter) will present a description of the Clinical Vocational Assessment Program (CVAP) at McLean Hospital, including a list of common referral goals and the Patient Performance Checklist. The remainder of this (chapter) will consider several facets of person-environment interactions relevant to the CVAP, with primary emphasis on the Open Door Thrift Shop program. Finally, a clinical case will highlight some of the concepts discussed.

It is difficult to predict the impact of psychiatric illness on a patient's ability to resume previously acquired competencies. To provide assessment in the critical area of work behavior, the McLean Hospital Rehabilitation Services Department offers a multi-faceted work activity: the Clinical Vocational Assessment Program. McLean Hospital is a private, non-profit psychiatric facility with a 328 inpatient capacity and approximately 900 patients registered in 11 separate outpatient clinics. The work activity program is available to both inpatients and outpatients. McLean Hospital is situated on 200 acres in a suburb 11 miles west of Boston, MA. Modeled after the European cottage system, there are 40 buildings, most clustered in the center of the campus. Two of the four work activity environments discussed are located in the Rehabilitation Building: the Food Service Training Program facilities, the Coffee Shop and Restaurant; and the Patient Library with the adjacent Clerical Training area. On campus, but located away from the center of hospital activity is the Greenhouse, and within a ten minute walk from the hospital is the community-based Open Door Thrift Shop.

FOOD SERVICE TRAINING PROGRAM

This program includes the basic coffee shop training component and the advanced restaurant segment. The Coffee Shop area and a 24-seat dining room serve as the location for the on-the-job training portion of the program. This fast food facility services the visitors, patients and staff of the McLean community. It is staffed entirely by rehabilitation management personnel who work in conjunction with the program supervisor to provide supervision and training for the patients. Classrooms, training kitchen, and reference library round out the facilities that complement the program. The on-the-job training segment of the program consists of 90 hours in the Coffee Shop working in one of the three following positions: counter person, grill and fry, salad bar. Participation is gradually scheduled from quiet to busy periods as the patient's ability and confidence increase. The ultimate goal of this phase of the program is to give the patient a basic knowledge and understanding with an entry-level degree of proficiency. The restaurant segment provides the patient an opportunity to learn fundamental vocational and interpersonal skills necessary for entry-level employment in the restaurant field or supports continuing in higher levels of education now offered in food service and the culinary arts field. The patients may experience one or all of the three different occupational categories: (1) Host/Hostess, (2) Waiter/Waitress, or (3) Cook.

LIBRARY-CLERICAL TRAINING PROGRAM

The Patient Library and adjacent clerical training room are the sites for this jointly supervised program. The Library stocks over 40 monthly periodicals, 3000 fiction and non-fic-

Table 30-1
Patient Performance Checklist

Production and Work Skills

Concentrates on Tasks	Accuracy in Use of Numbers
Follows Verbal Directions	Completes Tasks in Assigned Time
Follows Written Directions	Paces Own Time
Retains Directions Over Time	Consistent in Task Performance
Accuracy in Written Tasks	Plans Ahead in Task Assignments
Establishes Task Priority	Organizes Two or More Tasks
Able to Shift from Task to Task	Able to Learn New Tasks
Physically Coordinated for Task	Physical Tolerance (standing/sitting)
Can Work in a Noisy Area	Aware of Consumer Needs
Uses Tools/Equipment Properly	Handles the Unexpected

Cooperation

Discusses Work Problems with Supervisor	Works with Fellow Workers
	Willing to Redo Tasks

Motivation

When in Doubt, Asks Questions	Checks Own Work
Attempts Tasks Until Correct	Avails Self of Suggestion to Improve
Uses Independent Judgment	Sets Own Work Goals
Eager to Learn	Shares Improvement Ideas

Responsibility

Attends Regularly	Arrives Punctually
Notifies Work Area When Absent	Takes Breaks as Scheduled
Maintains Organized Work Area	Directs Others in Tasks
Follows Safety Procedures	Familiar with Environment of Area
Accepts Work Standards	

Work Traits

Separates Personal and Work Issues	Appropriate Dress/Hygiene
	Use of Verbal Communication
At Ease in Work Setting	Uses a Sense of Humor
Pride in Work Completed	Accepts Praise

tion books, vocational and career education reference books, and local and national daily newspapers. The area is open and available to patients, staff and visitors and typifies a small community reading room. The clerical area resembles a large office production environment with four secretarial work stations and two computer work stations. Files, shelves, tables, telephones, practice typewriters and other business machines complete the room. Each area has a distinct vocational skill development component; however, many of the task projects cross these boundaries. For example, inventorying new books involves labeling, cataloguing and shelving. These tasks are shared library and clerical efforts. The production of a patient newsletter also involves a broad array of patient endeavors. Article writing, layout design, editing, word-processing, and distribution are some of the singular tasks associated with the project. The program supervisor is able to match the patients' interests and pursuits with demonstrated skill proficiency. New skills can be learned, present skills evaluated, and former skills relearned. Environmental factors contribute to a patient's program choice and often the subdued atmosphere of the Library contrasts the busy task production in the clerical area. Both clerical and library tasks are largely individual skill efforts; typing or answering the telephone or reshelving books involve only the activity and the individual.

GREENHOUSE PROGRAM

The 60-foot greenhouse is located away from the center of hospital activity and overlooks a meadow and an apple orchard. Its quiet setting is conducive to the individual task efforts associated with horticulture. Specific tasks in the program include soil preparation, propagation of plants, continuous plant care, preparation, planting and care of gardens, and maintenance chores related to the facility. Along with those activities, several projects are organized throughout the year to introduce production oriented experiences. A sample of these projects is seasonal plant sales; supplying the floral arrangements for the evening Restaurant program, or wreath construction and sale during the Christmas season. This aspect of the program requires more cooperation among the patient participants and provides exposure to other vocational skills such as pricing, selling, and marketing. The program supervisor varies the assignment of tasks as well as the composition of group participants. As many as 15 people could be involved in one project or during one daily session 15 participants may be involved in very separate activities. A project may also be solely one individual's effort. Each circumstance is dependent on the patient's interest, rehabilitation treatment objective, and psychosocial tolerance level. The program space both indoors and outdoors permits this high level of flexibility. The variance in patients' functional abilities and behavioral manifestations can also be accommodated. If a patient can tolerate a half hour of attention to the activity then that individual could be assigned the task of watering the decorative plant foliage in a specific building. If a group of patients are addressing work-related production skills then the organization and implementation of a plant sale may be appropriate. A significant benefit to this program is the availability of employment in this field. The labor market is receptive to the temporary or part-time employment requirements of many of our patients.

OPEN DOOR THRIFT SHOP

The Shop program includes a full range of tasks from highly structured repetitive activities such as inventory sorting, pricing and tagging, and housekeeping assignments, to the less structured multi-step demands of window displays or the pronounced organizational and communicational requirements of cashiering. Task assignments are under the direction of the program supervisor and are specifically geared and modified to meet the individual's needs, with monitoring of psychosocial stimulation via the use of either upstairs or basement work locations. The overall treatment approach assesses not only areas for remediation but recognizes and utilizes the client's existing functional strengths. The basic objectives of the program are twofold: to permit formal and informal evaluation of clients' social, emotional, and basic vocational functioning; and to provide a transitional community setting for the habilitation or rehabilitation of work adjustment skills. General program expectations include a dress code which is appropriate to community retail standards, and the ability to maintain control over behavior disturbing to fellow workers and customers or to recognize impending loss of control and return to the hospital. Also, there is the expectation to arrange appointments that do not conflict with the established work schedule, to make arrangements for travel between the hospital and Thrift Shop, and a general ability to understand directions and maintain a minimum level of verbal communication.

PROGRAM STRUCTURE

Rehabilitation staff are responsible for referring patients to the Clinical Vocational Assessment Program (CVAP) and directly supervising each program site. The program supervisor plays a complex role. As a therapist, the supervisor observes the patient for a sufficiently protracted period to detect behaviors preventing adjustment to work. The therapist manipulates those conditions of work that will help the patient move toward a more adequate set of work behaviors. The patient is a vital and active part in this rehabilitation process: the patient chooses the specific CVAP placement, negotiates the treatment goals to be addressed, and participates in the evaluation of specific work-related behaviors. By emphasizing the negotiation and self-evaluation procedures designed in the CVAP, the patient is encouraged to own and control the experience. The Patient Performance Checklist focuses the treatment interaction for the program supervisor and patient. This multi-item behavioral protocol is filled out by the patient and supervisor together at regular intervals. There is a three-part rating scale: needs much improvement; needs some improvement; or, acceptable level of performance. It is around this concrete focus that important information is exchanged and reinforced: patient's goals and sense of progress, level of skill development, as well as attitudinal and emotional adjustment factors. It is the responsibility of both therapist and patient to justify their ratings of each work behavior with specific observations. The items on the evaluation protocol are generic to any job. The patient is encouraged to relate these items to organize and understand their experiences on previous jobs, to assess current performance in the hospital program, and to anticipate the types of demands he or she may encounter in his or her next vocational step.

The referring rehabilitation clinician continues to counsel the patient regarding adjustment and progress in the setting. The focus is kept on eventual transition to other less restrictive vocational opportunities. Since each program site varies in its occupational activity, the total program is unified around specific treatment objectives. The referring clinician specifies goals to be addressed over the course of placement. The 14 common goals for CVAP referral include:

1. Assessment of functional abilities, and social and emotional behaviors in a work setting.
2. Provide identification and discussion of interfering work traits.
3. Establish positive work identity.
4. Improve realistic self-assessment.
5. Increase interpersonal skills, both with coworkers and supervisor.
6. Transitional/preparatory experience.
7. Learn to assume responsibility.
8. Instruction in work skills/behaviors/work adjustment training.
9. Provide patient with successful work experience.
10. Learn to separate personal and work issues.
11. Capitalize on existing functional strengths and maintain self-esteem.
12. Vocational exploration.
13. Provide ongoing feedback regarding capabilities.
14. Patient-stated goal of eventual competitive employment.

APPLICATION OF ENVIRONMENTAL THEORY

The environmental themes conceptualized by Roann Barris (1982) provide a useful framework for understanding the clinical impact of the CVAP. Expanding on the model of human occupation, Barris focuses on three facets of person-environment transactions: (1) environmental characteristics that influence the volition subsystem and a person's decision to participate in a setting; (2) the influence of a setting's demands on the habituation and performance subsystems, and (3) factors which affect the individua's capacity to perform over an increased range of settings. Among those environmental characteristics which Barris considers influential to a person's desire to participate in a setting is that environment's arousal potential. She defines arousal potential as a composite of variables: psychophysical variables—the quality or intensity of physical stimuli; ecological variables or the meaning that event has to a person; and finally collative variables—properties of the setting, such as ambiguity, novelty, complexity, and incongruity. Barris views the collative variables as most likely to produce exploratory behavior and stresses that the therapist must determine an optimal level of arousal for each client. Too much or too little arousal may impede the urge to explore. Barris also proposes that when a setting's innate value and interest resonate with those of its client, then there is a greater likelihood of satisfying participation and thus the chance for a sense of efficacy in one's environment.

In viewing the 4 CVAP work sites from the characteristic of interests and values, it is clear that the environments pro-

vide a broad continuum of experience in these areas. In addition, not only do the settings provide quite different arousal experiences from one another, but within each setting there is varying ability to grade the intensity of such stimuli. At one end of the continuum lies the community-based Thrift Shop setting, which easily surpasses the other settings in terms of variety and intensity of psychophysical, collative, and ecological variables.

The Thrift Shop is a veritable bombardment of the sensory/perceptual apparatus; a person entering the shop is likely to be greeted by a cacophony of background street noises, shop telephone, shop radio, customer and worker voices, plus the visual experience of assorted clothing and housewares occupying every available floor, wall, and shelf space. Predictably, very few of the 80 patients who enter this program each year are neutral about its initial impact. Surprisingly, perhaps, the vast majority form an immediate positive cathexis based largely on the arousal factor. The very variety of the Thrift Shop's psychophysical properties lends itself to all of the collative variables complexity, novelty, surprise, incongruity, and ambiguity. Where else would one find the unlikely combination of objects, human and nonhuman, in one cluttered setting? For the many psychiatric patients whose interpersonal skills are shaky at best, the wide array of inanimate objects is often a safer start to relationships outside the hospital. The patient who likes clothing and finds comfort and competence in learning to price and tag, size, arrange garments on racks, and not incidentally set aside a few things for his or her own purchase is one example. The shop's motto "We have something for everyone," is as applicable to its patients' interests as to its customers', from dressing mannequins to truck work, to tinkering with mechanical objects in disrepair. The nature of the store, a recycling of used merchandise, its low prices, and the wide variety of task opportunities suggest a broad base of both interest and value appeal to patients.

Clearly, the Thrift Shop has some potent environmental characteristics, and for at least some referred patients these characteristics are noxious. The potential for too much arousal in this setting is obvious. The hypomanic patient whose volition subsystem may well direct him toward this kind of stimulation, nevertheless will often be unable to perform even previously acquired skills or engage in new learning.

In a sense, the manic patient is an individual whose volition subsystem has hypertrophied; he is filled with a drive toward enactment of his multiple interests and goals combined with an overblown sense-of efficacy, while his actual ability to perform, his level of skills lies at best in a state of splintered disarray, and at worst is nonexistent. For these patients the possible harmony between the volition subsystem and the Thrift Shop setting is pathological. Such patients are usually best directed toward a setting with less sensory overload, although an occasional hypomanic patient can make a satisfactory adjustment at the Thrift Shop by having his work space individually tailored. Thus, he might do tasks initially in the confinement of the supervisor's small office, in the back corner of the store removed from heaviest customer traffic, or in the basement location at a table facing the wall.

Another group of patients for whom the Thrift Shop environment is incompatible are those whose values do not include public service work, a belief in the ecology of recycling used merchandise or whose interests in a work subculture include a need for order, formality of dress, and high standards of cleanliness. There is invariably program failure for this group of clients whose values and interests are not well-matched to the Thrift Shop setting, with one curious treatment exception. One hospital unit at McLean which specializes in the treatment of severe obsessive-compulsive disorders, typically handwashing and bathroom rituals, has routinely insisted that all such patients participate in at least a brief stint at the Thrift Shop. The Thrift Shop environment becomes in effect, part of the behavioral flooding program of this unit whereby the individual is exposed to a massive amount of the feared item, such as dirt, dust, or human contamination. Thus, desensitization is achieved through continual overexposure, not only in the hospital ward setting, but in a community-based, "real-life" environment as well. It is perhaps a dubious distinction for the Thrift Shop that it succeeds in desensitizing individuals to less than sanitary conditions, but it is an interesting process to interpret from Barris' concepts.

At the time of interview at the Thrift Shop, the typical "hand-washer" is outraged at being referred and is exquisitely uncomfortable in the Shop, clear that the only reason for his or her presence is the absolute coercion of hospital ward staff. Yet by the end of most of these individuals' stays in the program, some resonation has occurred between the patients' volition subsystems and their environment. What happens? Initially the obsessive-compulsive patient is threatened and overwhelmed by the nature and level of arousal at the Thrift Shop. Deprived of the freedom to act defensively, albeit pathologically in the form of his or her compulsion, the patient feels frightened and out of control. But no longer able to maintain the same actions, the hand-washing for instance, a small break is made in the otherwise fixed vicious cycle for new feedback, and thus for a reorganizing of this new information by the individual. By itself, simply deterring the compulsive behavior is not enough. It is a combination of limiting the opportunity for the pathological action plus providing some successful competition for the individual's energy and attention, in a sense crowding out the obsessive ruminations with a more interesting agenda. Here lies the value of the Thrift Shop by virtue of its powerful arousal potential and the immediate chance to gain some measure of control over the environment through task performance.

To summarize, the compulsion is temporarily halted at the Thrift Shop, allowing the individual time and energy to perceive new information and demands for performance from a stimulating new environment, to organize and process such information and demands, and hopefully, to result in new actions and perceptions. By loosening the harsh constraints of obsessive-compulsive behavior, the individual may well find his urge to explore in the Thrift Shop setting awakened by the sheer variety of stimuli, his interests broadened, his sense of personal causation enhanced by the development of new vocational skills and routines.

In terms of its psychophysical variables, the library-clerical environment in this vocational model lies at the other end of the spectrum from the Thrift Shop. An orderly setting, it has no striking physical stimuli save the occasional multiple clicking of typewriter keys; even that noise level is well-muted by rugs. For the seasoned clerical worker, the setting would hold few impressive collative variables. Certainly for the novice, however the library-clerical environment could represent complexity and novelty. Probably the strongest arousal factor for this program resides in its ecological variables, the meaning of learning or relearning to type, using the computer, or filing. In short, the arousal potential of this environment is much less intense and varied than that of the Thrift Shop but certainly relative to the experience and perception of the entering patient. Unlike the Thrift Shop, the library-clerical program is a highly defined work subculture, with predictable environmental artifacts, task schedules, and work jargon. Given the specificity of its subculture, the match between this environment and the individual's interests and values would be vital. Without it, the person has little hope of program success.

Environmentally, the Coffee Shop and Greenhouse vocation programs lie somewhere between the polarities of Thrift Shop and clerical sites, and share some aspects of each. Like the clerical program, the Food Service Training Program has its circumscribed subculture. Again, the predictable artifacts exist: cash register, counter, grill, ice cream machine, and soda dispenser. Uniforms standardize the dress code and there is a vocabulary for ordering food items. The Coffee Shop and Restaurant possess considerable arousal potential; sounds, smell, temperature, and color, and a fair degree of complexity and novelty for the inexperienced referral. Both the Thrift Shop and Food Service sites are stimulating environments which can potentially exceed the optimal threshold of arousal for individuals, but are rarely guilty of insufficient arousal.

The Greenhouse program claims some of the order and predictability of the clerical setting, and a moderate degree of certain psychophysical variables, including a warm, moist climate, smells, tactile experiences, and color. The most striking arousal aspects of this setting are its novelty and ecological impact; the process of nurturing—whether plants or people—hardly a neutral event to most individuals. It is an environment which may be of value and interest to people both avocationally and vocationally and is usually perceived by patients as the least interpersonally competitive program.

In the remainder of Barris' paper on environmental themes, she considers several properties of the interaction with the setting, and an event called the trajectory of increasing occupancy. Press, or environmental demands is one property to consider in an individual's interaction with his environment. Press is defined simply as an expectation for a certain kind of behavior.

Just as arousal is the match between volition and environment, press is the match between environmental demands for performance and the system's ability to perform. Arousal tells us how likely a person is to attempt a performance; press tells us what the person is required to do and how likely he or she is to succeed. (Barris, p. 640)

The density of people in a setting is another property discussed by Barris with its implications for performance. Research findings around this issue suggest that individual responsibility and satisfaction are inversely correlated with the level of manning. Thus, in so-called undermanned environments, [with] fewer people than necessary to carry out normal group activities, there appear to be more desired opportunities available to each person and subsequently more chance to develop competence over a range of skills.

In relating some of these properties to the work-related programs at McLean, the concept of press is helpful in understanding the common discrepancy between descriptions of ward-based patient behavior and patient behavior in the CVAP placements. Patients may be reported engaging in a variety of pathological behavior on the ward (threatening, aggressive behavior, isolation, apparent hallucinatory activity) and yet nevertheless manage an hour or more of appropriate performance in a hospital work setting. Clearly the work placements may elicit expectations for performance which at least temporarily supercede more maladaptive behavior.

By their sheer physical set-ups, the library-clerical and food service areas connote some very clear expectations for behavior, whether it be the associated tasks of filing books, typing, or running the cash register. While the tasks of the Greenhouse and Thrift Shop may be less immediately clear and somewhat more varied, ranging from solitary to group or structured to creative, nevertheless there are strong task expectations for each of the work placements. This in contrast to the many ward-based environments where the main gathering place is a central foyer comprised primarily of chairs, ashtrays, and patients. That physical environment creates almost no press except one of absolute passivity, and in such a void of both structure and stimulation, it is little wonder that intrapsychic aberrations flourish. Of some interest in this regard is that the hospital-based work programs are sometimes negatively contaminated by their location on hospital grounds, in spite of the contrast of their own discrete settings. Thus, for some patients, the work program is not very "real," its expectations not to be taken seriously, since after all, it is only a hospital program. In essence, it appears that the press of the ward is simply generalized to the work site. Fortunately, with continued contact, most patients are eventually able to perceive the particular press of the work environment and adapt their behavior accordingly, but in a few cases termination has proved therapeutic as a means of ultimate feedback on behavior which fails to conform to the standards of the setting. The wearing of uniforms at the Coffee Shop certainly helps patients discriminate the press of the food service area. And the Thrift Shop, which is located 3/4 of a mile from the hospital, almost never suffers the blurring of its press with that of the hospital wards. In fact, the concept of press may explain why many long-term patients are often referred to the Thrift Shop as a means of interrupting the process of institutionalization. While still inpatients, these people can begin to experience community and work demands in a setting outside the hospital, and thereby ease the course of their transition.

One last comment remains in regard to press and the psychiatric patient. There seems to be a temporal component to this concept. That is, patients are often noted to make a satisfactory adjustment to one of the work settings for one or two hours, but after a certain amount of time their ability to meet the previous level of expectations declines. Fatigue may be a simple explanation. Where the physically disabled patient may evidence such fatigue in excessive perspiration or tremor, the ramifications for the psychiatric patient are often the gradual reemergence of pathological behavior, clearly a cue that the patient's physical and emotional tolerance has been reached, and that the originally optimal level of press is no longer optimal.

In terms of density characteristic, the general experience in the CVAP certainly corroborates Barris' notion that overmanning of an environment tends to restrict participation, while undermanning often encourages individual responsibility and satisfaction. There are, however, some interesting considerations related to overmanning and the functional mix of patients found at each of the work sites. The two work programs with the most multi-faceted press, the Thrift Shop and Greenhouse, have a great variety of task demands ranging from very structured and repetitive to highly creative within each setting. This permits a degree of overmanning that is not counterproductive. The Thrift Shop, for instance, could be effectively run by two full-time people. Yet both the Thrift Shop and Greenhouse tend to be heavily subscribed programs that are able to accommodate a daily census of 20 patients on overlapping schedules as long as the group reflects a diversity of functional levels. When the balance shifts to a majority of either high-functioning or low-functioning individuals, then the overmanning becomes more problematic. In both cases there would be difficulty in meeting the breadth of program needs and selected work would end up being duplicated ("busy work"), plus the supervisory burden increases. With the highly functioning majority there is the need to generate sufficient challenging opportunities; with the lower functioning there is the obvious requirement for more supervision and instruction. Fortunately, since all the work programs are open referral sites, there is rarely the problem of many clients simultaneously existing on one functional plane, if only because they enter at different times and thus have different amounts of experience behind them. For the food service and library-clerical areas with fewer but more structured and defined task expectations, overmanning almost always has negative consequences for the patients regardless of functional mix.

A few words about undermanning. While potentially a more therapeutic state could be created since participants would have greater opportunity to become involved, undermanning backfires in those programs with the public service component. When there is already pressure to get a product out, whether a hamburger or a sales slip, undermanning can create excessive pressure and ultimately impede performance of all but the most high functioning individuals.

The last concept that Barris covers in her consideration of environmental themes is the trajectory of increasing occupancy, or the theory that as people master performance expectations in one setting, they will usually seek new settings in which to both practice their acquired skills and increase their skill repertoire. Similarity between settings facilitates the transfer of behavior, but if they are too alike, if a person's life spheres have been too constricted or unchanging, then the opportunity for new learning and behavior will be limited.

The trajectory of increasing occupancy is very germane to this discussion of vocational rehabilitation with the psychiatric patient. On the one hand there is an effort to make each of the work programs a close simulation of its community counterpart to facilitate eventual transition by the patient; to promote success, however, the task demands made on each patient are carefully titrated, his daily schedule is limited, and community standards are selectively imposed. Thus, expectations for performance vary from patient to patient. It is always a delicate balancing act, and one which sometimes fails. There is the "truncated" trajectory, the patient who leaves when the work expectations, real or imagined, become too overwhelming, or the patient who leaves because he is bored or because the stigma of a hospital work placement is overpowering to him. There is also the "fizzled" trajectory, representing the patient who is never quite ready to leave, who makes a satisfactory adjustment to the safety and security of the work site as long as the hospital umbilicus remains intact.

The case study which follows illustrates some of the theoretical material discussed.

CASE REPORT

Bob is a bright, 29-year-old single male who experienced a three-year course of intensive psychiatric treatment, both as an inpatient and outpatient. He was hospitalized in a confused, agitated state with active suicidal ideation. The reported precipitating life stress was the added pressure of clinical assignments as a 4th-year medical student. His admission diagnosis was mixed affective disorder with a questionable temporal lobe seizure disorder. Since Bob possessed a medical background, the potential neurological explanation for his psychiatric condition became central to his acceptance of the problem. Medication trials and various neurological tests were compatible treatment interventions for this patient and his medically sophisticated family. Although Bob reported a history of learning disability in elementary school, his academic achievements were consistently successful. He maintained an interest in the arts and enjoyed athletics. His social relationships were few, although he maintained one child-

hood friend and did single out at least one other person in whatever environment he presently found himself. Dating relationships were extremely stressful.

While an inpatient for 2 years, Bob was active in directing his treatment program; his volition subsystem remained largely intact. He participated in the milieu structure, maintained an individualized physical fitness program, was a consistent member of a ceramic group and music relaxation group and was involved in a placement in the Food Service Training Program. The initial rehabilitation treatment goal is best stated in Bob's own words: "to learn to work better during periods of personal difficulty." All of the selected treatment environments were compatible with Bob's values and interests, called upon some of his previously learned skills and were sufficiently stimulating. An initial evaluation of his performance capacity revealed interfering behaviors to be (1) an inability to prioritize relevant information, (2) an overly self-critical attitude, (3) dependency on structures provided by school or family, and (4) generalized disorganization in the face of strong emotional stimuli. After a considerable period of time some of his maladaptive performance behaviors diminished; his task pace and accuracy improved, and overall concentration and performance stabilized. Interpersonal interactions continued to suffer from inconsistent behaviors idiosyncratic to his moods. At times he was withdrawn and at other times he was very sensitive and responsive to others. Equally inconsistent was his self-appraisal and his ease in exploring new situations.

Bob was discharged with the belief that only neurological follow-up was necessary. However, this proved insufficient. Within weeks after discharge, Bob quickly began to experience increasing social isolation and cognitive disorganization. Bob then contracted for a rehabilitation outpatient program and reentered individual psychotherapy. His reasons for participating in the outpatient program continued to highlight the central theme of medication trials but now included other needs such as a supportive environment, social network, and developing a sense of productivity. As an outpatient, he was determined to rehabilitate himself; again the volition subsystem proved to be a prime mover. He rejoined the ceramic group because of his attachment to the group leaders, became a member of two outpatient counseling groups, and started a nine-month involvement at the Thrift Shop. Bob quickly developed a proficiency in all of the Thrift Shop tasks. Though the Thrift Shop is an environment very different from Bob's previous work and school experiences, he immediately embraced the store's philosophy of recycling and selling inexpensive items particularly to people in need, and developed an interest in the vast array of merchandise available.

In a sense, the Thrift Shop became Bob's medical laboratory and an internship of a different order. The Shop's limitless variety of objects paired with Bob's imagination and creativity led to a sustained and productive level of arousal. Clearly, all of the environmental variables associated with arousal had an impact on Bob. He set up displays, repaired broken appliances, and was often able to find that special object to match a customer's special request. He helped to outfit a number of patrons looking for a unique Halloween costume. With the discovery of possible rare book acquisitions, Bob called numerous book dealers to appraise the worth of these finds. He composed an advertisement for an upcoming sale and suggested several store improvement ideas. One facet of the press of the Thrift Shop environment is to invite participation on many levels, and for this patient little prompting was needed to identify and fulfill many of the different demands presented. As Bob's sense of competency grew in this work role, he became eligible and applied for the Senior Clerk position at the Thrift Shop. This position is part of a transitional employment opportunity, and as such, requires a 20-hour commitment. He was responsible for knowing all Shop procedures, managing the store independently at times, closing out each evening, making deposits, training the vocational assessment patients, and handling customer requests.

Although a transfer of physical settings was not involved in Bob's movement to the Senior Clerk position, nevertheless the trajectory of increasing occupancy is represented here by all the additional responsibilities of the new position. Unlike the routine CHAP participation, Senior Clerk carries with it the expectation for a global understanding of the Shop program, as well as heavy emphasis on initiative and independent decision-making. Bob attained a high level of skill in the new position, though occasionally exceeded his authority and tended to over identify with staff, becoming too involved in the problems of the patients. His physical energy level tended to wax and wane; one day he might be enormously productive in reorganizing merchandise and on another day take little initiative around the store. Initially, Bob attributed the shifts in energy or any other dysfunction to his "unique and poorly understood" neurological problem. The inconsistencies were recognized and discussed using the Patient Performance Checklist. As Bob grew more confident and competent in his role, he perceived himself as more in control, and less a passive victim of some disease process. Gradually, the disparities in his performance diminished. At termination, Bob reported that the program experience was extremely beneficial because it gave him the opportunity to help others, to learn about himself and his various responses to situations, and to explore options for future employment. More importantly, he perceived himself as a rehabilitated person rather than a marginally functioning, neurologically disabled person. He could translate the sense of accomplishment as a productive store manager to exploring other career fields that were less conflicted and pressured than medical school.

SUMMARY

There are always a number of variables considered when a patient is referred to one of our work-related programs. The most compelling and prognostic factor, however is the patient's desire to participate, or the involvement of that person's volition system in choosing a setting. As Barris explains:

> Choosing a setting involves resonation between the volition subsystem and the environment. Arousal is a form of resonation between the urge to explore and feel control, and the novelty and complexity of the setting. The possibility of engaging in enjoyable behavior or fulfilling goals reflects resonation between the person's interests and values, and the environment. (Barris, p. 639)

Helping the patient to use his or her experiences in the work program to seek further vocational challenges is the task of the supervising clinician. Clarifying with the patient the purpose of his or her participation is critical and is reinforced during the evaluation sessions. The multi-item performance checklist focuses attention on those behaviors which either need to be improved or are positive attributes for the patient. This evaluation process helps to make the trajectory of increasing occupancy a cognitively reinforced experience; no longer are a person's past work history, current participation, and future vocational plans simply a series of discontinuous, discrete occurrences. The opportunities, qualities, and activities of each setting can be related to their impact on the patient's performance: identifying strengths and weaknesses, and using this information to establish a realistic vocational plan with the patient. A patient whose sense of efficacy is stimulated by a setting and whose values and interests coincide with the opportunities presented by that environment represents a therapeutic formula for success.

REFERENCE

Barris, R. (1982). Environmental interactions: An extension of the Model of Occupation. *Am J Occup Ther, 36*, 637-656.

CHAPTER THIRTY-ONE

Transitional Employment for the Chronically Mentally Ill

Jane L. Dulay and Mary Steichen

This chapter was previously published in Occupational Therapy in Mental Health, *2(3), 65-77. Copyright © 1982, Haworth Press. Reprinted by permission.*

A concept that is becoming increasingly popular in community-based treatment of the chronically mentally ill is that of transitional employment. Many discharged psychiatric patients find the transition from the hospital to the community difficult, particularly in the area of work. They find upon returning to the community that traditional job placements are not open to them. Although former patients often possess the necessary work skills to function on a job, they are unable to secure employment.

There are many factors contributing to the lack of opportunities available to the chronically mentally ill. These include a psychiatric history, a poor work history, a lack of recent job references, the inability to pass a job interview, and a lack of initiative in seeking employment. Transitional employment is a means of removing these barriers and aiding the former psychiatric patient toward becoming a functional member or the work force.

The first transitional employment program, referred to as TEP, was instituted in 1958 at Fountain House, a psychosocial rehabilitation program in New York City (Bean & Beard 1975). Since that time new programs have been developed in many community-based rehabilitation centers throughout the country. A 1996 survey by Fountain House found that there were 340 programs worldwide based on the Fountain House Model. (ICCD, 1996)

TEP offers discharged psychiatric patients an opportunity to become employed in the community, rather than in a sheltered work program, which traditionally has been the only type of employment situation available to them. TEP serves as the stepping stone between these sheltered work programs and competitive employment in the community. TEP contracts with businesses for positions within their companies. These positions are usually part-time, entry-level positions. TEP members rotate through these positions, holding a particular position for 6 months.

TEP offers the employing businesses a potentially never-ending supply of labor. The initial screening and interviewing for the positions and on-the-job training for each member assuming a position are provided by TEP staff members. As a major incentive to employers, the TEP staff guarantees the work shift will be covered in the event a member is unable to work on any day that he is scheduled.

Since these positions are reserved for TEP, the members are given an opportunity for employment regardless of their past psychiatric or work history. Many members who lack the confidence and initiative to compete for jobs in the community are given an opportunity to apply for a job that is readily available to them. After members have completed a TEP placement, they possess current work experience and a recent job reference which leaves them better equipped to enter the competitive job market.

The Towne House Creative Living Center, Oakland, California, (hereafter referred to as Towne House) is the only pre-vocational program in the San Francisco Bay Area that offers TEP to adults with a history of chronic mental illness (Hill, 1980). In 1980, the passage of state legislation, Bates Bill AB3052 (allocating state monies for community residential treatment system), provided the financial impetus for Towne House to expand its center-based, pre-vocational program and develop a TEP program. An occupational therapist was hired to develop and implement a TEP program similar to that of Fountain House, New York.

THE ROLE OF THE OCCUPATIONAL THERAPIST IN THE DEVELOPMENT AND IMPLEMENTATION OF A TEP PROGRAM

While designing the new pre-vocational component offering TEP as the major treatment service, the occupational therapist identified 3 key elements essential for a comprehensive rehabilitation program: 1) developing jobs for the chronically mentally ill in the business community, 2) developing criteria for entrance into the TEP program, as well as screening members for employment placement, and 3) providing a therapeutic link between the employment placement and Towne House via an ongoing support group for TEP members.

Job Development

Two important factors were considered for securing jobs in the business community: 1) assessing the special pre-vocational needs of the chronically mentally ill members who came to Towne House and 2) identifying appropriate employment placements which could provide the therapeutic conditions necessary for successful work performance of the TEP employee.

Of the 25 members who entered the TEP program in the first year, 64% were male, 36% were female; 44% had less than a high school education, 28% received only a high school education, and 28% received some college education. In terms of work experience, 44% had 0-5 months of work experience, and 56% had over 5 months of work experience. These figures reflect the results of a pilot study conducted by Howe in 1976 (Howe, Weaver, & Dulay, 1981). Her findings indicated that the prevocational program at Towne House appealed to young males with a high school education or less, who had never held a steady job, but valued paid work. All members had more than one psychiatric hospitalization prior to their involvement with Towne House and were receiving some type of financial assistance such as supplemental security income (SSI). 52% lived in supervised situations such as board and care homes, 14% lived with their families, 14% lived in semi-independent situations such as halfway houses and satellite housing, and 19% lived independently in apartments or hotels.

A review of the current job market indicated that the employment positions available and suitable for the Towne House members were the unskilled, entry-level positions that fell into three areas: janitorial, food services, and clerical. Companies which were most receptive to reserving job positions for TEP were those with job openings due to high turnover rates, absenteeism, and undesirable working hours such as weekend shifts, and were supportive of the mental health system.

A task analysis was conducted on each job secured for the program. The following conditions were observed to be important therapeutic indicators for successful work performance of the TEP members. Arrangements were made with the employer to adapt the TEP position to meet as many of the conditions as possible.

Type of activity. Structured, concrete, routine tasks that changed little from day to day gave the TEP employees a sense of competence early in employment.

Variety of techniques. Tasks that could be performed by a variety of methods with a minimum number of tools required to complete the task seemed to eliminate the pressure of the "right and wrong" way to do a task.

Rates of achievement. Tasks that allowed the TEP employee to perform at his (or her) own speed and that emphasized quality rather than quantity, decreased the pressure to work at a predetermined rate.

Space. An open, uncrowded work environment that was stable and relatively free of noise, decreased the possibility of overstimulation and distraction for the TEP employee.

Mental-motor coordination requirements. It has been expressed by TEP employees that sustained heavy physical labor, large gaps of inactivity requiring initiative and judgment to keep busy, or fine motor activities lead to frustration and feelings of inadequacy or exploitation by their supervisors. These feelings have been observed to trigger internal preoccupation and decreased attention span and concentration. Employers have, at times, interpreted this behavior as laziness or a tendency to daydream. Therefore, gross motor and simple cognitive level responsibilities such as sweeping, setting tables or collating papers are preferred and seem to provide the opportunity for concentration and an increase in attention span.

Social interaction. Interpersonal interaction seemed best when limited to one supervisor and two to three coworkers. Little or no public contact helped a TEP employee gradually learn to work and socially interact in an unsheltered, unsupported environment.

The occupational therapist, by adapting the work environment, plays an important role in assisting the chronically mentally ill attain their occupational goals. Johnson states that "occupational therapists have a contribution to make to most persons who, because of personal or environmental or social barriers, are unable to influence their environments in such a way as to enable them to fulfill their personal needs" (Johnson, 1971).

Currently, the TEP employment opportunities include janitorial positions at McDonald's restaurant, kitchen aide positions at a psychogeriatric nursing home, meal handler positions at senior nutrition sites, and clerical positions at a ticket agency.

The TEP job placements range from 2-4 hours a day, 1-5 days a week. The gradation of job responsibilities is according to the number of hours and days per week a TEP employee is physically and psychologically ready to handle.

Gradation of the number of hours in a work shift also serves to minimize a member's fears of termination from social security disability income or supplemental security income... [Readers are advised to check with the social security administration for current regulations]... The fear of losing disability or supplemental security income is a major work disincentive for the chronically mentally ill.

Screening Process

The occupational therapist agrees, as part of the contract with the employer, to send the most qualified person for the job. A five step screening process encourages members to apply for TEP job openings. At the same time, this screening process allows members who have unrealistic employment goals or who need more work adjustment to eliminate themselves at various stages of the process. Emphasis is on independent decision-making and a realistic appraisal of one's capabilities.

1. *Application.* TEP job openings are announced at the Towne House weekly member-run business meetings, posted on the bulletin board as well as advertised in the center newsletter. Interested members are requested to fill out the employment application required by the company. These employment applications also aid the occupational therapist in assessing a member's ability in reading, writing, and comprehension. At this time, members can join the TEP program. This requires an interview with the occupational therapist where a psychiatric and work history is gathered, and a commitment to attend the weekly support groups.

2. *Field Trip.* All applicants are required to take a field trip to the employment site via public transportation. This opportunity to become familiar with the transportation system, to see the actual work environment, and to meet the prospective supervisor and coworkers can aid a member in independently deciding whether he can meet the job expectations and/or if the job is a safe and meaningful work environment. At this point in the screening process as many as half of the applicants often decide not to continue.

3. *Work supervisor evaluation.* Most members applying for TEP placement are involved in the center-based prevocational program in activities such as recycling, landscaping, janitorial and food services. A recommendation, through the use of an assessment tool developed by the membership at Towne House, is requested from a member's work supervisor. This assessment tool evaluates a member's performance in work areas such as attendance, punctuality, ability to deal with authority, ability to get along with coworkers, ability to do a variety of jobs, and ability to follow directions (Howe, Weaver, & Dulay, 1981). Members who receive a high recommendation from their work supervisor are then selected to take a work sample evaluation

4. *Work sample evaluation.* The occupational therapist develops a work sample evaluation for each TEP segment. See Figure 1 for an example of a work sample evaluation. Patterned after the Bay Area Functional Performance Evaluation (Bloomer & Williams, 1979), each work sample is divided into three major parts. The main objective is to assess and predict work behavior and vocational potential.

Part I evaluates the member's ability to meet specific company requirements. For example, McDonald's does not permit beards. Is a member with a beard willing to shave it? A member is also evaluated on the ability to locate the company phone number, the use of the telephone, and the ability to remember the days and hours of his work shift.

Part II involves evaluation of the member's functional ability to carry out tasks similar to those that will be required on the job. The member's level of function is assessed in the following areas: (a) ability to paraphrase verbal instructions, (b) productive decision making, (c) organization of time and materials, and (d) ability to follow instructions leading to correct task completion.

The work sample concludes with a series of situational questions geared to assess a member's judgment in handling common problems or crises that may arise on the job.

A member who best meets all of the above screening requirements is chosen to be interviewed by the prospective employer. Once approved, a member completes two days of on-the-job training on a volunteer basis, and then is officially hired and placed on the company payroll. The TEP employee is paid the prevailing wages.

5. *On-the-job training.* The fact that the TEP staff will provide on-the-job training at no extra cost to the employer is a major selling point for involving the business community with the chronically mentally ill. Within the past year, TEP members who have successfully completed a placement have begun serving as TEP trainers, assisting the occupational therapist in teaching new TEP employees on-the-job responsibilities. A major reason for promoting this concept is that members related more readily to a peer rather than a staff member while learning a new job.

At the same time that a TEP employee is hired, another TEP member is also hired and trained to serve as a substitute in the event that the TEP employee cannot meet his or her work schedule. This provides the opportunity for members to learn reliance upon their peers rather than dependence on staff. The use of substitutes also promotes social networking among TEP members as they must know each other's phone number as well as where they can be reached during the day. It is the responsibility of the TEP employee to contact the substitute if he or she is unable to work a shift.

Once officially hired, a TEP member is asked to sign a contract drawn up by the occupational therapist. This contract clearly states the name of the supervisor, the length of employment, the requirements of the job and TEP program, and the names and phone numbers of the substitutes. A TEP placement is a maximum of 5 months. At the end of that time, the screening process is repeated. As part of the TEP program requirements the TEP employee is expected to continue attending the support groups.

TEP Support Groups

Whereas the actual job placement provides the opportunity for members to be engaged in a real work situation, the support groups, which meet three times weekly for 45 minutes, provide the crucial link for members to work on dealing with psychological problems and issues they face as they work to master occupational goals. It has been our experience that the psychotic defenses arising from psychological issues around the meaning of work are primarily responsible for a TEP member's inability to function successfully on the job, rather than an absence of specific work skills.

A model for day treatment and group therapy for chronic schizophrenics developed by Gootnick (1971, 1975) is used as the clinical orientation of the support groups. According to Gootnick the group structure provides a therapeutically safe environment for the schizophrenic to work on personal goals. The intense transference complications generated in individ-

NAME:
DATE:
RATER:

TEP PROGRAM
Towne House Creative Living Center
412 Monte Vista Ave.
Oakland, CA 94611

CLERICAL WORK SAMPLE EVALUATION

I. COMPANY REQUIREMENTS (if member able to answer YES to all questions proceed to tasks)   YES   NO
    1. Work a 6 hour shift _____
    2. Work on Saturdays _____
    3. Use public transportation to San Francisco _____

II. BASIC WORK SKILLS—I am going to give you a series of tasks to do that are similar to what will be required of you at Ticket Easy. I will first give you the instructions of the task. I would like you to summarize the instructions for me as you understand them and then proceed with the task. Are there any questions?

TELEPHONE USE

You will be working at Ticket Easy, located at 655 Stockton St., San Francisco. You may need to call them if you are unable to make it to work or will be late for work due to an emergency. I would like you to tell me how you would find out the telephone number of Ticket Easy. Do you understand the instructions?
If YES—would you summarize each step that I've asked you to do.
Go ahead and begin.
Any of the possibilities are correct:
Dial 411 for information _____ Look up in the telephone book _____
Have member do either one and check with the correct number: 421-6407
Why do you think I have asked you to do this task?

TIME

Your shift will be: Saturdays, approximately once a month from 10:00 am to 4:00 pm, with an hour lunch break. I would like you to tell me the days and hours of your work shift and how long of a break you have each day.
Do you understand the instructions?
If YES—would you summarize each step that I've asked you to do.
Go ahead and begin.
Why do you think I have asked you to do this task?

III. WORK TASKS—I will be timing you in the following tasks, so work as quickly, but accurately, as possible.

ATTACHING LABELS
Here are some address labels and ____ envelopes. I would like you to apply the labels onto the center of the front of the envelopes.

Do you understand the instructions?
If YES—would you summarize each step that I've asked you to do.
Go ahead and begin.
Why do you think I've asked you to do this task?

SORTING
Here is a stack of envelopes. I would like you to sort them into piles according to zip codes.
Do you understand the instructions?
If YES—would you summarize each step that I've asked you to do.
Go ahead and begin.
Why do you think I've asked you to do this task?

COUNTING
Here is a stack of cards. I would like you to count out 20. Do this 3 times.
Do you understand the instructions?
If YES—would you summarize each step that I've asked you to do.
Go ahead and begin.
Why do you think I've asked you to do this task?

IV. PROBLEM-SOLVING—I am going to describe several situations and would like you to tell me how you would handle each one.

1. It is Saturday morning and you have to go to San Francisco this morning to work. How will you go about getting to work?
2. You are in San Francisco, but you are lost. What would you do?
3. Your boss is the kind of person who likes to talk to you while you are working. He asks you what kinds of things you like to do. What would you tell him?
4. Your supervisor tells you you are working too slow. What would you do?
5. One of your co-workers is giving you a hard time. What would you do?
6. There is a large mailing to be done. You must complete 2000 mailings in 2 hours. What would you do?

Figure 31-1. Clerical work sample evaluation.

ual therapy that intensify conflicts of right-wrong, pleasing-displeasing, submission-defiance, dependence-independence, etc. and immobilize the patient from functioning are greatly diminished in the group experience. Thus, the group experiences in the TEP support groups provide opportunities for social relationships and for the identification with a group of peers who are experiencing similar psychological problems and achieving similar social and occupational goals.

To counteract the passive roles the chronically mentally ill assume in social and verbal exchanges and in making decisions, the emphasis in the TEP groups is on healthy, adult, member-to-member interaction, placing them in active, "doing" roles. The major role of the therapist is in minimizing member-to-staff interactions and acting as an observing ego, intervening only when the group members are unable to work as a group. For example, a common group occurrence that happens when a new member enters the group is that old group members will ignore the new member. One of the ways to address this issue would be for the therapist to ask the group if anyone noticed there was a new member in the group. Using this technique, the responsibility for social exchange is placed on group members to think and ask basic social questions such as, "what is your name, what brings you to join the TEP group, what kind of job are you looking for?", etc. As a result, members are in a position of practicing normal, everyday, social interactions which are critical for learning and integrating new skills or recovering lost skills.

When individual psychological issues surface, again the primary therapeutic feedback comes from the group members themselves. As members are exposed to each other's difficulties and disturbed thought processes as well as healthy resources, there are opportunities for reality testing concerning personal and occupational goals. Distortions that members have about themselves or others are often brought out and clarified, corrected, as well as consensually validated by their peers.

A case in point was a young man, C. R., who was officially hired for a janitorial position. His two days of volunteer on-the-job training proved he was capable of meeting the job requirements and the thoroughness of his work won the praise of the management. However, on the third day of employment, C. R. became increasingly anxious to the point where he was immobilized from walking through the door of his place of employment. He decided to quit his job. C. R. was encouraged to attend the group meeting to talk about this sudden change of attitude.

Members asked him why he did not want to work anymore. Was it because he did not like the work, or that the supervisors were mean to him? After much exploration, C. R. was able to express the notion that if he were to work and be successful, his mother would die. Some group members could empathize with this feeling and thought C. R. was making the right decision to quit his job. Others voiced the opinion that it was a ridiculous idea. If everybody thought that way, no one would be working today. One member shared with C. R. he used to think that if he worked his mother would die, too. However, he had to take the risk, and she has

not died yet. After hearing these shared experiences, C. R. was able to recall the time he had a volunteer job a year ago. His mother barred the doorway to prevent him from going to work. He also shared with the group that when he told his mother, who is his payee and controlled his money, that he had gotten a paid job, instead of being pleased she was upset with him for jeopardizing his SSI benefits. These experiences meant to him she did not want him to work, and that his working caused her to become upset and sick. C. R.'s ability to relate these thoughts to the group members demonstrated several significant steps for C. R.: his ability to trust the group to share his problems in reaching his goals; his ability to gain some control over his sense of omnipotence in the destruction of his mother; and the fact that the group did not act ruined like his mother because he wanted to work. As a matter of fact, after they had heard his reasons for quitting, they recommended he should stick with his job.

According to Gootnick (1975), "experiences in groups are responsible for enhancing the healthy part of the ego, that part of the schizophrenic ego involved with reality, so that defenses against the psychotic aspect of the self can be maintained. As a result, the patient's self-esteem is elevated and this leads to the ability to become involved with and relate to reality at a higher level." In TEP, this ability to become involved with and relate to reality at a higher level is demonstrated in several areas: increased care about personal appearance, increased social interaction with peers, moves to more independent living situations, and the ability to successfully complete a TEP job placement.

PERFORMANCE EVALUATION

Two performance evaluations are given by the immediate employment supervisor during a member's 5-month placement. The final written evaluation becomes a current job reference.

For many members who have never held a steady job, completing a 5-month placement is a major developmental achievement. Certificates of completion are awarded publicly at Towne House and photographs of the TEP members at work are displayed. Local newspaper announcements and articles have been helpful in creating a climate in the community that the chronically mentally ill can hold a job and be productive members of the community.

THE FUTURE ROLE OF OCCUPATIONAL THERAPISTS IN TEP PROGRAMS

It has been documented that occupational therapists have the skills and knowledge base to provide prevocational services to the mentally disabled (American Occupational Therapy Association, 1980). As more occupational therapists become involved in community-based programs, new therapeutic modalities need to be explored outside the traditional realm of treatment activities used in hospital-based treatment with the mentally ill. TEP can be an effective therapeutic modality in assisting the chronically mentally ill engage in productive, meaningful activity. This form of activity is not only age-stage specific, but also one of the few socially acceptable ways to integrate the chronically mentally ill into the community. Igi (1979) spoke of the need to provide "an arena that enables patients to acquire skills in a low stress environment and to experience a process they can replicate in their daily life to facilitate continued skill building and a sense of competence and mastery". TEP can be that arena as well as a cost-effective way to rehabilitate the chronically ill in the face of shrinking mental health funding. Finally, TEP is one of the rare opportunities open to a segment of the population who, because of their history of mental illness, have been denied the experience of gainful employment which is critical to being part of the mainstream of society.

REFERENCES

American Occupational Therapy Association. (1980). Position paper—the role of occupational therapy in the vocational rehabilitation process. *American Journal of Occupational Therapy, 34*(13), 881-883.

Bean, B. R., & Beard, J. H. (1975). Placement for persons with psychiatric disability. *Rehabilitation Counseling Bulletin, June,* 253-258.

Bloomer, J., & Williams, S. (1979). *The Bay Area Functional Evaluation.* San Francisco, CA: Rehabilitation Therapy Department, Langley-Porter Institute, U. C. S. F.

Hill, H. (1980). *Vocational rehabilitation services in the San Francisco Bay area mental health program.* Albany Press.

Howe, M., Weaver, C., & Dulay, J. (1981). The development of a work-oriented day center program. *American Journal of Occupational Therapy, 35,*(11), 711-718.

Gootnick, I. (1971). The psychiatric day center in the treatment of the chronic schizophrenic. *American Journal of Psychiatry, 128,* 4.

Gootnick, I. (1975). Transference in psychotherapy with schizophrenic patients. *International Journal of Group Psychotherapy, 25,* 4.

Igi, C. H. (1979). Apprenticeship: Skill building in the marginally disabled. Paper presented at the Mental Health Symposium of the Occupational Therapy Association of California, Los Angeles, California.

International Center for Clubhouse Development (ICCD), (1996). *1996 survey of clubhouses.* New York: Author.

Johnson, J. (1971). Consideration of work as therapy in the rehabilitation process. *American Journal of Occupational Therapy, 25,* (6), 303-308.

Social Security Amendments to the Social Security Act, 1936, Section 6714. The Trial Work Period, March 1979, and section T6400. Revised Earnings Guidelines for Evaluation or Substantial Gainful Activity, April 1979.

Transitional Employment Survey Memorandum 218. (1981). New York: Fountain House, Inc.

CHAPTER THIRTY-TWO

Building Employer Support for Hiring Persons with Psychiatric Disabilities

Richard M. Balser, Brenda M. Harvey, and Helaine Hornby

This chapter was previously published in the Mental Health Special Interest Section Quarterly, 21(4), 2-4. *Copyright © 1998, The American Occupational Therapy Association, Inc.*

For more than 15 years, the Maine Medical Center's Department of Vocational Services (Portland, ME) has been using innovative strategies for obtaining competitive employment for persons with disabilities. Two common themes have marked its approach: (a) enlisting the support of current and potential employers in whatever it does and (b) building natural supports in the workplace to minimize ongoing support costs and, more importantly, to normalize the job situation. In charting new territory in the employment of persons with disabilities, Maine Medical Center's latest efforts have focused on the most intransigent group, persons with serious psychiatric disabilities. (Only persons with schizophrenic or major mood and anxiety disorders, 18 to 55 years of age, who have been unemployed for at least 6 months, are allowed to participate in the federal project described in this [chapter].) Rates of unemployment for this group are a staggering high 85%, according to the National Institute on Disability and Rehabilitation Research (1992). Many factors contribute to their unemployment: (a) the effect of psychiatric symptoms and the unpredictably of the illness itself; b) the expectations of family members and the community; and (c) the barriers to employment created by employer discrimination as well as the absence of a readily available pool of jobs.

Fear and ignorance have traditionally characterized employers' responses to this group. To overcome employers' concerns as well as demystify the subject of mental illness, Maine Medical Center has formed a group for major employers in the greater Portland area. Called the Mental Health Employer Consortium (MHEC), the group meets every other month to learn about the subject of mental illness and how it affects behavior, how to deal with specific situations, and what can be done to accommodate persons with psychiatric disabilities on the job. Represented in the MHEC are major health and disability insurance companies, other hospitals, municipal governments, a supermarket chain, manufacturers, and a public university, among others.

This (chapter) provides initial observations about the workings of the MHEC and the staff members who support it. The (chapter) focuses on three areas:

1. The attitudes of employers toward hiring persons with serious mental illnesses
2. The role of employment specialists and occupational therapy practitioners in trying to bridge the gap between employers and persons with mental disabilities
3. Strategies used at job sites to increase the possibilities of employment for this most difficult-to-place group

ATTITUDES OF EMPLOYERS

Maine Medical Center's project evaluators polled employers to determine which factors raise concerns when they consider hiring persons with psychiatric disabilities. The four most important were (a) their ability to do the job, (b) the amount of time that would be required of supervisors, (c) the potential for absenteeism, and (d) interpersonal relationships. Table 1 displays various employment factors to the hiring decision in order of importance.

Employers noted that merely having a social conscience is not enough to sustain the interest of department heads in the long run.

Projects such as these must appeal to the employers' concerns about getting the work done without additional cost. Employers are concerned that the worker will be resented by other workers who may have to compensate for their absences or lack of productivity while on the job. Employers fear the person will not be able to assimilate and that they as supervisors will not know how to handle difficult situations, particularly when "patient privilege" is used to withhold information about the person's particular illness or how the illness might manifest itself. In addition to the MHEC itself, which works mainly with human resources staff members, Maine Medical Center has addressed some of the employers'

Table 32-1
Importance of Employment Factors in Hiring Decisions

Employment Factor	Very Important (%)	Somewhat Important (%)	Not Important (%)
Job performance	64	29	7
Supervisory support	53	27	20
Absenteeism	47	47	—
Interpersonal skills	38	62	—
Appearance	21	64	21
Rule infractions	20	33	47
Tardiness	21	50	29
Medical claims	—	3	64

concerns through the use of employment specialists and occupational therapy practitioners.

ROLE OF EMPLOYMENT SPECIALISTS AND OCCUPATIONAL THERAPY PRACTITIONERS

Two years ago, Maine Medical Center was awarded a major, multiyear grant from the U. S. Department of Health and Human Service's Center for Mental Health Services that has allowed Maine Medical Center to provide better staffing and support to the MHEC as well as to expand the clinical and vocational work performed with persons with mental illnesses. Specifically, the grant has added employment specialists and occupational therapy practitioners to the team who work with both the employers and the outpatients from the Department of Psychiatry at Maine Medical Center to obtain employment experience and placements.

Persons who have been unemployed for at least 6 months and who have schizophrenia or major mood or anxiety disorders are candidates for participation in the project. Participants are randomly assigned to one of two groups. Both groups receive family-aided assertive community treatment (FACT). This clinical strategy emphasizes a functional progression that includes support from and coordination with family members, early crisis intervention, and relapse prevention. Group goal setting, led by trained employment specialists as well as occupational therapy practitioners, is used to establish employment goals in conjunction with objectives set in the multifamily group. Both groups participate in activities designed to lead to employment. Those include the career exploration phase (cognitive testing and experiential exploration), the job matching and placement phase, and the post-placement support phase. Only one group, however, obtains job placements in companies that are members of the MHEC. Members of the other group may be placed anywhere. The theory behind the experiment is that

persons receiving both FACT and the employment interventions and companies in the MHEC will have better employment outcomes than persons receiving FACT alone.

In addition to testing the validity of the MHEC, one of the benefits of the project has been its ability to develop the role of employment specialists and occupational therapy practitioners in the context of community mental health services. The employment specialist functions as a broker. A stockbroker must understand the investment objectives of clients while knowing the attributes of the financial products he or she is trying to sell. The broker must make the appropriate match between the two to be successful. A real estate broker must know what will attract a house hunter to a particular property while being able to describe both the assets and the flaws of the home he or she is trying to sell. The employment specialist is a broker of people and jobs. He or she must have a sufficiently accurate grasp of the abilities and supports required of the person being placed while understanding the demands of the potential job needs of the employer. Employment specialists at the Maine Medical Center project appear to have mastered this duality. The employers with whom they work have described their greatest strengths as follows:

- *Learning the job.* Employment specialists make an effort to understand the business as well as the particulars of the job; they master the lingo of the trade and speak the employer's language.
- *Supporting the employee.* Employee specialists prepare and coach the employee about working in this particular environment; they provide support when the employee stumbles and serve as a "cushion" for the employee.
- *Bridging two worlds.* Employment specialists span the worlds of employers' needs and persons' frailties as well as strengths; they keep employers informed about what is happening. They can be called on night or day. As one employer stated, "It is helpful to know that the person was not just dropped off and told to do the job."
- *Helping with other employees.* Employment specialists provide counseling when employers have problems

with other employees whom they discover to have an emotional or psychological problem; sometimes they help to "save the job" for workers who in other times would have been dismissed summarily for behavior the employer could not understand or cope with.

- *Demystifing mental illness.* Employment specialists make mental illness less frightening by educating and supporting employers; they can represent the effort to other staff members and managers.

The employment specialist assumes a longer-term relationship both with the person being placed and with the employer than does the occupational therapy practitioner. The occupational therapy practitioner performs cognitive evaluations of the person seeking employment. These evaluations include learning style, the capacity to solve problems, memory, and ability to initiate and regulate goal-directed activity.

Armed with this specific information, the employment specialist can make a more precise presentation to the employer of the employees' strengths and limitations. The occupational therapy practitioner may evaluate the work environment so that the employer and employment specialist can prevent problems before they arise or make accommodations. Aspects such as lighting, the amount of stimulation in the environment, and the stress of the job duties are all considered by the practitioner.

Employers have noted these strengths in occupational therapy practitioners:

- *They speak with authority.* By performing a rigorous evaluation of the person's skill level, occupational therapy practitioners are able to speak with authority about the person's capabilities and potential problem areas as a worker.
- *They understand the work environment.* Occupational therapy practitioners observe the workplace with respect to productivity needs and processes; they comprehend what is required of a successful employee in that environment.
- *They advise supervisors.* Occupational therapy practitioners provide tangible assistance to supervisors in how to keep the worker focused; they troubleshoot other problems related to productivity and work processes.

STRATEGIES AT WORKSITES TO ENHANCE EMPLOYMENT

In addition to the role of the MHEC and the employment specialists and occupational therapy practitioners, the employers themselves have taken many steps to support persons with psychiatric disabilities on the job. Some of the most important are accommodations and education and training.

Accommodations

Employers make accommodations for their workers all the time, sometimes without thinking about it. When the worker has a psychiatric condition that has been disclosed, there is often a greater need for and greater awareness of adjustments in work scheduling or environmental makers. Among MHEC companies, the most common and most helpful accommodations include the following:

- *Differences in use of time* (e.g., allowing more time off, shorter but more frequent breaks, flexible hours.)
- *Restructured schedules* or avoiding having the person work at problematic times (e.g., not assigning the third shift to a person with clinical depression who is particularly vulnerable at night, avoiding the busiest time of day when work is particularly stressful.)
- *Extra support and supervision* or providing assistance either from the on-site supervisor or from someone outside the company. One of the most successful developments has been the establishment of employee assistance programs (EAPs). In many workplaces, there is an EAP confidential counselor available who can provide on-site support or a referral to external resources. Often, the EAP provides the gateway to other services, such as private counseling, substance abuse treatment, and community mental health care agencies.
- *Individualized assistance* (e.g., allowing a worker to keep water at the cash register to take medications, offering a map of the work site to help orient a worker, placing the worker next to a supportive employee.)

In addition, many employers provide mental health care benefits through their health insurance plans. Some employers use private vocational rehabilitation programs from which they recruit employees or work with the state vocational rehabilitation agency. MHEC employers are working diligently to spread the message that asking for accommodations is acceptable, and, in fact, they have learned that the accommodations often have benefits for both the worker and the company.

EDUCATION AND TRAINING

Many employers have gone far beyond a willingness to hire persons with psychiatric disabilities. One of the most noteworthy expressions of their commitment has been in the area of the training and education for coworkers, supervisors, and management. The formats have varied and have included panels, discussion groups, lectures, and interactive projects. The issue most often addressed is diversity, but lately there have been excellent programs on depression and disclosure. One example of this work is an insurance company's program entitled "A Day in the Life" (Unum Insurance Company, Portland, ME [www.unum.com]). It included 3 days of presentations and experiential activities covering all disabilities, including mental health. Two of the events focused on stigma attached to psychiatric disabilities and how to confront and eliminate it. Not only was the program well attended and well received by employees, but also it was publicized on television news, thus extending its educational effect to the general public.

PLANS FOR THE FUTURE

Great gains have been made in the years since the MHEC was first created. The following strategies have been identified to continue the growth of this effort.

- *Training and education* may be the most important strategies available. Through efforts in both the workplace and the community, more persons will have their biases erased and their misunderstandings corrected. More persons will see the great benefits for all concerned of tapping into this valuable resource of diligent and talented workers.

- *Trial employment and supported work* can develop a useful track record. Temporary and even, in appropriate circumstances, unpaid jobs can give a worker increased confidence and a chance to establish reliability. These jobs can show the employer how productive and valuable the worker can be.

- *Reaching more levels in the company* will help build support. Each member company has a single representative to the MHEC. Others must be exposed as well, with much attention paid to obtaining support from upper management in the company as well as from frontline managers. The current representatives are not in positions to create jobs but only to fill them. Employers at all levels must be educated on the idea.

- *Enhancing the role of employment specialists, occupational therapy practitioners, and other supports* can increase the likelihood that job placements will work. These resources are considered invaluable by employers because they demystify mental illness and provide tangible strategies for making workers productive. Employers want other supports as well to compensate for what they see for now as the additional risks they are assuming by hiring persons with mental illnesses. These supports may be financial, such as partial payment of salaries during the training period, or technical, such as providing advice when difficult situations arise.

Placing persons with serious mental disabilities on the path to employment has posed enormous challenges for family members, physicians, and assisting professionals. One group missing from this team has been employers themselves. Maine Medical Center has worked successfully with a consortium of employers who address issues as a group and who receive support at the worksite from employment specialists and occupational therapy practitioners. Combined with therapeutic treatment and family support for the person with disabilities, the employer consortium holds great promise for increasing the likelihood of employing persons with mental disabilities.

CHAPTER THIRTY-THREE

The Pros and Cons of Non-Traditional Practice

Ralph Adams

This chapter was previously published in Mental Health Special Interest Section Newsletter, 5-6. Copyright © *1991, The American Occupational Therapy Association, Inc.*

Numerous deterrents have been identified to explain the comparatively low representation of occupational therapists in non-traditional, particularly community-based, settings. Salaries are generally not competitive. The dearth of occupational therapists to serve as role models and provide peer support is frequently cited as a deterrent. Many therapists are unfamiliar with the structure and dynamic operation of non-hospital-based agencies and facilities. Furthermore, a clearly defined generic role delineation for occupational therapists in such settings is not available. Though none of these deterrents is insurmountable in itself, the whole complex of inhibiting factors can be quite intimidating.

The dog and pony show is a marketing institution, as is the slogan that affirms that "everything is negotiable." Admittedly, many non-traditional settings, particularly those designated as not-for-profit, offer lower and frequently non-competitive salaries. Administrators, however, are increasingly coming to realize that even not-for-profit organizations operate in a competitive market—a market in which "you get what you pay for" and "the benefit outweighs the cost." The adventurous occupational therapist is able to market personal competence and experience and the direct relevance of occupational therapy with an awareness that salary is negotiable. At the very least, one can suggest a term-fixed renegotiation based on demonstration of productivity and measurable service outcomes.

Though therapists in non-traditional settings frequently do not have other therapists physically present on-site, this does not mean that they are necessarily deprived of role models and peer support. Other professional team members may provide support and guidance in non-clinical areas. Networking with therapists involved in similar endeavors provides opportunity for mutual support and development. If one grants that the process of mentoring is somewhat analogous to professional parenting, then the importance of "quality time," rather than the physical presence of role models, deserves emphasis. Given efficient communication, mentoring can occur across state lines as readily as across the hall.

Though a particular setting may be unfamiliar, the client population generally is not. Granting the uniqueness of each individual, the basic human need for optimum self-actualization remains constant. Occupational therapists are uniquely equipped to address that need. An entrepreneurial therapist can clearly and assertively enunciate the role of occupational therapy as an essential component of rehabilitation. The ability to identify measurable and quantifiable objectives and outcomes and to provide a substantive rationale for specific interventions is second nature to occupational therapists. The vocabulary and thought processes that occupational therapists take for granted are generally not characteristic of the culture of many non-traditional programs. Yet funding sources and granting agencies have consistently begun to require their recipients to demonstrate in their initial proposals and subsequent documentation the type of clinical accountability that characterizes occupational therapy practice. The therapist who speaks the same language as the funding source and is comfortable in that role can readily be recognized as a valuable asset by an astute administrator.

The lack of a clearly defined role for occupational therapists in non-traditional settings might be viewed as an opportunity rather than a deterrent. Therapists in these settings have the opportunity to integrate skills and develop a broad array of competencies. These include program development, management, marketing, development of referral sources, training and supervision of staff, funding skills (e.g., grant writing), and business skills (e.g., budgeting, billing, and reimbursement policy awareness). In addition, therapists are able to personalize their professional roles in a challenging and rewarding way. Experienced therapists may feel that traditional settings do not always provide sufficient challenges, allow for innovation in treatment approaches, or encourage therapists to refine or diversify clinical and non-clinical competencies. Some non-traditional settings may appeal to assertive, experienced therapists because of the greater flexibility of those structures and the greater potential for defining one's personal professional role and identity in a way that is consistent with one's level of professional growth.

For the competent but less experienced therapist, accepting a lower-paying job in a non-traditional setting might be considered a career investment. It can be argued that the broader range of experience obtained in many non-traditional settings ultimately places one in a more competitive position in the employment market. A broad array of skills can be developed and honed in non-traditional settings in a comparatively short period of time. Therapists might need to educate themselves in certain areas, use consultants, and make lots of phone calls—but once the skills are developed, the therapists have become more marketable.

CHAPTER THIRTY-FOUR

Clinical Case Management: Expanding the Role of the Occupational Therapist in Mental Health Practice

Rita P. Fleming Cottrell

The mental health care system has changed dramatically. Deinstitutionalization, the consumer movement and managed care have resulted in an increased recognition of the need for community service alternatives to traditional, institution-based health care (Christiansen, 1996; Fidler, 1993/2000; Gibson, 1993; Schreter, 1993; Van Leit, 1996/2000; Walens, et al, 1995). The current realities of short-term inpatient stabilization, cost containment, and accountability to consumers requires the competent coordination of supportive services by a case manager (Bachrach, 1996; Fisher, 1996; Malloy, 1995). Occupational therapists who hope to become leading providers of mental health services, must adapt to these changes and challenges by developing competence in expanded roles within community delivery systems (AOTA 1996; Collins, 1996; Fidler, 1993/2000; Fine, 1996; Polatajko, 1996; Van Leit, 1996/2000).

The role of a case manager has been identified as key to the continuity of care in the community for persons with mental illness. It has been recognized as a critical, cost effective method to decrease recidivism, develop independent living skills, and improve the quality of life for those with mental illness (Brekke, et al, 1999; Felton, et al, 1995; Malloy, 1995; Solomon, 1992; Ware, 1995). Recognizing the demand for effective case management in a variety of health care areas, the AOTA has issued an official statement establishing the occupational therapist's role as a case manager (Dufresne, 1991). However, many occupational therapists may be hesitant to pursue professional opportunities in case management, citing concerns with role blurring and clinical competencies (Adams, 1993a; Adams, 1993b/2000; Hettinger, 1996; Krupa & Clark, 1995; Lysack, Stadnyk, Paterson, McLeod & Krefting, 1995). This chapter will address these concerns and clarify the role of the occupational therapist as a case manager and/or case management consultant within the practice specialty of mental health.

DEFINITIONS OF CASE MANAGEMENT

Case management is defined according to the role it plays within the health care system. It can be clinical or administrative. Kanter (1989) defines clinical case management in mental health "as a modality, ...(that) addresses the overall maintenance of the mentally ill person's physical and social environment with the goals of facilitating his or her physical survival, personal growth, community participation, and recovery from, or adaptation to, mental illness" (p. 361). Overall, clinical case management definitions emphasize continuity, quality of care and quality of life for individuals seeking service (Onyett, 1992).

As an administrative function, case management is defined as "a collaboration process which assesses, plans, implements, coordinates, monitors and evaluates options and services to meet an individual's health needs through communication and available resources to promote quality, cost effective outcomes" (Case Management Society of American, 1993, p.16). Whether case management in a managed care system achieves the goal of quality outcomes often depends upon the effectiveness of a clinical case manager. To be successful, a clinical case manager has to accomplish all that Kanter defined but do so in a cost-effective manner (Bachrach, 1996; Olsen, Rickles, & Travlek, 1995).

WHY CASE MANAGEMENT?

Current mental health treatment consists of short-term hospitalizations (often 3 to 7 days) for acute exacerbations of psychiatric symptoms and then discharge for follow-up care to community programs (Fidler, 1993/2000; Gibson, 1993; Schreter, 1993) Many individuals with grave illnesses which would have institutionalized them in the past, now reside in our communities. They often do not have adequate skills for community living (Kennedy, 1997).

In order to function in the community, mental health clients need knowledge and skills for daily living, environmental resources to meet needs and develop skills, and community supports to maintain their performance (Randolph, Balskinsky, Leginski, Parker & Goldman, 1997; Uttaro & Mechanic, 1994). These services must be provided along a continuum of care which is designed according to the diversity of functional levels of clients with mental illness (Schreter, Sharfstein & Schreter, 1997). While there may be community mental health programs available to assist clients in developing functional living skills, they are often limited, fragmented and/or difficult to access (Ellek, 1993/2000; Krupa & Clark, 1995). Complex referral and admissions procedures, long waiting lists, and arbitrary discharge dates, at the very least, complicate the process of receiving care, and at their worst can alienate the client from the mental health care system (Poirier, 1988; Randolph, et al, 1997). In addition, the harsh realities of living with a mental illness in the community can be overwhelming (Kennedy, 1997). Clients are frequently poor and rely on local, state, and federal services such as Supplemental Security Income (SSI), Medicaid, Section 8 Housing and food stamps (Adams, 1993a; Randolph, et al., 1997).

Meeting basic needs of food, shelter, clothing, and personal care on a monthly income of $366.00 can be a challenge for anyone. Waiting two hours in a crowded and noisy social service office for a "face to face" interview to determine eligibility for benefits can be intimidating to even the most confident applicant. Considering the effects of the symptoms of mental illness (e.g., social withdrawal, limited problem solving abilities, the "background noise" of hallucinations, residual and/or active delusions) on a person's ability to effectively negotiate these services, it is not surprising that so many patients "fall through the cracks", are repeatedly rehospitalized and/or wander the streets of our cities (Adams, 1993a; Ellek, 1993/2000). Clearly, many clients with chronic mental illness can not access and maintain these needed supports without assistance (Krupa & Clark, 1995; Randolph, et al, 1997). This is the primary role of the clinical case manager. A clinical case manager can provide the link between a client and the available services, assisting clients in developing skills for independent living (Clark & Fox, 1993; Moeller, 1991). Given the increased restrictions and complexities of the managed care environment, the skills of a clinical case manager are paramount to the maintenance of persons with mental illness within their communities (Malloy, 1995).

Consumers and their families have long recognized this need, vocalizing their demands for the integrative and supportive services of a case manager (Poirier, 1988). Consumers have asked for case management to help find, apply for, and obtain services and to help meet personal goals (Krupa & Clark, 1995). Families are demanding case management services to "assure them that their loved ones will get the services they need, when they need them, and will not get lost in

the system and be ultimately unserved" (Ashley, 1988, p. 499). When professional case managers are not available family members often serve as the on-line, defacto case manager. Professional clinical case management can relieve the burden of care for families whose resources are often stretched to the limits in providing long term care to their family members with mental illness (Intagliata, Willer & Egri, 1990; Winefield & Harvey, 1994).

Third party payers and legislative bodies want assurances that services funded are cost-effective and that they are provided efficiently and effectively to those who need them (Christiansen, 1996; Collins, 1996). Therefore, a clinical case manager must have a solid knowledge of managed care systems and develop competence in dealing with the realities of limited resources for health care (AOTA, 1996; Collins, 1996).

Current and future treatment of persons with mental illness will clearly be influenced by the outcome of insurance reform and managed care initiatives. It is hoped by leaders in mental health care and consumer/family advocates that the result will be a complete continuum of care in the community since emergency and in-patient care are so costly (Malloy, 1995; Schreter et al, 1997). Clinical case managers will be needed to move individuals with mental illness through this continuum of care (Clark & Fox, 1993).

WHY OCCUPATIONAL THERAPIST AS CASE MANAGER?

No one discipline or specific profession is identified in the literature as best suited for the case manager role (Krupa & Clark, 1995). Case management is not a profession in itself but an area of specialized practice within a profession (Fisher, 1996; Hettinger, 1996; Kanter, 1989). Bachrach (1992) states "case management draws personnel from the full array of service delivery professionals" [and is] "defined in terms of its functions, not on the basis of the professional training its practitioners undergo" (p. 209). Having diverse skills and the knowledge of a generalist rather than a specialist is preferred (Sullivan, 1981). Since occupational therapists are educated as generalists and the field requires a diversity of skills, occupational therapists are suitable professionals to provide case management services (Brinson & Kannenberg, 1996; Hettinger, 1996; Krupa & Clark, 1995; Walens et al, 1995).

Occupational therapy evaluation skills used to assess performance components, performance areas and performance contexts can be invaluable to the case manager role (Fisher, 1996; Lysack et al, 1995). Occupational therapy's emphasis on activities of daily living (ADL), independent living skills (ILS) and functional outcomes is tailor-made for the case management role for most clients with chronic mental illness have severe deficits in ADL and ILS (Dasler, 1993; Moeller, 1991; Uttaro & Mechanic, 1994). In fact, rehospitalization may be triggered by a breakdown in the performance of everyday tasks. Examples are clients with poor budgeting skills who didn't pay their rent which results in eviction and homelessness or clients with poor travel skills who miss appointments for medication renewal which leads to symptom exacerbation. The occuaptional therapy case manager can help such clients by providing concrete assistance, training, and advocacy in all areas of daily living (Berzon & Lowenstein, 1984; Lysack et al, 1995). Our ability "to provide services not simply based on talking, but on doing" is invaluable. (Crist, 1993, p. 170/2000, p. 149). The belief in promoting health and wellness and emphasis on quality of life through a collaborative approach are other occupational therapy attributes that are suitable to a case manager role.

Furthermore, several models of practice and frames of reference used in occupational therapy are relevant to case management work. For example, knowledge of "normal" developmental tasks and the effects of dysfunction on the developmental process can be useful in case management. Recognizing the "normal" issues a young adult with schizophrenia faces regarding autonomy, work, and independent living can help focus case management efforts on the client's capabilities and needs for vocational and residential services (Uttaro & Mechanic, 1994). Knowledge of development is also useful when working with clients who are parents (Mosey, 1986). For example, occupational therapists can teach parents what to expect at different stages of development or provide concrete suggestions for age-appropriate activities which can result in more effective parenting (Waldo, et al, 1993).

Learning theories and acquisitional frames of reference are also highly applicable to case management work. The teaching-learning process, and activity analysis, adaptation, and gradation are relevant to the practical, reality-based world of case management such as teaching daily living skills to clients (Crist, 1993/2000; Mosey, 1986). As Lamb noted the "most meaningful treatment with long-term patients is dealing with the realities and day to day issues of life and survival in the community" (1980, p. 763). The Model of Human Occupation (MOHO) provides a framework based on systems theory, for assessing a client's interests, goals, habits, roles, and skills and their interaction within the environment (Miller & Walker, 1993). It is relevant in case management to assess the client's "human system", as well as their social and environmental supports that facilitate order within this system. In addition, case management's "in vivo" approach within a client's home and community is compatible with the MOHO and acquisitional frames of reference.

The use of environmental adaptations to maximize functioning and compensate for disabilities is also emphasized in Allen's cognitive disabilities frame of reference (Miller & Walker, 1993). The use of observations and environmental assessments to evaluate what a client can and cannot do helps determine the adaptations, compensations, and supports needed for safe independent living. This information can help the occupational therapy case manager plan ADL training, make appropriate referrals to supportive living environments, and educate caregivers about the realistic parameters of a client's functional level.

Finally, the case management relationship is frequently long-term and very intense with the case manager common-

ly being viewed by the client as a surrogate parent (Bryan, 1990). Therefore, knowledge of psychodynamic and humanistic frames of reference is relevant in therapeutic interventions with the client (Mosey, 1986). Case managers need to be cognizant of, and able to deal with, psychodynamic issues, such as transference and countertransference, as well as skillful in using client-centered approaches and basic counseling skills (Bryan, 1990).

In recognition of the relevance of our philosophical base and professional knowledge and skills to case management work, the American Occupational Therapy Association (AOTA) has delineated the qualifications of therapists seeking to assume case manager positions. According to AOTA, occupational therapy case managers should be "advanced-level therapists (therapists with 5 years of experience, of which 3 years are within a specific practice arena) and [with] advanced skills pertinent to case management in the areas of management, communication, and systems (including medical, social, vocational, educational, and fiscal systems) (Dufresne, 1991, p. 1065).

The attainment of multiple years of experience and advanced practice skills is clearly desirable prior to assuming a primary role as a case manager. However, current trends in mental health service delivery and managed care may require that occupational therapists perform case management tasks, even if this role is not defined explicitly (Collins, 1996; Hettinger, 1996). Many "young" occupational therapists have found themselves (or will shortly find themselves) needing to provide services beyond their traditionally well defined occupational therapy practitioner role due to gaps in service delivery (Brinson & Kannenberg, 1996; Walens et al, 1995). Community-based programs are frequently understaffed and excessive caseloads may limit case management services to a 30 minute session once a month. The focus is then on crisis intervention and/or administrative issues, leaving little time available for independent living or quality of life issues. As a result, occupational therapists working in day treatment centers, sheltered workshops, transitional living programs, and other community-based settings are often called upon to provide the day to day support, training and advocacy a client needs to live in the community (Adams, 1993a). These are case management tasks but without the label of case management. Neglecting these tasks would indicate poor practice rather than a conflict in mixing roles (Lamb, 1980).

To meet the increased need for case management services in mental health practice, all occupational therapists should acquire a foundation in case management models, terms, principles and approaches early in their professional development, for their clients may not have the luxury of waiting 3-5 years while the therapist attains advanced practitioner status (Krupa & Clark, 1995). Entry-level occupational therapists can begin to perform certain case management tasks with supervision (e.g.: housing assessments and referrals for day treatment clients) (Lysack et al, 1995). All therapists can integrate their occupational therapy knowledge and skills into case management models and seek guidance and assistance from other professionals, as needed (Adams, 1993b/2000).

MODELS OF CASE MANAGEMENT

There are many models of case management. As Krupa and Clark noted "Evaluating attitudes, knowledge, and skills in relation to a specific case management model is the key to becoming an effective case manager" (1995 p. 21). Expanding one's role should not compromise one's fundamental professional identity (Lysack et al, 1995). The seven models discussed below are all interdisciplinary. They may be interagency or intra-agency and may overlap or combine with another model (Clark & Fox, 1993; Krupa & Clark, 1995).

Single Case Manager

In this model, a case manager works individually with clients, maintaining primary responsibility for all aspects of a client's case even as a client transitions through a system of care (Bachrach, 1992). This model allows for the development of a strong, therapeutic relationship and continuous collaborative treatment planning (Kanter, 1989). However, there is a risk of clients developing overdependence on the case manager with instability and/or regression developing when, and if, a case manager leaves. Case managers can also be at risk for burnout if a case becomes chronically difficult.

Sequential Case Managers

In this model, a series of case managers are available as clients move through a system of care. At each new point in the system a new case manager assumes primary responsibility for the client (Bachrach, 1992). The determination of who is the case manager is based on the client's primary need (e.g.: housing versus vocational). This model allows clients to receive case management services from the individual who is most knowledgeable about their primary area of need. This can be beneficial for clients with discrete needs; however, most clients with chronic mental illness have multiple needs over an extended period of time, limiting the suitability of the sequential model of case management for them (Intagliata, 1982).

Team Case Management

In this model, clients' needs are met by a team of three to four professionals, preferably of diverse backgrounds. Each professional brings their own expertise to the case, increasing the number of perspectives and specialties available to the client (Clark & Fox, 1993; Olsen et al, 1995). These varied viewpoints permit each team member to learn from each other. Thus this model can particularly benefit neophyte case managers. The team can also provide support to each other on difficult cases, thereby decreasing burnout (Bachrach, 1992). Having a therapeutic relationship with a team of case managers diffuses the intensity of these relationships and decreases the risk of over-dependency. However, the team must be cautious that this diversity of relationships does not diminish the team's decision-making power or result in "splitting" by the client.

Intensive Case Manager

This model provides the client with 24-hour on-call access to a case manager, 365 days per year. It is designed to meet the needs of clients with severe chronic mental illness at a high risk for recidivism. The intensive care manager (ICM) provides full support in all areas of concern in the client's home and community environment. An ICM's caseload is generally limited to 10 clients due to the intensity of their clients' needs. ICMs are organized into supervised teams that provide support for the "long haul" of maintaining these clients within their communities and preventing hospitalization (Mental Health Resource Center, 1990).

Assertive Case Manager

This model also combines a single case manager with team case management to provide an "in-vivo" approach in the client's home and community. It involves assertive outreach and frequent contacts like the ICM model; however, the assertive case management (ACM) model emphasizes a rehabilitative approach rather than a maintenance focus. ACM models are used in Programs of Assertive Community Treatment (PACTs) which have been initiated by several states to serve clients with chronic mental illness. These PACTs and ACM models use a problem-solving, rehabilitative approach to develop ADL and independent living skills (Bond, Miller, Krumwied and Ward, 1988; Solomon, 1992).

Cluster Case Management

In this model, case management services are provided to a group of clients at the same time (Bachrach, 1992; Harris & Bergman, 1988). Numerous direct service interventions (e.g.: completing food stamp applications) and psychoeducational topics (e.g.: how to get along with roommates) can be provided in a cluster model to increase efficiency. However, "caution must be exercised in using this approach" (for) "not every intervention or task is suitable for clustering and... not all patients respond favorably to group activities" (Bachrach, 1992, p. 210). On the positive side, cluster case management provides clients with a viable peer network that decreases social isolation, encourages collaborative problem-solving and develops social interaction skills (Harris & Bergman, 1988). Occupational therapists' experience in designing and leading therapeutic groups is a strong asset in adopting this model.

Case Management Assistants

In several of the models discussed above, carefully selected clients/consumers are trained to serve as assistants to the primary case manager. These assistants have firsthand knowledge of the effects of mental illness on function and are acutely aware of clients' concerns and needs. Case manager assistants can help break down the "us-versus-them" barrier that some clients develop. They can provide specific services like escorting clients to appointments enabling the primary case manager to devote time to more complex tasks. Most importantly, case manager assistants serve as role models, providing much-needed hope to clients (Felton et al, 1995).

System Case Management

This model emphasizes advocacy to help a client negotiate the system of care. The case manager serves as a "broker" of services, linking the client to needed services and addressing particular problems with systems as they arise (Clark & Fox, 1993; Lamb, 1980). It is a 1:1 approach like the single case manager model, but in the systems model the case manager is not concerned with all aspects of the client's care. Instead, the case manager identifies problems and refers clients to needed services. For example, a systems care manager would not provide counseling to a client but would refer a client to counseling services. This model is the most administratively focused (Lamb, 1980) and may be the least congruent with the occupational therapy philosophy of active engagement in doing with a client (Fidler, 1993).

CASE MANAGEMENT TASKS

As stated earlier, no one discipline is identified in the literature as best suited for a case manager role. Therefore, case management is often defined in terms of its functions and tasks. Seven of these tasks are described below.

1. *Comprehensive awareness of a client's needs:* This task is an expanded version of the occupational therapy evaluation process. It involves gathering information from the referral, intake interview, social history, mental status examination and all other assessments that are available in the client's files to identify client's assets, presenting problems, and needs (Gibson, 1993; Moeller, 1991).
2. *Collaborate with consumer to determine plan:* Based upon the above evaluation, the case manager collaborates with the consumer to identify his/her goals for treatment and determine the best plan for meeting these goals (Krupa & Clark, 1995). The treatment plan must also involve the identification of, and referral to, services and resources that will help the client meet his or her goals (Moeller, 1991).
3. *Identify and link consumers to the services they need:* Clients may need referrals to formal services (e.g.: vocational training, Section 8 housing, SSI) or informal supports (e.g.: food banks, shared housing, churches/synagogues). To provide referrals to needed services, a case manager must be aware of all resources available to clients in their geographic area (Adams, 1993a). This information is easily obtained through telephone books or the internet. National organiza-

tions, like the National Alliance for Mentally Ill (NAMI), have toll free numbers and readily provide information on local resources. Large communities, cities and state offices may have special directories describing their social services.

To increase the success rate of appropriate referrals, and to ensure inappropriate referrals are not made, a case manager should evaluate all services prior to referral to determine the service agency's admissions requirements, as well as the quality and nature of the services (Harris & Bergman, 1988). Once the service is determined appropriate for meeting a client's needs, the case manager assists the client in completing the application process (i.e., filling out forms, accompanying client to admissions interview). Key questions to consider when investigating a service are provided in Table 34-1.

While many of these questions can be answered through a review of an agency's literature and/or via a phone interview, visiting a program while it is delivering the stated service is helpful in uncovering discrepancies between literary descriptions and the actual delivery of service (Poirier, 1988). For example, a halfway house stated it accepted clients with deficits in self-care; when observations noted that only the best groomed individuals were residents. Clients with poor grooming were consistently denied acceptance to the program although these deficits were not noted as a reason for rejection. Case managers realized independent self-care was a prerequisite for acceptance even though it was not stated in the admissions criteria. Therefore, case managers worked with all prospective halfway house applicants on the development of self-care skills, prior to referral to this service.

4. *Monitor and coordinate the services provided:* Once clients are linked to the services they need, the case manager must monitor the services being provided to ensure their continued appropriateness. This requires ongoing evaluation of a client's response to services and continuous communication with service providers regarding a client's status (Fidler, 1993/2000). This task is similar to the occupational therapy reevaluation process (Mosey, 1986).
5. *Assist the consumer with daily problems and tasks:* Even when a client is effectively linked with a diversity of community services, the case manager is still the individual the client will turn to for assistance with daily problems and tasks. Home management, transportation, parenting, work and/or leisure activities can present difficulties to the client with mental illness (Kanter, 1989). Assisting consumers with these daily problems is familiar to occupational therapists (Gibson, 1993; Moeller, 1991).
6. *Advocate for the consumer:* Advocacy permeates all case management work (Schreter et al, 1997). Although occupational therapists are often involved in patient advocacy on treatment teams, the nature of case

Table 34-1
Investigation of a Community Service

Complete the following:

Name of agency:
Telephone number:
Location:
Accessibility of the agency to clients:
Types of services offered:
Referral sources for the agency:
Admission criteria:
Payment and reimbursement sources for services:
Waiting list (yes/no, length):
Characteristics of persons who are not eligible for the services:
Reasons for discharge from the services:
Potential frequency and duration of services:
Client responsibilities for continued participation in the services:
Family responsibility for the services:
Agency responsibilities for the client receiving services:
Goals of the agency:
Based on your findings, do you feel you could...

    a. Recommend the agency?
    b. Decide who would probably get admitted to the agency?
    c. Know what the client could expect, if admitted?
    d. Determine the reliability of the agency?
    e. Know when the client would be discharged from the agency?
    f. Modify your practice to prepare the appropriate clients for transfer to and/or sharing with this agency?
    g. Describe the case management type used by the agency?
    h. Discuss the effectiveness of the case management?

Reprinted with permission from Davis, L.J. & Kirkland, M. (1988). Module IV teaching resource: Investigation of a community service. *ROTE: The role of occupational therapy with the elderly-faculty guide* (pp. 453-544). Rockville, MD: AOTA.

---

management advocacy is more bureaucratic (Gibson, 1993). It requires the ability to negotiate several administrative systems and interagency policies and is critical when a client is turned down or rejected from a service or program (Ellek, 1993/2000, Krupa & Clark, 1995; Lysack et al, 1995). The reasons for denial or dismissal must be determined and attempts made to change a rejection into an affirmation (Poirier, 1988). Given the scarcity of some community services and the constraints of managed care, the advocacy task is of vital importance.

7. *Counseling:* The provision of 1:1, ongoing support is the task that is often most valued by the consumer. Mental illness can result in social isolation and loneliness (Kanter, 1989). Having a personal "cheerleader" in your corner to share your triumphs (no matter how small) and understand your worries (no matter how seemingly insignificant or overwhelmingly huge) can mean the difference between relapse and recovery. (Leete, 1993/2000; Ware, 1995) The skills learned during occupational therapy education such as therapeutic use of self, interviewing, the use of the teaching-learning process and effective group dynamics can be transferred to counseling and educating consumers and their families. Additional training may be needed to develop skills beyond entry-level abilities to deal with difficult situations (Krupa & Clark, 1995; Lysac, et al, 1995).

8. *Crisis intervention:* Even the best therapeutic relationship cannot avert the inevitable crises that occur in life such as deaths, evictions and crime. In addition, the culmination of normal life stresses combined with symptoms of mental illness can result in the exacerbation of an illness to a crisis level; therefore, crisis intervention is a task the case manager frequently performs (Intagliata, 1982). The development of crisis intervention skills requires additional training for occupational therapists seeking to become case managers (Krupa & Clark, 1995; Lysack et al, 1995). Fortunately, many community mental health centers provide crisis training for their staff and the Crisis Prevention Institute (1-800-558-8976) has excellent training resources available for purchase by professionals seeking to develop their crisis intervention

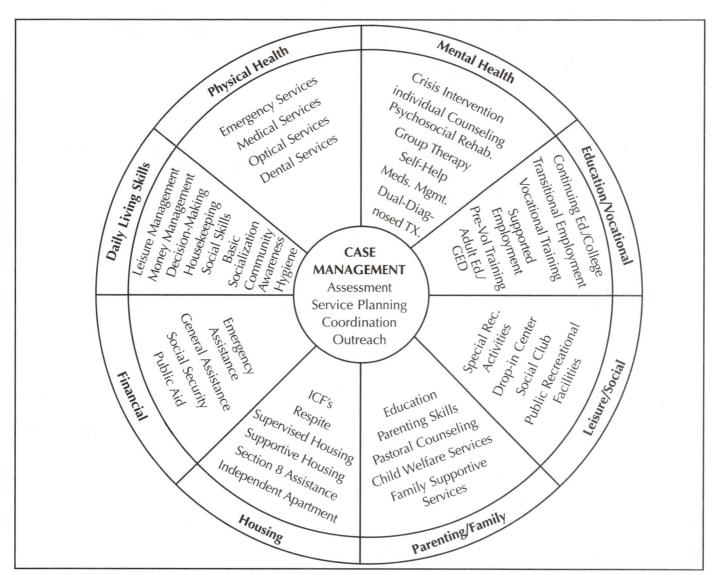

Figure 34-1. Community Services for people with mental illness. (Reprinted with permission from the Community Mental Health Board, Town of Oak Park, IL.)

skills. Crisis hotlines, victim service bureaus, emergency housing, and medical and psychiatric emergency rooms are available in most communities to provide a network for dealing effectively with crises.

9. *Evaluate functional outcomes:* Expertise in evaluating client's functional level and the outcome of treatment enables occupational therapists to readily assume this case manager task (Gibson, 1993) and meet managed care demands for accountability (Moeller, 1991).

10. *Reevaluate options, services, and outcomes:* Experience with the reevaluation process and treatment modifications are applicable to this task but expanding one's knowledge base about service options available in the community will enhance the occupational therapy case manager's ability to perform this task effectively (Lysack et al; 1995).

CASE MANAGEMENT AREAS OF CONCERN

The 10 tasks described previously are performed by the case manager with respect to eight main areas of concern (Moeller, 1991). As depicted in Figure 34-1, case management is the hub of service delivery with all other services being organized by and around the case manager. The effectiveness of case management intervention in each of these areas may depend on the case manager's ability to understand and respond to the cultural realities that influence their clients' lives. Case managers are most effective when they value and honor the social norms that prevail in clients' home communities (Krupa & Clark, 1995).

1. *Physical health:* Persons with mental illness require medical care for physical illnesses and routine preven-

tive care. However, clients' abilities to make, remember, and keep appointments may be hindered by their psychiatric symptoms (e.g., cognitive deficits) and/or by delivery system complications (e.g., MD refuses Medicaid, clinic has one month waiting list) (Adams, 1993a). Clients may also be unaware of the importance of physical symptoms and/or they may attribute physical symptoms to their mental illness and/or medication side effects. For example, a client complaining of increased thirst and frequent urination was unaware that these are potential symptoms of diabetes.

Our knowledge of the physical aspects of illness is a strong asset in helping clients with mental illness meet their physical health needs. Clients can be alerted to potential health risks, educated about preventative care, and be taught methods to manage illness and control symptoms (e.g., energy conservation). To increase efficiency, many of these tasks can be performed in a cluster case management model. Local health service organizations are resources for providing free consumer information packets and speakers to a group of clients (e.g., the Heart Association can provide information about dietary links to high blood pressure and heart disease, The Cancer Society can demonstrate breast self-examination techniques, and the Red Cross can conduct first aid workshops).

Given that most individuals with chronic mental illness are poor, finding competent and caring Medicaid providers to meet clients' physical health needs is a major case management task. Case managers must also be aware of Medicaid, Medicare, and private insurance eligibility criteria, benefits, and exclusions. This information is readily available from hospital benefits departments, managed care providers, State Departments of Social Services and the Social Security Administration.

2. *Mental health:* Prior sections of this (chapter) have highlighted major mental health areas of concern relevant to case management (i.e.: counseling, crisis intervention). Particularly relevant in this area are the behavioral observation skills that occupational therapists learn. Observations of subtle changes in behavior (e.g., poor hygiene) that may indicate symptom exacerbation prior to the occurance of a crisis and/or complete functional decompensation facilitates rapid intervention to provide needed supports and services.

Educating clients to manage their illness and medication(s) is another vital case management task (Keith, Starr & Matthews, 1993). The stress- vulnerability/coping-competence model (Liberman, 1988) is useful to teach to persons with chronic mental illness (Figure 34-2). This model recognizes the neurophysiological base of mental illness and the impact of socioenvironmental stressors, while emphasizing the importance of social support, skill development, medication(s) and rehabilitation programs (Liberman, 1988; Onyett, 1992). It is a model of empowerment that decreases

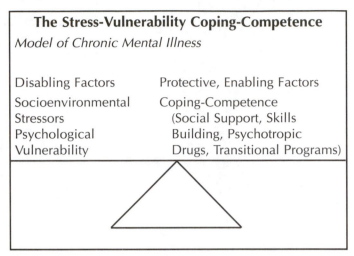

The Stress-Vulnerability Coping-Competence
Model of Chronic Mental Illness

Disabling Factors	Protective, Enabling Factors
Socioenvironmental	Coping-Competence
Stressors	(Social Support, Skills
Psychological	Building, Psychotropic
Vulnerability	Drugs, Transitional Programs)

Figure 34-2. The stress-vulnerability coping-competence model of chronic mental illness. (Adapted from: Liberman, R. P. (1988). Psychiatric rehabilitation of chronic mental patients. Washington, DC: American Psychiatric Press.)

stigma and fosters clients' active involvement in management of their illness (Leete, 1993).

Teaching stress management techniques to cope with mental illness and prevent relapse is critical (Hatfield, 1993). Referrals to peer run/consumer support groups (e.g., Recovery Inc.) "can be extremely valuable to clients by offering support, friendship, hope for the future and peer group modeling" (Leete, 1993, p. 280). Case managers can advocate for the development of local support groups to meet client's mental health.

3. *Educational/Vocational:* Services in this area of concern, which has been part of traditional occupational therapy, range across a continuum from pre-vocational training, to sheltered workshops, to transitional employment programs, to volunteer work, and to competitive employment with or without ADA accommodations (Crist & Stoffel, 1996/2000; Palmer and Gatti, 1993/2000) Referral resources include local adult education classes, community colleges, state offices of Vocational and Educational Services for Individual with Disabilities (VESID) and/or the Social Security administration's Plan for Achieving Self Support (PASS) program. VESID and PASS provide funding for education and/or vocational training expenses including tuition, books, equipment, uniforms, transportation and other related expenses. Additional vocational information is available from the President's Committee on Employment of Persons with Disabilities, the Job Accommodation Network (JAN), and the Dole Foundation (Cottrell, 1993)

To ensure educational/vocational service referrals are realistic, the client's work skills, behaviors and habits must be assessed. Program eligibility requirements and level of service are also evaluated to be sure they are within the client's capabilities. Given current limits on the availability of funding for educational/vocational services, a case manager must be certain a client is able to succeed in the program, for second chances are not guaranteed (Poirier, 1988). In addition, "failing" at school or work can diminish a client's confidence in his/her ability to progress. Knowledge of the Americans with Disabilities Act (ADA) can be very helpful in identifying reasonable accommodations that will enable a person with a mental illness to successfully perform the essential job functions of a student/worker role (Crist & Stoffel, 1996).

4. *Leisure/Social:* Clients with chronic mental illness often have significant leisure and social deficits (Woodside, 1993). Occupational therapists' repertoire of leisure and social assessments is useful for evaluating skill level in these areas. Their experience in helping clients develop basic social interaction skills is also useful in case management either on a 1:1 basis or in a group context through cluster case management (Crist, 1993/2000). Referrals to local community services (i.e., senior centers, psychosocial clubs, drop in-centers) can be made (Woodside, 1993/2000). Knowledge of public recreational facilities will aid clients on limited budgets as these facilities tend to be free and/or charge nominal fees (Poirier, 1988). Libraries, parks, museums, botanical gardens, and other public facilities provide environments in which it is socially acceptable to be alone. Clients may find these solitary and/or parallel leisure activities meaningful pursuits as they work to develop their skill level.

Local newspapers provide a wealth of information about leisure resources and events, particularly in the Friday/Weekend editions. Having clients read this newspaper can increase their awareness of local resources and provide a meaningful activity. Compeer Inc., a national program that matches trained volunteers with persons with mental illness to form a 1:1 peer/companion relationship, also can be employed to develop social and leisure skills. The partnerships meet once per week on a regular basis to do activities that are mutually interesting (e.g., go to a movie, browse a mall). Strong relationships often develop from this partnering, providing the person with mental illness a friend with whom to enjoy life (Poirier, 1988).

5. *Parenting/Family:* Occupational therapists' knowledge of roles and role strain is highly relevant to this area of concern. Having a person with mental illness in a family changes all family roles, as tasks and responsibilities are altered (Intagliata, Willer and Egri, 1988). A spouse is no longer a partner, a child is no longer independent (Bernheim, 1993/2000).

To work effectively with families who can serve as allies in the rehabilitation process, a case manager must recognize role changes and acknowledge the potential family burden of caring for a member with chronic mental illness (Bernheim, 1993/2000). This has been defined as the emotional, physical, and financial strain of care (Liberman, 1988). The reality of the long-term and often unpredictable course of chronic mental illness does lead to strain, even in the most supportive families (Intagliata, et al, 1990; Winefield and Harvey, 1994). Case managers can educate and support the family to maximize their adaptiveness. For example, one can use a psychoeducational model to develop a family's cognitive and behavioral skills for managing the manifestations of mental illness (Greenberg et al., 1993/2000). One can also identify positive functions the family can perform and actions to avoid (Intagliata et al, 1990; Liberman, 1988) (See Table 34-2). Occupational therapy skills in activity analysis, gradation, adaptation, and work simplification can be used to help families design meaningful activities that maintain the familial role(s) of the person with mental illness (e.g., Mom can't make the entire dinner but can make the salad). Our environmental assessment and modification skills are particularly useful in helping families maintain home environments that are supportive, but not over-stimulating. Most important, our abilities to address the functional effects of mental illness can facilitate the family's development of realistic expectations for their member with mental illness (i.e.: apathy and anergy does not mean a person is lazy; it does mean he/she needs increased time, support, and cuing to accomplish a task).

When a client is a parent, the additional concern is for the child. Parents must be able to meet their child's physical and emotional needs; communicate with and discipline their child; and participate in play and recreational activities, at an age-appropriate level (Mosey, 1986). While many persons with mental illness can be good parents, (either independently or with support), the chronicity and severity of mental illness often results in parenting skill deficits. Case managers must ensure the safety of the child by arranging additional supports (i.e., home care) and through parenting education. An occupational therapists' knowledge of child development can be particularly useful in helping a parent understand their child. Referrals to parenting skills classes and/or cluster case management to practice good parenting skills may be indicated (Waldo et al, 1993).

At times, even the best efforts of a client and the deepest love for a child is not sufficient for success in parenting. Extended families (i.e.: grandparents, siblings) may step in to raise the child. Case managers can provide support and information to these caregivers, and to clients to help them maintain an appropriate role within their child's life. If families are unable to provide the needed parenting, the case manager must network with child protective services to ensure the child is receiving adequate care. This may result in foster care placement and/or adoption (Waldo et al., 1993).

Table 34-2

Ways for Family Members to Assist in the Treatment and Rehabilitation of a Chronically Mentally Ill Relative

Functions to Serve	Traps To Avoid
Assist in locating, linking, and sustaining treatment and rehabilitation services	Over-involvement with ill relative, trying too hard to help and comfort
Supportive use of medication	Nagging or excessive criticism
Advocate for better services	Isolation from family and friends
Maintain tolerant and low key home atmosphere	Taking for granted small signs of progress
Reduce performance expectations to a realistic level	Expecting too much improvement too quickly
Encourage participation in treatment and low stress activities	Depriving self and other family members of fun, recreation, vacations, and personal activities

Reprinted with permission from Liberman, R. P. (1988). *Psychiatric rehabilitation of chronic mental patients* (p. 219). Washington, DC: American Psychiatric Press.

Again, the case manager must work with all parties to ensure the child's needs are met and the client's rights are maintained. Networking with legal aid societies can be invaluable to a case manager. Teaching clients activities and skills to use during their visits with their children can help ease the pain of losing custody. Feelings of loss and failure are common and can reoccur at different developmental milestones (Waldo et al., 1993). Support is critical for both the client and case manager. Supervision, team support, the National Alliance for Mentally Ill (NAMI) and Parents Anonymous are resources available for dealing with family and parenting concerns (Cottrell, 1993).

6. *Housing:* Finding, acquiring and keeping adequate, safe, affordable housing is often difficult, if not impossible for clients with chronic mental illness (Crowel, 1988; Kennedy, 1997). Although the Fair Housing Act and ADA prohibit discrimination against persons with disabilities, the societal stigma of mental illness still persists, limiting housing options for persons with chronic mental illness. The low income of these individuals decreases housing options further (Kennedy, 1997). In addition, the severity of their mental illness and deficits in independent living skills often results in homelessness. Outreach programs for the homeless and a continuum of housing options that have programming to meet the needs of varied functional levels are needed (Wilberding, 1993/2000). Case managers must be aware of all housing options and supports available in clients' communities (e.g., homeless shelters, group homes, single room occupancy (SRO) hotels, supportive housing, intermediate care facilities (ICFs), halfway houses, quarterway houses, adult foster care, Section 8 housing) (Schreter, et al 1997). The range of programming, structure, support, and safety can vary greatly in each of these settings; therefore, visiting potential housing will ensure it is realistic for a client, given his or her functional abilities (Crowel, 1988). The occupational therapist's skills of evaluating environmental demands and an individual's skills for independent living are pertinent to this area of case management.

Also pertinent is the occupational therapist's ability to teach needed home management skills which can be on a 1:1 basis, or in group through cluster case management (Wilberding, 1993/2000). Referral to a community mental health day treatment program for independent living skills training is another alternative. In addition, the development of social skills and assertiveness may be needed to enable a client to deal effectively with roommates and/or landlords. Case managers can assist in developing positive housing relationships by serving as an advocate to decrease potential housing discrimination and by serving as a supportive liaison between clients, their roommates, landlords, and/or housing staff (Adams, 1993a). Establishing stable housing is often the primary task of a case manager for lack of housing is a crisis that dominates all other areas of concern (Crowel, 1988; Kennedy, 1997).

7. *Finances:* Clients receiving case management services are generally reliant on public entitlement programs (i.e., SSI, welfare) and often have poor money management skills (Kanter, 1989). Several occupational therapy assessment tools include sections to assess money management skills. Budgeting skills can be developed either on a 1:1 basis or in a group format. Limited knowledge of public entitlement program requirements and procedures can be rectified through entitlement programs' consumer information brochures, telephone calls, or the internet (although hours of busy signals and phone tag may be a reality).

The process of obtaining and maintaining these benefits can be complex and overwhelming to anyone (Adams, 1993a; Kanter, 1989). Literacy, strict attention to detail, and assertiveness are basic requirements for success, but these skills are often lacking in persons with chronic mental illness. The transient living arrangements of many clients further complicates the obtainment and maintenance of benefits (Kennedy, 1997). Active advocacy is often required to ensure clients' financial needs are met. Case managers frequently must assist by completing numerous lengthy forms, gathering the required documentation for clients' benefits application(s), and/or accompanying the client to the required interview for benefits. Using family, peers and/or case manager assistants to provide this on-site support can be a cost-effective alternative (Bachrach, 1992)

Once a client has obtained benefits, the case manager must work with the client to establish a realistic budget to ensure bills are paid, food is bought and essential needs are met. Clients who live in supportive residences (i.e.: group homes) must learn to budget a monthly allowance of $30.00 - $50.00 to meet all personal needs (e.g.: toiletries, clothing, snacks, and cigarettes)—a definite challenge (Adams, 1993a). At times, to prevent evictions and/or other crises, case managers must become the client's legal "protective payee", controlling income until the client develops essential money management skills.

8. *Daily living skills:* Addressing this area of concern may be frustrating for non-occupational therapy case managers due to their lack of knowledge about the complexities of the underlying performance component skills needed to perform seemingly simple activities of daily living (ADL) (Goodman, et al, 1996). Numerous assessment tools are available to evaluate ADL skills and performance component assets and deficits, but many of these tools use simulated tasks, providing only baseline data. Valid and relevant information is more readily obtained if the ADL evaluation is conducted in the client's natural environment. Intervention must also be planned within the realities of the client's habitat (Goodman, et al., 1996). For example, clients may not have access to fully equipped kitchens; therefore all cooking is done on a hot plate or in an electric frypan. So evaluating and treating a client in a day hospital kitchen using a range and oven would be irrelevant (Walens, et al 1995). Occupational therapy skills in environmental assessment and modification, activity analysis, adaptation, gradation and work simplification are useful to managing this area of concern, but again, increased knowledge of community resources is needed to help clients develop and maintain their skills for community living. Teaching clients to use these additional resources (e.g., meals on wheels, Senior Center and school breakfast and lunch programs, soup kitchens and food pantries, transit half-fare cards, home energy assistance programs (HEAP), discount stores and thrift shops) can extend their money and improve their quality of life.

OCCUPATIONAL THERAPIST CASE MANAGER CONCERNS/ISSUES

Despite appropriate knowledge and skills, there are a number of relevant concerns and issues that must be addressed prior to the occupational therapist assuming a case manager role. These concerns include:

• *Role blurring or role overlap:* Rigid role delineation does not work in community mental health practice (Adams, 1993b) and it is the antithesis of case management. Clients' needs are too immediate and diverse and staffing is too limited for service to be provided by a series of well-defined specialists. In case management, each discipline brings its own perspective and skills to the case manager role, while actively learning from each other. This sharing of expertise is often nurtured in team case management with the resulting whole being greater than the sum of its parts. Occupational therapist case managers will perform tasks that may have been traditionally within the domain of another profession (e.g., obtaining benefits was the domain of social work, medication education was the domain of nursing), but many of these are realistically within occupational therapy's domain of concern as well. How can I work on ADLs if a client has no money or housing and is symptomatic due to medication noncompliance?

In addition, case management requires occupational therapists to expand their role beyond direct care clinical practice. Becoming a case management team leader, consultant or PACT director are primarily indirect roles which require a change in perspective and attitudes about the value of one's contributions (Jaffee, 1996). The ability to value indirect service and feel comfortable with role blurring is often dependent upon how secure an individual feels in his/her professional identity. Those who question their primary professional role should take time to solidify this identity in a supervised, structured setting prior to becoming a case manager (Krupa and Clark, 1995; Lysack et al., 1995).

• *Ethical dilemmas:* A case manager's primary responsibility is to the client and not to the case manager's employer; however, the employing agency has power over the case manager and can exert a great deal of influence. A case manager may be faced with the dilemma that what is in the best interest of a client may be counter to an agency's polices or beyond an agency's resources or non-reimbursable (Schreter, 1993). For example, many agencies deny acceptance to their mental health programs to persons with substance abuse histories while their addiction recovery programs deny acceptance to those with mental illness (Minkoff &

Drake, 1991). A case manager of a client who is mentally ill and chemically addicted (MICA) working for this agency is faced with an ethical dilemma in completing a program referral. If a client's complete history is revealed, the client is ineligible for service; yet, the omission of information is unethical. Resolving this dilemma requires Solomon-like wisdom and superb negotiating skills. Supervision, peer review and the agency's ethics committee can be used by case managers to resolve ethical dilemmas. The realities and limits of care must be shared with clients, while advocacy for change within a system of care is pursued (Christiansen, 1996).

- *Broker of services vs. primary therapist:* In some case management models, the case manager's main role is administrative; tasks include making referrals and coordinating services. Caseloads in this model tend to be large (i.e., 30-60 clients) (Clark & Fox, 1993). The case manager ensures clients follow through with referrals, and that the services provided are adequate and appropriate to meet clients' needs (Bachrach, 1992). The fact that other professionals are providing direct care can be difficult for occupational therapists who are used to being directly involved with their clients' care. Critiquing the appropriateness of working within this model, is useful in evaluating the congruency of it with our profession's philosophy and values (Fidler, 1993/2000).

- *Balancing ever increasing demands for occupational therapy:* When mental health agencies discover how well suited occupational therapists are for the case manager role, the demand for occupational therapy case managers increases. Occupational therapist case managers are asked to consult with other programs and case management teams while maintaining their own caseload (Gibson, 1993). To balance these demands occupational therapists can provide consultation and in-service training to groups of case managers on areas of greatest need (e.g.: self-care). The adoption of a cluster case management model can decrease the 1:1 caseload and allow the occupational therapist to provide service to groups of clients with similar areas of concern (e.g.: money management). Establishing an active clinical fieldwork program can increase occupational therapy personnel availability and decrease role strain, while netting the profession the secondary gain of having entry-level occupational therapists educated for community practice (Gibson, 1993; Lysack, et al, 1995).

- *Burnout:* The day to day realities of dealing with bureaucratic systems to meet the complex, multiple needs of clients with chronic mental illness can be overwhelming (Bachrach, 1992; Berzon & Lowenstein, 1984). Anti-burnout mechanisms can support case managers faced with difficult situations (Bachrach, 1992). They may consist of ongoing supervision and frequent team meetings to vent frustration, obtain support, and gain fresh perspectives (Intaglia, 1982). The

use of a portable phone when contacting agencies permits one to perform other tasks while being on hold for what often feels like perpetuity, thus decreasing stress. Individuals who have difficulty dealing with bureaucracy and ambiguity are not as well suited for the case manager role as those whose personal style welcomes the challenge of constant change and occasional chaos.

Diversifying the case manager's caseload to include clients with different needs and abilities can decrease the intensity of the workload. Matching a manager's special skills and interests to unique cases can renew sagging energy (Berzon & Lowenstein, 1984). Adopting case management models (i.e., team, cluster) which disperse responsibility among a number of individuals can also decrease stress (Clark & Fox, 1993; Intaglia, 1982). Case management assistants and "extenders" (i.e., peers, family, friends) can be enlisted to assist with certain tasks (e.g., accompanying a client to a medical appointment), diminishing the intense need to do it all. Field work students can also assist with tasks and provide new ideas and unbiased outlooks (Lysack et al., 1995). Most important, case managers can avoid setting themselves up for burnout, by recognizing that facilitating adaptation and enhancing quality of life, rather than achieving complete independent functioning, may be the most reasonable and appropriate goal for this population (Christiansen, 1996; Intaglia, 1982; Grady, 1997).

- *Counseling/education skills:* Forming a therapeutic relationship with a person with chronic mental illness is not easy, for severe impairment in social interaction skills is central to the illness itself (Woodside, 1993). A history of treatment failures and poor relationships can haunt the development of new therapeutic alliances. Helping clients acquire concrete services and doing structured activities with them are positive methods for developing trust (Harris & Bergman, 1988). At times, the 1:1 counseling and client and family education required in case management can become intense. Skill in managing difficult situations beyond one's scope (i.e., abuse cases, custody battles, evictions) can be developed through supervision, in-service training, and/or continuing education. Non-occupational therapy supervisors, publications and continuing education programs, can help broaden an occupational therapist case manager's perspective and developing competency.

- *Salary:* The relatively low paying salaries for case managers in most mental health care systems is often the biggest barrier to assuming this role (Walens et al., 1995). Occupational therapy assistants (OTAs) may find case management salaries more realistic but will need to work under the supervision of an occupational therapy. Case management team leader, director and/or consultant positions are valid positions for experienced occupational therapists and they provide more competitive salaries. One can begin a case management role on a part-time basis, in order to gain experience while maintaining a competitively salaried position at a more traditional setting. For example, combining a case management/ADL consultant position with home care practice can be financially acceptable and professionally rewarding. This job mix can also facilitate creativity and decrease burnout. In the meantime, the occupational therapist case manager/ADL consultant can measure improved functional outcomes for their clients, demonstrating the efficacy of his/her services (Landy & Knox, 1996). Marketing the occupational therapist's professional competence and the cost-effectiveness of occupational therapy services can result in an equitable income for an occupational therapist case manager (Adams, 1993b).

CONCLUSION

Occupational therapists can proactively face the challenges of a changing mental health care system by developing competence in case management. Expanding our role in community treatment and becoming core members of interdisciplinary teams has been viewed as essential to our professional growth, and possibly to our survival in a managed care system (Fidler, 1993/2000; Walens et al, 1995). Assuming leadership roles, including the case manager role, is an effective way to deal with the constraints of managed care while inspiring the health care delivery system to keep caring within practice (Peloquin, 1996). As Fine declared "occupational therapy practitioners must take a look around and take stock of the wealth of opportunities that will continue to unfold in mental health. If we, the purveyors of purposeful and meaningful activity, can not find purpose, meaning and promise for mental health practice in the opportunities and choices (available today), who can?" (1996, p. 22-23).

Occupational therapists who seize the opportunities available in case management will be rewarded on a professional and personal level. Professionally, case management offers a service delivery option that facilitates a strong collaborative therapeutic relationship which focuses on building strengths and addressing deficits in the individual's natural environment. Case management provides increased time for fostering change, enabling the therapist to witness long-term growth (Krupa & Clark, 1995). Case management is never boring, it is always changing, always stimulating. It requires creativity, a high level of autonomy, increased responsibility, continual learning and collaboration with a wide variety of individuals. Case management employs occupational therapy knowledge and skills on a more complex systems level, yet it remains a highly personal approach—a practice combination that can be very satisfying (Krupa & Clark, 1995; Lysack et al, 1995).

Personal rewards are derived from the pride and satisfaction gained in making qualitative differences in a person's life. Given that many occupational therapists enter our profession and pursue mental health practice due to their personal commitment to helping, the assumption of a case manager role can be very fulfilling (Harris & Bergman, 1988).

"The case manager has the opportunity to experience a full range of rewarding human emotions; joy, sorrow, pride, love, respect and trust, to name a few" (Krupa & Clark, 1995, p. 21).

Yerxa (1997) predicted that the 21st century "will begin an era of chronicity" (p. 613) and that there will be an "increased awareness of attending to the environment in which people actively live and work" (p. 614). Grady (1997) called for "more practice venues in the community where engagement in real occupation takes place" (p. 238) and Polatyko (1997) forecasted that occupational therapy practitioners will "take on many roles in enabling competence" (and) "use many and any tools"... "to enhance occupational competence" (p. 614). These predictions are highly congruent with case management principles and goals.

Occupational therapists who develop case management skills to supplement their traditional tools of practice can competently take on the role of case manager. This role expansion will enable occupational therapists to effectively serve clients with chronic mental illness in their community, in a caring and competent manner. Developing an individual's occupational competence through occupational therapy and case management can enable us to successfully meet the challenges of today's health care system and fulfill the potential of our next century of practice.

REFERENCES

Adams, R. (1993a). The role of occupational therapists in community mental health. In R. P. Cottrell (Ed), *Psychosocial occupational therapy: Proactive approaches* (pp. 165-167). Bethesda, MD: AOTA.

Adams, R. (1993b). The pros and cons of non traditional practice. In R.P. Cottrell (Ed.), *Psychosocial occupational therapy: Proactive approaches* (pp. 499-500). Bethesda, MD: AOTA. (See Chapter 33 in this text).

AOTA (1996). *Managed care: An occupational therapy source book.* Bethesda, MD: Author

Ashley, A. (1988). Case management: The need to define goals. *Hospital and Community Psychiatry, 39,* 499-500.

Bachrach, L. L. (1996), Managed care III. Whose business is patient care? *Psychiatric Services, 47,* 567-576.

Bachrach, L. L. (1992). Case management revisited. *Hospital and Community Psychiatry, 43,* 209-210.

Bernheim, K. F. (1993). Principles of professional and family collaboration. In R. P. Cottrell (Ed), *Psychosocial occupational therapy: Proactive approaches* (pp. 297-299). Bethesda, MD: AOTA. (See Chapter 45 in this text.)

Berzon, P., & Lowenstein, B. (1984). A flexible model of case management. In B. Pepper & H. Ryglewicz (Eds.), *Advances in treating the young chronic adult* (pp. 49-57). San Francisco, CA: Jossey-Bass.

Bond, G., Miller, L., Krumwied, R., & Ward, R. (1988). Assertive case management in three CMHCs: A controlled study. *Hospital and Community Psychiatry, 39,* 411-418.

Brekke, J., Ansel, M., Long, J., Slade, E., & Weinstein, M. (1999) Intensity and continuity of services and functional outcomes in rehabilitation of persons with schizophrenia. *Psychiatric Services, 50,* 248-256.

Brinson, M., & Kannenberg, K. (Eds). (1996). *Mental health service delivery guidelines.* Bethesda, MD: AOTA.

Bryan, C. M. (1990). The uses of therapy in case management. *New Directions for Mental Health Services, 46,* 19-26.

Case Management Society of American (1995). *CMSA Standards of Practice.* Little Rock, AR: Author.

Christiansen, C. (1996). Nationally speaking-Managed care: Opportunities and challenges for occupational therapy in the emerging systems of the 21st century. *American Journal of Occupational Therapy, 50,* 409-412.

Clark, R. E., & Fox, T. S. (1993). A framework for evaluating the economic impact of case management. *Hospital and Community Psychiatry, 44,* 469-473.

Collins, L. F. (1996). Excellence in a managed care environment. *OT practice* (pp. 20-22), Bethesda, MD: AOTA.

Cottrell, R. (Ed). (1993). *Psychosocial occupational therapy: Proactive approaches.* Bethesda, MD: AOTA.

Crist, P. (1993). Community living skills: A psychoeducational community-based program. In R. P. Cottrell (Ed), *Psychosocial occupational therapy: Proactive approaches* (pp. 169-175). Bethesda, MD: American Occupational Therapy Association. (See Chapter 19 in this text).

Crist, P., & Stoffel, V. (1996). The Americans with Disabilities Act of 1990 and employees with mental impairments: Personal efficacy and the environment. In R. P. Cottrell (Ed), *Perspectives of occupational therapy: Foundation and future of occupational therapy* (pp. 217-228). Bethesda, MD: AOTA.

Crowel, R. L. (1988). The integrated clinically managed housing network. In M. Harris & L. L. Bachrach (Eds), *Clinical case management* (pp. 63-78). San Francisco, CA: Jossey-Bass.

Dufresne, G. (1991). Statement: The occupational therapist as a case manager. *American Journal of Occupational Therapy, 45,* 1065-1066.

Ellek, D. (1993). The evolution of fairness in mental health policy. In R. P. Cottrell (Ed), *Psychosocial occupational therapy: Proactive approaches* (pp. 5-10). Bethesda, MD: AOTA (See Chapter 1 in this text).

Felton, C. J., Stasting, P., Shern, D. L., Blanch, A., Donahue, S. A., Knight E., & Brown, C. (1995). Consumers as peer specialists on intensive case management teams: Impact on client outcomes. *Psychiatric Services, 46,* 1037-1044.

Fidler, G. S. (1993). The challenge of change to occupational therapy practice. In R. P. Cottrell (Ed), *Psychosocial occupational therapy: Proactive approaches* (pp 15-19). Bethesda, MD: AOTA. (See Chapter 3 in this text).

Fine, S. (1996). The future of mental health practice. In M. Brinson & K. Kannenberg (Eds), *Mental health service delivery guidelines* (pp17-24), Bethesda, MD: AOTA.

Fisher, T. (1996). Roles and functions of a case manager. *American Journal of Occupational Therapy, 50,* 452-454.

Gibson, D. (1993). The challenge of adaptation: Shaping service delivery to meet changing needs. In R. P. Cottrell (Ed), *Psychosocial occupational therapy: Proactive approaches* (pp 11-14). Bethesda, MD: AOTA.

Goodman, M., Brown, J. A., & Deitz, P. M. (1996). *Managing managed care II: A handbook for mental health professionals* (2nd Edition). Washington, DC: American Psychiatric Press

Grady, A. P. (1997). Building inclusive community: A challenge for occupational therapy, 1994 Eleanor Clarke Slagle lecture. In R. P. Cottrell (Ed.), *Perspectives on purposeful activity: Foundation and future of occupational therapy* (pp. 229-240). Bethesda, MD: AOTA.

Greenberg, L., Fine, S. B., Cohen, C., Larson, K., Michealson-Bailey, A., Rubinten, P., & Glick, I. D. (1993). An interdisciplinary psychoeducation program for schizophrenic patients and their families. In R. P. Cottrell, (Ed), *Psychosocial occupational therapy: Proactive approaches* (pp. 305-310). Bethesda, MD: AOTA. (See Chapter 55 in this text).

Harris, M., & Bergman, H. C. (1988). Clinical case management for the chronic mentally ill: A conceptual analysis. In M. Harris and L. Bachrach (Eds), *Clinical case management* (p. 5-13). San Francisco, CA: Jossey-Bass.

Hatfield, A. B. (1993). Patient's accounts of stress and coping in schizophrenia. In R. P. Cottrell (Ed), *Psychosocial occupational therapy: Proactive approaches* (pp. 283-288). Bethesda, MD: AOTA. (See Chapter 40 in this text.)

Hettinger, J. (1996). Case management: Do occupational therapists have what it takes? Yes! *Occupational Therapy Week,* pp 12-14.

Intagliata, J., Willer, B., & Egri, G. (1988). The role of the family in delivering case management services. *New Directions for Mental Health Services, 40,* 39-52.

Intagliata, J. (1982). Improving the quality of community care for the chronically mentally disabled: The role of case management. *Schizophrenia Bulletin, 8,* 655-673.

Jaffee, E. (1996). Occupational therapy consultation in a managed care environment. *Occupational Therapy Practice,* 26-31.

Kanter, J. (1989). Clinical case management: Definition, principles, components. *Hospital and Community Psychiatry, 40,* 361-368.

Keith, S. J., Starr, S., & Matthews, S. (1993). A team approach to pharmocologic treatment of chronic schizophrenia. In R. P. Cottrell (Ed), *Psychosocial occupational therapy: Proactive approaches* (pp. 381-384). Bethesda, MD: AOTA.

Kennedy, R. (1997). Doors that offer hope may shut. *The New York Times,* pp. B1-B2.

Krupa, T. & Clark, C. C. (1995). Occupational therapists as case managers: Responding to current approaches to community mental health service delivery. *Canadian Journal of Occupational Therapy, 62,* 16-22.

Lamb, R. (1980). Therapist case managers: More than brokers of service. *Hospital and Community Psychiatry, 31,* 762-764.

Landy, C. & Knox, J. (1996). Managed care fundamentals: Implications for health care professionals. *American Journal of Occupational Therapy, 50,* 413-416.

Leete, E. (1993). The treatment of schizophrenia: A patient's perspective. In R. P. Cottrell (Ed), *Psychosocial occupational thera-*

py: Proactive approaches (pp. 277-282). Bethesda, MD: AOTA. (See Chapter 46 in this text).

Liberman, R. P. (1988). *Psychiatric rehabilitation of chronic mental patients.* Washington, D.C.: American Psychiatric Press.

Lysack, C., Stadnyk, R., Paterson M., McLeod, K., & Krefting, L. (1995). Professional expertise of occupational therapists in community practice: Results of an Ontario survey. *Canadian Journal of Occupational Therapy, 62,* 138-147.

Malloy, M. (1997). *Mental illness and managed care: A primer for families and consumers.* Arlington, VA: National Alliance for the Mentally Ill.

Mental Health Resource Center. (1990). *Intensive case management.* Albany, NY: New York State Office of Mental Health.

Miller, R., & Walker, K. F. (1993). *Perspectives on theory for the practice of occupational therapy.* Gaithersburg, MD: Aspen.

Minkoff, K. & Drake, R. E. (1991). *New Directions for Mental Health Services: Dual diagnosis of major mental illness and substance disorders.* San Francisco, CA: Jossey-Bass.

Moeller, P. (1991). The occupational therapist as case manager in community mental health. In R. P. Cottrell (Ed), *Psychosocial occupational therapy: Proactive approaches* (pp 183-185). Bethesda, MD: AOTA.

Mosey, A. C. (1986). *Psychosocial components of occupational therapy.* New York, NY: Raven Press.

Olsen, D., Rickles, J., & Travlek, K. (1995). A treatment team model of managed mental health care. *Psychiatric Services, 46,* 252-256.

Onyett, S. (1992). *Case management in mental health.* New York, NY: Chapman Hall.

Palmer, F., & Gatti, D. (1993). Vocational treatment model. In R. P. Cottrell (Ed), *Psychosocial occupational therapy: Proactive approaches* (pp. 211-219). Bethesda, MD: AOTA. (See CHapter 25 in this text.)

Peloquin, S. (1996). The issue is: Now that we have managed care, shall we inspire it? *American Journal of Occupational Therapy, 50,* 455-459. (See Chapter 68 in this text).

Poirier, S. (1988). Linking acute care with the community. In AOTA (Ed), *Acute care psychiatry: Practical strategies and collaborative approaches* (pp. 37-46). Rockville, MD: Author

Polatajko, H. J. (1996). Dreams, dilemmas and decisions for occupational therapy practice in a new millennium: A Canadian perspective. In R. P. Cottrell (Ed), *Perspectives on purposeful activity: Foundation and future of occupational therapy* (pp. 617-622). Bethesda, MD: AOTA.

Randolph, F., Balskinsky M., Leginski, W., Parker, L., & Goldman, H. (1997). Creating integrated service systems for homeless persons with mental illness: The ACCESS program. *Psychiatric Services, 48,* 369-373.

Schreter, R. K. (1993). Economic Grand rounds: Ten trends in managed care and their impact on the biopsychosocial model. *Hospital and Community Psychiatry, 44,* 325-327.

Schreter, R. K., Sharfstein, S. S., and Schreter, C.A. (1997). *Managing care not dollars: The continuum of mental health services.* Washington, DC: American Psychiatric Press.

Solomon, P. (1992). The efficacy of case management services for severely mentally disabled clients. *Community Mental Health Journal, 28,* 163-179.

Sullivan, J. P. (1981) (Ed). Case management. In J. A. Talbott, *The chronic mentally ill: Treatment programs and systems.* New York, NY: Human Sciences.

Uttaro, T., & Mechanic, D. (1994). The NAMI consumer survey analysis of unmet needs. *Hospital and Community Psychiatry, 45,* 372-374.

Van Leit, B. (1996). Managed mental health care: Reflections in a time of turmoil. *American Journal of Occupational Therapy, 50,* 428-434. (See Chapter 4 in this text).

Waldo, M. C., Roath, M., Levine, W., & Freedman, R. (1993). A model program to teach parenting skills to schizophrenic mothers. In R. P. Cottrell (Ed), *Psychosocial occupational therapy: Proactive approaches* (pp. 311-313). Bethesda, MD: AOTA.

Walens, D., Dickie, V., Tomlinson, J., Raynor, O. Y., Wittman, P., & Kannenberg, K. (1995). *Mental Health Special Interest Section Education Task Force Report.* Bethesda, MD: AOTA.

Ware, T. (1995). The value of case management for a consumer. *Psychiatric Services, 46,* 1231-1232.

Wilberding, D. (1993). The quarterway house: More than an alternative of care. In R. P. Cottrell (Ed), *Psychosocial occupational therapy: Proactive approaches* (pp. 127-138). Bethesda, MD: AOTA. (See Chapter 18 in this text.)

Winefield, H. R., & Harvey, E. J. (1994). Needs of family caregivers in chronic schizophrenia. *Schizophrenia Bulletin, 20,* 557-566.

Woodside, H. (1993). The day center and its role as a social network. In R. P. Cottrell (Ed), *Psychosocial occupational therapy: Proactive approaches* (pp. 329-332). Bethesda, MD: AOTA. (See Chapter 42 in this text.)

Yerxa, E. J. (1997). Dreams, dilemmas and decisions for occupational therapy practice in a new millennium: An American perspective. In R. P. Cottrell (Ed), *Perspectives on purposeful activity: Foundation and future of occupational therapy* (pp. 613-616). Bethesda, MD: AOTA.

CHAPTER THIRTY-FIVE

Old Answers for Today's Problems: Integrating Individuals Who Are Homeless with Mental Illness into Existing Community-Based Programs: A Case Study of Fountain House

Sara M. Asmussen, Joanna Romano, Paul Beatty, Larry Gasarch, and Susan Shaughnessey

This chapter is reprinted from Psychosocial Rehabilitation Journal, 18(1), 75-93 *by permission of the authors. Copyright © 1994. The authors would also like to note that this chapter would not have been possible without the support and insight of James R. Schmidt, retired Executive Director of Fountain House. Many thanks for your time and input.*

Homelessness in the United States has become a major problem for individuals and communities alike. Particularly at risk are individuals who suffer from major mental illnesses. As this group becomes more visible to the general public, different solutions are being discussed. One solution involves relaxing laws which protect "noncompliant" individuals against involuntary commitment (Belcher, 1988; Belcher & Ephross, 1989; Lamb, 1989, Miller, 1992). If this were to occur, reinstitutionalization, or warehousing, would be a very probable outcome. Apart from the obvious ethical and moral problems with such a plan, relaxing commitment laws would not offer individuals who are homeless any help (Kanter, 1989). Prior research has shown that the majority of adults who are homeless and mentally ill are not only discharges from mental hospitals, but also include individuals who lack community mental health services (Searight & Searight, 1988). Reinstitutionalization is even more abhorrent when we consider that the needs of the client and the available opportunities of community service agencies are frequently discrepant (Dattalo, 1990; Martin, 1990; Struening, 1987). Rehabilitation must be designed to meet the needs of the individual. As long as communities are not providing appropriate services for these individuals, relaxing commitment laws should not be considered as an option.

A more viable alternative to address the unmet needs of this group is to increase community services. Elements important to the successful implementation of community rehabilitation are 1) a well-functioning system of case management (Rife, First, Greenlee, Miller, & Feichter, 1991); 2) a relevant continuum of care (Lamb, 1990); and 3) extensive input from the client (Cohen, 1989; Berman-Rossi & Cohen, 1988; Moxley & Freddolino, 1991). Clearly, a comprehensive case management plan combined with a continuum of opportunities is necessary to achieve success. Cohen (1989) explains in detail the empowerment-oriented approach to engagement which has been proven to be effective with individuals who are homeless. Feelings of self-determination and autonomy result by allowing clients to participate fully in identifying needs, determining goals, and setting the terms of the rehabilitation process for themselves.

In a comprehensive summation, the Federal Task Force on Homelessness and Severe Mental Illness (NIMH, 1992) concluded that a combination of services are necessary to meet the needs of individuals who are homeless and plagued by mental illnesses. These services included: assertive outreach, integrated case management, safe havens, housing, psychiatric treatment, substance abuse treatment, health care, federal benefits, consumer/family involvement, legal protections, rehabilitation, vocational training, and employment assistance.

While providing all the services listed in the Task Force Report may seem impossible, services of existing agencies in the community could be integrated into a comprehensive system which could be individualized to meet the needs of each person. The purpose of this chapter is to describe a project which provided all these services through a comprehensive system of case management based on a consumer empowerment model. Individuals who are homeless, like individuals who are mentally ill, differ drastically from one another; therefore, a system of case management was designed whereby the individual determined which services he or she needed. The umbrella agency made sure that the case managers had access to all the opportunities which would be needed to help the clients.

PROGRAM DESIGN

This homeless project was implemented by Fountain House in New York City. Fountain House, an agency based on the Clubhouse Model of Vocational Rehabilitation, has a long history of integrating individuals with mental illnesses back into the community (Beard, Pitt, Fisher, & Goertzel, 1963; Community Adjustment, 1985; Malamud & McCrory, 1988; Noble, 1991). Currently, over 875 different clients, called members, are served in a variety of programs offered at Fountain House every month. These programs include a Prevocational Day Program, Residential Program, Evening/Weekend/Holiday Program, Member Education, High Point Farm Project, Employment Services, and support dinners for those at school, on part-time employment, full-time employment, and in housing. Fountain House is open 365 days a year and membership is not time limited; services are to be used as the individual needs them. If a member does leave the program and later wishes to return, easy reentry to the program is one of the benefits of membership. The goal of this project was to determine if these existing programs could be modified to serve the needs of individuals who were homeless and had mental illnesses. Below is a description of the changes which were instituted.

Assertive Outreach

In order to reach out to the most at-risk homeless individuals in the community, a Liaison Team was formed of existing clients (called members) and staff. This was an addition to the existing program and was a necessity to reach the most disabled individuals. The Liaison Team was further responsible for developing relationships with existing agencies who worked with individuals who were homeless. The team would visit these locations and members would talk with individuals who had mental illnesses, ascertaining their needs and discussing how Fountain House might help meet those needs. Previously, Fountain House membership had always been based on whether a person could attend the program on their own. The Liaison Team actually escorted people to Fountain House if they were unable to do this.

The first step upon joining the program was a period of orientation. As part of orientation, new members worked for one or more days in each of the 10 prevocational work units at Fountain House. Once a new member chose a unit, orientation was considered completed. An integral part of the program was that at no point in this outreach and orientation process were assessment or level of functioning instruments administered. The client flow charts in Figures 35-1 and 35-2 indicate the services received and movement through the program.

Case Management

Fountain House, as the umbrella agency, provided all case management services. The defining characteristics of case management within the clubhouse model are that members determine the: 1) work they do, 2) staff they work with, 3) number of necessary contacts, and 4) services they receive. Several dilemmas arose when trying to apply a straight case management model to this project. First, because of the need for a process of engagement, individuals could not just be assigned to a unit or case manager. The dropout rate would have been very high. Second, not all staff who work as case managers at the agency have the time or opportunity to visit shelters and reach out to homeless individuals in order to begin this process of engagement. And third, the Liaison Team could not serve as the case managers for all 201 individuals who joined through the project.

Normally there would be an intake and orientation process and then the individual would chose a unit on which to work. The case management would originate from this unit. However, the individuals who joined the program through this project needed more time in intake and orientation than was expected. Therefore, the engagement process started with the Liaison Team. For the most part, these individuals had needs which required immediate attention. Therefore, case management services began with the Liaison Team. It is important to note that case management was considered a process and not a person. Individuals could immediately begin receiving services and did not need to wait until the process of engagement was completed. In fact, using case management services as a tool of engagement was very effective. If someone needed a place to stay, a way to develop trust was to help them find housing and not wait until an official case manager was assigned.

The Liaison Team also conducted a basic needs assessment. Money was supplied from an Emergency Fund which was established specifically for this group. Clothes could be purchased from the thrift shop and showers and laundry facilities were available on site. The next step was to determine whether the individual needed immediate medical, psychiatric, or substance abuse services. If these services were needed, the individual was referred to the appropriate agency. The individual remained a member of Fountain House and eventually returned to the agency. Referrals were only made for specific problems, not for the purpose of discharging difficult clients.

The necessary paperwork for obtaining housing within the State of New York was started by the Liaison Team during orientation. Emergency housing, or safe haven, was provided in various ways. Several shelters provide beds for Fountain

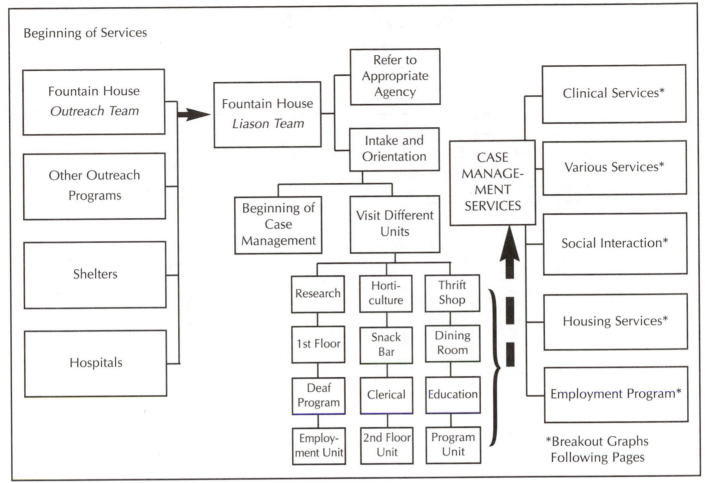

Figure 35-1. Fountain House flowchart.

House members; in exchange, the Liaison Team accepted referrals from these shelters. Rent for a room could be provided through the Emergency Fund. And finally, Fountain House has a large enough housing program that it was possible, on occasion, to provide temporary shelter.

Upon joining a unit, staff on that unit would take responsibility for the case management. If this unit connection did not work out, case management responsibilities were transferred back to the Liaison Team. Case management included a wide variety of services such as finding a clinic, seeing a doctor, obtaining housing, referrals to substance abuse clinics, and obtaining federal and/or state benefits. Other members often helped new members obtain these services. Employing this type of modified case management proved to be very effective. It impacted on the drop-out rate and the number of people who "fell through the cracks" of the system.

Rehabilitation

Despite the varying programs in which new members could become involved, all were centered around the voluntary Day Program at the clubhouse. The clubhouse was open from 9 a.m. until 5 p.m., Monday through Friday. Due to size, Fountain House is currently divided into 10 work units:

Research, Horticulture, First Floor (including a small bank), Snack Bar, Dining Room, Clerical, Education, Employment, Second Floor, and Program (including the Deaf Program, Thrift Shop, and Housing). The work which is conducted on each unit is performed by staff and members working together. Members are not paid; their work is voluntary. Work on units is used as a prevocational tool for preparing members for employment and is therefore real work, not "make work." This work experience is used as a stepping stone to paid employment. This same process was available to project participants. A modification which was implemented was the use of the Evening/Weekend/Holiday Program as a drop-in center. Individuals who were unable to attend the Day Program would have a place to go where case management services, food, and socialization were all available.

Vocational Training and Employment Assistance

After the member had worked on a unit at the clubhouse, the opportunity to try work through Fountain House's Employment System was made available. Members decided when they were ready to try work. There were no fixed periods of adjustment and no formal assessments concerning job

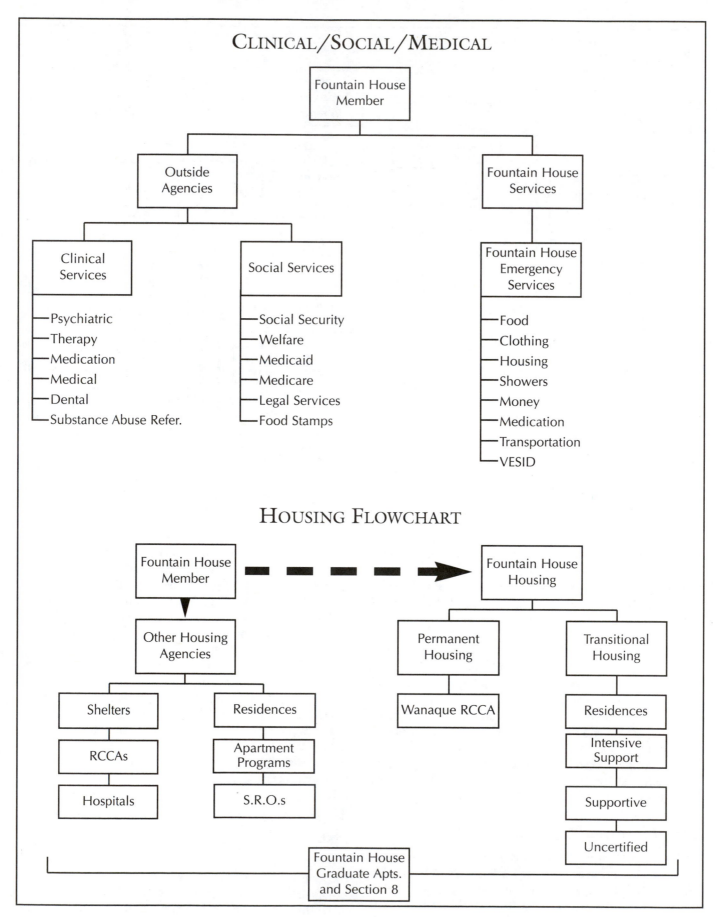

Figure 35-2. Various services provided.

readiness, since "symptoms of illness may be present without disability" (Lovell, 1992). Many participants had left other programs due to the restrictiveness of rules; therefore, this system was designed to be flexible. Participation is not viewed as a program of one-time, irreversible steps. People may have to return to a more supported level of employment due to the cyclical nature of mental illness.

Expanding the employment system for homeless individuals included accounting for those who are severely underprepared for employment. This group included individuals who had never worked, work minimally, or refused medication and/or therapy. The Employment System was composed of Group Placements for people who needed the most support; TE (Transitional Employment) for those who needed to develop work behaviors; and Independent Employment (IE). This systematized process of rehabilitation has been shown to be effective (Asmussen & Beatty, 1991) and can be implemented into any facility providing employment opportunities for this group.

GROUP PLACEMENTS

Despite the success of TE, there is an identifiable group of severely disabled clients who are not utilizing TE. To remedy this, positions were secured where a variation on the structure of the TE setting enabled some of these individuals to work successfully. The variation involved more flexible hours, a setting where a group of members worked together, and intensive on-site staff presence was available. Examples of the type of work done on group placements include wrapping packages at Saks Fifth Avenue at Christmas time, envelope insertion for proxy votes for Prudential Securities shareholders meeting, and running the indoor mail delivery system at DMB&B. Group Placements are the ideal vehicle for initially engaging individuals who are homeless because of the staff presence and because the group, not individual, productivity is measured. This allowed individuals who were not work-ready to get an experience working.

TRANSITIONAL EMPLOYMENT (TE)

On TE placements, members work on paid, part-time, unsubsidized positions in an employer's regular place of business. Most individual TE placements involve working four hours per day, five days a week for six months. The members are paid directly by the company and appropriate tax deductions are withheld. After on-site training, members go to the job unaccompanied and work individually, integrated among the company's regular employees. All placements belong to Fountain House; it is the Fountain House staff who decides which member fills a position. All placements pay at least minimum wage and the member is paid the same prevailing wage as a non-handicapped individual in the same job. A Fountain House staff person or a member who has had the job previously, trains the new member on the job for two to

five days. Following the training, the TE placement manager keeps in contact with the company on a regular basis and provides fill-in coverage if the member on the placement is absent from work. Jobs on TEs ranged from mail room clerk to high level data entry positions.

Even though the members work five days a week, they are expected to attend the clubhouse for the remainder of the day—obtaining a TE placement is not the end of a process, but rather the beginning; the ultimate goal is independent employment. This allows for the discussion of work related issues with the support of the other members and staff. This is particularly relevant for this group of individuals because they needed more supports in order to remain in the community. When a member completes a TE, there is ample opportunity for this individual to go to another TE or to begin working with the Employment Unit to obtain an independent job.

INDEPENDENT EMPLOYMENT (IE)

This program assisted members in preparing resumes, learning interviewing procedures, and organizing job searches. Once independent employment is obtained, off-site support services are available. These services are utilized for everything from helping to resolve social issues to obtaining housing and medical treatment. By offering this type of employment variety, each individual's rehabilitation goals can be customized to his or her abilities. Very few participants used these services, probably due to the short time period.

SCREENING MEMBERS FOR EMPLOYMENT

The manner in which individuals who were homeless were chosen for Group or TE Placements was very informal. Anyone who expressed a desire to work and was able to meet the hygiene requirements was selected for employment at the Group Placement level. Group Placements were organized so that individuals who would normally not be able to work because of behavior, or low production, could obtain employment. While production speed is very important, other members of the group who are faster can make up for the low production rate of an individual. Members were chosen to go on TE if 1) they expressed a desire to work; and 2) their prior work performance on their units or Group Placements was good.

Consumer/Family Involvement

Family involvement is of course welcomed; however, with this particular group family members were rarely available. There was an effort made to reunite families who were no longer together due to the person's mental illness or homelessness. Consumer involvement was central to the success of the project. Members who were formerly homeless them-selves were on the Liaison Team. In terms of the day-to-day functioning of the program, members did the large majority of the work which was necessary to keep the agency running.

Legal Protections

There was not much need for this service with the people in this project. This outcome is probably not generalizable to the rest of the country. Legal services were used for illegal evictions and obtaining federal benefits. Fountain House staff workers and members are trained in these two areas so that the attorneys were only used as a back-up. When legal repre-sentation was needed, the MFY Legal Services provided assis-tance. This is a non-profit organization of attorneys who work pro bono in the community to help those who are destitute.

Housing Options

In New York City affordable housing is difficult to obtain. The Housing Program at Fountain House was designed so that individuals were placed in living arrangements which met their present needs. Support services were available so that individuals were able to live at the highest possible level of independence. To achieve this end, a wide range of housing options were used, from residences, which are staffed 24-hours, to supported independent apartments where mem-bers hold their own leases. While not every agency is able to run a housing program, it is possible to connect with other housing programs in the community, a resource which Fountain House staff also successfully employed.

Initial housing placements for this project were made when a new member first joined the program. The decision was based on input from the member, staff, other members, shelter staff, and doctors. Once an individual was placed in a living situation, it became clear quite quickly whether it was an appropriate placement. If the member was placed in an environment which was too independent, interventions were instituted. When the individual was moved into a situation which was too supportive, a move to a more independent level of housing was instituted.

Linkages With Other Agencies

The networks which developed between Fountain House and other agencies were very important. No one agency can provide all services; therefore, existing facilities in the com-munity were used to provide specialized support for mem-bers. Extensive networks have been developed with shelters and other places homeless individuals congregate. In return, these facilities provided other homeless Fountain House members with food and shelter. Hospitals were an important part of the network because many of the project participants were in need of medical and psychiatric services.

Linkages with the federal, state, and city agencies and serv-ices were centered around agency funding and client benefits. These agencies and services included: the Social Security Administration (SSA), Food Stamps, Public Assistance, Medicaid, Medicare, New York State Office of Vocational and Educational Services for the Individual Who's Disabled (VESID), Human Resources Administration (HRA), New York City and State Offices of Mental Health (NYC & NYS OMH), U.S. Department of Housing and Urban Development (HUD) and the U.S. Department of Labor (DOL).

Tracking the number and types of linkages was one of the original goals of this project; however, this proved to be impossible. Because case management is viewed as a function and not a person, it was too cumbersome to track all con-tacts. After two years it was possible to document, through paper trails, linkages with 54 other agencies which were used to meet the intensive needs of this group of individuals. To give an example of the number of contacts, Table 35-1 exhibits the number and types of contacts which were made for one person in a 21-month time period. This individual was in need of more services than most of the participants, but the information regarding contacts is very good. Further, it provides a picture of the commitment which is necessary if an agency chooses to work with individuals who are mental-ly ill and homeless.

INITIAL PROGRAM OUTCOMES

Project Participants

All participants were homeless and had major mental ill-nesses. All participants were approached during the time period from June 1990 to May 1992. For the purpose of this project homelessness was defined as any person who lacked a regular place to live or was living in a place not designed for human habitation. The main goals of the project were to get people into a clubhouse program and help them obtain employment and secure housing. The eligibility require-ments for membership in the clubhouse are as follows:

1. The person must be over 16 years of age.

2. The person must have a diagnosis of chronicity and psy-chosis or a history of severe psychiatric disability.

3. Substance abuse must not be the primary presenting problem (i.e., individuals who have abuse problems will not be excluded if there is a psychiatric diagnosis).

4. The person must not have an ongoing history of violent or criminal behavior.

Measures and Data Collection

Demographic data and psychiatric and work histories were collected for all subjects who attended Fountain House. These data were collected initially at intake and then updated and are still being completed as information is received from shelters, hospitals, and doctors. Information was kept on daily attendance, employment, and changes in housing sta-tus. Caseworkers also provided the research team with monthly updates on the services participants received and

Table 35-1
Linkages With Other Agencies

Type of Agency	Telephone	Letters	In Person	No Beds	Hospitals
Liaison Team	13		4		
Shelters	15	2	1		
Human Resources Ad.	1	2			
Psychiatric Services	11	2	4	1	1
Substance Abuse Services	43	11	25	8	8
Medical Services	18	3	21	2	7
Department of Aging	2				
Housing Services	22	8	10		
Social Security Admin.	12	8	5		
Legal Entities	4				
Police	3	1	4		
Outreach Teams	3		1		
Emergency Rooms	5				9
EMS (Ambulance)	2		5		
TOTAL	154	37	80	11	25

perceptions about what obstacles kept a non-working member from employment. When a member was employed, information was collected on the type of job, hours worked, wage, and employer.

Initial Outcomes

The project proved to be an effective means of stabilizing a population which has traditionally been underserved and neglected. 201 (88%) of the 228 undomiciled individuals contacted by the Liaison Team joined Fountain House. During Year 1, 128 individuals were invited to join the program. In Year 2, 100 individuals were invited to join. Of the Year 1 participants, 101 (80%) continued in the program during Year 2. 100% of these participants were suffering from major mental illnesses, while 34% had additional substance abuse problems. The demographic information for people who joined is in Table 35-2.

By the end of the second year of the project, 85 (42%) of the participants took part in Group Placements or TEs, and 9 (5%) went on to Independent Employment. It was also found that the longer a person remained in the program, the more likely they were to go to work. Fifty percent of the individuals from Year 1 who continued in the program for Year 2 (N=101) went to work, versus 35% of the individuals who started the program during Year 2 (N=100). Participants remained on the job for an average of 19.2 weeks Participants who did not work remained in the Day Program for as long at they wished. Some will eventually try work, others may just attend the program never working for a salary.

Housing changes proved difficult to analyze. This was due to the issue of what constituted a housing "upgrade" and what constituted a "downgrade." For example, someone who moved into a permanent housing situation, had a relapse, and returned to a supportive living environment would be counted as a "downgrade." However, when the nature of mental illnesses is considered, having long-term support is the most important factor. This individual would of course eventually move back into a more permanent setting when he or she was ready. This should not be considered a "downgrade" but rather a process by which people with this illness achieve independence and integration. At this point the most useful way of presenting housing shifts is to look at the number of upgrades from the streets and shelters. Table 35-3 simplifies the data for the 201 individuals who joined the program.

CONCLUSIONS

As tempting as it is to simply follow a cookbook version of how to implement a Homeless Project into existing agencies by accounting for all the necessary components of such a project, there are several assumptions which need to be analyzed before developing such a program. These assumptions have been found to be not only useful but crucial to the success of the project at Fountain House.

First, there must be money for emergencies. This sounds trivial, however, when someone needs something, one very effective way of establishing a relationship with that person is by providing short-term help. If someone is seeking housing or employment and this is not an immediate possibility, food, shower, and a safe place to sleep can be provided. The otherwise disenfranchised person begins to develop a sense of trust. Based on this trust the person might return to the program again, eventually leading to attendance in order to receive rehabilitation services. These funds should not in any way be tied to attendance or adherence to rules, but as an aid to help the individual meet some immediate need.

Table 35-2
Demographic Information

Demographic	(N)	(%)
Gender		
Male	110	55
Female	91	45
Age		
< 21 Years	0	0
22-30 Years	34	17
31-40 Years	67	33
41-50 Years	62	31
51-65 Years	34	17
> 65 Years	2	1
Unknown	2	1
Race		
White, Non-His.	81	40
Black, Non-His.	75	37
Asian/Pac. Islander	5	3
Hispanic	21	10
American Indian	6	3
Other	6	3
Unknown	7	4
Marrital Status		
Single	137	68
Married	6	3
Sep/Div/Wid/Unk	58	29
Highest Education		
No Degree	53	26
High School/GED	65	32
Further Education	63	31
Unknown	20	10

Table 35-3
Housing at Intake and End of Project

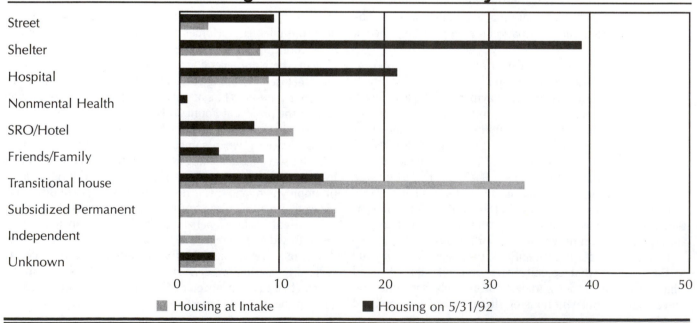

Street
Shelter
Hospital
Nonmental Health
SRO/Hotel
Friends/Family
Transitional house
Subsidized Permanent
Independent
Unknown

0   10   20   30   40   50

▨ Housing at Intake   ■ Housing on 5/31/92

Second, no assessment instruments need to be given at any point of the program. There are no accurate instruments in the field currently. Any program can create its population by accepting into the program only those who pass certain assessments. However, that still leaves a large population of unserved individuals who are homeless. This group may indeed need our help the most. The object of the program should not be to assess people out, but to reach out to the most destitute.

Third, consumers must be involved in every step of the rehabilitation process. This includes the design, implementation, and execution of the project. They must have a forum through which their concerns can be stated and heard. Consumers must also be allowed to choose the staff they work with, the type of work performed, and the amount of contact, if any, they need with staff. This can be a problem if case management is viewed as a specific individual or team. What kind of a choice does a consumer have if he or she is assigned a case manager? Consumers are quite capable of telling staff what it is they need and want. By implementing case management as a process, people will attend a voluntary program and will develop their own support systems among peers. These support systems have been shown to help the individual remain in the community (Martin & Nayowith, 1988).

Fourth, the environment or atmosphere of the program must be welcoming. The physical environment must be clean, well lit, well furnished, comfortable, inviting, and in general a place you would want to spend time. This is particularly important when working with a group of individuals who are many times treated as invisible and unimportant. The physical environment will then become a place to which people choose to return.

Fifth, there must be opportunities to work for wages with the understanding that many individuals may not be ready for traditional work settings. Even though most individuals who joined this project did not have any aspect of their lives in order, the vast majority looked forward to participating in work as soon as possible. Normally, nine out of the ten people participating in orientation expressed the desire to return to, or start, work. The emphasis in orientation was centered around getting back to work, as much as it was centered around the basic needs of shelter, food, and clothing.

Sixth, there must be long-term follow-up and support for this particular group (Lovell, 1992). If the environment is welcoming enough, people will develop their own support networks. The agency can facilitate this by having a system whereby people are welcomed back after long absences, and not dropped from the roles for non-attendance. An individual may not attend the day program when first approached for a variety of reasons, such as severity of symptoms, fear, substance abuse, or not viewing the program as relevant to his or her needs. By providing no time-limits on membership, the individual has the opportunity to attend at any time. This also provides the long-term support and base that some individuals may require to overcome barriers in their lives.

Seventh, services individualized for each person is essential. Each person has different needs, aspirations, and resources. Therefore, the type of help they receive should be based on these factors. Again, this can only be achieved if case management is seen as a function and not as an individual. No one person can meet all the needs of another person. When individualization occurs, people are more apt to use the services of the program and thus continue to return. Rehabilitation can be effective only when the person attends.

Eighth, it is known that individuals struggling with both homelessness and mental illnesses will leave a program if that program is not perceived as meeting their needs. The term "consumer" implies that the person is a paying customer. Agencies should design programs around the question "would people pay to be here?" This question is not that far-fetched when viewed in light of the fact Social Security, OVR, Medicaid, and Welfare are all looking at voucher systems as means of payments to agencies providing services. The term "consumer" should not be used as a euphemism for mental patient, but in the true sense of the definition.

And finally, program administrators must be willing to make these changes within their agencies. Many times agencies are run on strict attendance schedules, forcing people to take medication, see psychiatrists, and attend group therapy. People with mental illnesses who are homeless are currently not in any programs because the rules and structures were found to be irrelevant (Lovell, 1992); therefore setting up more programs which exclude the same people is not helpful.

Overall, homelessness is an area in which existing agencies can make a tremendous impact. However, making an impact will require agencies and communities to understand that people cannot always live by the "right" rules. We, as providers, must put aside our views of the "correct" courses and responses. Homeless individuals have as much right to decide which services are appropriate for them as do housed individuals. As service providers, we need to continually separate our own belief systems and their ensuing punishment responses from the individual standing in front of us.

Note

This work was funded by the Stewart B. Mckinney monies through the Department of Labor. Matching funds were provided by the Samuel & May Rudin, Hearst, Frances & Edwin Cummings, Herman Goldman, Mental Illness, and St. James Church Foundations. The authors would like to thank James R. Schmidt, retired Director of Fountain House, for his leadership and insight during the development of this project.

References

Asmussen, S. M., & Beatty, P. (1991). *The development, analysis, and cost effectiveness of an employment system* (Contract No. 13-P-10032-2-02). Washington, DC: Social Security Administration.

Beard, J. H., Pitt, R. B., Fisher, S. H., & Goertzel, V. (1963). Evaluating the effectiveness of a psychiatric rehabilitation program. *The American Journal of Orthopsychiatry, 33*,4, 701-712.

Belcher, J. R. (1988). Are jails replacing the mental health system for the homeless mentally ill? *Community Mental Health Journal, 24,*3, 185-195.

Belcher, J. R., & Ephross, P. H. (1989). Toward an effective practice model for the homeless mentally ill. *Social Casework, 70,* 7, 421-427.

Berman-Rossi, T,. & Cohen, M. B. (1988). Group development and shared decision-making working with homeless mentally ill women. *Social Work with Groups, 11,*4, 63-78.

Cohen, M. B. (1989). Social work practice with homeless mentally ill people: Engaging the client. *Social Work, 34,*6, 505-509.

Community adjustment. (1986). Evaluation of the clubhouse model for psychiatric rehabilitation, IX. *Rehab Brief: Bringing Research into Effective Focus,* pp. 1-4.

Dattalo, P. (1990). Widening the range of services for the homeless mentally ill. *Administration and Policy in Mental Health, 17,*4, 247-256.

Kanter, A. S. (1989). Homeless but not helpless: Legal issues in the care of homeless people with mental illness. *Journal of Social Issues, 45,*3, 91-104.

Lamb, H. R. (1989). Involuntary treatment for the homeless mentally ill. *Notre Dame Journal of Law, Ethics and Public Policy, 4*(2), 269-280.

Lamb, H. R. (1990). Will we save the homeless mentally ill? *American Journal of Psychiatry, 147*(5), 649- 651.

Lovell, A. (1992). Classification and its risks: How psychiatric status contributes to homeless policy. *New England Journal of Public Policy,* 247-263.

Malamud T. J., & McCrory, D. (1988). Transitional employment: A community model for the vocational rehabilitation of individuals with prolonged mental illness. In J. Ciardiello & M. Bell (Eds.), *Vocational rehabilitation of persons with prolonged mental illness* (pp. 150-162). Baltimore, MD: Johns Hopkins University Press.

Martin, M. A. (1990). The homeless mentally ill and community-based care: Changing a mindset. *Community Mental Health Journal, 26*(5), 435-447.

Martin, M. A., & Nayowith, S. A. (1988). Creating community: Groupwork to develop social support networks with homeless mentally ill. *Social Work with Groups, 11*(4), 79-93.

Moxley, D. P., & Freddolino, P. P. (1991). Needs of homeless people coping with psychiatric problems: Findings from an innovative advocacy project. *Health and Social Work, 16*(1), 19-26.

National Institute of Mental Health. (1992). *Outcasts on main street: Report of the federal task force on homelessness and severe mental illness* (DHHS Publication No. ADM 921904). Washington, DC: U.S. Government Printing Office.

Noble, J. H. (1991). *The benefits and costs of supported employment for people with mental illness and with traumatic brain injury in New York state* (Contact No. C-0023180). Buffalo, NY: Research Foundation of the State University of New York.

Rife, J. C., First, R. J., Greenlee, R. W., Miller, L. D., & Feichter, M. A. (1991). Case management with homeless mentally ill people. *Health and Social Work, 16*(1), 58-87.

Searight, H. R., & Searight, P. R. (1988). The homeless mentally ill: Overview, policy implications, and adult foster care as a neglected resource. *Adult Foster Care Journal, 2*(4), 235-259.

Struening, E. L. (1987). *A study of a residence of the NYC shelter system.* New York, NY: New York State Psychiatric Institute.

Occupational Therapy Evaluation and Intervention in an Employment Program for Homeless Youths

Kathleen Kannenberg and Debra Boyer

This chapter was previously published in the Psychiatric Services, 48, 631-633. *Copyright © 1997, the American Psychiatric Association.*

Beginning in 1995, we helped initiate a demonstration project in Seattle that employs homeless youths and that includes an occupational therapist as part of the program staff. The use of an occupational therapist in an employment setting for homeless youths is a unique approach to addressing clients' developmental and functional deficits, and it tests several assumptions about the service needs of high-risk youth.

The employment program, called the Working Zone, promotes normal developmental processes for homeless youth. In this (chapter) we outline the rationale for using occupational therapy in this setting, briefly describe the program, and discuss the occupational therapy evaluation and intervention process. A case study illustrates the type of information collected in the occupational therapy evaluation and describes an occupational therapy intervention.

WHY OCCUPATIONAL THERAPY IN THIS SETTING?

Several studies have documented a high prevalence of child abuse and neglect, particularly sexual abuse and assault, in the histories of homeless youths.[1-9] Services for high-risk adolescents, such as employment programs, alternative schools, substance abuse treatment, and housing programs, are likely to include a large proportion of clients with trauma histories. Outcome data on programs for street youths are sparse, but many report limited success, particularly with youths who lacked adequate nurturing in early childhood and were maltreated. For example, a study conducted in Seattle in 1986 indicated that only about a third of street youths successfully left the street in a two-year period.[3]

Despite a variety of intervention services, significant numbers of homeless youths persist in dangerous behaviors and unstable living situations. They often appear incapable of change or of availing themselves of resources provided to them. Services are seldom designed to adequately address the sequelae of maltreatment manifested in disrupted developmental progress, basic functioning, and adaptive capacity.

Relatively little attention has been given to the impact of abuse on sensory, motor, and physical development, which underlies more complex social and emotional functioning.[10] Clinical and research literature on abuse and trauma supports the idea that the ongoing problems of homeless youths may be related to the impact abuse has had on their developmental competencies and current coping and functioning skills. It suggests that interventions with adolescents who clearly display social and emotional problems should also address concurrent problems associated with developmental and functional deficits. Thus when the Working Zone program was planned, an occupational therapist was included on the staff to address the developmental issues of youth through both program design and individual evaluation and intervention.

THE SETTING AND THE THEORETICAL FRAMEWORK

The Working Zone is a collaborative project designed to serve the employment needs of homeless youths ages 15 to 22. Funded by the Department of Housing and Urban Development and the Seattle Housing and Human Services Department, it is a project of the University District Youth Center, a drop-in center for homeless youths. Both the youth center and the Working Zone are administered by the Center for Human Services, a private, nonprofit agency in Seattle.

Clients are referred to the Working Zone by case managers in programs serving homeless youths in the Seattle area. The program focuses on developing participants' employability and job skills in order to improve their housing status. Participation in the program is not time limited; some clients leave the program and come back.

The employment program model is based on a developmental, or occupational behavior, frame of reference. Young people are considered to move through a sequence of developmental stages in different areas of human function.[11] Normal development is orderly, predictable, sequential, and cumulative and evolves by building on previous skill acquisitions. Among the important concepts in an occupational behavior orientation are that play experiences are a prerequisite to mature work behavior; that occupational choice is a developmental process; that individuals fill a succession of roles in their lives, including the role of worker; and that skills are interdependent and are achieved in a progression from simple to complex.[11,12]

The ability to work is often seen as a primary indicator of mature adult functioning.[13] Vocational development begins in childhood. A major goal of socialization for children is to develop work attitudes, goals, and behaviors. Youths who have physical, developmental, or emotional disorders often do not develop the foundation of skills necessary for these tasks.

Homeless youths, with their frequent histories of trauma, have generally lacked normal play experiences and have not had control over their environment, which is critical to the human need for mastery. They have found that their basic needs are not met, and they have a poor self-concept and a decreased sense of self-efficacy. A dominant theme for these youths is failure to acquire critical skills that are normally developed in non-abusive homes through the natural developmental process.

Because these youths don't master normal developmental tasks and lack basic competencies, they frequently experience failures, which are often considered their fault or are viewed as resistance or lack of motivation. These developmental deficits lead to other failures, which are compounded by the youths' inability to make decisions in the increasingly complex situations they face.

Expectations for youths at the Working Zone are based on the hierarchical stages of play specified in the occupational behavior approach.[14] In the transition from childhood to adulthood, an individual undergoes the important process of occupational choice: exploration, tentative choice, and realistic definite choice. In the first stage, humans learn how to work through a sequential process beginning in exploratory play, where children are motivated by curiosity and novelty to play, explore objects in the environment, and learn about individual abilities and limitations. The goal of this stage is for individuals to feel safe and supported, discover interests that motivate them to continue engagement in work experiences, and explore the role of worker.

The next stage is skill building, in which an individual practices newly developed work skills, habits, and interpersonal behaviors in an effort to achieve mastery, develop competent work behaviors, and acquire an identity as a worker. In the final stage of occupational choice, the individual interacts with the environment; the emphasis is on meeting standards of quality and production, demonstrating work habits and skills acceptable in a competitive work environment, identifying realistic areas of interest, and moving toward a definitive occupational choice.

Expectations or outcomes for youths at the Working Zone's employment sites follow this same sequence, although youths may enter the program at any of the three vocational stages. The program includes a variety of work opportunities that provide safe, supportive, yet realistic work settings, such as manufacturing ceramic tile mosaics, gardening, producing a newspaper, and street cleaning. They allow youths to explore interests and provide them with the right amount of challenge to develop competency and promote achievement in the worker role.

OCCUPATIONAL THERAPY EVALUATION AND INTERVENTION

In the employment program, the occupational therapist provides both direct and consultative services, making evaluations and designing interventions. Occupational therapy evaluation identifies a youth's current functional status and his or her stage in the developmental sequence. Occupational therapy interventions are then designed to facilitate each youth's step-by-step mastery of the interrelated skills needed to move through the developmental sequence until the level appropriate for the youth's chronological age is reached or until no further development is possible.[15]

Each participant entering the employment program is referred for an occupational therapy evaluation to obtain information about his or her level of vocational development and performance strengths and deficits and to determine whether fuller assessment or intervention is necessary to support the youth's successful performance as a worker. The data collection process consists of an interview, structured clinical observations, administration of the Jacobs Prevocational Skills Assessment (JPSA),[14] an analysis of the data from other team members, and record reviews or acquisition of collateral information when available. The JPSA is a work-related assessment tool developed for adolescents; it consists of a series of structured work tasks designed to assess performance in specific work-related skill areas.

If results of the screening indicate a need for further assessment, additional standardized tests are administered or a job-site analysis of the youth is done. Results of all assessments are analyzed and used as the basis for recommendations for assignment to specific work sites or supervisory strategies. Interventions include adapting the job task or the job's physical and social environment to increase the likelihood that the youth will succeed, teaching the youth compensatory strategies such as asking for a break if frustrated by the task, and using specific skill development strategies to help the youth learn appropriate work skills and interpersonal behaviors.

A Case Study

Jean is a 17-year-old who was living in a shelter and has a sporadic work history. She had been enrolled in a Working Zone gardening employment site before occupational therapy was implemented in the program. Although she appeared motivated to work and earn money in order to maintain housing, she was unable to sustain interest in the work or meet basic expectations for performance, and ultimately she quit.

Several months later, she re-entered the employment program. This time she received an occupational therapy screening, which included an interview, a brief vocational history, and administration of the Jacobs Prevocational Skills Assessment. Results of the JPSA indicated she had multiple performance deficits in the areas of fine motor coordination, eye-hand coordination, attention to detail, problem-solving, organizational skills, ability to follow directions (especially written directions), task focus, and work-related interpersonal skills. She reported significant academic deficits, saying that she had received special education services before dropping out of school. The results of the assessment interview and Jean's vocational history indicated that she had a very strong interest in cooking.

Because Jean was clearly at risk for continued failure in work, additional assessments, including the Quick Neurological Screening Test,[16] were made. The results indicated possible neurological deficits, including deficits in fine and gross motor coordination and balance and in auditory and visual perception and memory. These deficits indicated she required extra time to write or to complete fine motor tasks and to process information and respond. She also demonstrated difficulty with social skills, including initiating and maintaining conversations, and with social problem solving, such as picking up nonverbal cues and understanding social nuances. Among her strengths were cooperativeness, a strong desire to be a cook, consistent work habits, a stable transitional housing placement, and willingness to receive help at the job site.

The occupational therapy evaluation results were used to develop an individualized employment plan. Jean was enrolled in a 12-week training program at a local cooking school. Recommendations were made for how the school's supervisors could increase Jean's chances of succeeding in the program, such as by providing step-by-step directions and demonstrating them, keeping their questions and comments short and direct, requiring only short and simple responses from her, allowing her extra time to complete work tasks, requiring her to pay careful attention to detail or to complex steps, having her repeat or demonstrating correct procedures for her with students who were supportive and friendly.

At this point, at eight weeks, Jean has nearly completed the program. She demonstrates dependability, punctuality, and good attendance; she is able to ask questions when she needs clarification; and she is ready to begin a job search.

Jean is typical of the youths seen in such social service settings in her personal history, her response to services, and other characteristics. If her deficits had not been addresssed, she would have failed in this or any other employment program.

Her case illustrates the importance of integrating occupational therapy theory and practice into the employment program. Jean's stage of vocational development was a transition from skill and habit development to occupational choice. Because she was placed in a job site congruent with her interests, she was able to sustain her motivation. Recommendations for adaptations supervisors could make at the work site to facilitate her performance enabled her to be successful at work.

Conclusions

Assessments and strategies for promoting functional competencies among homeless youth are not generally provided in traditional social service settings. The positive effects of counseling and other services that are offered may not be maintained because they do not address underlying developmental issues.

Developmental lags in the sensorimotor, cognitive, and psychosocial domains mean youths still cannot make decisions, solve problems, or think logically despite our attempts to counsel, feed, clothe, house, and employ them. Occupational therapy offers a unique theoretical perspective as well as interventions and strategies for addressing this gap in services. Occupational therapy provides an additional perspective and resource for addressing the stubborn and perplexing problems of homeless youth. Working in concert with mental health and social work approaches, the occupational therapy practitioner is a significant contributor to this area of social services.

References

1. Boyer D. (1989). Male prostitution and homosexual identity. *Journal of Homosexuality, 17,* 1-4.

2. Boyer D. (Ed). (1988). *In and out of the street life: Readings on the intervention with street youth.* Portland, OR: Tri-County Youth Consortium.

3. Boyer D. (1986). *Street exit project: Final report* (Grant 90-CT-0360 from the Administration for Children, Youth and Families, Department of health and Human Services). Seattle, WA: Youth Care.

4. Janius, M., McCormack, A., Burgess, A., et al. (1987). *Adolescent runaways: Causes and consequences.* Lexington, MA: Lexington Books.

5. McCarthy, B., & Hagan J. (1992). Surviving on the street: The experiences of homeless youth. *Journal of Adolescent Research, 7,* 412-430.

6. McCormack, A., Janus, M., & Burgess, A. (1986). Runaway youths and sexual victimization: Gender differences in an adolescent runaway population. *Child Abuse and Neglect, 10,* 387-395.

7. Stiffman A. (1989). Physical and sexual abuse in runaway youths. *Child Abuse and Neglect, 13,* 417-426.

8. Yates, G., MacKenzie, R., Pembridge, J., et al. (1988). A risk profile of runaway and non-runaway youth. *American Journal of Public Health, 78,* 820-821.

9. Trickett, P., McBride-Chang, C. (1995). The developmental impact of different forms of child abuse and neglect. *Developmental Review, 15,* 311-337.

10. Mosey, A. C. (1981). *Occupational therapy: Configuration of a profession.* New York, NY: Raven.

11. Matsutsuyu, J. (1989). Occupational behaviour approach. In A. S. Allen, P. N. Pratt. (Eds.). *Willard and Spackman's occupational therapy for children.* St. Louis, MO: Mosby.

12. Pratt, P. (1989). School work tasks and vocational readiness. In A. S. Allen & P. N. Pratt. (Eds.), *Occupational therapy for children.* St. Louis, MO: Mosby.

13. Jacons, K. (1991). *Work-related programs for children and adolescents in occupational therapy: Work-related programs and assessments.* Boston, MA: Little, Brown.

14. Creighton, C. (1985). Three frames of reference in work-related occupational therapy programs. *American Journal of Occupational Therapy, 39,* 331-334.

15. Mutti, M., Sterling, H., & Spalding, N. (1978). *Quick neurological screening test.* Novato, CA: Academic Therapy Publications.

CHAPTER THIRTY-SEVEN

Occupational Therapy Interventions for Homeless, Addicted Adults with Mental Illness

Tina Barth

This chapter was previously published in the Mental Health Special Interest Section Newsletter, 17(1), 7-8. *Copyright © 1994, The American Occupational Therapy Association, Inc.*

Now that the mental health provision system in the United States is being reconsidered and reworked, I believe that this is a chance for occupational therapists to expand the use of their skills and training in ways other than direct patient treatment. Many occupational therapists are wonderful at running shelters and day programs, and they are excellent program planners. As systems thinkers, occupational therapists can be valuable to the mental health system.

I work for a private, not-for-profit agency that was founded 23 years ago to help keep homeless, vagrant adults from freezing to death on the streets of the Bowery in New York City. The agency tries hard to have as few qualifying requirements as possible for services. For example, although the continuing day treatment program is designated as a program for persons with mental illnesses and chemical additions, it accepts persons who do not have chemical addictions. A mental illness is a qualifying criterion, and addiction is not an exclusionary criterion. In the alcoholism programs, alcoholism or related problems are qualifying criterion and mental illness is not an exclusionary criteria. The functional capacity as well as diagnosis is considered as grounds for admission.

Clients may also be HIV positive and symptomatic. They may be on probation or parole, or enter the agency as part of alternative sentencing. Some may require detoxification and then mental health services. They may be found in serious distress on the streets, and agency members may work with clients for several months in the streets before convincing them that they could use some services. Clients are also referred from the state and city hospital systems.

The Reception Center and the Alcoholism Crisis Center together form a specialized station for homeless persons. No clients are admitted to the station from institutional settings.

This concept is an experiment in New York state. Part of the station has existed for 14 years as a detoxification program, to sober up persons from alcohol and drugs. It is not a medical facility. If a person undergoing detoxification from a drug exhibits a certain range of symptoms, he or she is transferred to a local hospital. The remainder of the station is a shelter for homeless adults who have mental illness and often are addicted. Because the station is not a medical facility or a program funded by Medicaid, it is available to anyone who meets the admission criteria. The person's fundability is not a consideration at admission. Our population often does not have insurance, identification, or sometimes legal immigration status. The station also services persons who actively avoid all types of institutional settings out of fear of being locked up.

SUCCESSFUL INTERVENTIONS

To understand the basis for successful interventions with homeless adults who are socially disaffiliated and have chronic mental illnesses and addiction, it is necessary to first present three basic ideas: use of the acronym MICA to categorize persons with mental illnesses and chemical addiction, self-trust, and engagement.

First, I dislike the concept of classifying persons as MICA because I believe that clients are cheated with that label. Persons who are fully mentally ill and fully addicted need the complete range of both sets of service integrated properly (Minkoff, 1989). Too often, I have seen clients who need intensive work with their addiction not get it at all or else their teams stop short of any confrontation out of the mistaken belief that persons with a mental illness do not have enough ego strength to tolerate an intervention. When treatment is incomplete, the clients are supported through the emotional crisis but enabled to continue using substances. They are also crippled by the knowledge that there is something wrong, and it is so terrible that even the clinical people cannot discuss it openly. Avoidance leading to strengthened denial becomes the behavioral model (Moyers, 1988).

The second basic idea is self-trust. If someone has a mental illness and addiction, it is extremely important to talk about what the psychotropic medication does for him or her. Why does the person take the medication? What is its effect? When he or she abuses a substance, what is he or she seeking? How useful is it? What are the side effects and the downside of using the substance? It is important to put all of the answers to these questions on the table and to involve the client in looking at them clearly. When a client can admit to a problem, the problem actually exists, and the search for a solution can begin. Clients who take responsibility for their maintenance will begin to see themselves as capable and powerful enough to safely make decisions about their own lives. Often, when clients come to the shelter, they do not believe that this is true. They have been told over and over that they are not capable, that they should just take their medication and perform their activities with no questions. Supporting the questioning and tying it to reality is the basis of helping a client to develop self-trust.

The third idea, engagement, can be summed up in a favorite mental picture that this agency uses with its clients. Staff members tell clients, "When you came to us, you were running away from something that is painful, such as a hurt or loss or great fear. You were looking back over your shoulder and running away from this thing as fast as you could." However, clients are told, if they are successful with treatment, they will come to believe that there is something good in front of them that is worth pursuing and that is attainable. They will have enough trust to turn away from the bad thing behind them, look forward, and move toward the thing that they can have. Soon the hope of attaining that thing will become more important than the fear of what they are running from. This process is known as engagement at this facility because of the belief that real change does not occur and real rehabilitation does not begin until a client is engaged in the hope of recovery based in reality and is confident that he or she is capable of moving forward and looking ahead.

ASSESSING THE CLIENT

The shelter assesses many areas of function in persons with mental illness and addiction. An excellent summary of these assessment concepts was examined in detail by Sandra Watanabe (1968), who based her writings on her experiences as an occupational therapist in the home treatment service of a state hospital.

The first concept is life space, or the actual physical world of the individual person as well as his or her perception of it and emotional reaction to it (Watanabe, 1968, p. 439). In a client who has psychoses, the world view can be narrowed as a defense mechanism, and it is difficult to plan a life without

a broad view of the world. The next concept is mastery, or the ability to conceptualize the life space and use it (p. 440). The hallmark of mastery is coping skills. The third concept is life tasks or personal and social regular activities, including activities of daily living and roles such as job identity (p. 442). A client can be committed to a role as well as get satisfaction from it. Some of our clients will never be employed, but may eventually achieve fairly permanent stipend placement two or three days a week, with the expectation that they will report there on a regular basis as if it were a fully paid job. The last concept is responsibility, the operationalization of self-trust (p. 441). It is the client's ability to select goals that will satisfy him or her and fit within a culture. This is the basis of engagement, which I described earlier.

As an occupational therapist, I can operationalize these concepts, look at the client's functional capacity, and evaluate the living and day programs to which the client may be referred. I can slowly and carefully interview the client and spend time on projects and skill building. This information assists in accurate selection of viable placement options.

WORKING WITH CLIENTS WITH ADDICTIONS

When I was first learning occupational therapy, I was told that my clients would want to consume my services, that they would be happy to be in my company, and that people sought out and used psychiatry voluntarily. In 1976, when I began working with persons with addictions, I realized that this was not true.

It was a question of motivation. The first group I worked with, who had addictions but not mental illnesses, were coerced into treatment. No one was there voluntarily. When I set up a tile project, they picked up the tiles and flipped them at me. I gave them some ice cream sticks to make boxes from, and they snapped the sticks.

People with addictions enter treatment because they have no choice. They are coerced. If they could find a way to continue to use substances and simultaneously get rid of whatever is coercing them (i.e., family members, pain, fear of death), they would.

How is it possible, therefore, to provide consistently successful treatment? The solution lies in the approach. I believe that honesty is the key. At this agent, clients are told that if they want to actively voluntarily participate in putting their lives back together, then the first thing they will need is the full and voluntary use of their physical central nervous system. Because a person who is stoned, high, or withdrawing from drugs does not have full use of his or her sensorium, the first step in treatment must be detoxification or restraint from a particular drug. The same is true with psychotropic medication. Until clients are free from acute physical or mental stress and have the most use of their minds possible, they are really not in the best position to work in their own behalf or to make judgments for themselves.

Clients who are not in a good position for self-care (e.g., a person who has picked up a substance and returned to the shelter) are not allowed to make decisions for themselves. If they wish to stay at the shelter, they stay in-house until they are clean and dry, or they leave and do not come back. Staff members at the shelter explain that unless they have use of their steering equipment, they cannot drive the car. Many of the clients understand this metaphor and are relieved to have the terms put simply, clearly, and practically.

If we are honest, direct, and work on a day-to-day practical level with our clients, we can help them recognize their successes. If we confront their addiction at the same time we also generate hope, then we assist our clients in believing that they can move toward something worthwhile.

ANNA AND THE SLIVER OF SOAP

At the Reception Center shelter, clients are helped to express who they are without socially alienating other members of their own culture. They learn that they can be part of a culture without giving up parts of themselves, as illustrated by Anna and her sliver of soap.

Anna, who appeared to be in her early 50s, used to live on the F train, one of the longest subway lines in New York City. One day, Anna was feeling unwell because she had a bad chest cold. She got off the F train at the Bowery stop, wandered around, and encountered one of our street teams. When Anna was brought to the shelter, she was having conversations with herself.

When technicians and staff members tried to help her take a shower, Anna raised an immense fuss. I could not figure out why she was upset, because she had seemed to be looking forward to washing and getting clean clothes.

The problem was Anna's piece of soap, a sliver that was only about 2 1/2 in. long. She carried it between her breasts and refused to get it wet. She would not part with this little sliver of soap although the technicians offered to give her a whole new bar to keep.

As an occupational therapist and the supervisor on duty, I entered the situation, thinking, "In Anna's life space, what is so special about this sliver of soap? It obviously is not just a sliver of soap because she will not exchange a large bar of soap for it. Well, there is only one way to figure it out. Ask a psychotic woman from the streets who is steaming."

I asked Anna what the soap was, and she told me that she had taken it from her daughter's house the last time she saw her. Anna carried the soap between her breasts because she was busty, and it stayed there securely. The heat of her body made the soap give off a pleasant odor that helped her get through daily life. It comforted and reminded her of her daughter. Her daughter was no longer speaking to her because when Anna was drunk, she would get loud and obnoxious. The daughter finally told Anna that she had had enough, and Anna believed her. This soap was really the last little piece that Anna had of her daughter.

A coping strategy was organized. Staff members gave the soap a new home, in a soap dish box with holes in the bottom. Anna could carry the box around with her and lock it in a locker when she went on day trips or at night. Gradually, Anna left the soap in the locker more often, first overnight, then two or three days in a row. Eventually, she left it permanently.

Before I could understand the whole range of Anna's problems, it was crucial that I first identify and understand what the soap meant to Anna. For me, that process is the essence of occupational therapy.

A professional person who wants to be taken seriously by peers will dress in society's expected costume, a suit and tie or a dress and nylon stockings. When Anna put her sliver of soap in a box, she was taught the equivalent of putting on a suit or nylons and pumps. In other words, she learned how to express who she is and at the same time move through a culture. I believe that because occupational therapists are trained to think about and work on problems of this type, they are excellent choices to assist clients in growing through problems. Such skills could be invaluable if applied to administrative areas in the mental health system of the future.

REFERENCES

Minkoff, K. (1989). An integrated treatment model for dual diagnosis of psychosis and addiction. *Hospital and Community Psychiatry, 40,* 1031-1036.

Moyers, P. A. (1988). An organizational framework for occupational therapy in the treatment of alcoholism. *Occupational Therapy in Mental Health, 8*(2), 27-46.

Watanabe, S. (1968). Four concepts basic to the occupational therapy process. *American Journal of Occupational Therapy, 22,* 439-445.

CHAPTER THIRTY-EIGHT

Occupational Therapy Intervention with Homeless Women

Paula Chaparas Kearney

This chapter was previously published in Occupational Therapy Practice, 2(4), 75-81. Copyright © 1991, Aspen Publishers, Inc.

Connie is 19 years old, extremely paranoid, and has been expelled from numerous shelters because of a tendency to act out violently. When first approached by occupational therapists at the Dinner Program for Homeless Women in Washington, DC, Connie was reluctant to join the occupational therapy group. Consequently, she was provided with a craft activity to work on in her own space. She would approach the therapists when she had a question or required more supplies. Eventually, Connie was able to join in group activities, initially sitting on the periphery and later becoming an active, integrated member of the group. Connie is one of a growing number of homeless women who could benefit from receiving occupational therapy services.

This (chapter) describes a generic program designed to meet the needs of homeless women who attended a dinner program. There are many opportunities for occupational therapists interested in working with homeless people in general and homeless women in particular. These opportunities exist no matter what the area of practice specialization. The needs of this population span all ages and are physical as well as psychological and social in nature. This (chapter) also describes a model for inclusion of this type of experience into occupational therapy curricula.

Unlike the traditional notion of the skidrow, middle-aged or elderly male alcoholic or the "crazy" bag lady, homeless people constitute a heterogeneous group with varied factors leading to their homeless status and different needs as a population.[1-6] Families, most of them headed by women, are increasingly in the ranks of the homeless population. This trend is expected to continue.[7] The "feminization of poverty" is a recent phenomenon that has received much attention. Many homeless women report leaving their homes secondary to domestic violence, including wife battering and sexual abuse.[8] Studies suggest that factors leading to homelessness include lack of housing, unemployment and poverty, deinstitutionalization, and domestic violence and abuse.[5] Substance abuse is also a major factor leading to homelessness.

Estimates of the prevalence of mental illness in the homeless population vary. These estimates range from a low of 15% to a high of 90%.[4] Women currently comprise two thirds of the chronically mentally ill population in the United States.[9] Yet there is a paucity of research regarding the service needs of mentally ill women. Additionally, many programs base their treatment of women on societal stereotypes:

Rehabilitative programs often encourage women to assume relatively dependent roles and to be either unemployed or employed in such domestic pursuits as housecleaning and babysitting.... By contrast, programs for men tend to focus on their eventual readiness for competitive employment.[9(p9)]

In a drop-in center for homeless people gender-related role expectations were described by Strasser:

No services were asked from women, although cooperation with procedures was expected.... [Men] were often expected to contribute some service as well as to follow routine. Women not only entered for meals ahead of all men, sick, injured, or well, but occasionally women who arrived late for meals were served, while men would be turned away if late. The service is regarded... as "lady's privilege".[(9p9)]

As professionals who are concerned with adaptive role assumption, occupational therapists may be instrumental in decreasing the bias in the delivery of psychiatric services to mentally ill homeless women.

The homeless have varied needs. A study by Breakey et al[5] on homeless men and women in Baltimore showed a high incidence of psychiatric and medical disorders in this population. Grunberg and Eagle described a processor "shelterization," which is a result of shelter living. This shelterization, similar to institutionalization, is marked "by a decrease in interpersonal responsiveness, a neglect of personal hygiene, increasing passivity, and increasing dependency on others."[10(p525)] The authors stated "that many of the homeless lack the most basic social skills. They cannot manage their money or entitlements and cannot take care of simple personal needs (haircuts, laundry, food preparation)." [10(p525)] What discipline is better suited to address these areas? Different interventions are appropriate for different situations. The mentally ill homeless have different needs from the situationally homeless.

SETTING

The Dinner Program for Homeless Women is housed in a church in Washington, DC. Volunteers prepare dinner for the women. The doors open at 4:00 PM, and dinner is served at 6:00. The program was designed to provide the women who attend with meaningful structured activity in the time before dinner. The women who attend the program are representative of the heterogeneity of the homeless population. They come from all walks of life, are all ages, and have varying degrees of psychiatric pathology. This program was coordinated by the cochairs of the Mental Health Special Interest Section of the District of Columbia Occupational Therapy Association with the thought that this would be an effective means to meet the state association goal of increasing the visibility of occupational therapy in the community while providing valuable service to a needy population.

The cochairperson decided that it would be feasible to provide occupational therapy services once a week. Initially, members of the state association were used to staff the program. Gradually, occupational therapy students from Howard University in Washington, DC, were used to assist. This enabled the students to become enlightened about the critical need experienced by and the vast rewards of servicing this population.

PROGRAM

In application of the Model of Human Occupation[11] to the population of homeless women, one can observe potential deficit in each of the performance subsystems. The volitional subsystem consists of personal causation, valued goals, and interests. Although many of these women have valued goals and interests, personal causation is of particular concern with this population. Personal causation refers to the belief that one "has skills that she can use effectively, that she is personally in control, and that she will succeed in the future in whatever she chooses to do."[12(p148)]

Homeless women are seldom presented with the opportunity to anticipate successful outcomes to their actions. In fact, the opposite is more likely. Environmental factors such as lengthy application forms and the need for a mailing address often present bureaucratic barriers and closed doors to any attempt to alleviate their homeless status.

The habituation subsystem consists of the internalized roles and habit patterns that constitute being homeless. The primary occupational role becomes that of surviving in the streets. Habits are based on survival and the availability of community resources. For example, a homeless woman's daily schedule may begin when she is told she has to leave a shelter in the morning. She may then go to a park for a couple hours until a soup kitchen opens for lunch. After lunch, she may wander the streets until the dinner program opens in the evening. She may then enter a warm store until a shelter opens in the evening, only to repeat this sequence in the morning.

The performance subsystem is often significantly deficient in this population. Many homeless women have numerous skill deficits in the areas of motor, process, and communication performance. These deficiencies may, in fact, have led to the women's homeless status in the first place. This program was designed primarily to address this area. It is hoped that once the skills are developed or compensated for, successful habituation of a productive role may be accomplished. Once productive roles are established, a sense of personal causation may be achieved.

In attempting to devise an occupational therapy program that would best meet the needs and match the goals and interests of this diverse population, the therapists designed a survey to determine the interests of the women who attended the program. The survey was distributed to willing participants. If a woman was unable to read, the survey was read to her. The survey results showed that the women would be most interested in participating in craft activities.

As noted in an earlier publication,[13] there were specific criteria for the selected activities. Each activity was intended to be time limited, to provide a success experience, to provide a useful end product, and to enhance interaction and expression of emotion.

Due to the transient nature of this population, the composition of the group could be entirely different on any given week from the previous week. Therefore, each activity should be able to be completed in one group session.

A success experience is particularly important when working with this population. When one considers the numerous frustrations and failures experienced by this group of people, the ability to provide someone with the opportunity to feel masterful can be significant.

Providing a useful end product allows group members to retain evidence of their ability to be effective. This is also a population that generally does not own many material possessions. Examples of useful crafts include leather change purses and belts, pomanders to keep personal belongings smelling fresh, articles that can be given as gifts, or items such as centerpieces for the tables at the dinner program.

Activity should enhance interaction and expression of emotion. Women in this setting tend to be withdrawn and often sit by themselves with little interaction. When engaged in an activity that encourages interaction, they often brighten, become less suspicious of each other, and recognize each other as a source of support. For example, when engaged in a Valentine's day project, the group was faced with the decision of what type of banner they wanted to make to decorate the facility. The group decided that they would cut hearts out of felt and write the name of someone important to them. The names on the banner ranged from those of rock stars to those of children who were no longer in their custody. The discussion that ensued was significant, with many of the group members realizing they had much in common and offering their support to one another.

Activities were generally conducted in one of two formats. The activity was either a group project, in which group members worked together on a common task, or the activity was parallel, with group members working on separate individual tasks.

Group tasks were effective in fostering interaction and the ability to collaborate effectively with others and in increasing trust in each other. Examples of successful group tasks included holiday decorations and banners; making toys for needy children; and nail care, in which the participants manicured each other's nails. Group tasks can serve practical purposes such as enhancing facility appearance while providing concrete evidence of the group's ability to work together in a constructive manner.

Parallel activities enabled participants to make something of their own in which they could take pride. They could keep the end product of their effort, give it away as a gift, or use it at the facility. Discussion may center around the common experience of the group members, what the participants plan to do with the completed project, what skills are required to work on the project, and what feelings were experienced while engaged in the activity. Examples of successful activities of this nature include making and mailing greeting cards, making jewelry, and making decorative items to serve as centerpieces for the facility.

PROGRAM GOALS

The program goals directly relate to function in the community. These goals are the building blocks that lead to adaptive role function. Program goals include: (1) to increase a sense of trust in others, (2) to develop a sense of competence and mastery over the environment, (3) to decrease isolation and to facilitate appropriate interpersonal interaction, (4) to practice basic task skills, (5) to generalize skills practiced in this setting out in the community.[13(p6)]

1. Increasing a sense of trust in others is of particular importance with this population. When one considers the victimization experienced by many of the women, it is not surprising that trust would be an issue. Not only have many of the women fled from violence at home, but they also are vulnerable to violence on the streets. Group activities may foster a sense of trust in health care providers and encourage trust in each other. Establishing a sense of trust is important because if one does not trust others, one will never be able to reach out for assistance or make contacts to attain gainful employment.

2. Developing a sense of competence and mastery over the environment is a gradual process. A lifetime of adversity and frustration is not quickly undone. Therefore, the ability to complete a leather belt, work effectively as a group member, or socialize appropriately with another person can be significant.

3. Decreased isolation and appropriate interaction occurred naturally when the women were involved in the activities. The isolation that was prevalent in this setting was remarkable. The women who attended the program frequently sat by themselves, or if they sat at a group table there was little interaction. Much of the interaction that did occur was inappropriate. Many of the women were intrusive or delusional or actively responding to internal stimuli. When in a group setting, social skills can be modeled and practiced. Group members are forced to interact by nature of the group setting and shared materials.

4. Basic task skills may be practiced in this setting. These skills include the prevocational skills that are necessary for appropriate job functioning. Some of these skills are maintaining attention and concentration, dealing with frustration, and fine and gross motor skills.

5. Finally, through participation in this program, the skills practiced in this setting may be generalized into the community. Many of the women who participated in the occupational therapy groups went on to provide assistance with the meal preparation. Perhaps from there it was possible to receive job training or apply for a position. Although engaging in a therapeutic craft group may not place the women directly into gainful employment or locate suitable housing for them, it is important not to underestimate the impact that such an experience may have. This population often experiences failure and frustration in the community and frequently rejects assistance from health care professionals. Therefore, it is important to acknowledge the steps that lead to the ability to gain the confidence to make a telephone inquiry about a job or complete a housing application. Hopefully, this program enabled some of its participants to take that step into the mainstream of society.

INCORPORATION INTO OCCUPATIONAL THERAPY CURRICULA

Exposing students to the experience of providing occupational therapy services in community settings with underserved populations serves a two-fold purpose. Valuable community service is provided while enlightening future occupational therapists to the rewarding and challenging opportunities that exist in the community. Additionally, this experience may be used to explore the importance of having empathy in dealing with occupational therapy clients. Providing occupational therapy services in the community should by necessity be a requirement for occupational therapy curricula if the discipline is to keep up with the trend of community health care delivery. By exposing students to this experience, occupational therapists serve their profession. Hopefully, through exposure to unconventional community practice areas, occupational therapy students will proactively identify new frontiers for practice in the future. The following model

Table 38-1

Course Objectives: Community-Based Health Care

1. Recognize the impact of cultural factors, attitudes, motivation, and personality structure on role behavior.

2. Recognize the role of prevention in maintaining a balance of self care, work, and leisure.

3. Recognize the impact of socioeconomic, political, and cultural systems on health across the developmental spectrum, particularly as they affect minority and underserved populations.

4. Demonstrate effective interpersonal skills, interactions with clients, peers, supervisors, and other professionals.

5. Demonstrate knowledge of theoretical approaches related to activity, performance, and adaptation.

6. Develop a plan identifying the approach, method, and environmental changes to maximize performance.

7. Demonstrate instructional skills in teaching activities to clients.

8. Recognize and use nonverbal cues effectively in interpersonal and group interaction.

9. Define and prioritize clinical problems.

10. Demonstrate awareness of body language and identify ways to use it when interacting with peers, patients, and colleagues.

11. Demonstrate effective listening skills with patients and colleagues.

12. Demonstrate understanding of the advocacy process as it affects health care legislation and the access of individuals to health care.

13. Demonstrate a commitment to advocacy for underserved populations—the poor, the homeless, and other marginal groups of people.

Source: Course objectives from Community-Based Health Care, Howard University, Washington, DC, Prof. Sally Hobbs Jackson, Fall 1988.

illustrates how an experience such as this was incorporated into an occupational therapy curriculum.

Initially, occupational therapy students from Howard University became involved with the Dinner Program for Homeless Women as a student association project. This involvement evolved into two courses at the junior and senior level entitled "Community Based Health Care" and "Special Problems in Occupational Therapy." Both of these courses incorporated the experience of assisting with occupational therapy groups at the dinner program as part of the course requirement. Course objectives for the senior-level course may be found in Table 38-1. These objectives are pertinent goals for future occupational therapists, regardless of what area of practice is selected. This setting provided an opportunity to practice these skills and receive feedback from clinicians while providing a valuable community service.

Initially, the students appeared overwhelmed by the experience. They were hesitant to approach the women and required encouragement to do so. However, once the students had experienced one occupational therapy group, they generally appeared more comfortable in this setting. Many of the students expressed increased empathy and interest in working with this population. The following quote is from a paper by one of the students enrolled in one of these courses:

This experience sensitized me to the individuals beneath the bulky coats and the shopping bags and to some of the stresses they live with day to day. For instance, they are often fatigued and are in constant danger. I am more aware of the fact that homeless people do not share the simplicities in life that I take for granted. In addition, I am also more concerned about homeless people and the quality of their life and the fact that they are growing in number every day.

Experiences such as this should be incorporated into more occupational therapy academic programs. For it is through service to the needy that one attains empathy. This is also an opportunity to educate the general public about the merits of occupational therapy. Those who might not otherwise have had any exposure to occupational therapy may have an opportunity to experience the virtue of this discipline in the community and observe its value in a multitude of settings with many varied populations.

Many opportunities exist for occupational therapists in all areas of specialization to provide treatment to the growing population of homeless women. Services may be designed to enhance motor, cognitive, social, parenting, vocational, or community living skills. As a discipline that focuses on skill development and adaptive role function, occupational therapy can provide a unique service to this population. Occupational therapists need to proactively identify such populations for the discipline to thrive in the future.

References

1. Belcher, J. R. (1988). Are jails replacing the mental health system for the homeless mentally ill? *Commun Ment Health J, 24,* 185-195.

2. Belcher, J. R. (1988). Defining the service needs of homeless mentally ill persons. *Hosp Commun Psychiatry, 39,* 1203-1205.

3. Belcher, J. R. (1989). The homeless mentally ill and the need for a total care environment. *Can J Psychiatry, 34,* 186-189.

4. Belcher, J. R., & DiBlasio, F. A. (1990). The needs of depressed homeless persons: Designing appropriate services. *Commun Ment Health J, 26,* 255-265.

5. Breakey, W. R., Fischer, P. J., Kramer, M., et al. (1989). Health and mental health problems of homeless men and women in Baltimore. *JAMA, 262,* 1352-1357.

6. Santiago, J. M., Bachrach, L. L., Berren, M. R., Hannah, M. T. (1988). Defining the homeless mentally in a methodological note. *Hosp Commun Psychiatry, 39,* 1100-1102.

7. Hagen, J. L. (1987). Gender and homelessness. *Social Work, 32,* 312-516.

8. Stoner, M. R. (1983). The plight of homeless women. *Sac Seru Rev, 57,* 565-581.

9. Strasser, J. (1988). Overview of service delivery issues. In L. L. Bachrach, & C. Nadeison. *Treating chronically mentally ill women.* Washington, DC: American Psychiatric Press.

10. Grunberg, J. & Eagle, P. F. (1990). Shelterization: How the homeless adapt to shelter living. *Hosp Commun Psychiatry, 41,* 521-525.

11. Bruce, M. A. & Borg, B. (1987). Occupational behavior frames of reference. *Frames of Reference in Psychosocial Occupational Therapy.* Thorofare, NJ: SLACK Incorporated.

12 Oakley, F., Kielhofner, G., & Barris, R. (1985). An occupational therapy approach to assessing psychiatric patients adaptive functioning. *Am J Occup Ther, 39,* 147-154.

13. Del Vecchio, A. L. & Keamey, P. C. (1990). Homeless women's dinner program: Adapting traditional interventions to a nontraditional environment. *Ment Health Spec Int Sect Newsl, 13,* 2-4.

CHAPTER THIRTY-NINE

Domestic Violence: Implications and Guidelines for Occupational Therapy Practitioners

Christine A. Helfrich

Occupational therapists treat victims of domestic violence in many different settings. Often, the therapist is not aware that her client has been touched by domestic violence. This may be due to not understanding what domestic violence is, or not knowing how to look for it. Some therapists may even question if it is appropriate for occupational therapists to treat victims of domestic violence. The focus of this chapter will be to present why it is not only appropriate, but absolutely necessary, to recognize and treat survivors of domestic violence. At the conclusion of the this chapter the reader will be able to:

1. Define domestic violence
2. Understand the scope of the problem of domestic violence
3. Describe how to screen for domestic violence
4. Identify how to intervene with survivors of domestic violence
5. Describe the role of occupational therapy

WHAT IS DOMESTIC VIOLENCE?

Legal definitions of domestic violence vary from state to state; however, most definitions incorporate similar information. Readers should consult their state's Domestic Violence Act for a complete definition. For the purposes of this chapter the following definition will be used:

Domestic violence is any act carried out with the intention of physically or emotionally harming another person who is related to you by blood, present/prior marriage or common-law marriage, having (or having had) a child in common, or having (or having had) a dating relationship. This also includes a person with a disability and their personal assistant. Domestic violence includes physical abuse, sexual abuse, emotional abuse, economic abuse, destruction of property or pets, and stalking. (Illinois Domestic Violence Act of 1986)

This definition includes partner abuse, elder abuse, child abuse, and abuse of individuals with a disability by their personal assistant who is not a relative. It is beyond the scope of this chapter to address each type of abuse as the dynamics of partner, elder, child, and disabled abuse differ; however, much of the information will be applicable to all groups. Unless otherwise indicated, this chapter will consider the domestic violence victim to be an adult female and the perpetrator to be an adult male.

As described in the definition there are six types of domestic abuse.

- *Physical Abuse* includes hitting, punching, kicking, biting, being thrown or tied down, choking, smothering, burning, threatening to use a weapon, refusing to help her when she is sick or injured, or driving recklessly to frighten her.
- *Emotional Abuse* includes verbal abuse, intimidation, threats, isolation, restricting her activities, humiliation, insults, ignoring her needs, lying, or breaking promises.
- *Sexual Abuse* includes forcing her to have sex, hurting her during sex, using weapons intravaginally, orally, or anally, coercing her to have sex without protection, criticizing her sexually, or flaunting extra-marital affairs.
- *Economic Abuse* includes taking her money, keeping her from getting or keeping a job, or making her ask for money.
- *Destruction of Property or Pets* includes breaking property or her favorite objects, hurting or killing her pets or giving away objects.
- *Stalking* includes following her, placing her under surveillance, or any conduct which places her in reasonable apprehension of immediate or future bodily harm, sexual assault, confinement, or restraint.

The types of abuse described indicate a continuum of behaviors and actions that may not always be indicative of abuse. In every relationship there are disagreements and quarrels. Who defines what abuse is? The general rule is to allow the woman to define whether or not an act is abusive. The health care practitioner's role is to educate the woman regarding the legal definition of abuse and inform her of legal and practical options (Sassetti, 1993). She must then make a decision of what she will do based on the information she has been given. The victim of abuse only has to experience one type of abuse to be identified as a victim and protected under her state's domestic violence act. At the end of this chapter the legal and ethical implications for the occupational therapist will be discussed.

WHO ARE THE VICTIMS OF DOMESTIC VIOLENCE?

The only risk factor for becoming a victim of domestic violence is being female (Sassetti, 1993). In 95% of domestic violence cases the woman is the victim. Contrary to many myths and stereotypes, domestic violence is not partial to demographics, age, socioeconomic status, race, or ethnicity. However, there are several events that occur in a woman's life that place her at higher risk for becoming a victim of abuse (American Medical Association, 1992). These include:
- History of being abused as a child
- Beginning cohabitation with a partner
- Legally marrying
- Pregnancy (Increases the risk by 25%!)
- Separation from military service (self or partner)
- Loss of a job (self or partner)
- New signs of independence by the woman (i.e., new job, return to school, graduation from school)
- Separation or divorce

Each of these life events threatens the status quo of the current relationship. This may require a renegotiation of roles between partners, which is the dynamic believed to increase the risk for abuse. In most abusive relationships the partner has a strong need to be in control. His control is in jeopardy during times of change in the relationship. The woman's risk of being abused does not end when she leaves the relationship. In fact, she is at most risk for being killed after she has left her abusive partner (Russell, 1995).

In addition to the direct victims of domestic violence, (the actual target or recipient of abuse), there are also indirect victims. Indirect victims are those individuals who have witnessed the abuse of another family member or whose lives are directly impacted by the abuse of a family member. This includes children who were present while their mother was being abused. The children may encounter psychological (depression) or behavioral (aggression) effects or they may be affected by the decisions that are made as a result of the abuse (loss of custody). In order to escape the abusive relationship the family may need to go into a shelter or move away. The child is forced to change schools, meet new friends, lose or change their contact with the other parent, and adapt to a new environment and lifestyle. While this is occurring, the child is trying to integrate a myriad of feelings and experiences with a mother who is doing the same to adjust to the effects of the violence.

WHAT ARE THE EFFECTS OF DOMESTIC VIOLENCE?

Domestic violence has both short- and long-tem effects on the individual and her children. Short-term effects of domestic violence may include emotional or physical injury or disability, interference with role function, economic difficulty and homelessness. Long-term effects may include continued physical or mental disability, loss of role identity, loss of family ties and support systems, loss of employment, homelessness, and in the most severe cases death may ultimately occur. Most studies looking at the medical effects of domestic violence only address the immediate, acute effects; studies that explore the long-term consequences related to disability are needed.

SCOPE AND RELEVANCE OF DOMESTIC VIOLENCE AS A HEALTH PROBLEM

Up to 4 million women are abused each year with as many as 2 million suffering serious injury and 2,000 to 4,000 suffering death at the hands of their husbands, boyfriends, or former partners (Keller, 1996). Research indicates that domestic violence may be the leading cause of injury to women, resulting in more injuries that require medical intervention than rape, automobile accidents, and muggings combined (Council on Ethical and Judicial Affairs, AMA, 1992). These statistics have led to the identification of violence as a public health epidemic.

Within the larger problem of violence and injury are trends of special concern. These include domestic violence against women and children, abuse of the elderly, and abuse and neglect of those with a disability. While no accurate estimate of the scale of domestic violence is available, imputations based on available evidence suggest a problem of considerable magnitude. For example, approximately half of all homicides involve individuals known to each other (Reiss & Roth, 1993) and abuse is the leading cause of death among infants and children (Peterson & Brown, 1994). According to the National Crime Victimization Survey, approximately three-fourths of all violent events (e.g., rapes and assaults) involve an intimate or relative (U.S. Department of Justice, 1994). Injury is more likely to be sustained when assault involves an intimate, underscoring that domestic battery is a major vector for injury among women (Rosenberg & Mercy, 1991). Women, children, and the elderly appear to be at heightened risk for violent injury and a principal dynamic appears to be domestic abuse (U.S. Department of Justice, 1997). The Centers for Disease Control (CDC) estimated that 34% of American women are assaulted each year. (CDC, 1993).

Studies indicate that approximately 30% of all women who visit emergency rooms have injuries related to on-going partner abuse (Abbott, et al., 1995; Dearwater, et al., 1998; Centers for Disease Control and Prevention, 1993). Of these battered women using emergency rooms, only 5% have been identified by staff as victims of domestic violence (Goldberg & Tomlanovich, 1984; Randall, 1990).

There are a number of reasons why battered women have gone unidentified. Studies have divided the reasons into three general areas: a) health care providers' reluctance to screen for domestic violence, b) women's reluctance to disclose domestic violence, and c) lack of staff training for how to screen for domestic violence.

Reluctance to Screen for Domestic Violence

Health care providers have offered a wide range of impediments to identification of abuse. There has been a tradition within the health care system of interpreting domestic violence as a private matter, or a "taboo topic" (Hoff, 1992; Keller, 1996). Many professionals also hold the belief that battered women may be masochistic, and fall into a pattern of "blaming the victim" (Gremillion & Kanof, 1996; Holtz & Furniss, 1993; Keller, 1996).

Providers may also label victims as "difficult patients" when they appear to be passive, hostile, anxious, depressed, hysterical, or engaging in substance abuse (Holtz & Furniss, 1993; Kurz, 1987). Providers are more likely to respond to a battered woman when they see the woman as a "true victim," for example, a woman with a pleasant personality who claims to be taking action to leave the violent relationship (Kurz, 1987). Health care professionals also report that the identification and referral of battered women involves too much of their time and, because they may underestimate the prevalence of abuse, they may not look at it as a worthwhile investment of time (Gremillion & Kanof, 1996). Becoming involved with an abused patient may have a psychological impact on the providers, especially if they have been involved in partner or spousal abuse themselves (Gremillion & Kanof, 1996; Quillian, 1996). Other reasons why health care professionals fail in identification may be a concern over offending the patient, a feeling of powerlessness to respond, a fear of being involved with the law, concern over misidentification, and a reluctance to not see domestic violence as a medical issue (Ferris, 1994; Neufield, 1996).

Women's Reluctance to Disclose Domestic Violence

Women also may fail to spontaneously self-disclose a history of abuse for numerous underlying psychological, social, and institutional reasons. Abused women may fear bodily harm or death from the perpetrator if they disclose the abuse.

Many abused women also present with psychological vulnerability and low self-esteem and may be embarrassed or ashamed of the abusive situation (Rodriguez, et al., 1996). Abused women may feel a sense of family responsibility, fulfilling the traditional gender role of protecting the spouse, and fearing intervention in the family by the authorities. The perceived and real difficulties of single parenthood and economic insecurity may also be reasons why abused women do not identify themselves. Many battered women may not self-identify themselves as abused because they do not understand the definition of domestic violence (Keller, 1996; Rodriguez, et al., 1996).

Staff Untrained to Screen for Domestic Violence

A significant reason why many professionals do not appropriately identify these women is a lack of knowledge and training regarding domestic violence (Neufield, 1996). Training in domestic violence and in how to make routine inquiries to determine probable domestic violence is still rare in health care settings, even those that tend to see high proportions of women experiencing abuse (Keller, 1996).

Although most existing domestic violence data are derived from emergency department studies, these studies may not present a representative sample of the general population of battered women (Sugg & Inui, 1992). Victims of domestic violence also seek services in primary care clinics and physician's offices. Battered women account for 14% to 28% of women attending primary care clinics (Gin, Rucker, et al 1991; Rath, et al., 1989). Women who are abused visit their primary care physician more often than women who are not abused (Elliot & Johnson, 1995). Cases seen in these settings most often do not involve recent physical trauma but rather present with stress-related illnesses and complaints such as chronic pain, sleep disturbances, frequent headaches, and abdominal and gynecologic problems (Koss, et al., 1991). It is of note that most research in medical settings has taken place in urban emergency departments where poor, minority populations are likely to go for primary care. This may inflate the prevalence of domestic violence for minority groups (Holtz & Furniss, 1993).

Occupational therapists are also reluctant to identify or work with victims of domestic violence. Consistent with the literature on other health care providers, Johnston (1998) found that occupational therapists' knowledge about domestic abuse correlated directly with their attitudes about occupational therapy's role with victims. In a study of over 200 practicing occupational therapists, Johnston (1998) found that therapists were able to correctly answer only 65% of basic knowledge questions related to the identification and treatment of domestic violence victims. Sixty-eight percent of therapist respondents stated that did not feel adequately prepared to identify victims of domestic abuse. However, 88% indicated that they have a low acceptance of violence towards women, which is a finding consistent with occupational therapy's code of ethics. The individual therapist's level of knowledge about wife abuse was directly correlated to the degree of caring attitude they expressed about victims of abuse and to their views about the role that occupational therapy should have with victims of abuse. Other factors that contributed to more knowledge of abuse or a more positive attitude towards working with abuse victims included being female, being abused as a child, or receiving formal instruction regarding domestic abuse. These factors are consistent with studies of attitudes of other health care professionals. The level of education received by occupational therapists regarding wife abuse was very low. Only 35% reported having received any formal instruction on this topic. Each reader of this text will be contributing to a change in the field of occupational therapy where more practitioners are informed about domestic violence.

IDENTIFICATION OF VICTIMS OF DOMESTIC ABUSE

Cycle of Violence

Women who are in abusive relationships experience a range of experiences with their partners. This range has been described by Lenore Walker (1994), in her classic text *The Battered Woman*, as the Cycle of Violence. The Cycle of Violence has three phases.

- *Phase 1: Tension Building.* During this phase there is arguing, blaming, and tension in the relationship.
- *Phase 2: Battering.* This is the phase where the violence actually occurs. The violence may include physical violence such as slapping, choking, kicking, use of weapons, sexual abuse, and verbal threats and abuse.
- *Phase 3: Contrition.* This is the calm period after the abuse where the abuser denies the violence, apologizes, provides gifts or special treatment to the victim, and promises the abuse will not occur again.

This cycle represents a pattern of behavior that repeats itself. Each phase repeats, changing in relevant emphasis and severity over time. The battering phase will occur more frequently and phase of contrition will be of shorter duration. In other words, as time goes on the battering increases in severity and occurs more frequently. The other phases may still occur but will lose their emphasis in the life of the relationship. This is why intervention with victims of domestic violence must occur. If the cycle is not interrupted, it is likely to eventually result in death. Intervention is most likely to be effective immediately after the battering phase. At that time the woman's defenses are down and she feels most vulnerable. She is most aware of the impact of violence on her ability to function. As she moves into the contrition phase she begins to feel stronger and more supported by her partner and may have more difficulty identifying the abuse as a problem. This difficulty will be discussed further under the heading "Reasons Women Stay in Abusive Relationships."

Physical Indicators of Abuse

In most cases the women seen in occupational therapy who are victims of domestic abuse will be there for other reasons. Therefore, it is important, not only to know what questions to ask to screen for victimization, but also, to know what visible signs to look for. Common physical indicators of abuse include (King & Ryan, 1989; Moss & Taylor, 1991):

- *Bruises* in unusual places (back of the arm or on the breasts) or at various stages of healing indicating a repetitive pattern of injury.
- *Burns* caused by cigarettes, ropes, or "dry burns" caused by irons or stoves, particularly in unusual places (the back) or of prolonged severity.
- *Lacerations* to the facial area (lips, eyes) or genitals.
- *Orthopedic injuries* that do not fit the individual's developmental level or explanation (spiral fracture to the arm explained by falling down stairs).
- *Head & facial injuries* such as subdural hematomas (caused by shaking or hitting), absence of hair, retinal and jaw injuries.
- *Internal injuries* including injury to an unborn fetus caused by external trauma to the stomach area.

Occupational therapists are often in a position to see these physical indicators because of the nature of their relationships with clients. Occupational therapy evaluates what a person can *do*, not just what they *say they can do*. Therefore, in the course of evaluating a woman's ability to complete activities of daily living, she is more likely to visibly expose injuries that would not be visible to a social worker, asking about her discharge plans. The occupational therapist, upon seeing an unusual injury, is challenged by what to do with that information. It is common to dismiss an injury or bruise as insignificant or not out of the ordinary. Many of the injuries listed above could also occur through accidents. So, how does the occupational therapist decide if the injury warrants further exploration? The following questions may help to clarify the therapist's level of concern about the possibility that an injury is abuse-related:

- Is the type of injury consistent with the explanation of the cause? (Black eyes don't usually occur from running into a wall.)
- Is there a central pattern to the injuries? (Torso, breasts)
- Are there bruises that are in various stages of healing? (Bruises change color over a period of time.)
- Is the woman trying to keep the injury hidden? (Wearing long sleeves in the summer to cover up lacerations on her arm.)
- Does the woman become dismissive or defensive when questioned about the injury? ("It's nothing." Or "It was just an accident!")
- Is the injury consistent with the woman's developmental level?

Psychological and Behavioral Indicators

It is difficult to identify psychological and behavioral indicators of abuse. Part of the difficulty arises from the fact that the indicators are often the same as the effects of domestic abuse on one's psychosocial functioning described earlier such as guilt, self-doubt, denial, fear, dissociation, anger, shame, and helplessness (Stark & Flitcraft, 1996). These indicators may also be present in women who have suffered other types of psychological trauma. In order to avoid errant labeling of women, the occupational therapist is encouraged to ask questions directly leading to understanding if abuse has played a role in the life of the individual. One way to think about how to assess the role of abuse in someone's life is to frame questions around the Model of Human Occupation (Kielhofner, 1995). Using the Model of Human Occupation as a guiding framework, questions are recommended in the following domains:

1. Environment
   - Safety of physical and social environment
   - Physical and social supports
   - Physical and social threats

2. Roles
   - Past and current roles
   - Desired future roles
   - Impediments to role fulfillment
   - Supports for role fulfillment

3. Habits
   - Amount of daily structure
   - How is daily structure determined?
   - Desired changes to daily structure

4. Volition
   - Sense of internal control
   - Belief in skills
   - Self-appraisal of skills
   - Values related to independence and parenting
   - Interests which are independent from the abusive partner
   - Interests which the woman has been unable to pursue

5. Mind/Brain/Body Performance Subsystem
   - Skills needed for functional performance independent of partner
   - Physical or cognitive impediments to leaving abusive partner

Direct Questions About Abuse

After trust has been established with the woman, the therapist is in a better position to question her directly about her experiences with abuse. The therapist can then ask directly if the woman is being abused, what type of abuse is occurring, and how she feels about her situation. It is not uncommon for a woman to deny being abused and then minutes later to disclose that her partner "pushes her around" once in awhile. This doesn't necessarily mean that the woman is *deliberately* denying that she has been abused. Instead, it often indicates

a lack of knowledge on her part that the behaviors she is describing are abusive. Women who were raised in abusive homes may not identify behaviors as abusive because they are experienced as normative to her. For these reasons, it is often not useful to initially ask a woman if she is being "abused." Focusing questions around being safe or being threatened may result in clearer answers.

In any area of practice the therapist must consider who else is present when questions regarding safety or abuse are being asked. Questions must never be asked in front of the person suspected of being the abuser. Asking questions in front of the abuser may place the woman at greater risk for being abused further. Even if she denies the abuse, the abuser may accuse her of leading the therapist to ask her about it. In some settings, such as home health, finding a place to speak confidentially will be very difficult. The occupational therapist may need to be creative in order to create a context in which she can speak to the woman privately.

HOW TO RESPOND TO ABUSED WOMEN

One of the primary reasons that occupational therapists and other health care providers are reluctant to ask about abuse is that they don't know what they will do with the information once they get it (Johnston, 1998). How the therapist responds to a disclosure of domestic abuse has legal, ethical, and practical implications. There are several levels on which to respond to the knowledge that a patient or client is a victim of domestic abuse, which range from direct treatment of the abused woman to providing referrals to other health care providers.

- *Mandatory Reporting:* Some states have mandatory reporting laws. The laws range from the need to report suspected abuse to those that only require reporting in cases where a deadly weapon was used. Each reader should consult the Domestic Violence Act and Occupational Therapy Practice Act of his/her own state.

- *Provide Information:* Occupational therapists have an ethical responsibility to inform women of their treatment options. This would include options for maintaining the safety needed to pursue treatment. Therapists should be aware of local domestic violence crises line numbers. Therapists should also be able to direct women or assist them with obtaining basic information on safety and the availability of resources to her and her children. The National Domestic Violence Hotline number is 1-800-799-SAFE (7233).

- *Inform Treatment Team Members:* The therapist should ask the woman who else she has disclosed her abuse to. If the occupational therapist is the first person to whom she is disclosing, the therapist should encourage the woman to disclose to other members of the treatment team. If she refuses to do so, the therapist must handle this information like any other medically relevant information. The therapist must involve other members of the team; however, judgment must be used in how the information is shared, to ensure the woman's safety. She must be kept safe while she is in treatment. If the abuser learns that she has told health care providers about the abuse, she may no longer be safe in the hospital. In this case, it may be necessary to transfer her elsewhere where her location will not be disclosed. It is important for the occupational therapist to consider the level of education and attitudes of others on the team. If they are not educated about domestic violence and the dynamics which occur between a woman and her abuser, they may not be aware of how to handle such information. It is vitally important that the information not get back to the abuser.

- *Build Support System:* The woman who is being abused is very likely to be isolated from supportive friends and family. She may have isolated herself to hide the abuse, which may feel embarrassing or shameful. Or, the abuser who does not allow her to have contact with others may have isolated her. In either case, she will need to rebuild a support system in order to heal and continue on with her life. The occupational therapist can refer her to support groups and agencies, which specialize in treating adult victims of domestic abuse. Most of these agencies also either provide services for children or will provide referrals for the children.

- *Direct Treatment:* Occupational therapy treatment that directly addresses the issues of domestic abuse may include developing skills needed for successful role performance of desired roles, independent living skills, environmental adaptations, exploration of new roles, educational, pre-vocational or vocational treatment.

- *Therapeutic Use Of Self:* The occupational therapist who identifies the abuse or to whom the abuse experience is disclosed to will also need support. Hearing about another's experience of being abused can be simultaneously difficult, frightening, and interesting. The information must not be held as a secret by the therapist. It is important to process these experiences to provide effective care. Each individual will experience hearing about abuse differently depending on his or her personal history related to abuse. Those experiences must be understood and integrated before the therapist can effectively intervene with abused women.

REASONS WOMEN STAY IN ABUSIVE RELATIONSHIPS

Despite offering information or interventions to a woman, she may not accept it when it is offered. The refusal of assistance can be frustrating to occupational therapists;

however, the therapist should not feel his/her efforts have been futile. The average woman leaves her abusive partner five to seven times before staying away (Russell, 1995). There are a variety of reasons that a woman may refuse assistance and choose to stay in, or return to, an abusive relationship (NiCarthy, 1982, 1987).

1. *Economic Pressure:* She may feel she can't support herself and/or her children alone.
2. *Belief he will change:* She may strongly believe that he will stop being abusive or that she has the power to change him.
3. *Fear:* If he has threatened to kill her if she leaves, she may be terrified that he will find her, especially if he is extremely violent or has carried out threats in the past.
4. *No place to go:* She may have no place where she can stay safely if she leaves.
5. *Love:* Women are often raised to expect to make sacrifices when in love. She may feel trapped by her own emotions.
6. *Fear of being alone:* Living alone at night may be more frightening to her than living with the abuser.
7. *Concern for the children:* She may feel she doesn't have the right to separate the children from their father and tried to keep the family together.
8. *Guilt:* She may feel she is causing the abuse and is to blame.
9. *Concern for the abuser:* She may feel responsible for his future and his happiness and believes leaving him will destroy him.
10. *Pressure by others:* She may be pressured by friends, family, clergy, or children to forgive him and make things work out.

This range of experiences contributes to why the woman has difficulty leaving the relationship. It is important for the therapist to know that even if an intervention is initially refused, the intervention may still have an impact on the woman's life. She may remember the intervention or return to the information provided, weeks, months, or years later—when she is ready to accept it. Women have called crisis lines and arrived at emergency shelters with referrals from all types of sources (Helfrich, 1997). As information providers, occupational therapists cannot always know when a client will use the information provided.

SUMMARY OF THE ROLE OF OCCUPATIONAL THERAPY

Occupational therapists are likely to see victims of domestic violence in all settings in which they work. In adult physical dysfunction settings, individuals may be seen who are in treatment secondary to an injury caused by domestic violence. These injuries may include head traumas, spinal cord injury from gunshot wounds, burns, orthopedic injuries, or facial or internal injuries. Pediatric therapists may see either parents or children as victims of domestic violence. Parents may miss appointments with their children to hide the results of injuries either to themselves or their children, or they may appear unmotivated to follow through with a home program for their child because the situation at home does not allow them to complete assigned exercises or activities. In mental health, clients often have long histories of abuse, but the fact that they may currently be in an abusive situation is often overlooked. In the community and home health, elders may be encountered who are being abused by family members or caregivers and are unable to help themselves.

In all of the above situations the client presents with similar issues that are very important for the occupational therapist to consider. The abuse may be thought of as an environmental stressor that interferes with occupational functioning. The impact of the abuse on the individual's environment may be so great as to interfere with all aspects of functioning in some way. This chapter described what domestic abuse is and provided background information needed by an occupational therapist to understand its impact on function.

REFERENCES

Abbott, J., Johnson, R., Koziol-McLain, J., & Lowenstein, S. (1995). Domestic violence against women: Incidence and prevalence in an emergency department population. *Journal of the American Medical Association, 273*(22), 1763-1767.

American Medical Association (1992). American Medical Association Diagnostic and Treatment Guidelines on Domestic Violence. *Archives of Family Medicine, 1*, 39-47.

Centers For Disease Control and Prevention. (1993). Emergency Department Response to Domestic Violence. *Morbidity and Mortality Weekly Report, 42*(32), 617-620.

Council on Ethical and Judicial Affairs, American Medical Association. (1992). Physicians and domestic violence: Ethical considerations. *Journal of the American Medical Association, 267*(23), 3190-3193.

Dearwater, S., Coben, J., Campbell, J., Nah, G., Glass, N., McLoughlin, E., & Bekemeier, B. (1998). Prevalence of intimate partner abuse in women treated at community hospital emergency departments. *Journal of the American Medical Association, 280*(5), 433-438.

Elliott, B.A., & Johnson, M. M. P. (1995). Domestic Violence in a Primary Care Setting. *Archives of Family Medicine, 4*, 113-119.

Ferris, L. E. (1994). Canadian Family Physician's and General Practitioners' Perceptions of Their Effectiveness in Identifying and Treating Wife Abuse. *Medical Care, 32*(12), 1163-1172.

Gin, N. E., Rucker, L., Frayne, S., Cypan, R., & Hubbell, F. A. (1991). Prevalence of domestic violence among patients in three ambu-latory care internal medicine clinics. *Journal of General Internal Medicine, 6*(4), 317-322.

Goldberg, W. G., & Tomlanovich, M. C. (1984). Domestic violence victims in the emergency department. *Journal of the American Medical Association, 251*, 3259-3264.

Gremillion, D. H., & Kanof, E. P. (1996). Overcoming barriers to physician involvement in identifying and referring victims of domestic violence. *Annals of Emergency Medicine, 27*(6), 769-773.

Helfrich, C. (1997). *Homeless mothers experience of transitional housing: An ethnographic study.* Unpublished Dissertation. Ph.D. Public Health Sciences-Community Health, The University of Illinois at Chicago.

Hoff, L. (1992). Battered women: Understanding identification and assessment. *Journal of the American Academy of Nurse Practitioners, 4*(4), 148-155.

Holtz, H., & Furniss, K. K. (1993). The health care provider's role in domestic violence. *Trends in Health Care, Law & Ethics, 8*(2), 47-51.

Illinois Domestic Violence Act of 1986, P.A. 82-621, §101.

Johnston, J. L. (1998). *Knowledge and attitudes of occupational therapy practitioners regarding wife abuse.* Unpublished Master's Thesis. Chicago, IL: Rush University.

Keller, L. E. (1996). Invisible victims: Battered women in psychiatric and medical emergency rooms. *Bulletin of the Menninger Clinic, 60*(1), 1-21.

Kielhofner, G. (Ed.) (1995). *A Model of Human Occupation: Theory and Application* (2nd Edition). Baltimore, MD: Williams & Wilkins.

King, M. C., & Ryan, J. (1989). Abused women: Dispelling myths and encouraging intervention. *Nurse Practitioner, 14*(5), 47-58.

Koss, M. P., Koss, P. G., & Woodruff, W. J. (1991). Deleterious effects of criminal victimization on women's health and medical utilization. *Archives of Internal Medicine, 151*, 342-347.

Kurz, D. (1987). Emergency department responses to battered women: Resistance to medicalization. *Social Problems, 34*(1), 69-76.

Moss, V. A. & Taylor, W. K. (1991). Domestic violence: Identification, assessment, intervention. *AORN Journal, 53*(5), 1158-1164.

NiCarthy, G. *Getting free: A handbook for women in abusive relationships.* Seattle, WA: The Seal Press, 1982.

NiCarthy, G. *The ones who got away: Women who left abusive partners.* Seattle, WA: The Seal Press, 1987.

Neufield, B. (1996). SAFE questions: Overcoming barriers to the detection of domestic violence. *American Family Physician, 53*(8), 2575-2580.

Peterson, L., & Brown, D. (1994). Integrating child injury and abuse-neglect research: Common histories, etiologies, and solutions. *Psychological Bulletin, 116*, 291-298.

Quillian, J. P. (1996). Screening for spousal or partner abuse in a community health setting. *Journal of the American Academy of Nurse Practitioners, 8*(4).

Randall, T. (1990). Domestic Violence Intervention Calls for More Than Treating Injuries. *Journal of the American Medical Association, 264*, 939-940.

Rath, G. D., Jarratt, L. G., & Leonardson, G. (1989). Rates of Domestic Violence Against Adult Women by Men Partners. *Journal of the American Board of Family Practice, 2*(4), 227-233.

Reiss, A. J., & Roth, J. A. (1993). *Panel on the understanding and control of violent behavior.* Committee on Law and Justice, Commission on Behavioral and Social Sciences and Education, National Research Council. Washington, DC: National Academy Press.

Rodriguez, M. A., Quiroga, S. S., & Bauer, H. M. (1996). Breaking the silence: Battered women's perspectives on medical care. *Archives of Family Medicine, 5,* 153-158.

Rosenberg, M. L., & Mercy, M. A. (1991). *Violence in America.* New York, NY: Oxford University Press.

Russell, M. (1995). Piercing the veil of silence: Domestic violence and disability. *New Mobility,* 44-55.

Sassetti, M. (1993). Domestic violence. *Primary Care, 20,* 289-305.

Stark, E., & Flitcraft, A. (1996). *Women at risk: Domestic violence and women's health.* Thousand Oaks, CA: Sage Publications.

Sugg, N. K., & Inui, T. (1992). Primary care physician's response to domestic violence. *Journal of the American Medical Association, 267*(23), 3157-3160.

U.S. Department of Justice. (1994). *Selected findings from the Bureau of Justice statistics: Elderly crime victims—National Crime Victimization Survey,* March, NCJ-147002. Washington, DC: Bureau of Justice Statistics, Office of Justice Programs.

U.S. Department of Justice. (1997). *Changes in criminal victimization—National crime victimization survey,* April, NCJ-162032. Washington DC: Bureau of Justice Statistics.

Walker, L. E. (1994). *The battered woman syndrome.* New York, NY: Springer.

CHAPTER FORTY

Occupational Therapy in Forensic Psychiatry

Victoria P. Schindler

INTRODUCTION

Forensic psychiatry is defined as "the branch of medicine dealing with disorders of the mind in relation to legal principles and cases" (Nolan & Nolan-Halley, 1990, p. 649). Although forensic psychiatry has been viewed as a specialty in the realm of psychiatric services, the reality of current (and probably future) mental health care is that as the number of criminal acts increases, the number involved in the criminal justice system and the mental health system also increases. Individuals who have had contact with the criminal justice system are seen in all types of correctional facilities and in non-forensic in-patient and out-patient mental health settings. Heath care professionals working in all of these settings need to be knowledgeable of the basic workings of the forensic system and need to have adequate information to provide the safest and most therapeutic treatment possible. This chapter aims to provide an overview of this information by addressing:

- A brief history of forensic psychiatry
- A description of forensic settings
- A description of a forensic population
- The role of occupational therapy with a forensic population
- A description of an occupational setting
- Case studies

BRIEF HISTORY OF FORENSIC PSYCHIATRY/LEGAL PRECEDENTS

The precedent for forensic psychiatry was established in the British courts in 1843 as the M'Naghten rule. This rule derives from a famous case in England involving Daniel M'Naghten.

For years Mr. M'Naghten suffered from the delusion that he was being persecuted by the Prime Minister of England, Sir Robert Peel. As a result Mr. M'Naghten planned to kill Mr. Peel. Instead, Mr. M'Naghten mistakenly shot and killed Mr. Peels' secretary. Mr. M'Naghten was later adjudicated insane and committed to a hospital. This began a great debate about criminality and insanity. As a result, the M'Naghten rule was established. This precedent-setting rule states that individuals are guilty by reason of insanity if they have a mental disorder which rendered them unaware of the nature, quality, and consequences of the act, or if they are incapable of realizing that the act was wrong. This rule determined criminal responsibility in many States in the United States until 1954, when the Durham rule was established in the District of Columbia Court of Appeals. In the case of Durham vs. the United States, it was established that an individual is not criminally responsible if the unlawful act was the product of mental disease or defect. This rule was later amended in 1955 by a group of legal scholars constituting the American Law Institute, and was written into the criminal code in many states. This legal standard is still the guiding principle for determining criminality and maintains that an individual is not responsible for an alleged act if, because of mental illness, the individual is unable to appreciate the wrongfulness of the act or adhere to the requirements of the law (Freedman, Kaplan, & Saddock, 1980; Gutheil, 1995).

DESCRIPTION OF FORENSIC SETTINGS

The history and development of forensic settings is closely linked to the history and development of traditional psychiatric settings. Original psychiatric facilities were known as lunatic asylums. Populations consisted entirely of individuals on involuntary status and little differentiation was made between those individuals who had committed crimes as a result of their mental illness and those who had not (Goldman, 1994; Gutheil, 1995; Lloyd, 1995). In the United States, individuals with mental illness who were too troublesome were often sent to jail. This sparked a movement for prison reform, and in 1826, the Boston Prison Discipline Society initiated legislation to investigate conditions in the jails in Massachusetts. The Society determined that mentally ill individuals occupied many of the jail cells, and quickly sponsored legislation to establish the Worcester State Hospital, which opened in 1833. This established a precedent for public sector care of individuals with serious mental illness (Surles & Shore, 1996).

Currently, individuals involved in the forensic system can be found in state forensic hospitals, state psychiatric hospitals, jails, prisons, and in community settings.

State Forensic Hospitals

State forensic hospitals are maximum-security settings under the jurisdiction of the state department of mental health services. Because of the maximum-security environment, individuals with serious offenses (e.g., murder, manslaughter) are referred to these facilities. Individuals in state forensic hospitals are usually under court order to address one of the following:

- Evaluate and/or restore to competency to stand trial
- Comprehensive treatment for individuals found Not Guilty by Reason of Insanity (NGRI)
- Comprehensive treatment for individuals found Guilty but Mentally Ill
- Evaluation and treatment for individuals with mental illness in the state's prisons and jails

Definition of Terms

Competency to Stand Trial—If, because of mental illness, an individual is unable to understand the nature of his/her legal charges and/or is unable to cooperate with legal counsel, the individual is determined to be incompetent to stand trial. It is the responsibility of the treatment team at the forensic state hospital to evaluate for competency and restore to competency if necessary (Freedman, Kaplan, & Saddock, 1980; Curran, McGarry, & Shah, 1986; Gutheil, 1995; Dressler & Snively, 1998).

Not Guilty by Reason of Insanity—A socially harmful act alone does not constitute an offense. The act must be deliberate in nature. If an individual, at the time of the commitment of an offense, has a mental disease or defect that renders him/her incapable of understanding the criminal nature of his/her offense and incapable of determining right from wrong, the individual can be found not guilty by reason of insanity (Freedman, Kaplan, & Sadock, 1980; Curran, McGarry, & Shah, 1986; Gutheil, 1995; Dressier & Snively, 1998). It is then the responsibility of the state forensic hospital to provide comprehensive treatment. Many individuals determined to be not guilty by reason of insanity are transferred to progressively less-restrictive settings (including

non-forensic settings) and eventually to the community as they are restored to sanity.

Guilty but Mentally Ill—Some states use this commitment status to address an individual who is mentally ill, but whose mental illness did not preclude him/her from understanding the criminal nature of the offense. Once sufficient treatment for the mental illness has been provided, the individual is transferred to a correctional setting to complete a prison term (Gutheil, 1995).

Individuals with mental illness in state prisons and jails—States that do not have comprehensive mental health services in their jail and prison system use the services provided at the state forensic hospital for defendants or inmates with mental illness. Usually the individual will be court ordered to the forensic facility for stabilization of the psychiatric condition. Once stabilization is achieved, the individual is returned to the sending facility (Dressler & Snively, 1998).

State Psychiatric Hospitals

An individual with a less serious offense (e.g., simple assault, shoplifting) due to mental illness is committed to a locked unit of a state psychiatric hospital as opposed to a state forensic hospital. Additionally, when an individual with a more serious offense in a state forensic hospital is court-ordered to a less restrictive environment, he/she is usually transferred to a state psychiatric hospital (Curran, McGarry, & Shah, 1986).

Jails

City or county jail is usually the point of entry for the individual with forensic charges. Lack of community support combined with the cognitive and social deficits lead many individuals with mental illness to commit crimes. A common scenario is one in which a homeless individual with mental illness commits robbery in order to obtain food or shelter. This results in arrest. Often, after initial assessment in the jail, the individual is transferred to a forensic hospital for evaluation for competency or for stabilization. For an individual remaining in the jail, the system for psychiatric care varies from state to state. Some states offer comprehensive mental health services while others offer almost no services at all. It is estimated that at least 30,700 severely mentally ill individuals are in jail (Steadman, 1990; Torrey, et. al, 1992; National Alliance for the Mentally Ill [NAMI], 1996).

Prisons

State or federal prisons incarcerate individuals found guilty of criminal activity. Although prisons are intended for individuals who have committed crimes but are not mentally ill, it is estimated that at least 60,000 severely mentally ill individuals are in prisons (NAMI, 1996). Prison environments are destructive to most goals of rehabilitation, and active treatment is rare or non-existent. Little positive activity is provided, and inmates are removed from their families and social support systems. The safety and control measures of prison are contrary to the normal routine and activities of everyday life (Freedman, Kaplan, & Saddock, 1980; Steadman & Cocozza, 1993; Dressler & Snively, 1998).

Community Settings

Individuals committed to forensic hospitals and state psychiatric hospitals usually progress to non-forensic community settings once they have received adequate, successful treatment for their mental illness. Here, individuals continue in therapy under court supervision and hopefully return or begin the activities associated with a normal life (Curran, McGarry, & Shah, 1986; Wasyliw, Cavanaugh, & Grossman, 1988; Heilbrun & Griffin, 1993; Dressler & Snively, 1998).

DESCRIPTION OF A FORENSIC POPULATION

In some ways the forensic client is not very different than any other client with a diagnosed mental illness. Diagnoses such as schizophrenia, bipolar disorders, substance-related disorders, and depression are common in forensic clients. However, the forensic client does differ in other ways. Often the forensic client has been severely mentally ill for many years and the mental illness has been untreated or undertreated. Additionally, the forensic client usually has social deficits, and many forensic clients are also diagnosed with antisocial personality disorder and have histories of assaultive, dangerous behavior. Many forensic clients are also isolated from their family and social supports and have been victims of abuse and neglect during their childhood (Curran, McGarry, & Shah, 1986; National Institute of Mental Health, 1991; Dressler & Snively, 1998). Recently, sex offenders have also been court-ordered to the forensic system. Although many of these sex offenders do not have a diagnosed mental illness, their repetitive sexual criminal acts have resulted in their commitment to the mental health system (Curran, McGarry, & Shah, 1986; Applebaum, 1997). Additionally, since many individuals with mental illness are homeless or live in inadequate community settings as a result of deinstitutionalization, the number of individuals committing crimes and entering the forensic system is constantly growing (Steadman, 1990; Torrey, et. al, 1992; NAMI, 1996).

THE ROLE OF OCCUPATIONAL THERAPY WITH A FORENSIC POPULATION

Occupational therapy with the forensic client must first seek to establish therapeutic rapport. Individuals involved in the criminal justice system often have a profound sense of distrust—especially of persons in positions of authority.

Before progress can be made, trust must be established and feelings of anger controlled (Mosey, 1986; Curran, McGarry, & Shah, 1986).

Occupational therapy also assists in the comprehensive evaluation of forensic clients. In addition to evaluating performance skills in the areas of a client's life roles, occupational therapy contributes to assessments regarding competency, dangerousness, and malingering. With all of these evaluations, information is usually aggregated by the client's psychiatrist and presented to the client's attorney, the prosecuting attorney and the judge. Ultimate decisions regarding competency or insanity of an individual at the time of an offense are legal—not psychological decisions (Curran, McGarry, & Shah, 1986).

Although the competency evaluation is completed by a psychiatrist or psychologist and entails specific legal questions and procedures, occupational therapy assessments can serve as an adjunct to this process. A competency assessment addresses a client's ability to understand the roles of the individuals in court (e.g., judge, jury, defense attorney, prosecuting attorney) and the client's ability to cooperate with higher attorney (Curran, McGarry, & Shah, 1986; Gutheil, 1995). A client's ability to successfully complete and cooperate with a competency evaluation can be supported or refuted by the client's cooperation and completion of occupational therapy assessments, especially assessments that target cognitive and social domains. For example, a client who is able to learn and complete multi-step activities would be expected to learn the basic differences in roles and functions among the various individuals in a courtroom.

Predicting dangerousness is a very important but difficult evaluation task for the forensic practitioner. Although there is no definitive formula or rule to predict dangerousness, and studies of previous predictions show low success rates (Curran, McGarry, & Shah, 1986; National Institute of Mental Health, 1991), it is nevertheless important to progress toward increasing accuracy in predicting dangerousness. Although forensic psychiatrists, psychologists, and social workers use specific statistical and clinical evaluations to predict dangerousness occupational therapy practitioners can assist in this process. Evaluation and documentation of a client's response to a frustrating task, a difficult social situation, or need to follow rules of an occupational therapy program can offer important information concerning an ability to appropriately address everyday, stressful situations.

Forensic evaluations also address the issue of malingering. Malingering is the intentional falsifying or exaggerating of one's physical or psychological condition for self-gain (American Psychiatric Association, 1994; Curran, McGarry, & Shah, 1986; Gutheil, 1995; Dressler & Snively, 1998). Some forensic clients intentionally exaggerate their psychiatric illness or falsify information regarding their illness in order to avoid criminal charges or a prison sentence. Although forensic psychiatrists, psychologists, and social workers use specific clinical evaluations to assess malingering, occupational therapy practitioners can assist in this process, too. Documentation regarding a client who claims to not be oriented to time or place and not know the name of his/her psychiatrist but can follow directions for a multi-step task or win a chess game can provide support for a diagnosis of malingering.

Occupational therapy programs with forensic clients have many goals similar to those of programs for other clients with psychiatric illnesses. Forensic clients benefit most from concrete, reality-based programs that assess and improve skills in the areas of family and friend interactions, job or school performance, self-care, and recreation. (Stein & Brown, 1991; Axer, Johannsen, & Kopelowicz, 1995). Of course, the areas mentioned above,—competency, dangerousness, and malingering— separate the forensic client from the typical client with a psychiatric diagnosis, and must be continually assessed and treated. Nevertheless, forensic clients must be able to practice and test their skills in everyday life situations (Derks, Blankstein, & Hendrickx, 1993) since many forensic clients will eventually return to the community.

Occupational therapy programs in forensic environments must also be painstakingly aware of issues concerning safety and security. With a forensic population there is always a concern that clients may suddenly become assaultive or destructive. Limiting setting or negative attitudes conveyed by staff can lead to provocation. It is important for staff to be firm, but also truthful and calm with forensic clients. Occupational therapists should be constantly aware of their surroundings and trained in methods to address crisis situations and violent clients (Lloyd, 1995, Dressler & Snively, 1998). Elective staff training has been developed to address techniques of verbal and physical intervention, and the therapeutic use of seclusion and restraint (Applebaum & Dimieri, 1995; Maier, 1996).

The physical environment of a forensic facility can present many challenges to typical occupational therapy programming. Locks, gates, bars, alarms, and uniformed staff give the appearance of a correctional, as opposed to a therapeutic, environment. Due to safety and security concerns presented by everyday objects and tools (e.g., forks, scissors) in a forensic environment, creating a therapeutic environment can be challenging. With an adult forensic population, it is important to use age-appropriate and gender-appropriate activities, but limitations on the types of materials can limit the variety of therapeutic media. Strict policy and procedures must be implemented for all sharps for accountability and supervision during use (Dressler & Snively, 1998). Specific sharps cabinets hold a limited and constantly monitored inventory of scissors, screwdrivers, and hammers. Direct care staff, assigned to work with the occupational therapy staff, assist in this security process. All occupational therapy staff is trained in verbal and physical intervention techniques to carefully subdue and restrain the violent client and to observe escalating behavior in order to intervene prior to a full crisis.

A DESCRIPTION OF AN OCCUPATIONAL THERAPY PROGRAM IN A FORENSIC SETTING

The occupational therapy program described in this chapter is part of a multidisciplinary rehabilitation program. The other programs include vocational rehabilitation, recreation, creative arts, and education. Since occupational therapy addresses all performance skills within life roles, the occupational therapy practitioners in this forensic setting emerged as the natural leaders and coordinators of the initial rehabilitation assessment and referral process.

As soon as the patient is determined by the treatment team to be psychiatrically stable (this may be 1 to 2 days after admission), he/she will be referred to an occupational therapist. The occupational therapist then conducts a rehabilitation screening and an occupational therapy evaluation. In addition to contributing to an assessment for competency, malingering, and/or dangerousness, the occupational therapy evaluation addresses all performance components (cognitive, sensory-motor, and psychosocial functioning) within an individual's occupational performances (work/school, play/leisure/recreation, self-care, and family interaction) (Mosey, 1986). Performance components and occupational performances are viewed within an individual's past, present and expected environments, but for forensic clients these environments may differ greatly from traditional environments. For example, if an individual is expected to return to a jail or prison upon discharge, the unique aspects of these environments must be considered at the time of evaluation. Jails and prisons have ample non-productive time in which inmates are in their cells or large dayrooms with little to do. Does the individual have adequate cognitive and psychosocial skills to adequately cope with the difficult role of inmate? Can these skills be improved to facilitate better adjustment to this role? Can these skills also be improved to address the temporary or permanent loss of other roles such as worker? Based on the findings of the assessment process, the occupational therapist refers the client to occupational therapy programming and any or all of the appropriate multidisciplinary programs to address the client's unique needs.

The occupational therapy program consists of four tracks: daily living skills, reality orientation, prevocational skills, and life management. Each track is organized into three levels to accommodate clients with low, moderate, and high levels of functioning. For example, in the prevocational track, the group for individuals with low functioning skills has only five members and uses short-term, 2 to 3 step easy, success-oriented craft activities (e.g., rubber doormats) to construct and sell at a craft fair. The clients with moderate functioning skills participate in a volunteer group in which they complete work for community organizations (e.g., collate mailings). In this way the clients are able to establish a positive connection with the community. The newsletter group, developed for the clients with the highest functioning skills, produces a newsletter for the hospital population. Worker roles, such as writer, computer operator, editor, are explored.

Sensory-motor, psychological, social, and cognitive performance components are addressed within the performance areas of work/school, leisure/recreation, family interaction, and self-care. For example, in the prevocational groups, a client's former and future work roles are determined. Based on the work roles the client has held in the past and the work role he/she hopes to attain in the future, skills required for that role are addressed. Since vocational rehabilitation coordinates a workshop and patient worker program in the facility, clients can progress to a work role in the reasonable future. Another attainable role in a forensic setting is that of a friend. Due to the nature of their crime or the fact that they committed a crime, many forensic clients are estranged from family and friends in the community. It is important for them to develop new friendships and to interact with others who are experiencing similar legal situations or psychiatric illnesses.

Friendships can help to maintain a commitment to progress. Occupational therapists can assist clients to recognize and develop the skills, such as communication skills, that are needed for success in this role. Friendships can then be developed with other clients.

CASE STUDY—M

M is a 27-year-old male found not guilty by reason of insanity for robbery, 1st degree, of a house. Prior to committing the crime, M had become tense, paranoid, hostile and threatening.

M graduated from high school, and served in the Marines from 1988 to 1992, but was discharged due to unauthorized absences. M has a minimal work history, primarily in construction, and was unemployed at the time of the crime.

M is the oldest of three children. His parents and brothers are living, but M was living with his girlfriend of 3 years at the time of the crime. He was never married and has no children. There is no history of mental illness in his family.

During his early 20s, M was in and out of jail for theft charges. He was also hospitalized once at age 22 for depression. He admits to abusing alcohol, LSD, and cocaine since age 15.

After remaining in jail for 9 months, M was found not guilty by reason of insanity on his charges and was court-ordered to a forensic hospital. Upon admission he was irritated, demanding, and paranoid. He possessed poor impulse control and seemed unpredictable. He was refusing medication. He was diagnosed with Schizoaffective Disorder and Antisocial Personality Disorder.

Initial occupational therapy assessments found M to be independent in activities of daily living skills, able to attend and concentrate for up to one-hour and follow multi-step directions. He was oriented and all sensorimotor functions were within normal limits. Although he was somewhat comfortable with his peers, he was paranoid and suspicious of

treatment team staff. Due to his interest in resuming a work role in the future, he was referred to the occupational therapy prevocational group.

From the start he was able to follow multi-step directions after initial set-up. He attended closely to details. As he became comfortable, he became more cooperative and friendly with group members and occupational therapy staff. His tasks increased in complexity and he was able to progress to helping his peers. As he achieved consistent success in the prevocational group, he worked with the occupational therapist to secure a position in the vocational rehabilitation program. In this program he progressed from a piece-rate worker in the sheltered workshop to foreman. After several months he was discharged to a state hospital where he continued to pursue his work role.

CASE STUDY—L

L is a 43-year-old male committed to a forensic hospital to evaluate for competency to proceed to trial and for sanity at the time of the offense.

L has a long history of criminal activity dating to his childhood. At age 10, L was charged with larceny and sent to a school for juvenile offenders. From age 10 to 18 he was ordered to this school four times. At age 19 he was charged with robbery and sentenced to a chain gang. After his release he lived with an aunt whom he subsequently assaulted with a meat cleaver. While serving a 10-year sentence in prison for this assault, he stabbed a sleeping inmate in the eye and burned another inmate with matches. L also has a history of assaulting nurses. Prior to this hospitalization, he assaulted a nurse at a state psychiatric hospital by fracturing her nose. It is this charge of aggravated assault that is the subject of the current competency evaluation.

L's psychiatric history is also extensive. He was first diagnosed with schizophrenia at age 22. In addition to experiencing severe, acute psychotic episodes with extreme paranoia, he has also been described as impulsive and explosive without regard for consequences. Over the years he has been treated with nine different types of antipsychotic medications; his response has been limited, and he has periods of non-compliance. L also has a history of alcohol and drug abuse.

L has a very limited school and work history. He attended special education classes until he quit school in the 8th grade at age 18. His IQ was determined to be 64, which resulted in a classification of Mild Mental Retardation. Although he attended a trade school where he learned welding and bricklaying, his longest job was for 9 months as a truck driver. He has not been gainfully employed since 1974.

L was born the third of 10 children. His mother was diagnosed with schizophrenia and was frequently hospitalized in a state psychiatric facility until her death in 1977. His father remarried, but was in and out of prison and served prison time for murder.

L was admitted to the Intensive Treatment Unit where he was placed in seclusion under observation. He was suspicious, paranoid and hostile. He was diagnosed with Schizophrenia, Paranoid Type, Mixed Substance Abuse, Mild Mental Retardation, and Antisocial Personality Disorder. However, he responded to a different regime of medication to a point at which he was able to participate in the evaluation process.

Initial occupational therapy assessments found L to be disheveled and unkempt. He sat alone and would not engage in productive activity. He appeared to be responding to internal stimuli and was distrustful of the staff. He was extremely isolative and would not engage in conversation with peers or staff. His cognitive skills were very limited and he appeared to be illiterate. Due to his need to develop basic cognitive and social skills, he was referred to occupational therapy.

Significant cognitive and social deficits were demonstrated in the occupational therapy groups. He was unable to concentrate for more than 10 minutes, needed assistance with the set-up of the tasks, and had difficulty following simple directions. He was extremely quiet with a flat facial expression and gave only short, quick responses when addressed. L remained in the occupational therapy program for 15 months. During this time he engaged in a variety of long-term projects consisting of constructing items for bi-annual craft sales. At the time of discharge he was able to concentrate for a full one-hour group session and follow multi-step directions and work independently. He was pleasant and cooperative with peers and staff. Although he never became very talkative, he did initiate brief conversations with peers and staff. He agreed to assist the therapist when asked. As he progressed through his treatment, he was able to rely less on the therapist and more on himself in order to have his needs met.

During this hospitalization, L was found competent to stand trial. The improvement noted in his cognitive functioning in occupational therapy corresponded with his ability to understand the roles and functions of the individuals in the courtroom and the improvement noted in his interpersonal functioning corresponded with his ability to cooperate with his attorney. Currently L is awaiting his trial.

SUMMARY

This chapter provided a brief history of forensic psychiatry, a description of forensic settings, the role of occupational therapy with a forensic population, an example of an occupational therapy program in a forensic setting, and two case studies demonstrating the successful use of occupational therapy with forensic clients.

With the number of forensic clients growing, occupational therapy practitioners will be working with forensic clients in a variety of inpatient and outpatient settings. It is therefore important for occupational therapists in all practice areas to understand the unique needs of this population. Although many clients are ultimately discharged from forensic settings, underlying issues leading to criminality (e.g., poverty) may remain. It is important to address these needs at all lev-els of intervention and to maintain any improvements resulting from treatment.

REFERENCES

American Psychiatric Association. (1994). *Diagnostic and statistical manual of mental disorders* (4th edition). Washington, DC: Author.

Applebaum, P. S. (1997). Law & psychiatry: Confining sex offenders: The Supreme Court takes a dangerous path. *Psychiatric Services, 48,* 1265-1267.

Applebaum, P. S. & Dimieri, J. D. (1995). Law & psychiatry: Protecting staff from assaults: OSHA steps in. *Psychiatric Services, 46,* 333-338.

Axer, H., Johannsen, C., & Kopelowicx, A. (1995). Implementation of psychiatric rehabilitation in a forensic facility. *Psychiatric Rehabilitation Journal, 19*(2), 69-72.

Curran, W. J., McGarry, A. L., & Shah, S. A. (1986). *Forensic psychiatry and psychology.* Philadelphia, PA: F. A. Davis.

Derks, F. C., Blankstein, J. H., & Hendrickx, J. J. (1993). Treatment and security: The dual nature of forensic psychiatry. *International Journal of Law and Psychiatry, 16,* 217-240.

Dixon, J. W., & Rivenbark, W. H. (1993). Forensic treatment in the United States: A survey of selected forensic hospitals. *International Journal of Law and Psychiatry, 16,* 105-116.

Dressler, J., & Snively, F. (1998). Occupational therapy in the criminal justice system. In E. Cara, & A. MacRae (Eds.), *Psychosocial occupational therapy: A clinical practice* (pp. 527-552). New York, NY: Delmar.

Freedman, A. M., Kaplan, H. I., & Saddock, B. J. (1980). *Comprehensive textbook of psychiatry/II* (2nd edition). Baltimore, MD: Williams & Wilkins.

Goldman, H. H. (1994). Sesquicentennial anniversary supplement, 1844-1994. Supplement to *American Journal of Psychiatry.*

Gutheil, T. Legal issues in psychiatry. (1995). In H. I. Kaplan & B. J. Saddock (Eds.), *Comprehensive textbook of psychiatry/VI* (pp. 2747-2766). Philadelphia, PA: Williams and Wilkins.

Heilbrun, K. & Griffin, P. A. (1993). Community-based forensic treatment of insanity acquitees. *International Journal of Law and Psychiatry, 16,* 133-150.

Lloyd, C. (1995). *Forensic psychiatry for health professionals.* London, England: Chapman & Hall.

Maier, G. J. (1996). The role of talk down and talk up in managing threatening behavior. *Journal of Psychosocial Nursing and Mental Health Services, 34*(6), 25-30.

Mosey, A.C. (1986). *Psychosocial components of occupational therapy.* New York, NY: Raven Press.

National Alliance for the Mentally Ill [NAMI]. (1996). Hope for those who require long-term care? The forgotten population. *National Alliance for the Mentally Ill [NAMI] Advocate,* 13.

National Institute of Mental Health. (1991). *Caring for people with severe mental disorders: A national plan of research to improve services.* Department of Health and Human Services Publication

Number (ADM) 91-1762. Washington, DC: Superintendent of Documents., U. S. Government Printing Office.

Nolan, J. R., & Nolan-Halley, J. M. (1990). *Black's law dictionary* (6th edition). St. Paul, MN: West Publishing.

Steadman, H. J. & Cocozza, J. J. (Eds.). (1993). *Mental illness in America's prisons.* Seattle, WA: The National Coalition for the Mentally III.

Steadman, H. J. (Ed.). (1990). *Effectively addressing the mental health needs of jail detainees.* Seattle, WA: The National Coalition for the Mentally Ill.

Stein, E., & Brown, J. D. (1991). Group therapy in a forensic setting. *Canadian Journal of Psychiatry, 36,* 718-722.

Surles, R., & Shore, M. F. (1996). The public sector-private sector interface: Current issues, future trends. *New Directions for Mental Health Services, 72,* 71-79.

Torrey, E. F., Stieber, J., Ezekiel, J., Wolfe, S. M., Sharfstein, J., Noble, J. H., & Flynn, L. M. (1992). *Criminalizing the seriously mentally ill.* Washington, DC: Public Citizen's Health Research Group and the National Alliance for the Mentally Ill.

Wasyliw, O. E., Cavanaugh, J. L., & Grossman, L. S. (1988). Clinical considerations in the community treatment of mentally disordered offenders. *International Journal of Law and Psychiatry, 11,* 371-380.

CHAPTER FORTY-ONE

Psychosocial Occupational Therapy in School-Based Practice: Opportunities for Impact

Wendy C. Hildenbrand, OTR

In today's occupational therapy circles, discussion focuses on changing health and human services with particular concern about legislative mandates impacting service delivery and resulting in reimbursement challenges, staffing reorganization and, in many cases, the reduction in occupational therapy personnel. This conversation is happening at a time when our profession is further clarifying the scope of practice for occupational therapy, thereby presenting a challenge to historically defined practice parameters and offering opportunities for practitioners to broaden practice impact in traditional and emerging service arenas. Understandably, the threatening nature of these issues and actions has many practitioners feeling vulnerable in their practice. Indeed, the uncertainty of such professional change can breed anxiety; however, the change process also supports personal rejuvenation and renewed professional focus.

As an occupational therapist "specializing" in mental health and working with adolescent and adult populations in an acute psychiatric unit of a general hospital, I saw neverending opportunities for observation of the functional implications of psychosocial dysfunction and/or psychological compromise. Of particular interest were the young people who were struggling with issues of self-identity, self-efficacy, and self-management in daily living. These experiences solidified my passion for acknowledgement of and attention to psychosocial issues as they impact a person's ability to participate, to their desired level of satisfaction, in meaningful life occupations. For me, an additional experience within this setting was the process of hospital-wide "restructuring" and "rightsizing of hospital resources" – an administrative exercise that would mandate personal and professional change.

As a "mental health" practitioner with a particular interest in children and adolescents and in need of direction, I began to contemplate the "real" world that existed for young people outside of the acute hospital setting. The review that followed suggested that there were opportunities for therapeutic impact that went beyond addressing acute psychosocial crisis needs and invited involvement in daily routines that provide structure and facilitate growth for children, such as classroom settings and school systems. Following discussion with colleagues in this practice arena, a concern surfaced that it was possible, and in some places likely, that psychosocial issues are not thoroughly considered in assessment of and intervention with children in the schools. The implications of *not* identifying psychosocial issues in children serviced by occupational therapy or the inability to address these areas of concern once identified are significant. Although not intentional, inattention to this core occupational therapy principle appeared to limit the scope of service to be provided as well as the child's range of potential for success in the school environment. With new insights and a new agenda, I accepted a traditional school-based occupational therapy appointment where I was assigned to work with elementary and secondary students.

THE EDUCATIONAL PROCESS

There were many transitional steps and cognitive adjustments made during my ensuing practice shift. These transitions included the move from the hospital environment to a school-based setting and an adjustment from crisis and disability management to daily ability management. Additionally, there were necessary transitions in thinking that took place among colleagues as we joined together for this exploratory journey into the world of "psychosocial occupational therapy."

Regarding my own "education," it became clear very early that there was much to learn about school-based service delivery models, intervention strategies, and team expectations. In my attempt to grasp these practice challenges, I developed competencies through structured observations, discussions, readings, and seminars. In spite of the learning curve that I was living, I was comforted in knowing that I had a unique professional contribution to bring to others and this practice environment – the passion for acknowledging and addressing psychosocial factors as they impact performance. It became apparent quickly that I was considered the "expert" in psychosocial issues and child and adolescent psychiatric and/or behavioral disorders, with the expectation being that I would share experiences and insights that would enlighten and educate others. In receiving requests to share information and reveal my psychosocial "tricks of the trade," it became evident that the lack of attention to psychosocial issues was not due to devaluing their importance but was due to limited experience and tools regarding the area of psychosocial assessment and intervention. Additionally, there was much uncertainty about how to present psychosocial concerns as relevant and within the scope of occupational therapy practice in the school setting. Just how were we as occupational therapist to "frame" the problem so that other team players, including family members, would recognize the occupational therapy connection considering their historical expectations of and experiences with occupational therapy in the schools? This question provided focus as we collectively explored how to articulate psychosocial concerns and infuse interventions as occupational therapists within this service delivery system.

As part of the educational process, the "new" talk regarding psychosocial issues became familiar dialogue instead of a novel concept. Addressing first things first, we responded to concerns that the "expected" therapy service in this arena had not included attention to psychosocial issues and that some colleagues might view such focus as "not in my practice area." Florey (1989), in raising the issue of "treating the whole child" (p. 365), presented a critical reminder that "psychosocial principles in occupational therapy treatment have been and continue to be a cornerstone of entry level practice" (p. 365). Unfortunately, the pervasive presence of psychosocial principles in occupational therapy practice and in our professional preparation is often overlooked or capsulated as the core of the mental health specialty area instead of core to our profession's foundation and future. In school-based practice, many referrals are initiated because of handwriting or other fine motor problems, delays in developmental task mastery, or the "something's not quite right with this kid" concern. When addressing the whole child, it is important to recognize that these children and adolescents also experience feelings of inadequacy, difference, and exclusion that can then lead to negative self-worth, inappropriate interpersonal skills, ineffective self-management, and inadequate role performance. Fortunately, our department had acknowledged the reality that children, with and without the challenges of psychiatric diagnoses or emotional interruption, are striving to master the developmental milestones associated with psychosocial growth and competence as well as academic skills development needs. While an incorporated concept for most, this definitely challenged the comfort zone of others and provided an educational forum to support our professional broadening.

In an effort to define psychosocial intervention needs for children receiving our services, it was necessary to define what was meant when claiming to want more emphasis on a psychosocial treatment agenda as a part of our services. From early discussions, we determined that we must first define psychosocial, perhaps beginning with what it does not mean. This philosophical exchange was important in that it provided an opportunity for individuals to distinguish between psychosocial dysfunction or issues and psychiatric conditions or symptoms. It could be suggested that it was frequent misinterpretation within multiple practice settings that prompted the introduction and acceptance of the AOTA Position Paper specifically outlining and separating the "psychosocial core of occupational therapy" (AOTA, 1997/2000). It states that "the psychosocial dimensions of human performance are acknowledged as fundamental in all aspects of occupational therapy, whether practice occurs in settings such as the classroom, rehabilitation center, hospital, nursing home, or community" (p. 869). The Position Paper further remarked that "there is a difference between the psychosocial foundations of occupational therapy and the specialty of mental health practice," a specialty area where there is "the application of core and specialized knowledge to those individuals with a diagnosis of mental illness" (p. 869). This distinction was critical to transitions within our department and helped provide clarity in our message. For additional clarification of psychosocial constructs, we turned to AOTA Uniform Terminology for Occupational Therapy and found psychosocial skills and psychological components were defined as "the ability to interact in society and to process emotions."

Further exploration of the subcategories (psychological, social, self-management) provided initial discussion points while also stimulating recognition of the need for expanded identification of psychosocial skills and abilities.

After establishing our common ground, we began the process of an informal departmental review of practice models and/or frames of reference, problem areas, and intervention approaches that were being referenced in therapy. Through this process, we uncovered a great collective strength as we found that many identified psychosocial issues were being addressed in ongoing treatment sessions. A collective weakness was the lack of documentation regarding psychosocial issue recognition and intervention by occupational therapy practitioners. We found that identified psychosocial issues and/or observed progress regarding these issues were not indicated in staffings, individualized education program (IEP) meetings, goal and objective statements, or in other formal discussions of a child's needs and problems. This was contrary to the frequent informal exchanges that would take place regarding a child's behavioral needs and emotional well-being. It was concluded that if we were to be recognized as a contributor in this area, we were going to have to be more visible, vocal, and invested in maintaining a presence in the psychosocial intervention realm.

The need for increased psychosocial visibility was addressed in several ways starting with the expansion of our internal Occupational Therapy Functional Assessment data form to highlight areas of interpersonal skill, social participation and self-management within the school environment. Departmental discussion of frames of reference allowed for broader understanding and use of assessment measures, including the Coping Inventory (Zeitlin, 1985), to help frame coping exchanges, identify coping effectiveness and target intervention approaches and the Sensory Profile (Dunn, 1999) to support understanding of sensory response and its effect on performance and environmental engagement. While these were useful tools in identifying performance issues, often the most informative assessment data came from classroom observation, task analysis, and analysis and utilization of assessment findings presented as a part of testing required for determination of special education and/or related service eligibility.

Regarding documentation, we challenged our own comfort zone regarding goal setting, intervention planning and presentation of psychosocial concerns in formal forums. We also challenged the system to recognize and embrace the depth of contributions that were to be made by an occupational therapist treating a "whole child." Meetings to construct a child's Individualized Education Program, having often described our contribution to be a "motor report," included a more comprehensive summary that included psychosocial assessments and/or concerns. Admittedly, some of our initial efforts to think out of our designated "box" met some resistance with suggestions that our observations and insights had already been covered in another's report. This helped to firm our commitment to educate administrators, teachers, related service providers, and family members about occupational therapy service provisions in the psychosocial arena. The ability to articulate the rich value of occupational therapy as a critical player in enabling successful experiences in daily life tasks would ensure a continuing presence in traditional school-based practice, as well as highlight the expanded impact to be made by occupational therapy when supported in efforts to practice outside of the traditional therapy "box."

THE EXPERIENTIAL PROCESS

We committed ourselves to the process of recognition of psychosocial problems as contributors to occupational performance deficits and/or challenges in school settings and identified opportunities for impact in three areas including (1) responding to psychosocial issues, (2) reframing psychosocial dysfunction, and (3) addressing psychiatric concerns. These three areas of opportunity are highlighted in the following stories of Mandy, Tony, and Andy.

Responding to Psychosocial Issues

"Mandy," a rising 14-year-old ninth grader, excelled in her academic performance yet struggled daily with the effects of juvenile rheumatoid arthritis. Bone growth was delayed, joint mobility and stability were seriously impaired, and her endurance with activity or task was limited. She had been involved in multiple therapies, including occupational therapy, for most of her life and parents viewed continuing therapeutic intervention as critical in maintaining performance components of strength, mobility, and range of motion. Recognizing that service delivery in the educational setting was very different from the medical model in how it necessitates treatment; these "clinical" concerns expressed by parents were considered inappropriate by some and presented quite a challenge to all. Therapy in school settings must be "educationally relevant" meaning that for medical conditions or disabilities to be considered in the determination of service needs, such conditions must clearly interfere with the student's ability to benefit from individualized plans and programs as well as their ability to adequately perform within the educational setting. Mandy's academic success and progress toward future goals to "letter in academics" and pursue a career as a doctor suggested that her academic performance had not been negatively impacted by her physical complications. In fact, her problem-solving abilities and resourcefulness had served her well, as she was able to secure accommodations and adaptations to support her limitations.

However, when truly assessing her ability to respond to the environmental and social needs that are implicit in the high school arena, as well as her future goals, it was clear that there were other issues that had not been overtly identified or formally addressed. Interpersonally, Mandy had difficulty maintaining friendships because of her immature social skills and social expectations. She verbalized her needs and opinions, but was often demanding or sarcastic in her requests. She presented with minimal accountability for management of her arthritis-related health maintenance needs. Limited acceptance of responsibility for the consequences of her behavior interfered with her ability to acknowledge or act on the need for personal change. Recognizing the reality of and potential for future personal and professional difficulties, it was easy to discuss these presenting concerns with the student, the parents, and other team members. Prior to this meeting, it was suggested that identifying psychosocial issues as problems for occupational therapy intervention was risky; however, the risk saw benefit when the parents stated that they were "glad someone is finally addressing this (the interpersonal and psychosocial concerns) with her." Certainly, we continued to address Mandy's physical maintenance needs and worked to ensure that adequate environmental and compensatory supports were in place to support her success. It was the introduction of frank exchanges about psychosocial concerns, along with suggested intervention approaches and the noted improvement in social performance and self-responsibility outcomes that was viewed as welcome change in programming.

Reframing Psychosocial Dysfunction

"Tony," a very active 6-year-old first grader, quickly became identified in his classroom as the "handful," a label that was accented by his "special" seat next to the teacher's desk at the front of the room. Tony was very fidgety, in constant motion while seated, would often drop his school supplies and tools on the floor, and would often fall to the floor himself in his efforts to retrieve items seemingly to meet his internal need for movement and additional sensory input. He struggled to focus on school-related tasks, had difficulty understanding and/or following directions, and would often receive unsatisfactory reports regarding his academic output, social conduct, and interpersonal skills. His attempts to interact with peers and adults were typically thwarted by his poor recognition of personal space, his limited ability to allow delayed gratification and his inability to self-monitor and self-regulate his personal needs. In his efforts to join others in conversation or play, he would bump, poke, touch, talk loudly, and aggressively introduce himself into a group, only to be told to quit, go away, or be met with threats of "I'm going to tell the teacher." Consequently, he would isolate himself, entertain himself (sometimes through destruction of his own or others' property), or chastise himself for being "bad" and not being a friend to other children.

For the occupational therapist that assessed and worked with Tony, it was very evident that this child had sensory seeking needs and integration problems that were interfering with his classroom success as well as limiting his social participation opportunities. The academic/interdisciplinary team members believed he could benefit from intervention targeting the refinement of sensory processing and integration systems. For the parents, already skeptical about "team" recommendations and sensitive to the expressed rationales, they were certain that the problems observed in the classroom were due to teacher, environment, and curriculum structure deficits. To them, it seemed that everyone was telling them much more about what was wrong with their son than what was right with their son. Needless to say, our discussion with the parents about their child and his "sensory integration deficits" and our desire for occupational therapy involvement with Tony was very abstract and threatening. In our final efforts to secure necessary services for this child, it was simply stated that we hoped to "increase his ability to understand the needs his body has and to help him learn to manage himself around other people and in the places he wants to be." It was further stated that we were hopeful that this internal change and external awareness would help him to "do better in school and to make more friends." Of everything discussed with the parents, "making more friends" was most meaningful and representative of their desires for their child. "Reframing" the child's current problems and future outcomes allowed for acknowledgement and acceptance of the child as one with potential for satisfying and successful life engagement.

The process of reframing, recognized as "a process of coming to see a person or a situation in a new way because one has changed the framework, the lens, through which one views that person or situation", provides an opportunity for revision of perceptions (Niehues, Bundy, Mattingly, Lawlor, 1991). It was not until we were able to jointly "reframe" not only the problem, but the target outcome as well, that we were able to agree about his therapeutic need and a focus or target performance outcome for therapy intervention. Through this more positive and hopeful frame, we were able secure therapeutic services and were able to target and address the psychosocial concerns of both the child and his parents.

Addressing Psychiatric Concerns

"Andy," a 7-year-old second grade student diagnosed with attention deficit hyperactivity disorder, received academic services from within his behavior disorder classroom placement. Initial therapy department assessments indicated that he had overall deficits in visual-perceptual, fine motor, and gross motor skills. Required district evaluations (such as IQ testing) identified marginal cognitive capabilities, and developmental/educational markers not met presented a picture of gross delays in academic skill mastery. Classroom observation highlighted significant organizational and attentional difficulties related to his heightened distractibility. Social inadequacies, including poor interpersonal skills and ineffective self-management, resulted in Andy having very few friends. Across educational contexts, his response to redirection fluctuated and teachers remarked that he often appeared to attend to internal stimuli as if he was "not with us." In spite of recent medication trials, he had been in a "fog" that had limited his child development, life participation, and day-to-day enjoyment.

While it was painfully clear to everyone involved with Andy that his needs were many, it was peculiarly familiar to me as his problems and behaviors seemed to cluster as potential symptoms of larger, unidentified psychiatric concerns. During a discussion with his classroom teacher, the possibility of sensory/perceptual processing abnormalities and/or auditory or tactile hallucinations as possible explanations for his overt behaviors was explored. It appeared that my experience working with children and adolescents with psychiatric conditions brought added credibility to our shared observations and interpretations. For the teacher, the validation of her own silent questions provided a sense of confidence in her recognition of "issues that were outside of the education arena" yet were in critical need of attention if this child was to grow from his academic experience. Referrals were made, results reviewed, recommendations offered and, in the end, Andy's psychiatric diagnosis was revised, as was his medication regime. This required support and educational updates for those that lived and worked with him daily; however, it was outwardly apparent that the behavioral and pharmacological changes were making an impact in his availability to learning and his readiness to engage in school tasks. He was now able to stay seated in a classroom for task completion, was able to focus and follow directions and sequences, and

Table 41-1
Examples of Psychosocial-Focused Goals/Intervention Approaches

	Problem Areas	*Occupational Goals*	*Intervention Approaches*
MANDY	Interpersonal skills	Mandy will communicate needs and ideas without sarcasm when interacting with adults and peers to support development of friends and social networks.	Communication Log – to allow for thought formulation, feedback and planning.
			Future forecasting regarding career goals and communication needs.
			Coordination and preparation of own birthday luncheon with peers and staff.
	Adjustment to disability	Mandy will initiate and complete stretch and range routines on 5 of 7 days weekly to encourage recognition of and responsibility for disability management.	Stretch and range home program, including exercise parameters and reinforcers, developed jointly for home and school.
TONY	Peer interaction	Tony will participate in structured play with two same age peers without touching others to encourage appropriate peer contact and play inclusion.	Provide structured peer play with support and reinforcement for boundary recognition and social self-management.
	Sensory self-regulation	Tony will verbally express internal discomfort and/or need for environmental change to allow for self-regulation and social participation.	Consult with teacher to construct and make available modulating sensory experiences within the classroom.
			Provide education for parents regarding sensory issues/needs and management strategies for home and community.
ANDY	Social participation	Andy will sustain social contact with peers in group contexts to support relationship building and environmental registration.	Initiate a "therapy buddy" system with schoolmates to assist with acquisition of social skills and peer support.
			Consult with PE class teacher to idenify peer/partner or leadership opportunities.
	Reality-based attention	Andy will contribute to discussion with reality-based comments to encourage task focus and support active learning.	With peers, engage in task group (e.g. current events board or "class portrait" collage) with end product for display in classroom.

was able to initiate and respond to interactions with his peers and adults. After a year of restructured support and programming, Andy shared with me, smiling, that "I can read now and I have friends, too!" Later academic reevaluation provided objective support, through standardized testing and scores, for the many reports of his improvement in the educational and social performance arenas.

In all three cases, our attention to these issues (Table 41-1) was acknowledged, supported and welcomed by counselors, teachers, and special education coordinators as well as parents and children. As a result, we increased the sensitivity to student's psychosocial needs and heightened the awareness of occupational therapy's willingness and readiness to address these concerns.

OBSTACLES AND OPPORTUNITIES

The practice formation that was experienced individually and collectively did not come without struggle and challenge to our efforts to broaden perceptions of occupational therapy practice. Knowing the potential for obstacles, it was important to gather support inside and outside of the immediate occupational therapy department, including that of the special education administration of the school district. Fortunately, this maiden adventure was housed within a progressive school district that supports innovative programming for students. Regardless, a key factor in the eager reception to the idea of more active and overt identification of psychosocial issues was the opportunity to establish early groundwork. This preparatory process allowed for self-assessment regarding skills, knowledge base, and comfort level regarding psychosocial issues and intervention. The educational process became a forum for discussion, thereby generating interest and identifying ideas for intervention and approaches of benefit to the psychosocial needs of children and adolescents. Responsibility for change and investment in the process were additional and necessary benefits.

In spite of the initial work that had been done, there remained a need for assurance regarding the pragmatics of "how will we do that too?" There was a concern expressed by some that they were unsure how to do it or were not sure they could fit it into the already tight therapy time. It has been my belief that psychosocial issues are recognized and intervention approaches happen, but the therapeutic assessment (often through observation of performance and interaction) or response to intervention (perhaps redirection, change in structure, or behavioral approaches) is often not documented or otherwise reported. Instead, they might be minimized as part of the therapeutic process and dismissed as routine. Therapeutic use of self and the ability to address an individual's psychosocial needs and emotional well-being are skills to be embraced, not set aside or buried "underground." This tendency to disregard our psychosocial contribution means lost opportunities in many practice arenas. Solid efforts to identify and articulate these therapeutic exchanges could actually support and solidify our position as providers in the psychosocial domain. In raising individual awareness, incorporation of psychosocial strategies into intervention became manageable and more easily recognized as an extension of what was already being done rather than implementation of a burdensome requirement.

STRATEGIES FOR SUCCESS

Our internal preparation enabled us to respond with energy and focus to our own charges to strengthen and expand the psychosocial presence of occupational therapy in the school setting. Commitment to this departmental effort allowed discussion of successes as well as challenges along the way. Suggestions for successful integration of psychosocial occupational therapy approaches within school-based practice are provided in the following collective tip summary affectionately titled…

THE "ABC'S"

A—Accept discipline differences and similarities. Both provide opportunities for interdisciplinary discovery and collaboration

B—Broaden your own vision of occupational therapy practice, then help others see your vision

C—Create opportunities. Suggest change in a student's individualized education plan (IEP), suggest partnerships around common outcome goals (co-teach social skills with classroom teacher), be willing to incorporate other's ideas with your and transform into demonstration projects. Be creative in what you create.

D—Document psychosocial concerns and intervention responses. Record of attention to these issues and effectiveness in intervention supports our position in this arena.

E—Educate everyone and know that you will do so more than once. Teachers, administrators, other "related service" staff, parents, do not typically connect psychosocial issues with occupational therapy practice. Help them make this connection!

F—Familiarize yourself with the function and focus of other disciplines, the parameter and policy issues of the setting, "traditional" expectations of team members

G—Generate interest and ideas. Talk, discuss, pose provocative questions, and provide doable suggestions and solutions. Action will often follow.

H—Humor helps to mediate problems, maintain perspective, and relieves stress.

I—Innovative thinking and practice involves risk. Plan, prepare and proceed.

J—Judge not, particularly when entering a practice environment that is new to you. There is much to be learned before we have all of the answers!

K—Knowledge is a powerful thing! Prepare yourself through continued education and experience. Engage in scholarly activity. Conduct clinical research based on practice questions. Share your knowledge!

L—Listen! Many opportunities are disguised as another person's venting or the repeated discussion of a "problem" student(s) in need of services, our services. Be open and responsive to these opportunities.

M—Mainstream yourself! Don't be afraid to be present and visible in building activities. Provide therapy in classrooms. Discuss psychosocial concerns across settings (PE, Art, Recess, Reading, etc.). Let them know who you are and what information/ intervention suggestions you have to offer.

N—Negotiate for what you want. Special interests and specific skills can still be matched to student and classroom needs within a school or district. (The chance to work with adolescents and with children with behavior disorders was important to me. Negotiation made this a reality.)

O—Occupation, yes, engagement in meaningful occupation, is essential in our efforts to address psychosocial issues affecting an individual's emotional well-being. Opportunities for engagement in relevant life tasks are available daily within this setting!

P—Prioritize. Admittedly, it would be great to say that psychosocial issues are the most critical issues to address for each child, however this is not always the case. It is just as important to recognize when to rest the psychosocial banner as it is to raise the banner. The success of the child in the school setting with regard to daily life performance is *the* priority. To recognize this is a strength.

Q—Question yourself. This is good way to maintain clarity and truth in your professional objectives and focus. When questioning yourself, be sure to be truthful in your responses. Challenging and critiquing yourself can be much less painful than assessments from others.

R—Reward successes. Whether a subtle change in student ability or significant change in departmental programming, recognition of successful efforts helps to support continued effort and enthusiasm

S—Support each other. Growth and change can be both stimulating and stressful. Be available with ears and genuine interest.

T—Try, Try, and Try Again! Be prepared for hesitancy or rejection when introducing an alternate viewpoint for performance challenges. Others might not be as ready as you are for expanded thinking and practice. Plant the seeds and tend the garden!

U—Unite with varied disciplines as partners in daily practice. Traditionally, we join with teachers and other special education personnel in problem solving and educational planning. Join with social workers, school counselors, and community outreach liaisons as well. They "fit" well with our focus on life participation.

V—Volunteer where psychosocial expertise is an asset. Participate on behavioral plan committees. Co-lead or lead the groups that present behavioral challenges for the teachers and paraprofessionals. Present an in-service about the "psychosocial core" component of occupational therapy practice and occupational performance.

W—Welcome the role of a "Generalist." In embracing and presenting your full range of skill as an occupational therapist, you will become more available to a wider range of opportunities. Your "specialist" abilities will be enhanced rather than extinguished as you become recognized for your attention to the whole person.

X—Mas! Winter break... enough said!

Y—Yesterday is no longer available to you. Learn and grow from your experiences. Explore options and possibilities. Give all you have in the present. Prepare for future professional directions you might entertain.

Z—is for Zebra! Yes, Zebra in the sense that you will probably be viewed as an "animal of a different color." Personal commitment and professional expertise regarding psychosocial occupational therapy is not the norm in school-based practice. Your difference in focus will help bring about a difference in outcomes!

REAPING REWARDS

Given time to reflect on the implemented changes and the effects of this transition in thinking about psychosocial occupational therapy practice, I feel encouraged about the successes and hopeful about the ability to address future challenges and opportunities. It is not uncommon to hear discussion of psychosocial issues or to see identification of psychosocial goals and treatment strategies on a child's IEP. Therapists are more confident in their presentation of psychosocial issues and are responding to and seeking out opportunities to educate others about psychosocial issues and intervention, including the importance of addressing a person's overall psychological well-being. Additionally, there is respect for mental health practice as a specialty and a heightened recognition of the influence of the psychosocial core of occupational therapy. The coordinator of the occupational therapy department offered this comment, summing up the change in intervention effectiveness and impact, saying "We treat our kids more deeply now." This means we made a significant difference, however, there is still much work to be done. We must look around us every day for opportunities to bring psychosocial occupational therapy into the forefront of practice rather than allow this core foundation concept to be devalued or disregarded. When we recognize and embrace these opportunities, we will find ourselves face to face with opportunities for impact.

REFERENCES

American Occupational Therapy Association. (1997). The psychosocial core of occupational therapy position paper. *American Journal of Occupational Therapy, 51,* 868-869. (See Appendix A in this text.)

American Occupational Therapy Association. (1994). Uniform terminology for occupational therapy–Third edition. *American Journal of Occupational Therapy, 48,* 1047-1054. (Reprinted in Cottrell, R. P. (1996). Perspectives on purposeful activity: Foundations and future of occupational therapy (pp. 651-665). Bethesda, MD: AOTA.)

Dunn, W. (1999). *The sensory profile.* San Antonio, TX: The Psychological Corporation.

Florey, L. L. (1989). Nationally speaking: Treating the whole child: Rhetoric or reality? *American Journal of Occupational Therapy, 43,* 365-369.

Hildenbrand, W.C. (1997, September). Meeting the challenge of psychosocial shifts in service. *Mental Health Special Interest Section Quarterly,* pp.1-3.

Niehues, A., Bundy, A. C., Mattingly, C. F., Lawlor, M. C. (1991). Making a difference: Occupational therapy in the public schools. *Occupational Therapy Journal of Research, 11,* 195-210.

Zeitlin, S. (1985). *The coping inventory.* Bensonville, IL: Scholastic Testing Service.

CHAPTER FORTY-TWO

School-Based Occupational Therapy for Students with Behavioral Disorders

Sally Schultz

This chapter was previously published in Occupational Therapy and Psychosocial Dysfunction, *173-196. Copyright* © *1992, Haworth Press.*

As a result of the Education for All Handicapped Children Act (EHA), also known as Public Law 94-142, occupational therapy became identified as an "education-related service" for special education students (Federal Register, 1975). School systems began to rapidly employ occupational therapists, and today, schools are the profession's second most frequent employer (American Occupational Therapy Association [AOTA], 1986; Chandler, 1990). While the number of occupational therapists in public schools has increased dramatically, the scope of practice has expanded little. Contemporary school-based therapists serve four categories of handicapped students: mentally retarded, multihandicapped, learning disabled and orthopedically impaired (Dunn, 1988; Occupational Therapy News, 1985). These are the same groups of students served by occupational therapists prior to the passage of the EHA (Brown, 1989; Dunn, 1988; Gilfoyle & Hays, 1979; Kalish & Presseller, 1980; Kinnealey & Morse, 1979; Royeen, 1986; Royeen & Marsh, 1988).

Florey (1989) stated that in recent years occupational therapy has essentially ignored the psychosocial needs of children. She questioned whether the current focus among pediatric therapists on sensory-motor dysfunction has not essentially eliminated services to children who do not have physiological problems. Although occupational therapy was a pioneer in developing function-based programming for children in psychiatric hospitals (e.g., Edelman, 1953; Gleave, 1947; Llorens, 1962; Rabinovitch, Bee & Outwater, 1951; Scheimo, 1949; Vander Veer, 1949), few school-based therapists currently serve the student with a behavioral disorder (Robert Wood Johnson, 1988).

Occupational therapy recognized the importance of individualized programming for the student with a behavioral disorder long before "mainstreaming" and the individualized education plan was conceptualized. However, as stated by Adelstein, Barnes, Murray-Jensen, and Baker-Skaggs (1989), the public schools have failed to provide the occupational therapy services for students with behavioral disorders unless they have accompanying organic etiologies.

This chapter contains four main sections: (a) a discussion of three factors that have led to the infrequency of occupational therapy for students with behavioral disorders; (b) an inter-disciplinary review of literature which supports the need for occupational therapy with students who have behavioral disorders; (c) the essential constructs on which to develop a school-based occupational therapy program for students with behavioral disorders; and (d) guidelines for implementing an occupational therapy program based on these constructs.

For purposes of clarity, the term, "behavioral disorder" is used in this chapter. Although a variety of labels are used in the literature to describe students with behavioral disorders, "behavioral disorder" is the term preferred by the Council for Children with Behavioral Disorders and other noted special education scholars (Huntze, 1985; Kauffman, 1986) and other recognized special education leaders (Braaten, Kauffman, Braaten, Polsgrove & Nelson, 1988).

FACTORS CONTRIBUTING TO INFREQUENT OCCUPATIONAL THERAPY

Several factors can be identified which have resulted in occupational therapy being underutilized as a related service for students with behavioral disorders. Three of these factors are discussed: (a) allegiance by the occupational therapy profession to the medical model; (b) generalized confusion about the role of occupational therapy in the schools; and more specifically, (c) inadequate understanding (among special educators, school counselors and occupational therapists) of how occupational therapy is used to address the educational needs of students with behavioral disorders.

Allegiance to the Medical Model

White (1971) cautioned that some occupational therapists have had difficulty abandoning their psychoanalytic roots for a function-oriented perspective. He urged therapists to become as committed to increasing the patient's feelings of competency, as they are to analyzing the patient's conflicts, limitations and anxieties. Matsutsuyu (1971) shared White's perspective. She stated that the traditional psychiatric treatment model (i.e., practice based on Freudian theory) is focused on the patient's etiology and deficits, not potential. In contrast, occupational therapy is philosophically grounded in the positive aspects of the human condition. Occupational therapists have historically focused on using the patient's strengths to enhance functional potential. The traditional psychoanalytically driven hospital setting is philosophically incongruent with the occupational therapist's perspective and therapeutic goals. Consequently, the occupational therapist who practices in the psychiatric arena often finds it necessary to modify both beliefs and methods of intervention to accommodate the prevailing medical model.

Confused Role in School-Based Setting

The school-based occupational therapist must assimilate into yet another model. The educational model may be even more foreign than the psychiatric. It is not surprising that there is confusion between therapists and educators as to the overall purpose of occupational therapy as an education-related service (Baron, 1989; Bloom, 1988; Brown, 1989; Coutinho & Hunter, 1988; Creighton, 1979; Hightower-Vandamm, 1980; Langdon & Langdon, 1983; Ottenbacher, 1982; Royeen & Marsh, 1988; Stephens, 1989). In one survey (Brown, 1989), the results revealed that educators perceived the occupational therapist's role in parent training as being just as important as providing direct services. Few (17%) of the occupational therapists in the survey agreed. Other studies revealed that many educators believed that occupational therapy was no more than a duplication of services already in place (Bloom, 1988; Ottenbacher, 1982).

Occupational Therapy for Psychosocial Dysfunction

The casual observer of psychosocial occupational therapy typically sees only the activity in progress. The observer assumes the patient is being engaged in a task to escape problems, to have something to do, or to learn a hobby to be continued upon discharge. The observer must be educated to see beyond the superficial and develop an understanding of the complex nature of occupation and its relationship to emotional well-being and psychosocial development in children (Llorens & Rubin, 1962).

OVERVIEW OF PRESENT PROBLEM

The above three factors have contributed to the infrequency of occupational therapy with students that have a behavioral disorder. Although occupational therapists frequently provide services for school-age patients in the psychiatric setting, it is apparent that occupational therapy has not successfully bridged the gap between hospital-based and school-based practice. Forness (1988), a renowned authority in the education of students with behavioral disorders, stated that the related services have done little to demonstrate the need for their special interventions. Another noted special education scholar, Weintraub (1988), lamented the paucity of services provided to students with behavioral disorders. He asserted that this group of students is the most underserved and inadequately served handicapped population.

REVIEW OF INTERDISCIPLINARY LITERATURE

Special education programming for students with behavioral disorders has been based on one of three models of intervention: psychoeducational, ecological, and behavioral. Each of these models has enjoyed periods of widespread acceptance. Adherents to each model have demonstrated efficacy and have compiled a significant body of knowledge (Grosenick, George & George, 1987). While some special educators have advocated allegiance to one of these models, others call for an expansion of both theory and technique. Braaten (1983), Coombs (1986), Hobbs (1967), Rhodes (1987), Van Til (1983) and others, have stated the need for an integration of compatible special education theories as well as greater interdisciplinary collaboration.

The concepts and assumptions which underlie occupational therapy provide a natural foundation from which to generate an interdisciplinary, holistic approach to serving the needs of students with behavioral disorders. However, there is no model for practice that articulates such occupational therapy intervention.

Transdisciplinary Constructs

A review of the literature in education, psychology, and occupational therapy was conducted. The research question was to determine whether transdisciplinary constructs were consistently present which would: (a) lend interdisciplinary support for an occupational therapy program for students with behavioral disorders; and (b) serve as basic guidelines for developing an interdisciplinary model specific to this population and environment. The following synthesis of education, psychology, and occupational therapy literature provides the results of the literature review.

Each of these three bodies of literature has an extensive knowledge base on functional behavior. The review of literature in education, psychology, and occupational therapy revealed seven constructs relevant to the research question; each of these constructs were consistently present within the respective bodies of knowledge. These constructs are as follows:

1. Importance of meaningful occupation of time
2. Use of the exploratory environment
3. Need for socially interdependent learning
4. The innate urge toward competency
5. Impact of perception on performance
6. Adaptation as the vehicle for functional development
7. Function as the by-product of the occupational adaptation process

Meaningful occupation of time. According to Reilly (1974) occupation is the process of being engaged in meaningful tasks relevant to the phenomena of everyday living. Work, play and self-care occupations constitute the continuum of occupational behaviors. Reilly based her treatment approach on the assumption that an improvement in occupational behavior competencies positively affects individual role performance. She championed the fundamental occupational therapy perspective that human beings are by nature occupational and have an innate urge to be occupational competent.

There has been a similar thread in both education and psychology literature that demonstrates a recognition of the importance of occupational development as an essential aspect of learning. Kilpatrick (1914) stated that if the academic content has meaning to the student, i.e., immediate application to current life situation, the student is eager to engage in the learning process. Erickson's (1950) stage of industry versus inferiority is consistent with the concept that school should be occupationally relevant. Holt (1967) incorporated the project method into his teaching techniques. He espoused providing the student the opportunity to initially engage with the learning task in a playful and self-directed manner. Didactic instruction followed occupational exploration. From a developmental learning perspective, the tasks identified by Havighurst (1972) emphasized activities pertaining to work, play, and self-care as necessary for growth. Van Til (1983) encouraged educators to embrace the concept of personal relevance to identify the appropriate direction of education for students with behavioral disorders. His account of working with correctional students provided examples of making academic content relevant to everyday life, to elicit student enthusiasm and motivation to learn. Rhodes (1987) called for greater consistency between academic content and everyday occupational experiences.

The exploratory environment. An exploratory environment is one in which the individual has the opportunity to acquire and refine skills through creative activities. It is a setting that promotes experimentation without risk of failure. The learning that occurs, through the process itself, is the product

(Kielhofner, 1983). The influence of the environment in educating students with behavioral disorders has been aptly demonstrated by educators in the work of Hewett (1980), Hobbs (1967), and Rhodes (1972). An exploratory learning environment expands the concept of environment beyond the physical setting. It embraces both the student's internal and external environment and the potential the student has to act upon the environment (Kielhofner, 1983). As Rhodes (1987) stated, educators need to become aware of the child's potential to create his or her own environment. An exploratory setting offers the student a naturalistic arena in which internal and external environments can unite and be experienced in the here and now. Exploratory learning is a self-directed intrinsically motivating process (Hobbs, 1967). Exploration is implicitly rewarding in that it yields an avenue to move from a state of disorganization and confusion to a more satisfying organized existence (Kielhofner, 1983). The exploratory environment is a setting that can help the student with behavioral disorders become more competent in integrating both material and symbolic phenomena (Hobbs, 1967).

Socially interdependent learning. The importance of a group approach in changing behavior has a well documented history. From the pioneers in psychological group processes, such as Anderson's (1936) group occupational projects and Slavson's (1947) activity groups with children, to contemporary educational interventions, the "group" remains the recommended mode of teaching students with behavioral disorders. Though group appears to be necessary, it is not a sufficient example, while social skills curricula are found to be effective in the learning setting, generalization appears to be poor. The behaviors learned are often not displayed in the regular classroom, the lunchroom, or on the school bus. The most common obstacle to effective mainstreaming of students with behavioral disorders is their poor ability to get along with others (Schloss, Schloss, Wood, & Kiehl, 1986).

Another education scholar, Hobbs (1967), stated that only through group interaction toward a social reality can the student acquire different ways to adapt. For new behaviors to become integrated into the student's adaptive response pattern, the learning must be experienced as a socially relevant phenomena. A function-oriented group, such as articulated by occupational therapists Schwartzberg, Howe, and McDermott (1982), may better meet the student's social need by involving the student in working with others to carry out real-life tasks. Such an approach is consistent with Slavson and Schiffer's (1975) work using task oriented groups with children who displayed severe behavioral disorders. They found that it is the experience of interacting with others, along with increased activity competency, that has the corrective effect on personality.

Urge toward competency. The belief that human beings have a drive toward competency emerged as one of the most prevalent concepts in the literature reviewed. White's (1959) seminal article cajoled educators and psychologists to embrace another dimension of the human personality. He lamented that psychology and education has focused treatment interventions on external motivators and ignored the most critical aspect of human change, intrinsic motivation. Occupational therapy has historically emphasized intrinsic motivation. Florey (1969) defined intrinsic motivation as the experience of internal pleasure and satisfaction derived from productive activity. Intrinsic motivation creates the desire to participate in independent action.

Hobbs' (1982) description of project Re-Ed emphasized the need to develop the students' competency in terms of what the student finds personally rewarding. Hewett's (1980) engineered classroom approach also incorporated the concept of internal motivation as the necessary step to achieving functional competencies. As another well-known educator stated, reinforcement doesn't lie in a piece of candy or gold star but in the actual doing of the activity (Bruner, 1964). According to Florey (1969), the occupational therapy is effective because it taps the individual's intrinsic motivation to master the environment. However, educators often say that motivation appears to be lacking in the student with a behavioral disorder. Other educators have stated that if nurturing the student's intrinsic motivation was the driving force in academic programming, the student would be naturally inclined to engage (Holt, 1967). He concluded that motivation would not be a problem.

Impact of perception on performance. DeCharms (1968) developed a theory of motivation based on the concept of personal causation. He determined that the belief in one's ability to impact the environment results in how one actually behaves. Rhodes (1987) added an additional dimension to understanding the power of the child's perceptions. He encouraged educators to teach the student how to be a generator of information rather than merely a receiver. He stated that what the student thinks is projected onto the environment and that this results in a modification of that environment. Hobbs (1967) emphasized the importance of successful experiences in building the perception of competence. White (1971) stressed that therapists should become equally as sensitive to the perception of competence as we are to defense mechanisms and behavioral manifestations. Fidler and Fidler (1983) also emphasized the influence of perception on performance. They addressed the link between the initial mental image of the action objective and the action that ultimately occurs. They stated that performance of the action then creates a subsequent mental image influencing future performance. Fidler and Fidler concluded that one's ability to act and subsequent performance is an interdependent phenomenon. As Kielhofner (1983) stated, perceptions provide an internal map of the world and one's potential to act upon it. The actor builds a perception of competency as a result of the doing processes. The student with a behavioral disorder is often limited perceptually and frequently denied experiential opportunities to create a positive self-image as a competent and performing person.

Adaptation as the vehicle for development. The concept of adaptive functioning has become increasingly prevalent in special education literature addressing students with behavioral disorders. Sparrow and Cicchetti (1987) stated that the adaptive behaviors of the student with a behavioral disorder

may be the most crucial element of development. They proposed that while intelligence and achievement scores are valuable for classification purposes, they are inadequate measures on which to base educational programs. Sparrow and Cicchetti encouraged an emphasis on adaptive functioning to measure the student's progress. Their beliefs are consistent with Hobbs' (1975) insistence that it is the student's typical performance which is a more accurate gauge of potential than aptitude. Sparrow and Cicchetti stated that assessment should focus on communication, daily living skills, socialization and motor development. They studied the adaptive functioning of students with a behavioral disorder compared to normal children. They found that the normal children averaged almost two standard deviations higher in their adaptive functioning. Overall, the students with behavioral disorders scored lower in socialization and displayed three times as many maladaptive behaviors as the normal children studied. Occupational therapists have addressed adaptation as a developmental process. Kielhofner (1983) stated that adaptability is promoted through experiences that provide the opportunity to explore, develop competencies and experience mastery over the environment. Rogers (1983) stated that adaptability is what enables the individual to meet environmental demands. The individual's adaptive potential is limited by personal experiences, perceptions of capacities and opportunities.

Function as determined by role performance. The ability to function is most meaningfully measured in terms of role performance requirements, not specific behaviors (Kielhofner, 1983). Functionality is developmental and varies with setting, age, and culture (Sparrow & Cicchetti, 1987). For the student a functional assessment should assess peer relations and use of leisure time in addition to other traditional adaptive functioning competencies. The roles of the student are those of student, friend, worker, and family member. A focus on role performance to measure function provides an expanded definition of functionality (Kielhofner, 1983). While diagnostic categories provide valuable information, they tell little about daily functions. The concept of role establishes the link between the individual behavior and the respective environment (Ferris, 1964). Role theory embraces behavior as the product of self and one's role. The behavior is thus as much the result of interacting roles as it is skill deficit or personality. In programming for students with behavioral disorders, role performance has received far less attention than specific skill acquisition.

Some special educators (Schloss, Schloss, Wood and Kiehl, 1986) have questioned whether effectiveness studies are asking the right question. They suggested the more salient question is whether the change in target behavior results in an improved social status, not increased manageability in the classroom.

Integration of the Constructs into a Model

It is proposed that the seven transdisciplinary constructs discussed in the above synthesis of literature form a valid

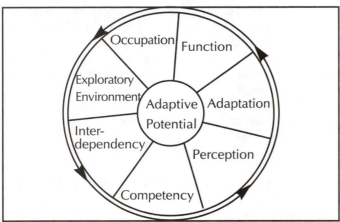

Figure 42-1. Constructs of Occupational Activity Grouping.

framework for the design of an occupation-based therapy model for students with behavioral disorders. The proposed therapy model is referred to as the Model for Occupational Activity Grouping-Students with Behavioral Disorders (SBD). The model is based on a synthesis of the seven interdisciplinary constructs identified in the literature review. An occupational therapist is suggested as the preferred professional to implement programming based on the model. Programming could be carried out by a certified occupational therapy assistant or other professional personnel under the direction of an occupational therapist. The Model for Occupational Activity Grouping (SBD) may be used as a guide to: (a) develop a special independent curriculum or learning module, (b) incorporate an additional component in the existing social skills curriculum, (c) or as an on-going group therapy intervention.

This model is designed to provide an additional dimension to traditional special education programming for students with behavioral disorders. Current programming is typically limited to behavioral management and offers little opportunity for the development of students' unique interests and competencies (Bauer & Sapona, 1987). The proposed model focuses on nurturing the positive element of the student with a behavioral disorder.

MODEL FOR OCCUPATIONAL THERAPY ACTIVITY GROUPING—STUDENTS WITH BEHAVIORAL DISORDERS

Essential Conditions

The essential conditions of the model are as follows:
1. The program must be implemented in a setting conducive to experiential group learning.
2. The primary modality of the program is the introduction of occupational activity (Schkade & Schultz, 1990) presented in an exploratory atmosphere.

3. Interaction will be fostered that promotes the social interdependency and individual relative mastery of the group members.

These three conditions set the stage for the student's unique competencies to be nurtured. It is proposed that new occupational experiences will have both an internal and external effect leading to improved occupational adaptation (Schultz & Schkade, 1991) and enhanced student role performance. Figure 42-1 presents the cyclical nature of the essential constructs of Occupational Activity Grouping-(SBD).

OCCUPATIONAL ACTIVITY GROUPING—ASSUMPTIONS AND CONSTRUCTS

As with any theoretically based model, certain assumptions and related constructs underlie and direct the interventions. For the proposed model, the assumptions reflect the interdisciplinary constructs upon which the model is based. These six assumptions are as stated below:
1. Occupational competencies in work, leisure/recreation, and self-maintenance are developmentally acquired (Havighurst, 1972; Kielhofner, 1983; Reilly, 1974).
2. An exploratory environment is one that is consistent with the individual's abilities, developmental needs, interests, age and roles (Hewett, 1980; Reilly, 1974).
3. Social competency is one of the primary developmental tasks of the student (Hobbs, 1982; Rhodes, 1972; Slavson, 1947; Slavson & Schiffer, 1975).
4. Adaptation is a function of the interaction of environmental factors, internal perceptions, and exploratory activities (Hewett, 1980; Hobbs, 1982; Kielhofner, 1983; King, 1978/1996; Rhodes, 1987).
5. As adaptive potential becomes actualized, the student acquires an internal sense of mastery further substantiated by external recognition. Both internal and external factors nurture the student's urge toward increased competency (Reilly, 1974; Sparrow & Cicchetti, 1987; White, 1959).
6. Development of individual adaptive potential will better enable students to gain social acceptance as they perform in their student role (Kielhofner, 1983; King, 1978; Reilly, 1974; Sparrow & Cicchetti, 1987).

These six assumptions are represented by the constructs contained in Figure 42-1. The arrows show the developmental progression of therapeutic intervention and the results of such intervention. Occupational Activity Grouping begins with the student's adaptive potential and is designed to actualize that potential through real-life experiences.

Viability and Validity of the Model

The Model for Occupational Activity Grouping-SBD presents the occupational therapist with a holistic framework for treating the occupational dysadaptation of students with behavioral disorders. Although occupational therapists have not traditionally addressed this student group, the literature strongly suggests that special educators will welcome new interventions for this special education population. The model remains to be tested; it is asserted that face validity has been established in that it is grounded by beliefs that are valued by not only the occupational therapy discipline, but also special education and psychology.

IMPLEMENTING OCCUPATIONAL ACTIVITY GROUPING-SBD

Population

This model for practice is intended for use with those students who are labeled (according to the EHA regulations) "seriously emotionally disturbed" by school districts. This label describes students who display one or more of the following characteristics over a long period of time and to a marked degree, adversely affecting educational performance: (a) an inability to learn which cannot be explained by intellectual, sensory, or health factors; (b) an inability to build or maintain satisfactory interpersonal relationships with peers and teachers; (c) inappropriate types of behavior or feelings under normal circumstances; (d) a general pervasive mood of unhappiness or depression; or (e) a tendency to develop physical symptoms or fears associated with personal or school problems (Education of Handicapped Children, Federal Register, 1977). These students typically have a low tolerance for rules, limits and directions and respond to perceived demands by acting out. They may also be depressed and withdrawn. Academic deficits and low motivation for school tasks are common. Poor social skills are an ever present problem. Students with severe behavioral disorders are typically served in self-contained classrooms. Individual carrels are often used to reduce distractions. Students with behavioral disorders are usually not actively included in school activities. The Model for Occupational Activity Grouping-SBD has the potential to address educational needs underserved by special education. Occupational Activity Grouping may provide a holistic intervention that will better enable the student with a behavioral disorder to benefit from special education.

Group Composition and Frequency

The model is inherently flexible. It allows for the divergent needs of the acting-out, the withdrawn, or the depressed student. It can be modified to fit the developmental needs of the different ages among students with behavioral disorders. The model encourages the creation of heterogeneous groups of students having various manifestations of behavioral disorders. Diversity in student's personality, interests, and problem-solving style lends itself well to this model. Age differences of two to three years should not hinder the group and may in fact generate a desirable environment. Adolescent groups, however, may function best if they are limited to the same sex. Sexuality concerns may jeopardize the therapeutic climate with this age group. The group sessions must be conducted with enough frequency to develop group cohesion. It is suggested that students meet for a minimum of two class sessions per week; daily groups are recommended.

Initiating the Group

The ideal group is begun with two or three higher functioning students with behavioral disorders. These two or three students should tend to model appropriate behaviors learned from the group leader for new students as they are added to the group. No more than two new members should be added weekly. The group should not exceed seven members with one facilitator or ten members with two facilitators.

Setting

The specific site for the group is not of particular importance. The therapy group can be implemented within almost any physical setting. Specifics of the physical space do not have a direct relationship to the purpose of the occupational activity group. The group may be housed in one environment (e.g., the school wood shop, art room, home economics room, science room, greenhouse), or the group may rotate to different settings as indicated by group interest or logistical constraints. The most basic intent of the occupational activity group is to provide the experience of learning as a group. This is not dependent upon a specified set of materials or physical space.

Therapeutic Relationship

The most crucial elements of occupational activity grouping are the facilitator and the method of intervention. In the Model for Occupational Activity Grouping-SBD, the group leader assumes a facilitative posture (Bauer & Sapona, 1987) and is present to encourage individual and group problem-solving. The facilitator is not present to teach the proper technique or way to do the occupational activities, but to help the student arrive at the highest level of relative mastery (Schkade & Schultz, 1990). The term, relative mastery, goes beyond the "ability to do the task" and implies that mastery is a phenomenological event that is characterized by three components: effectiveness, efficiency and satisfaction to self and others. It is proposed that the therapeutic climate produced by a facilitative approach provides the best opportunity for the student with a behavioral disorder to experience relative mastery (Schkade & Schultz, 1990).

Relative mastery is the product of both occupational readiness training and occupational activity. Evaluation of the student's initial level of occupational performance will indicate how much support the therapist needs to provide through occupational readiness (Schultz & Schkade, 1991). The therapist's role is to create a therapeutic climate using appropriate media, modalities, and therapeutic use of self that will enable the student with a behavioral disorder to have greater relative mastery of the occupational challenges that are part of the educational environment. The occupational activities that are presented to the student are not "taught" but provided in an atmosphere where personal meaning and investment can be explored.

Therapeutic Programming

The therapeutic program should approximate the student's age, developmental level, and social, physical and cultural environment. The activities that are included in the therapy program should be normalizing. For students in the early elementary age group the typical program would focus on incorporating media and activities which are part of the child's everyday life. For example, an independent living skills program of about six weeks duration could be introduced by the occupational therapist for students with behavioral disorders. Based on individual student's interests and competency, the therapist would facilitate a progressive series of group experiences focused on independent living. The program would begin with basic kitchen skills, food preparation, nutrition, and grocery shopping. Once the essential occupational training had occurred, knowledge and skill would be put into practice through occupational activities which require not only competency, but elicit adaptive responses from the group members. The goal would be to help each student develop: (a) basic competency in the occupational activity; (b) independent problem-solving skills, (c) cooperative work ability, and (d) adaptive responses to challenges experienced during the occupational activities. The therapist should design interface programs for the student's classroom and home environments. It is critical to extend therapy beyond the confines of the particular "treatment setting." The outcome effect of the therapy program would be objectively measured in terms of: the student's responses within the therapy environment; generalization of the therapy into the classroom setting; and feedback from parents on responses at home. Generalization from therapy is the best indicator that occupational adaptation has occurred.

Similarly, a program for the high school student may also emphasize independent living skills. The components of occupational readiness, occupational activity, relative mastery, and occupational adaptation would remain constant factors; only the specific techniques, media, and experiential methods would change.

The therapy programs for Occupational Activity Grouping can range from producing an "underground newspaper," to theatrical or musical productions, to gardening, to community volunteer work, or to furniture refinishing. The only barrier to programming is the knowledge and creativity of the occupational therapist.

CONCLUSION

Occupational Activity Grouping may remove some of the educational barriers experienced by students with behavioral disorders. Such students are frequently prevented from engaging in necessary social competency-building activities, e.g., the school newspaper; team sports, talent shows, and creativity contests, due to their behavioral problems or as disciplinary action. Occupational Activity Grouping could provide therapeutic experiences in such age-appropriate school-based activities that may yield a vital educational benefit. As Holt (1967) stated, the arts, and other productive activities exercise the brain as well as the eye and the hand. Arts, crafts, and skilled trades, for example, are rich in opportunities to develop problem-solving ability necessary for academic success and social functioning.

Based on the literature review, a therapeutic program guided by Occupational Activity Grouping would expand the curriculum for students with behavioral disorders. Such a therapeutic program could create an environment wherein the student is artfully facilitated in exploratory learning that will develop competencies that are directly related to student's role performance.

DISCUSSION

It is incumbent upon educators of students with behavioral disorders to recognize that the diverse needs of their students require a broad and collaborative theoretical base. Current programming for this population is inadequate and incomplete. It is also incumbent upon occupational therapists who are interested in treating psychosocial dysfunction to move from hospital-based practices and to provide earlier intervention that may more effectively meet the needs of students who are at risk for both severe academic dysfunction and social maladaptation as adults.

This (chapter) articulates a rudimentary model for occupational therapy services for students with behavioral disorders. Occupational Activity Grouping is proposed as an addition to the special education curriculum. It addresses the most basic needs of students with behavioral disorder to experience learning as a pleasurable, meaningful activity. Occupational Activity Grouping may provide the setting for the student to not only develop the skills essential to benefit from special education but the opportunity to reinforce, in a naturalistic environment, those competencies acquired in special education. Occupational Activity Grouping may develop the student's underlying adaptive potential by engaging him or her in meaningful, self-directed activities to awaken intrinsic social interest and the urge to become competent. While a few school settings have incorporated some of the constructs presented in this (chapter) into present programming, they have tended to do so intuitively; knowing that certain kinds of activities and learning experiences are rewarding to disenfranchised students. However, occupational therapists have had little involvement in the creation or implementation of such programs.

This (chapter) was written to provide a theoretical foundation for an interdisciplinary school-based program focused on the relationship between intrinsic occupation and the desire to learn. Basic guidelines were stated to encourage implementation and to provide a consistent framework from which to initiate a pilot project and design a research plan to measure the outcome effect of Occupational Activity Grouping for students with behavioral disorders.

REFERENCES

Adelstein, L., Barnes, M., Murray-Jensen, F., & Baker-Skaggs, C. (1989, December). A broadening frontier: Occupational therapy programs for children and adolescents. *Mental Health Special Interest Section Newsletter, 2.*

American Occupational Therapy Association (1986, September). Member data survey. *Occupational Therapy News,* 11-12.

Anderson, P. (1936). Project work-individual group therapy. *Occupational Therapy and Rehabilitation, 15*(4), 265-269.

Baron, K. (1989). Occupational therapy: A program for child psychiatry. *Mental Health Special Interest Section Newsletter,* 1, 8.

Bauer, A., & Sapona, R. (1987). Facilitating communication as a basis for intervention for students with severe behavioral disorders. *Behavior Disorders, 13*(4), 280-287.

Bloom, D. (1988). Perception of faculty members in special education concerning occupational therapy services in schools: A pilot study. *The Occupational Therapy Journal of Research, 8,* 104-113.

Braaten, S., Kauffman, J., Braaten, B., Polsgrove, L., & Nelson, C. (1988). The regular education initiative: Patent medicine for behavioral disorders. *Exceptional-Children, 55,* 21-27.

Braaten, S. (1983). Preface. *Programming for Adolescents with Behavioral Disorders, 1,* 1-8.

Brown, E. (1989, September). Survey targets areas for improvement in school based occupational therapy. *OT Advance,* 2.

Bruner, J. (1964). *Toward a theory of instruction.* Cambridge, MA: The Belknap Press of Harvard University Press.

Chandler, B. (1990). School systems. *OT Week, 7,* 10.

Coombs, A. (1986). Curriculum Development. *ASCD and the humanist movement: ASCD in retrospect.* Alexandria, VA: Association for Supervision.

Coutinho, M., & Hunter, D. (1988). Special education and occupational therapy: Making the relationship work. *American Journal of Occupational Therapy, 42,* 706-712.

Creighton, C. (1979). The school therapist and vocational education. *American Journal of Occupational Therapy, 33,* 373-375.

DeCharms, R. (1968). *Personal causation.* New York, NY: Academic Press.

Dunn, W. (1988). Models of occupational therapy service provision in the school system. *American Journal of Occupational Therapy, 42,* 718-723.

Edelmen, A. (1953). Some observations on occupational therapy with disturbed children in a residential program. *American Journal of Occupational Therapy, 7,* 113-117.

Erickson, E. (1950). *Childhood and society.* New York, NY: Norton Press.

Federal Register. (1975).

Federal Register. (1977).

Ferris, R. (1964). *The discipline of sociology: Handbook of sociology.* Chicago, IL: Rand McNally.

Fidler, G., & Fidler, J. (1983). Doing and becoming: The occupational therapy experience. In G. Kielhofner (Ed.), *Health through occupation.* Philadelphia, PA: F. A. Davis.

Florey, L. (1969). Intrinsic motivation: The dynamics of occupational therapy theory. *American Journal of Occupational Therapy, 23*(4), 319-322.

Florey, L. (1989). Nationally speaking-treating the whole child: Rhetoric or reality? *American Journal of Occupational Therapy, 43,* 365-368.

Forness, S. (1988). Planning for the needs of children with severe emotional disturbance: The national education and mental health coalition. *Behavior Disorders, 13,* 127-132.

Gilfoyle, E., & Hays, C. (1979). Occupational therapy roles and functions in the education of the school-based handicapped students. *American Journal of Occupational Therapy, 39,* 222-224.

Gleave, G. (1947). Occupational therapy in children's hospitals and pediatric services. In H. Willard & C. Spackrnan (Eds.), *Principles of occupational therapy* (pp. 141-174). Philadelphia, PA: Lippincott.

Groseniek, J., George, M., & George, N. (1987). A profile of school programs for the behaviorally disordered: 20 years after Morse, Little, & Fink (1964). *Behavior Disorders, 12,* 3.

Havighurst, R. (1972). *Developmental tasks and education.* New York, NY: Longmans.

Hewett, F. (1980). *The emotional, disturbed child in the classroom: The orchestration.* Boston, MA: Allyn and Bacon.

Hightower-Vandamm, M. (1980). Nationally speaking-the perils of occupational therapy in several special arenas of practice. *American Journal of Occupational Therapy, 34,* 307-309.

Holt, J. (1967). *How children learn.* New York, NY: Pitman Publishing.

Hobbs, N. (1967). Helping disturbed children: Psychological and ecological strategies. *American Psychologist,* 1105-1115.

Hobbs, N. (1975). *Issues in the classification of children* (Vol. 1 & 2). San Francisco, CA: Jossey-Bass.

Hobbs, N. (1982). *The troubled and troubling child.* San Francisco, CA: Jossey-Bass.

Huntze, S. (1985). A position paper of the Council for Children with Behavioral Disorders. *Behavioral Disorders, 10,* 167-174.

Kalish, R., & Presseller, S. (1980). Physical and occupational therapy. *Journal of School Health, 50,* 264-267.

Kauffman, J. (1986). Educating children with behavioral disorders. In R. Morris & B. Blatts (Eds.), *Special education: Research & trends.* New York, NY: Pergamon.

Kielhofner, G. (l983). *Health through occupation.* Philadelphia, PA: F. A. Davis.

Kilpatrick, W. (1914). The Montessori system examined. In H. Suzzalo (Ed.), *Riverside education monograph.* Cambridge, MA: The Riverside Press.

King, L. (1978). Toward a science of adaptive responses-1978 Eleanor Clark Slagle Lecture. *American Journal of Occupational Therapy, 32*(7), 429-437. (Reprinted in Cottrell, R. P. (1996). Perspectives on purposeful activity: Foundations and future of occupational therapy (pp. 81-89). Bethesda, MD: AOTA.)

Kinnealey, M., & Morse, A. (1979). Educational mainstreaming of physically handicapped children. *American Journal of Occupational Therapy, 33,* 365-372.

Langdon, H., & Langdon, L. (1983). *Initiating occupational therapy programs within the public school system: A guide for occupational therapists and public school administrators.* Thorofare, NJ: SLACK Incorporated.

Llorens, L., & Rubin, E. (1962). A directed activity program for disturbed children. *American Journal of Occupational Therapy, 16,* 287-289.

Llorens, L., Rubin, E., Braun, J., Beck, G., & Beall, C. (1969). The effects of a cognitive-perceptual-motor training approach on children with behavior maladjustment. *American Journal of Occupational Therapy, 23*(6), 502-512.

Matsutsuyu, J. (1971). Occupational behavior-A perspective on work and play. *American Journal of Occupational Therapy, 25*(6), 291-294.

Occupational Therapy News. (1985). *American Occupational Therapy Association, 7,* 10.

Ottenbacher, K. (1982). Occupational therapy and special education: Some issues and concerns related to Public Law 94-142. *American Journal of Occupational Therapy, 36,* 81-84.

Rabinovitch, R., Bee, I., & Outwater, B. (1951). The integration of occupational and recreational therapy in the residential psychiatric treatment of children: A symposium. *American Journal of Occupational Therapy, 5,* 1-8.

Reilly, M. (1974). *Play as exploratory learning.* Beverly Hills, CA: Sage.

Rhodes, W. (1972). *Study of child variance: Conceptual project in emotional disturbance* (Vols. 1-4). Ann Arbor, MI: University of Michigan Press.

Rhodes, W. (1987). Ecology and the new physics. *Behavior Disorders, 13*(1), 58-61.

Robert Wood Johnson Foundation. (1988). *Serving handicapped children: Special report* (No. 1). Princeton, NJ: Author.

Rogers, J. (1983). The study of human occupation. In G. Kielhofner (Ed.), *Health through occupation.* Philadelphia, PA: F. A. Davis.

Royeen, C. (1986). Nationally speaking-evaluation of school-based occupational therapy programs: Needs, strategy, and dissemination. *American Journal of Occupational Therapy, 40,* 811-813.

Royeen, C., & Marsh, D. (1988). Promoting occupational therapy in the schools. *American Journal of Occupational Therapy, 42,* 713-717.

Schloss, P., Schloss, C., Wood, C., & Kiehl, W. (1986). A critical review of social skills research with behaviorally disordered students. *Behavioral Disorders, 12,* 1-12.

Schkade, J. & Schultz, S. (1990). *Occupational adaptation: An integrative frame of reference.* Unpublished manuscript.

Schultz, S., & Schkade, J. (1991). *Occupational adaptation: Implications for treatment.* Unpublished manuscript.

Schwartzberg, S., Howe, M., & McDermott. R. (1982). A comparison of three treatment groups in facilitating social interaction. *Occupational Therapy in Mental Health, 2,* 1-16.

Slavson, S. (1947). *The practice of group therapy.* New York, NY: International Universities Press.

Slavson, S., & Schiffer, M. (1975). *Group psychotherapies for children.* New York, NY: International Universities Press.

Sparrow, S., & Cicchetti, D. (1987). Adaptive behavior and the psychologically disturbed child. *Journal of Special Education, 21*(1), 89-100.

Stephens, L. (1989). Occupational therapy in the school system. In P. Clark & A. Allen (Eds.), *Occupational therapy for children* (2nd Edition) (pp. 593-611).

Van Til, W. (1983). Programming for youth in secondary schools and the community. *Programming for Adolescents with Behavior Disorders, 1,* 1-8.

Weintraub, F. (1988). The council for exceptional children commitment. *Behavior Disorders, 13,* 138-139.

White, R. (1959). Motivation reconsidered: The concept of competence. *Psychological review, 66,* 297-333.

White, R. (1971). The urge towards competence. *American Journal of Occupational Therapy, 25*(6), 271-274.

CHAPTER FORTY-THREE

Occupational Therapy in a Multidisciplinary Psychiatric Home Health Care Service

Stacey D. Azok and Jeffrey Tomlinson

This chapter was previously published in the Mental Health Special Interest Section Newsletter, 17(2), *1-3.*
Copyright © 1994, The American Occupational Therapy Association, Inc.

The Visiting Nurse Association (VNA) of Cleveland has been providing psychiatric home health care services since 1988 and in 1991 added an occupational therapist to its team. The psychiatric home health care team had been comprised of nurses and social workers with previous psychiatric experience. Nurses were case mangers and coordinated all services, and social workers provided family and couple counseling, as well as referrals to community resources. Because several team members had experience with occupational therapy in mental health care and knew what occupational therapy offered, the marketing of occupational therapy services to the VNA was easier to accomplish than it would have been otherwise.

From the beginning of the occupational therapist's employment, one resource was identified that helped define occupational therapy services in mental health care. The American Occupational Therapy Association's Uniform Terminology for Occupational Therapy (AOTA, 1989/1996), a nationally recognized document, provided a clear, concise delineation of the occupational therapist's areas of expertise. This definition of occupational therapy practice parameters was quickly accepted by the team members and helped them to understand further what occupational therapy could offer to the clients they served in mental health care. The fundamental difference between other professions and occupational therapy was occupational therapy's rehabilitative approach. Each professional, including the occupational therapist, brought his or her own expertise to the team in a manner that complemented the others, thus creating a balanced program for the clients in mental health care.

The populations served by occupational therapy during the first year that the occupational therapist was on the team ranged from 25 to 94 years of age. Conditions included major depression, bipolar disorder, schizophrenia, and anxiety dis-

orders. In a period of 13 months, the occupational therapist worked with approximately 30 to 40 clients. To qualify for home health care services, clients had to be determined to be homebound. This determination was often established when psychosocial symptoms and functional deficits affected be client's ability to leave the home. Use of these considerations in determining who is homebound may be new for home health care teams accustomed to using the more traditional criteria associated with physical disabilities. The psychosocial symptoms and deficits included severe anxiety, immobilizing depression, memory impairments, agoraphobia, impaired judgment, impaired safety awareness, and paranoid delusions. Usually, the case manager-nurse first identified the need for occupational therapy services. However, during the weekly team meetings, other team members, including the occupational therapist, played roles in identifying this need. The case manager then requested a written referral from the psychiatrist to initiate the occupational therapy services.

The occupational therapist first conducted a comprehensive evaluation or as much of the evaluation as a client was able to tolerate during the first visit. Usually evaluations were completed within the first two 1-hour sessions, but additional information on functional tasks was collected in subsequent treatment sessions. Conducting evaluations in the home allowed the therapist to assess clients' actual functional abilities in their living environments, rather than drawing inferences based only on clinical observations. Barriers, absence of materials, disorganized spaces, and malfunctioning tools could be identified, and changes or adaptations could be made to enhance performance.

During a home visit, the occupational therapist could often meet with family members or caregivers. These contacts allowed the occupational therapist to collect further information on the client's functional status and information

COGNITIVE

Oriented to: ☐ NT   ☐ Person   ☐ Time   ☐ Place   ☐ Situation

Concentration/Attention Span: ☐ NT   ☐ 0-5 min.   ☐ 5-15 min.   ☐ 15-30 min.   ☐ 30-60 min.

	WFL	IMP min / mod / max	NT	Memory:	WFL	IMP min / mod / max	NT
Integration of Learning:				Short-Term:			
Judgement:				Long-Term:			
Frustration Tolerance:				Sequencing Ability:			
				Organizational Skills:			
Ability to Follow Directions: ☐ NT				Problem-Solving			
Responds to: ☐ Physical Cues				Generalization of Learning:			
☐ Demonstrative Cues							
☐ Verbal Cues							
☐ Written Cues				Other: _____			
Able to execute: ☐ 1-Step Directions				Comments: _____			
☐ 2-Step Directions				_____			
☐ 3-Step Directions							
☐ 4-Step Directions							

Figure 43-1. Excerpt from the cognitive section of the Occupational Therapy Mental Health Assessment for the Visiting Nurse Association of Cleveland (1992). Note: NT=not tested, IMP=impaired, WFL=within functional limits.

on variations in that functional status over time. This communication with the family also provided information on how the family perceived and responded to the client's behaviors, symptoms, and disabilities.

A complete occupational therapy evaluation included an assessment of performance components (i.e., sensorimotor, cognitive, and psychosocial skills) and an assessment of specific performance areas, including activities of daily living (ADL), work skills, and leisure skills. Following is an excerpt from the cognitive section of the Occupational Therapy Mental Health Assessment developed in 1992 for the VNA of Cleveland by Stacey Azok, OTR/L, and Terra Turner, OTR/L. This section of the form is used to communicate to other professionals the client's cognitive skills at the time of assessment (Figure 43-1).

A check-off format like the evaluation excerpt in Figure 1 is advantageous because it can be completed by the occupational therapist in a timely manner and provides an organized, easily read presentation for other team members. The completion of this type of form should always be supported, either in the comments section or in the evaluation summary, with a brief description of the effects these impairments have on the client's functioning.

The VNA of Cleveland had a variety of distinct occupational therapy goals. Following is a summary of six goal areas offered to the clients.

1. Client will identify problems in ADL, home management, work, and leisure performance and follow through with activities that address these problems.
2. Client will identify and follow through with adaptive coping strategies.
3. Client will develop and follow through with a plan to maintain a balance of ADL, home management, work, and leisure tasks.
4. Client will concentrate on and pay attention to tasks.
5. Client will use compensatory strategies for cognitive impairment.
6. Client will initiate and follow through with activities to prepare for community reintegration.

The setting of a goal and engagement in treatment activities should be a collaborative or negotiative process for the occupational therapist and the client. Treatment activities and goal completion may be done independently by the client or with the assistance of the therapist or family members. Occupational therapy treatment interventions provided in the home included training in ADL, home management, work skills, and use of adaptive equipment; adaptation of the home environment; exploration to determine enjoyable vocational or leisure tasks; planning and monitoring of performance in vocational or leisure tasks; education on resources and supports available; instruction in time management skills; instruction in the use of public transportation; training in social skills and coping skills; and provision of activities that facilitate self-expression. Clients and caregivers also received instruction in problem-solving skills; compensatory strategies for cognitive or sensorimotor deficits; energy conservation, work simplification, and body mechanics; relaxation; and home exercise.

When family members or caregivers were available in the home, they collaborated with the occupational therapist and became extensively involved in the client's treatment. This involvement included therapist input to family members on how to assist the client to be more independent and collaboration in problem-solving and adaptations, leading to the therapist's modeling of more effective responses and interventions with the client. As mentioned, the family members and caregivers also offered the occupational therapist information related to client functioning between therapy sessions. This collaboration between the therapist, the client, and the family made the clients and family members more inclined to repeat treatment activities when the therapist was absent and to transfer newly acquired skills to related tasks.

Coordination of the treatment plan and all services, including the planning of new services, required extensive communication among all the members of the mental health team. Members held weekly team meetings and communicated by phone or voice mail on an ongoing basis to maintain continuity of care.

As always, services did overlap. Some overlap of services was necessary to reinforce essential aspects of the client's care and to ensure coordination. However, there was always a need for a clear definition of what the occupational therapist could provide, as distinct from the other team members. The occupational therapist's role can be defined as follows: The occupational therapist focuses on activity analysis and functional abilities, and considers comprehensively the effects that psychosocial, cognitive, and sensorimotor skills have on functional performance.

As is the case for all other providers, documentation of the initial assessment, treatment interventions, and improvement in the client was essential for the Medicare intermediary to reimburse for services. The most important aspect of this documentation was to show a measurable improvement in functioning.

CASE STUDY

The following is a case study of one client who received occupational therapy services for remediation of a psychosocial disability primarily due to mental health problems. J. F., a 74-year-old married woman, had been diagnosed with major depression and parkinsonism, secondary to basal ganglia degeneration. She was referred to occupational therapy because of an impaired daily living routine and decreased functioning in self-care, home management, and leisure skills. The client also had difficulty with motor skills such as ambulation and standing tolerance. The client had become dependent on her husband and her home health care aide.

This dependency had become a severe stressor for the husband, who was becoming increasingly agitated with his wife and unable to care for her effectively. This in turn was straining the marital relationship.

The occupational therapist visited this client for 13 sessions over a 9-week period. Treatment goals focused on the client being able to perform ADLs with supervision but without physical assistance from caregivers, perform home management tasks with minimal assistance from others, and engage in two or three leisure activities. The occupational therapist provided ADL training; education in energy conservation, work simplification, and relaxation techniques; and exploration and planning of leisure activity interests. Because of the client's depression and anxiety, there were motivational and attitudinal aspects of the client's performance that the occupational therapist needed to address. The therapist encouraged discussion of self-esteem issues, identifying activities that were particularly motivating to the client and achievable short-term goals.

At each session, goals were reviewed with the client and reinforced. The husband also participated in or observed most of the sessions and actively cooperated in the goal setting. The husband gave feedback to the occupational therapist on which leisure goals were realistic in light of the client's previous performance. When goals were set, the occupational therapist educated the husband on the reasons for certain activities and the importance of the goals. This communication with the husband, along with the husband watching the client make progress in each session, helped enlist the husband's support in the client's treatment. In addition, the nurse-case manager and the social worker provided family counseling to help the couple adjust to the client's present state. The husband participated in the preparation for activities by going out to buy supplies the client needed. With the occupational therapist's encouragement, the husband gradually learned to be less protective in ADL with the client. The husband also reported the client's activities and progress to the occupational therapist.

Next, the husband started to participate in various leisure activities with the client. In addition to working with the husband, the occupational therapist encouraged the home health care aide to allow the client gradually to do more for herself. At the termination of occupational therapy services, each treatment goal had been achieved. The client was able to perform self-care and many home management tasks with greater independence, and she was once again involved in leisure pursuits that brought her pleasure. These gains ended the client's dependency role with the husband and home health care aide.

This case study is one brief description of how occupational therapy interventions regarding the mental health aspects of a disability can have a dramatic effect on a client's functioning within the home. In addition to enhancing the quality of the client's life, the occupational therapy interventions can help the family caregiver experience great relief from the client's extensive dependence on care. This gives family members more time to spend with the client in leisure or social activities, or more time to pursue their own interests and needs.

CONCLUSION

The occupational therapist was well received as a contributing member of the multidisciplinary mental health care team at the VNA of Cleveland. At present, the program is expanding, and to meet the needs of its clients, it is seeking more occupational therapists and occupational therapy assistants who work in mental health.

ACKNOWLEDGMENT

This article was based primarily on Stacey D. Azok's clinical experience at the Visiting Nurse Association of Cleveland, 2500 East 22nd Street, Cleveland, OH 44115.

REFERENCES

American Occupational Therapy Association. (1989). Uniform terminology for occupational therapy (2nd ed.). *American Journal of Occupational Therapy, 43,* 808-815. (Reprinted in Cottrell, R. P. (1996). Perspectives on purposeful activity: Foundations and future of occupational therapy (pp. 651-665). Bethesda, MD: AOTA.)

Azok, S., & Turner, T. (1992). *Occupational Therapy assessment for the Visiting Nurse Association of Cleveland* (Available from the Visiting Nurse Association of Cleveland, 2500 East 22nd Street, Cleveland, OH 44115.)

Consultation: A Vital Skill for Occupational Therapists

Peggy Wittman

This chapter was previously published in Occupational Therapy in Health Care, 10(2), 65-71. Copyright ©1996, *Haworth Press.*

INTRODUCTION

A new graduate stops by to say 'hi' to a faculty member and shares that she is really excited about her new job in a local school system. She is especially happy that she has just talked her supervisor into cutting her caseload from eleven different schools to seven! Another student has just returned from a mental health fieldwork I experience in a site serving 150 clients with substance abuse problems which has never had an occupational therapist on staff. He has been encouraged by site staff to help write a grant for new programming which would include funding for occupational therapy consultation services. Occupational therapists are being hired in record numbers to provide comprehensive services to nursing homes, home health agencies, and school systems. Simultaneously, it is anticipated that in order to survive in the current community-based mental health care system, the direct, hands-on service model of providing occupational therapy services to mental health clients will soon become a thing of the past to be replaced by a consultative, indirect service model (Adams, 1990/1993; Bruhn, 1993; Klugheit, 1994; Nielson, 1993; Quinn, 1993). "Many predict that the role of physical and occupational therapists will shift from that of hands-on-provider of care to that of evaluator, educator, consultant, supervisor, and specialist" (APTA, p. 3). As Nielson (1993) states, "Working within the community mental health system shifts the occupational therapy emphasis from direct involvement with clients to a more indirect role... We must give up the idea that the only way to be an occupational therapist is to perform occupational therapy, and that the indirect roles of consultant, case manager, or program administrator do not lessen the impact of occupational therapy" (p. 2).

While supervision skills will also be needed by occupational therapists, this (chapter) differentiates between supervision and consultation. Jaffe (1996) maintains that management, administration, and supervision "all have authority and control" (p. 27). Consultation, on the other hand, is a facilitative process designed to assist in problem solving. As such, consultants have no power to make final decisions, implement services, administer programs, supervise staff, or treat patients and there is no guarantee that the consultant's ideas will be accepted (p. 27).

The need for cost-effective services in a managed care environment will force many health care professionals to change the way they deliver, and indeed think about, what they do. Occupational therapy will be no exception. A recent study done in Canada (Lysack, Stadnyk, Paterson, McLeod, & Kresfting, 1995) indicates that 85% of therapists working in community-based practice settings describe their principal job roles as consultants/educators. Current trends including the use of non-licensed personnel, patient-focused care, and interdisciplinary service delivery models will continue to mandate the need for occupational therapists to develop and effectively use consultation skills.

LITERATURE REVIEW

A review of the published literature yields writings which address several primary issues about consultation in general. Many textbooks (Goodstein, 1978; Jaffe, 1992; Pendleton, Schofield, Tate & Havelock, 1984; Rieman, 1992) discuss models, or theories, about consultation and describe various ways in which consultation can be both conceptualized and implemented. Jaffe (1988), Mitra (1994), and Nesbit and Johnson (1993), describe examples of effective consultation from a case perspective while other literature (Clark, 1986; Harchik, Sherman, Sheldon, & Strouse, 1992; Peck, Killen & Baumgart, 1989; Petti, Cornely, & McIntyre, 1993) reports the results of quantitative studies on effectiveness. Babcock and Pryzwansky (1983) explored preferences for type of consultation and found that educational professionals preferred a collaborative model of consultation over other indirect service models. Phillips and McCullough (1990) discuss ways to implement such collaborative efforts. Watson (1986) describes the use of psychiatric liaisons in hospital programs; her article may be especially relevant to those occupational therapists who practice in acute care mental health settings and are involved in assisting their colleagues on rehabilitation units to incorporate psychosocial evaluation and treatment into client care. And finally, Dutton (1986) describes how to design a consultation contract for use by occupational therapists.

THE CAPLAN MODEL OF CONSULTATION

While the literature mentioned above provides a plethora of general information including some useful "how to" techniques, if occupational therapists are to successfully practice in the community mental health care system, an overall model of consultation is necessary as a framework for the further development of specific skills. One such conceptual model is Caplan and Caplan (1993). Originally written in the early 1970s following the establishment of community mental health programs, these four fundamental types of consultation are still relevant to occupational therapists seeking a theoretical model with the potential for practical application. Discussed previously in the occupational therapy literature by Baxley (1994/2000), these four types are again described below in order to provide a reference point for formulating the type of consultation which may be needed and effective in given situations.

In *client-centered case consultation*, the consultant's work relates to *the management of a particular case or group of cases*. The consultant helps by using specialized knowledge and skills to make an expert assessment of the client's problem and to recommend how the consulted should deal with the case. The primary goal of the consultation is for the consultant to communicate to the consultee how this client can be helped. A subsidiary goal is that the consultee may use experience with this case to improve his/her knowledge and skills, so that he/she will be better able in the future to handle other similar problems. This is probably the most common type of consultation in which occupational therapists are involved. The occupational therapist who is asked by a classroom teacher for assistance with a special needs child, a nurse for help with a nursing home resident's behavioral problems, or the psychologist in a partial hospitalization program for assistance with a participant's discharge plans, are all examples of this type of consultation.

Consultee-centered case consultation is the type of consultation in which the consultee's problem relates to the management of a particular client, but instead of the consultant working directly with the client, the main focus is on *understanding the consulted difficulty with the case* and working with the individual to remedy the problem. The purpose of this consultation is to improve professional competency so that the consultee can directly help the client and

future clients with similar problems. The occupational therapist who does not see the client in the above examples but instead works only with the classroom teacher, the nurse, or the psychologist to provide them with intervention strategies, therapeutic techniques to try, and perhaps knowledge about a particular problem, diagnosis, or theory is doing this kind of consultation.

Program-centered administrative consultation involves work with a problem in the area of planning and administration; how to *develop a new program or improve an existing one*. The consultant helps by using his/her knowledge of administration and systems, as well as knowledge of particular kinds of theory and practice techniques to prescribe an effective course of action for a client or group of clients. This type of consultation is becoming more and more necessary as occupational therapists address the needs of populations of people who for economic, political, and other reasons do not have access to direct, individualized occupational therapy services and yet need rehabilitation. The work of occupational therapists to assist community agencies in the development of partial hospitalization, aftercare, and out-patient programs in facilities or settings with few professionally trained staff members exemplifies this kind of consultation.

Finally, *consultee-centered administrative* consultation has a focus on *problems of programming and organization* instead of on dealing with a particular client. The consultant's primary goal is to understand and help remedy organizational problems which will enable the consultee to develop and implement effective plans to accomplish the mission of the organization more effectively. An occupational therapist employed by a private mental health care facility to work with the management team in assessing programming needs for the entire client population is doing this type of consultation.

Obviously, in many cases an occupational therapist may use all four types of consultation in performing her/his job while in other cases, he/she may employ primarily one or two types of consultation. For example, an occupational therapist employed by a mental health center which provides partial hospitalization, intensive out-patient, and home health services might provide client-centered case consultation. Assessing the abilities of several dually diagnosed clients to live independently in the community and then giving ideas about appropriate activities for other staff to do is an example of this type of consultation. The occupational therapist could also provide consultee-centered case consultation to other staff members responsible for doing home visits by sharing some general ideas about how to adapt home environments to assist a client with organizational skill deficits. Simultaneously the occupational therapist consultant might provide program-centered consultation to the out-patient treatment team in helping them develop a daily program for clients with substance abuse problems. And finally, the occupational therapist might provide administrative consultation by assisting managers in the mental health center develop a way to measure customer satisfaction, determine appropriate functional outcome goals for specific populations, and/or do a needs assessment related to clients' abilities to perform daily living skills.

Conclusion

In conclusion, in conjunction with changes in the health care system, especially the advent of managed care, occupational therapists must develop skills for extending services in order to provide care to the many clients who desperately need and should receive them. A working knowledge of consultation theory is a first step in this process. Consultation skills are rapidly becoming a necessary, perhaps even entry level, skill for occupational therapists, especially those who wish to begin or continue to practice in mental health.

References

Adams, R. (1990). The role of occupational therapists in community mental health. *Mental Health Special Interest Section Newsletter, 13*(1), 1-2. (Reprinted in Cottrell, R. P. (1993). Psychosocial occupational therapy: Proactive approaches (pp. 165-167). Bethesda, MD: AOTA.)

Babcock, N. L., & Pryzwansky, S. B. (1983). Models of consultation: Preferences of educational professionals at five stages of service. *Journal of School Psychology, 21*, 359-366.

Baxley, S. (1994). Options for community practice: The Springfield Hospital model. *Mental Health Special Interest Section Newsletter, 17*(1), 3-5. (See Chapter 17 in this text.)

Bruhn, J. (1993). Potential Patterns. *Journal of Allied Health, Summer*, 293-301.

Caplan, G., (1970). *Theory Practice of Mental Health Consultation.* New York, NY: Basic Books.

Caplan, G. & Caplan, R. B. (1993). *Mental Health Consultation and Collaboration.* San Francisco, CA: Jossey-Bass.

Clark, M. J. (1986). Factors enhancing the success of consultation. *Nursing Administration Quarterly, 10*, 1-8.

Dutton, R. (1986). Procedures for designing an occupational therapy consultation contract. *American Journal of Occupational Therapy, 40*, 160- 166.

Goodstein, L. D. (1978). *Consulting with human service systems.* Reading, MA: Addison-Wesley Publishing Company, Inc.

Harchik, A. E., Sherman, J. A., Sheldon, J. B., & Strouse, M. C. (1992). Ongoing consultation as a method of improving performance of staff members in a group home. *Journal of Applied Behavior Analysis, 25*, 599-610.

Jaffe, E. (1988). The occupational therapist as a consultant: a model of community consultation. *Occupational Therapy in Health Care, 5*, 87-106.

Jaffe, E. (1992). *Occupational therapy consultation: Theory, principles, and practice.* St. Louis, MO: Mosby.

Jaffe, E. (1996). Occupational therapy consultation in a managed care environment. *OT Practice*, 26-31.

Klugheit, M. (1994). An appreciation for the role of occupational therapy in community mental health treatment. *Mental Health Special Interest Section Newsletter, 17*(1), 1-3.

Lysack, C., Stadnyk, R., Paterson, M., McLeod, K., & Kresfting, L. (1995). Professional expertise of occupational therapists in community practice: Results of an Ontario survey. *Canadian Journal of Occupational Therapy, 63*, 139-147.

Mitra, A. L. (1994). Occupational therapists as consultants: A Canadian perspective. *Gerontology Special Interest Section Newsletter, 17*(2), 1-4.

Nesbit, J., & Johnson, C. (1993). Facilitating transition from hospital inpatient to community resident for mental health clients: A consultative model. *Occupational Therapy Practice, 4*(4), 54-S9.

Nielson, C. (1993). Occupational therapy and community mental health: A new and unprecedented turn. *Mental Health Special Interest Section Newsletter, 16*(3), 1-4.

Peck, C. A., Killen, C. C., & Baumgart, D. (1989). Increasing implementation of special education instruction in mainstream preschools: Direct and generalized effects of nondirective consultation. *Journal of Applied Behavior Analysis, 22*, 191-210.

Pendleton, D., Schofield, T., Tate, P., & Havelock, P. (1984). *The consultation: An approach to learning and teaching.* New York, NY: Oxford University Press.

Petti, T. A., Cornely, P. J., & McIntyre, A. (1993). A consultative study as a catalyst for improving mental health services for rural children and adolescents. *Hospital and Community Psychiatry, 44*, 262-265.

Phillips, V. & McCullough, L. (1990). Consultation-based programming: Instituting the collaborative ethic in schools. *Exceptional Children, 56*, 291-304.

Quinn, B. (1993). Community occupational therapy in Canada: A model for mental health. *Mental Health Special Interest Section Newsletter, 16*(2), 1-4.

Rieman, D. W. (1992). *Strategies in social work consultation: From theory to practice in the mental health field.* New York, NY: Longman Publishing Croup.

Watson, L. J. (1986). Psychiatric consultation-liaison in the acute physical disabilities setting. *American Journal of Occupational Therapy, 40*, 338-342.

Humanistic and Holistic Approaches in Occupational Therapy Practice

EDITOR'S NOTE

Occupational therapy is a caring holistic profession. Caring and holism are firmly rooted in our historical heritage, our professional philosophy, and our art of practice (Burke & Cassidy, 1996; Gillfoyle, 1980; King, 1980; Mosey,1986; Peloquin, 1996). Occupational therapists care by helping people maximize their capabilities, adapt to their losses, and engage in satisfying, productive activities—utilizing their assets and minimizing their limitations (Devereux, 1991; Mosey, 1986).

Traditionally, occupational therapists collaborated with the individual, facilitating the ability to do for him-or-herself (Devereux, 1996). As Gage and Polatajko (1995) note, today, occupational therapy practice must be client-driven for this type of practice "is one where the professional looks to the client to be an active participant, without abdicating professional responsibility" (p. 117). Current practitioners need to consider all aspects of the individual, personally, socially, culturally and spiritually, to provide holistic care. Recent trends in health care have seriously challenged occupational therapists ability to maintain this tradition of caring and holism. Managed care and other external constraints have limited intervention time, often resulting in reductionistic, economically driven care. (Burke & Cassidy, 1996; Fine, 1998; Howard, 1996).

On the other hand, increased consumer demands for quality care, the growth of wellness and prevention models, an enhanced emphasis on quality of life, and the development of client-centered approaches are supportive of sustaining the art of caring and holistic occupational therapy practice, (Baum & Law, 1998; Christiansen, 1996; Freidland & Renwick, 1993; Frese, 1998). Therapists who align themselves with these movements will find strong support for the individuation of intervention. Therapists practicing in more market-driven environments will need to assertively work to balance their client's individual needs with current market demands. (Baum & Law, 1998; Burke & Cassidy, 1996; Fine, 1998; Howard, 1996).

To do so, therapists must actively and continually work on their helping skills. Certification establishes competence in a field of knowledge, but competence must be permeated with caring to have any relevant meaning or lasting effect (Davis, 1998; King, 1980; Borg & Bruce, 1997). The chapters in this section clearly describe the vital role caring, empathetic, helping relationships play in facilitating therapeutic change within individuals. Although we cannot truly know the client's experience, it is hoped that reviewing the personal dimensions of the individual and their perspectives on therapy will increase awareness, understanding, and empathy for clients, thereby enhancing the readers' helping skills.

This section's first chapter by Turner, provides a strong contrast between helping and non-helping relationships. Turner reflects on her personal experiences as a hospitalized psychiatric patient, which ranged from disastrous, dehumanizing, and hopeless to successful, respectful, and life-affirming. Turner clearly identifies characteristics from both ends of the helping continuum. Her vivid descriptions provide readers with a renewed appreciation of the value of respect, kindness, and collaboration in therapeutic relationships and of the need for well-designed, goal-directed treatment programs.

The importance of caring and competence in therapeutic relationships is strongly supported in the next chapter by Leete, who chronicles her 20-year battle with schizophrenia. Leete's personal account describes the characteristics of helping relationships and therapeutic programs that enabled her to maintain hope, accept her illness, and pursue a fulfilling and productive life. Her descriptions of beneficial approaches are highly relevant to occupational therapy practice. Patient education; structured, goal-directed activities; support groups; community residences; vocational training; stress management; and social and independent living skills training are all advocated by Leete as vital for gaining control over one's illness and life. As occupational therapists skilled in these areas, we can work in collaboration with clients to develop their ability to cope with their illnesses and to attain a satisfying quality of life.

Hatfield continues this exploration of coping and adaptation to schizophrenia in chapter 47, which reviews a number of narratives written by clients about their illnesses. Based on these personal accounts, Hatfield identifies four internal sources of stress for persons with schizophrenia. She provides poignant, realistic, first-hand examples for each stressor and identifies coping strategies used by clients in dealing with these stressors. This presentation is highly relevant to occupational therapy, as the identified stressors can have significant functional impact on a person's task, social, and occupational performances. The clients' expressed need for structure and predictability in the external environment is also relevant to the occupational therapist who wants to assist individuals in adapting to their illness in a functional manner.

The next chapter in this section presents a research study that is also pertinent to occupational therapists who want to increase their understanding of the individual's perspective of his or her illness. The authors found that individuals with schizophrenia are aware of early warning signs that their illness may be exacerbating, and that almost all of the clients take action to manage these increasing symptoms. The most frequent symptom-management actions employed by this study's sample group were activity-based. Adding new activities, focusing on existing activities, and getting busy were adaptive strategies identified that are relevant to occupational therapy practice in mental health.

The ability of individuals to adapt and cope with potentially devastating illnesses and events is further explored in Chapter 49, by Fine. This inspiring Eleanor Clarke Slagle lecture examines the concepts of resilence and human adaptability in the face of major adversity and trauma. Fine provides several theories and various perspectives on stress, coping and resilence. Her analysis of the personal and social meaning of trauma is intertwined with the poetry and statements of individuals who have experienced chronic or terminal illness, physical and mental disabilities, abuse, torture, improvishment, the Holocaust and other disasters, and yet, remained resilient. According to Fine, occupational therapists must resist solely framing their practice according to the economics of the health care system. We must base practice on an understanding of the unique personal experiences of our clients, for function simply cannot be separated from feelings.

The vital importance of considering all aspects of the individual is further explored in this section's final chapter on holism in mental health practice by Hemphill-Pearson and Hunter. They discuss the historical roots of holistic medicine, philosophical principles of holism and the characteristics of holistic approaches. A holistic health practice model for occupational therapy is presented and a case study is provided to illustrate the application of holistic principles. According to these authors, a founding principle of the profession of occupational therapy was that the mind, body, emotions, spirit and environment were interrelated. Embracing this fundamental belief in today's specialized practice environment is essential to providing holistic care that meets the full spectrum of individual needs.

While all occupational therapists learn early in their professional education that occupational therapy is concerned with the whole person, this holistic view of practice is often unfortunately dichotomized into the practice areas of physical disabilities and mental health (Friedland & Renwick, 1993; Slaymaker, 1986; Yerxa, 1996). Academic coursework and clinical fieldwork are frequently represented as either a physical disabilities or a mental health learning experience.

While this split may be realistic for presenting many content areas (i.e., diagnostic criteria, specific evaluation, and intervention methods), it is vital for occupational therapists to remember the continual need for a holistic approach in all areas of practice (Fine, 1991; Pendergast, 1991; Slaymaker, 1986; Yerxa, 1996). People do not fit into a physical disabilities or a mental health peghole for we are not just round or square pegs. We have innumerable dimensions, multiple facets, and great depth. These characteristics do not disappear upon clinical diagnosis.

The adolescent with a spinal cord injury, the parent with multiple sclerosis, the artist with Acquired Immune Deficiency Syndrome (AIDS), the retired executive with hemiplegia—all face major disruptions in their lives and uncertain futures. These traumatic changes cannot be addressed purely from a physical perspective. While muscle strength, range of motion, sensation, and perception are vitally important to evaluate and treat, they alone are not sufficient. One also needs to consider the person's age, personality, coping style, values, interests, and goals in order to design a meaningful and relevant treatment program and to be able to motivate the individual to participate in this program. The adolescent may want to explore school and career options, while the parent may be more concerned with maintaining a familial role within the home. The artist with AIDS may view maintaining a modified, productive work schedule that utilizes creative skills as vital, while the retired executive may want to develop avocational interests to fill the "empty" days. These psychosocial issues must be considered to ensure that occupational therapy uses its full potential to help each individual attain and maintain a satisfying and meaningful quality of life.

It is my hope that the readings in this section will facilitate the development of increased understanding, empathy, and respect for each individual's experience and a renewed commitment to developing therapeutic helping relationships and holistic programming, (even in environments that are unsupportive of, or perhaps antagonistic to, these approaches).

In closing, I would like to remind readers that being caring and holistic does not equal being perfect. Therapists are human, and all of our therapeutic relationships or interventions will not always be ideal, especially in challenging practice settings. Sharing our humanity is what is vital to a helping relationship. Perfection is not the goal; mutual growth is. The quote below from Schulman reflects on the benefits of maintaining humanity in a therapeutic relationship. Questions for further consideration follow to facilitate the introspection and self-analysis skills that are essential to developing and maintaining caring, therapeutic relationships and a holistic approach.

Each of us brings our own personal style, artistry, background, feelings, values, beliefs, and so on, to our professional practice. Rather than denying or suppressing these, we need to learn more about ourselves in the context of our practice, and learn to use ourself in pursuit of our professional functions. We will make many mistakes along the way, saying things we will later regret, having to apologize to clients, learning from these mistakes, correcting them, and then making more sophisticated mistakes. In other words, we will be real people carrying out difficult jobs as best we can, rather than paragons of virtue who present an image of perfection.

As we demonstrate to our clients our humanness, vulnerability, willingness to risk, spontaneity, honesty, and our lack of defensiveness (or defensiveness for which we later apologize), we will be modeling the very behaviors we hope to see in our clients. Thus, when workers or students ask me: "Should I be professional or should I be myself?", I reply that the dualism implied in the question does not exist. They must be themselves if they are going to be professional. Fortunately, we have the whole of our professional lives to learn how to effect the synthesis. (Schulman, 1984, p. 15)

Questions to Consider

1. What are my needs to be helpful? What motivates me to engage in therapeutic relationships? How do I benefit from this process?

2. What are my helping strengths? What can I uniquely offer a client?

3. What are my values and beliefs? My sociocultural background? How do these influence my ability to help others?

4. What are my helping limitations? Are there individuals or topics that make me feel uncomfortable or vulnerable? How do I handle these feelings therapeutically? Am I open to feedback and supervision on issues that make me uncomfortable?

5. Do I look for strengths and assets in clients, as well as for their problems and limitations? How do I relate assessments to my clients?

6. What are the characteristics of helping relationships and therapeutic programs? How do I design my occupational therapy interventions to maximize these therapeutic characteristics? How can I facilitate patient collaboration with goal setting and treatment implementation?

7. What are the potential functional effects of the four stressors identified by Hatfield on an individual's task, social, and occupational skills?

8. How can occupational therapy assist patients in coping and adapting to their illnesses and pursuing satisfying, productive lives? What do patients seem to value and need most? How can I join with a patient to meet these needs? How can I support an individual's resilience?

9. Think of your current lifestyle; your roles, daily activities, values, interests, and goals. Now, imagine you are diagnosed with Multiple Sclerosis (MS). Your symptoms include fatigue, diminished endurance, decreased muscle strength, incoordination, and blurred vision.

a. What would be your reaction to this diagnosis? How would the significant people in your life react to your acquired disability?

b. How would your life change? What effect would your symptoms have on your current lifestyle?

c. What would be important psychosocial issues facing you as you adjusted to a physical disability?

d. What role adjustments and activity adaptations would you need to make due to your decreased functional abilities? How would MS impact your ability to perform work, leisure, and family role tasks?

e. What impact would MS have on your view of yourself as a sexual, lovable person?

f. How would the course of MS, with its exacerbations and remissions, affect your future goals?

g. What are your physical and sociocultural environmental concerns, constraints, and supports? What resources would you utilize to assist you in adjusting to a disability?

h. How would you like to be approached by an occupational therapist? What treatment activities and programs would be most relevant, interesting, and valuable to you? What would you want to work on in occupational therapy to attain and maintain a satisfying quality of life?

10. Imagine you are working in a busy, inpatient physical rehabilitation setting. You want to approach patients holistically, but you feel restricted by reimbursement constraints, strict documentation standards, and a limited length of treatment time.

a. Why bother? Why is it important to consider psychosocial issues with a non-psychiatric, physically disabled patient population?

b. What are the psychosocial reactions and behavioral manifestations that may be exhibited by a person with a physical disability? How might these influence the occupational therapy evaluation and intervention process?

c. How would incorporating psychosocial issues into your evaluation procedures assist you in setting relevant goals and planning appropriate treatment for your patients with physical disabilities?

d. What are the psychosocial issues that can influence a patient's motivation to engage in a treatment program? How can an occupational therapist increase a patient's interest and motivation to engage in physical rehabilitation?

e. How can a busy, overworked occupational therapist meet all of a clients needs and goals? How do you personalize needs and goals? How do you work on two things at the same time?

f. What resources are available to assist you in meeting the individuals psychosocial needs while in your treatment setting? What are the aftercare support services and professional resources available for referral to a client upon discharge from this setting. How can you ease the discharge process and transition back home and into the community? How can you ensure that your clients are leaving your setting with the skills and knowledge needed to empower them to pursue satisfying and productive lives?

11. What are current barriers to providing holistic care? How can I advocate for holistic intervention programs that consider all aspects of the individual in a system of care that is often market-driven and reductionistic?

REFERENCES

Baum, C., & Law, M. (1998). Nationally speaking: Community health: A responsibility, an opportunity, and a fit for occupational therapy. *American Journal of Occupational Therapy, 52,* 7-10.

Borg, B., & Bruce, M. A. (1997). *Occupational therapy stories: Psychosocial interaction in practice.* Thorofare, NJ: SLACK Incorporated.

Burke, J. P, & Cassidy, J. C. (1996). Disparity between reimbursement-driven practice and humanistic values of occupational therapy. In R. P. Cottrell (Ed.), *Perspective on purposeful activity: Foundation and future occupational therapy* (pp. 595-598). Bethesda, MD: American Occupational Therapy Association.

Christiansen, C. (1996). Nationally speaking: Managed care. Opportunities and challenges for occupational therapy in the emerging systems of the 21st century. *American Journal of Occupational Therapy, 50,* 409-412.

Davis, C. M. (1998). *Patient-practitioner interaction. An experimental manual for developing the art of health care* (3rd Edition). Thorofare, NJ: SLACK Incorporated.

Devereux, E. B. (1991). Occupational therapy's challenge: The caring relationship. In R. P. Cottrell (Ed.), *Perspectives on purposeful activity: Foundation and future of occupational therapy* (pp. 319-325). Bethesda, MD: American Occupational Therapy Association.

Fine, S. B. (1991, August 22). Holistic approach includes mental health [Letter to the Editor]. *OT Week,* 46.

Fine, S. B. (1998). Surviving the health care revolution: Rediscovering the meaning of "good work." *Occupational Therapy in Mental Health, 14*(1/2), p 7-18.

Frese, F. J. (1998). Occupational therapy and mental illness: A personal view. *Mental Health Special Interest Section Quarterly, 21*(3), 1-3.

Friedland, J., & Renwick, R. (1993). The issues: Psychosocial occupational therapy: Time to cast off the gloom and doom. *American Journal of Occupational Therapy, 47,* 417-471.

Gillfoyle, E. (1980). Caring: A philosophy of practice. *American Journal of Occupational Therapy, 34,* 517-521.

Howard, B. S. (1996). How high do we jump? The effect of reimbursement on occupational therapy. In R. P. Cottrell (Ed.), *Perspectives on purposeful activity: Foundation and future of occupational therapy* (pp 587-594). Bethesda, MD: American Occupational Therapy Association.

King, L. J. (1980). Creative caring. *American Journal of Occupational Therapy, 34,* 522-528.

Mosey, A. C. (1986). *Psychosocial components of occupational therapy.* New York, NY: Raven Press.

Peloquin, S. M. (1996). The patient-therapist relationship: Beliefs that shape care. In R. P. Cottrell (Ed.), *Perspectives on purposeful activity: Foundation and future of occupational therapy* (pp. 319-325). Bethesda, MD: American Occupational Therapy Association.

Pendergrast, N. (1991). Holistic approach includes mental health [Letter to the Editor]. *OT Week,* 46.

Slaymaker, I. H. (1986). A holistic approach to specialization. *American Journal of Occupational Therapy, 40,* 117-121.

Yerxa, E. J. (1996). The social and psychological experience of having a disability: Implications for occupational therapists. In L. W. Pedretti (Ed.), *Occupational Therapy: practice skills for physical dysfunction* (4th Edition) (pp. 253-274). Baltimore, MD: Mosby.

CHAPTER FORTY-FIVE

The Healing Power of Respect: A Personal Journey

Irene M. Turner

This chapter was previously published in Occupational Therapy in Mental Health, *9(1), 17-22. Copyright © 1989, Haworth Press.*

It was unnecessary; it was unfeeling; it was humiliating; it invaded my privacy; it made me feel very embarrassed; I felt like slightly less than a child; and there was nothing I could do about it.

I was being admitted to a locked unit of a long-term psychiatric clinic. My belongings were searched, then locked away, and I was stripped and dressed in bed clothes—those horrible green hospital-issued "smock things" that tie in the back with two ill-spaced and sometimes nonexistent ties. Thus clad and dehumanized I was sent to "mingle with the other patients." At that point, they wanted to talk to me about as much as I wanted to speak to them, which was not at all, and at the very first opportunity I retreated to my small room. At least I could hide my face in the privacy of my own space. But not for long! Soon my appointed therapist appeared to talk to me, give me a physical examination, and have me draw some pictures for her. A relationship began that should have helped me during the following months, but on the contrary, it made me feel even worse about myself. How could I believe, at that time, that I was worth anything if my therapist insisted on calling me Mrs. Turner even though I told her it was important for me to be Irene? She did not speak to me in the hall unless I spoke first, and then it was always a formal "Hello, Mrs. Turner." During our therapy sessions, she constantly wrote notes and did not look at me; after 10 months of biweekly meetings she almost acknowledged my personhood by giving me a formal handshake and wishing me well as I was leaving the hospital.

Some positive relationships helped during the time I spent there. I interacted well with fellow patients, and I discovered that some staff members genuinely cared about their work and wanted to help me just because I was me. Two members of my treatment team, one my primary nurse and the other a mental health worker, were very supportive. They helped by listening to me, often by giving firm reprimands when I became self-destructive, sometimes by just sitting and holding my hand for a short time. The mental health worker forced me to try to concentrate by playing card games or Scrabble with me. The nurse picked out some knitting yarn and a pattern for me and helped me knit a sweater—often watching close by for several hours as I struggled to concentrate. Two senior staff members who played oboes for a hobby allowed me to play piano with them, and this helped keep me in touch with reality and gave me the opportunity to do something I enjoyed. We three gave several brief recitals for patients and staff. These relationships were especially meaningful to me, in part because many of the activities which were supposed to be of help to me were not fulfilling my needs.

Some of the activity therapies I felt to be insulting. I was insulted partly because of my own perfectionism and rigidity, I am sure, but nonetheless my feelings were real and based on some real shortcomings. Activities such as art therapy and leisure crafts were pitifully lacking in supplies. Searching through the sparse, somewhat chaotic supply of art or craft materials added greatly to my sense of confusion and lack of focus and direction. Often after I found the supplies I wanted I was not able to complete a project because of inadequate time. Storage for unfinished work was not available. Dance therapy did give opportunity for some exercise, but it also made my self-esteem spiral downward. The skips, leaps, hops, and runs were done with a partner or in sequence, like follow the leader, while others watched. I always felt clumsy and uncoordinated, and I hated to attend. Music therapy met none of my needs. Song sheets were distributed so that we could make singing selections, but I was not familiar with many of the songs, and I felt frustrated. I realize that I was reacting negatively because of my musical training, but not having musical notes to accompany the words was disconcerting. I was not able to express my feelings through music as I had once been able to do. I experienced each session as a much too casual, inadequately planned, sing-along. The most meaningful activity at that time consisted of two separate but short sessions in creative writing—something I had never tried before. These sessions were taught by volunteers and when they left, I felt strangely abandoned because they had cared about what they were doing, they had come prepared, and they had tried to help me discover something about myself through use of the written word. Both leaders had treated me with respect and never made me feel like "just a mental case." At the time, I felt keenly the difference between being treated with respect and being merely "treated."

I know that I am an unusually sensitive person and suffer from low self-esteem, but my unhappiness did not come entirely from within. The thread binding together so many of my experiences in that hospital was lack of respect. I received the message that it was all right to offer me activities in ill-equipped, cluttered areas. After all, "I was too mentally ill to notice." I began to care less about myself, to take less care of myself, and to take little pride in what I did. It was likely that I would be unable to finish a project because of time limitation, and any feedback would be extremely minimal. My sense of accomplishment, or even a desire for accomplishment, dwindled. When some activity therapy staff gave the impression that it was not important for them to prepare for groups, I began to feel less important as a person. At one point, I tried to stop going to these activities, but I was made to feel like a naughty, rebellious child for suggesting such a thing. At that time, I had an unhealthy need to please people at any cost. I returned to the groups, participated in them, and felt increasingly more depressed. Not wanting anyone to know how truly ugly and unworthy I felt, I tried to bury my feelings.

During 10 months of hospitalization I had taken several different types of antidepressants. None of them seemed to work very well, however, and my doctor decided that I should take nothing. I had the feeling that I never stayed on one medication long enough to test its effectiveness. No one discussed the meds with me, so I never knew what to expect, and I believed that no one cared enough about me to explain how the meds should work, why I took them, and why I was taken off them. I thought the doctors did not want me to get well.

My self-esteem continued to deteriorate. I felt that I was a "mental patient" who was making no contribution to family or friends. I felt incapable of doing anything well, and the staff gave me the impression that they really did not care about helping me. I felt hopeless, and I had little faith in the treatment I was receiving. Although I felt less like living than before I entered the hospital, I began to prepare for discharge. I tried not to mention suicide, and I talked positively about returning to work because I did not want the staff to know my true feelings about my job. In reality, I hated it and dreaded going back to my office. I feared facing my coworkers almost to the extent of feeling paralyzed. After remaining in that long-term hospital for almost a year, I was discharged having fear, inadequacy, helplessness, and hopelessness as my constant companions. There was no follow-up support, aftercare, or suggestions made about any support groups in the community. There had been no discharge planning group of any kind in the hospital. I just left.

The return to work was, in many ways, worse than I had imagined. Although my friends tried to treat me naturally, they could not, and acquaintances treated me with such condescension that I retreated from everyone. One younger employee, for example, offered to show me the way to the cafeteria, in spite of the fact that he knew I had worked in the building for over five years. I was utterly miserable. I received very little support from friends at work and, with the exception of my therapist whom I saw once a week, no support from the psychiatric community.

The transition from hospital to work was more difficult because of some confusion about my job assignment when I returned to the office. For four weeks, I sat at a perfectly clear desk and did nothing but answer a few phone calls. There was no opportunity for me to show my peers or my immediate supervisor that I was capable of functioning in the workplace. When I tried to describe my feelings about having no real work to friends, they merely laughed and said they would like to have "my kind of problem." I sat, did nothing, and felt progressively worse about myself. I, too, began to believe I was crazy and unable to do minimal tasks. By the time someone in authority intervened and began to prepare a new job assignment, I had already determined that I would not go back to that office with its empty desk and no work. I just wanted to die.

One of the activities I still found meaningful was playing the organ regularly for worship services at a small church. Some members of that congregation, and most especially my minister, were supportive and very concerned about me. Their watchfulness over me intensified as they identified increasing depression in me. I felt more hopeless than ever, so I planned to kill myself by taking an overdose of pills with vodka. However, my minister had been making frequent telephone calls to check on me, and he and another friend managed to enter my home when I did not answer the phone and prevented me from taking the entire supply. They took me to the psychiatric wing of a general hospital. I remember very little about that admission process except for a vague memory of thinking it very strange that my friends were with me as a nurse was trying to get me to answer some simple questions, while I wanted only to go beck to sleep. Later, when I became fully awake, I was dismayed to discover that I was in the maximum security section.

During the five weeks I stayed there, my contact with life outside that ward was very restricted. My meals were served in a small sitting area next to the nurses' station. I was encouraged to watch television for very short periods each day, but I could not tolerate the shallowness and stupidity of most programming, so often I just stared into space when other patients wanted to watch a program. I could not go to the craft area to work on projects, nor participate in any groups held away from the restricted area. At one point, I had asked if someone could bring a small craft project to the sitting area for me, but there was no one to supervise one-to-one, so I was not allowed to do anything with my hands. The head nurse had suggested that I read some books, and when I protested that the sitting area was too noisy, she permitted me to read in my room during certain hours (it was considered safe because my closet was locked and all toilet articles, even my toothbrush, were kept at the nurses' station). I knew I could not concentrate enough to read, but I seized the opportunity to go to my room. I held a book in my hand for hours and when a nurse checked on me every fifteen minutes or more often—I tried to remember to turn a page. I was allowed to have only one visitor—my minister— because others upset me too much. He could not come often, but when he did come I was greatly helped and comforted.

I felt like a prisoner. I was awakened each morning at a certain time, my meals were served at a certain time, I went to bed at a certain time. And in between those certain times I sat in a plastic covered chair in full view of the staff person assigned to me. I was extremely depressed.

Since I had not been able to respond to treatment in the length of time it was possible to stay at that hospital, my doctor decided to transfer me to a different long-term hospital. The memory of my earlier experiences was very fresh, so I was prepared for the worst.

My first impression as my minister, two other friends, and I drove into the hospital grounds was one of spacious serenity. In spite of my resistance, I had a brief glimpse of the security this place could offer me. A bit later my friends and I were shown into a quiet room to await my new therapist. The quietness and the spaciousness were surprises because they were so different from the noisy cluttered hallway I expected since that was my earlier experience. It seemed to matter to the staff of this hospital that my admission be as easy as possible. I appreciated those moments with my friends because even though my thoughts were in turmoil I knew they cared about me. I was so afraid that I was to spend the next few months among people who did not care. The only thing I knew about this new place was that I was to have a woman as a therapist. During that short waiting period I speculated about what she would be like.

My speculations did not prepare me for the doctor who was assigned to me. My spirits took a nosedive when she entered the room. She was beautiful! I saw a woman so impeccably dressed that I was sure she must be uncomfortable. She seemed aloof, stiff, and stone-like. When she began to speak I was completely convinced that she could never help me. How could she help me if I could not understand her Italian accent? After a short interview, she took me to the unit where I was to live. I received the first hint of how wrong my first impressions were during my first hour there. I had appreciated the fact that she took me to the unit and did not send me with some other stranger. Then she did an amazing thing. The mental health worker who was searching my luggage for sharp or other dangerous objects was going to remove a picture of my daughter because it was in a glass frame. When I started to cry, my doctor said I could keep the photograph. It was such a small but tremendous statement, affirming my personhood—my ability to think and feel and react like any normal mother. I am convinced that it was at that moment that I took my first tentative step toward helping this extraordinary woman help me. A relationship which has profoundly affected my life had begun when my doctor left me—with my daughter's picture—I felt very alone. But I was relieved to discover that from the first

I could wear my own clothes. And in spite of the fact that I was restricted to the sitting room, I did not feel so isolated. The other patients respected my need to adjust to the unit, and thus did not intrude, but offered their friendship and willingness to help. For the moment, the gesture was as significant as doing something specific. The staff members were friendly and tried to make it easier for me to relax.

That evening I was introduced to the first of many, many "hall meetings" and observed how milieu therapy works. We twenty patients plus the staff on duty met for approximately an hour and discussed a variety of things, including housekeeping issues (keep the coffee area cleaner), reminders of activities for the weekend (a dance, of all things!) and also "agenda items." These agenda items turned out to be issues concerning people, and my heart sank when I heard my name put on that agenda. My fear was exaggerated, however. My peers merely wanted to welcome me and give me the opportunity to speak if I wanted to do so. Beyond introducing myself, I had nothing to say and was not pushed to say more at that time. As I listened to the rest of the discussion, I learned that the patients really cared about each other and shared their feelings of support, concern, encouragement, disappointment, anger. When I heard the feedback from those patients, I felt more of a sense of belonging than I had experienced in quite some time. It was ever so small, but coupled with kindness from my doctor, I was beginning to feel something other than a desire to die.

My first several weeks in the hospital were very difficult. I was not restricted to the sitting room the entire time, but I was restricted to the unit since I was still extremely depressed and suicidal. Nevertheless, I felt "bound in," and I believed that I was receiving my just punishment because I was such an evil, unworthy person. I did not want to talk to the other patients, nor did I want to share my true feelings with the staff. I thought that if I simply remained quiet, everyone would assume that I was feeling better, and this would result in early discharge. The staff members were very patient with me. I resented their intrusions and their restrictions, but, at the same time, I dimly recognized their actions as evidence of caring and support. Someone sat with me when I could concentrate on a project, such as an embroidery sampler, which I enjoyed although I was not allowed to keep the needle or scissors. I began to feel less like a prisoner because I was given some freedom and because the staff seemed to respect me and care about my getting well. One mental health worker, in particular, was thoughtful enough to take me for brief walks outside in the fresh air. I appreciated visiting the vegetable and flower gardens and feeding the rabbits near the greenhouse.

The occupational therapist made some suggestions about things I could do while I remained on hall restriction. She brought some small projects which were simple, and I appreciated just being able to have something to do with my hands. I remember coloring with magic markers and feeling good about the lovely designs which took form. Even as I did these things, I felt support from people who were beginning to be important to me—my doctor often stopped by to make comments, my occupational therapist complimented me, and other patients appreciated my giving them a colorful card. The sense of connections with others was a good feeling.

At the appropriate time, the occupational therapist introduced me to an activity program which was to enhance tremendously the benefits I was gaining from psychotherapy. At first I was most skeptical, because on paper it looked a great deal like the program to which I had been exposed previously. However, a larger variety of activities was offered at this hospital, and I wanted to attend those which the occupational therapist and I had decided would be meaningful. Having input into the final choice of activities was important for my self-esteem, because it implied that what I thought and did as an individual mattered. Thought and concern were given to my selections, and I received the message that I would not be haphazardly assigned to an activity and then "baby-sat" for the time I spent there.

"Referred groups" consisted of ongoing activities to which I was referred for specific treatment objectives, and I was expected to attend them regularly. From that group I helped to choose dance therapy, leathercraft, ceramics, and art therapy. "Skill development groups" consisted of self-selected activities which rotated on a monthly basis, and were designed primarily for leisure. From this group I selected activities such as knitting, creative writing, and nature hikes. "Open activities" involved supervised activities such as swimming, crafts, and beachball volleyball, which were available to all patients. All of these activities were good for me, but some were more significant than others.

I remember being told while I was making a leather notebook that I was too intense: I needed to accept the fact that my design would be good enough and I could accept it even if it were not perfect. I had learned early that to be acceptable I had to please, and in order to please I had to be as nearly perfect as possible. I was always my own strictest judge, and when I did not meet my own standards, my self-esteem plummeted. Because of those feelings, the group leader continued to encourage me to relax and take pride in what I was doing— even with the flaws. Finishing that notebook reminded me that "good" is all right, too, and if that is so with a leather notebook, it could be so for other things in life.

My dance therapist and fellow patents in dance therapy helped me to lose some of my feelings of inadequacy and low self-confidence. The origin of some of these feelings centered on the belief that my musical talent had disappeared. One day my dance therapist sat on the floor and encouraged me to feel the rhythm of the music with my body by moving in any way I felt comfortable. She held my hands and rubbed them in an attempt to make me aware of their importance and their strength. I shall remember the moment for years to come because she respected me and tried to help me rediscover and accept my best qualities.

Perhaps the most important activity for me at the time was art therapy. Initially, I protested being referred to that group because I am not an artist! I could not imagine how I could benefit from drawing pictures of which I would be ashamed. I soon discovered that being artistic was not a prerequisite to reaping benefits from art therapy. One extremely important thing, especially in the beginning, was the fact that there were enough art materials with which to experiment. I was not forced to draw. I could choose to do so, but I could also select other options. As my art therapist guided me in learning to express some of my deepest feelings, I found expression through the use of watercolors, acrylic paints (a special favorite of mine), finger paints, collages, and modeling clay.

When the art therapist introduced me to scribble art, something special happened. My skepticism again came to the fore when she suggested that I loosen up my arms by swinging them around and that I shake my hands to completely relax them. However, by that time I had developed some trust in her and had gained a small understanding of the real value of art therapy. Although it was not difficult to close my eyes and make scribble lines on a piece of construction paper, I believed I would never be able to see images or forms. To my amazement, the lines, angles, squiggles, and circles began to take shape. From the very depths of my feelings pictures formed on the paper with such clarity that it often frightened me. Those scribbles were very valuable to my progress. Often during the following weeks I took the scribbles with me to psychotherapy sessions, since there were times I had been able to express feelings in those scribbles which I had never been able to verbalize. It was helpful to put the pictures on the floor, admit that they meant something to me, and begin to explore their meaning with my doctor. At times I felt that a major breakthrough had been made as a result of discussing the scribbles.

On several different occasions, I had discussed with the occupational therapist my desire to enter a referred group in interpersonal skills. She discouraged my participation in it at that time because she felt that I was not ready for the kind of confrontation which took place there. I had a great deal of difficulty accepting her statement and thought that she disliked me. I began to misinterpret other things the occupational therapist said and did. I allowed myself to be hurt and felt that I had done something wrong. Feelings of rejection were evoked when I could not understand the reason she referred another patient to interpersonal skills ahead of me.

Later, when I was ready, I was referred to the interpersonal skills group which was honest, confrontive, supportive, and caring. I learned to communicate more effectively by observing myself and others as we talked together, as we listened to each other, as we gave nonverbal messages by body language, expressions, or eye contact and tried to understand the complex and often incongruous relationship to the verbal ones we shared. As the weeks passed, I was grateful for the fact that my enrollment in that group had been delayed until I was able to hear the feedback given to me without being devastated by it. Again I was reminded that people genuinely cared about me and had my best interest in mind when decisions about my schedule were made.

During the long months of hospitalization I was a member of the patient organization, Patient Activities Committee (PAC), which planned evening and weekend activities for fellow patients. Our responsibilities entailed selecting, organizing, providing leadership during the activity, and evaluating these events. Involvement in PAC helped me to remember that there was a community outside the hospital and that I would be discharged to that community when I was ready. Working with fellow patients to help make our plans become reality gave me the opportunity to improve my interpersonal skills in a supportive environment.

For a long time, I served PAC as secretary to its executive body, thus enabling me to use my secretarial skills, and I felt a real sense of accomplishment when I had completed the weekly typing assignments. On the other hand, it gave me little opportunity to work closely with other patients, so I approached the PAC Coordinator to ask about filling the vacant leadership position of co-chairman. She said she did not think it was wise because I still needed to learn some important things about relating to others in a task-oriented situation.

At first it was difficult for me to accept those comments, and it was hard not to feel a sense of personal rejection. However, the important thing about that conversation and the resulting decision to remain as secretary was that at no time was I treated without respect. On the contrary, this respect given to me was, I feel, the basis for my developing a sense of trust which resulted in my ability to listen and try to change. I knew I needed help, and I trusted the Coordinator enough to believe that she could help.

She did! I learned many things from her, but two things are noteworthy. She repeatedly reminded us that while we as patients experienced ourselves as different from nonpatients, the so-called "normals," this was more a function of our feelings of isolation rather than reality. She frequently quoted from Harry Stack Sullivan, "We are all more simply human than otherwise." Recognizing that fact helped me have a sense of connectedness to the outside world. Secondly, she helped all of us examine those of our behaviors which tended to separate us from others and rejoiced with us as we made progress in correcting those behaviors. What a marvelous asset to my psychotherapy that woman was.

I was receiving psychotherapy, and many of the problems which had brought me to the hospital were being addressed in my activities. However, I also began to realize that there was care and concern for me as a total person and not just as a mental patient. Therefore, it did not surprise me to learn that there was a hospital chaplain, and I appreciated the fact that religious services were provided regularly for patients. During the early weeks of my hospitalization, I had not felt comfortable enough with my own feelings about the church to attend those services, but my doctors suggested that I do so. My academic training had been in organ and church music, and my professional involvement with the church was of long standing. Once again being a part of a communal worship service met many of my deepest spiritual needs. After I had attended a few services, my doctor further suggested that I make an appointment to speak with the chaplain. I did so, but I had such anxiety, fear, skepticism, and doubt about the usefulness of such a meeting that I almost canceled the appointment. I am so grateful that I did not do so, because the chaplain also became a special "significant other" in my

life. My sessions with him were very important. Some of my fear of men, especially ministers, began to disappear, and my self-esteem grew with his acceptance of me. I often took my "scribbles" from art therapy to discuss with him. Together we explored the pictures' meaning, and the insight I gained helped me understand the origin of many of my fears. He gave me a sense of security and stability, and he often gave me very direct advice. He told me once, "When you feel like harming yourself, pick up a pencil or pastel chalk to use rather than a knife or a razor." It worked!

There was hope for me, because I was beginning to believe there was hope. That tiny grain of hope needed nurturing, and I was gratefully amazed as I moved closer and closer to a discharge date that I received support from many staff members.

A vocational counselor, who helped me plan how to reenter the work force, administered some vocational tests and discussed their findings with me. We discussed the job market, updated my resume, and addressed the questions of revealing my psychiatric hospitalization or changing occupations. In preparation for work, I was given a work therapy assignment in the hospital. Work expectations were discussed, and my performance was evaluated. Vocational counseling and work therapy did not take away all the fear of returning to work, but it helped prepare me. My work therapy assignment was one which used the secretarial skills I planned to use when I left the hospital. Being regular in attendance, and being on time, both to start work and to end work, were goals I was expected to meet.

The transition to work outside the hospital began before I was discharged. Fortunately I was able to obtain a part-time job in a small law office which suited my needs and interests. Although I enjoyed the job, even though it was stressful at times, I was grateful that I could return to the hospital after my work day and talk about what had happened. Receiving valuable feedback helped my transition from the hospital.

The discharge planning group in which I participated was helpful in a special way. During my stay in the hospital I had been focused inward. The practical side of living had not concerned me for many months. In this group, we focused on living arrangements, budgets, meal planning, entertainment, dealing with family and friends, and handling free time. The occupational therapist who led the group made valuable specific suggestions to each patient about groups or activities in the community. She gave me the name and schedule of a community chorus which I joined in order to use my musical talents as well as to make some social contacts. I remember reflecting during the discharge planning group that I would not be "just leaving" this hospital as I had left the other hospital months earlier.

Leaving and saying goodbye were things that were very difficult for me because they provoked feelings of abandonment. I was encouraged, along with every other patient who left, to set aside specific times for saying farewell to the patients on my hall, to individual staff members, and to members of activity groups which I attended. The process of actually saying goodbye did take some planning and coordinating of schedules, but the help I received was worth the effort. I discovered that it was all right to say goodbye. It did not mean that I was being abandoned or that I was being rejected because I was not perfect enough to please everyone. Nor did it mean that there was no one to care about me any more.

This part of my discharge process was both sad and happy. I would miss a group of good friends, but I would take with me many lessons learned from them: lessons about caring, for others and for myself; lessons about acceptance, of others and myself; lessons about honesty, with others and myself; lessons about listening without feeling personally attacked.

Discharge planning is one important thing. The actual discharge is enormously different! I was petrified. Even though I knew my plans were well made I had gigantic doubts about my ability to implement them. Many of my worst fears from my past reappeared to haunt me. I could not trust my own feelings, but fortunately I trusted the hospital staff and they had faith in me. Their attitude often gave me the courage I needed.

My tenure as an inpatient ended on a beautiful day in May 1987. Going through the locked door of the hall which had been my home for so many months created an extraordinary mixture of emotions. I was happy, but a bit sad; I was eager, but a little uncertain; I was confident, but somewhat insecure; I was prepared, but I also had doubts; I felt alone, but I knew I still had the support of the hospital staff to help during the transition period. That support continued to be very important to me. I was extremely fortunate to be able to work as a volunteer in the Activity Therapy Department of the hospital after my discharge. The work consisted of secretarial duties similar to those I had as a paid employee outside the hospital, but the difference in the two jobs was significant. In the hospital, I had feedback and support from several sources but especially from my supervisor who had known me during the long months of my hospitalization.

During the hours when I was doing my volunteer job, my supervisor did not discuss therapy issues but only issues related to my work habits. I learned so much about the way I functioned in a work-related environment. For the most part, my work skills were solid, but I needed honest feedback and suggestions about the way I worked with people—my supervisor, my peers, people I might need to supervise. Because of my volunteer job I became better prepared for working independently outside the hospital.

My relationship with the hospital chaplain continued to be most important. He gave me honest, straightforward and caring feedback and encouraged me to explore how I felt and to verbalize feelings clearly. He also encouraged me to use my musical training by playing the organ for worship services for the patients. I believe that in this way I made a small contribution to the life of the hospital.

During that transition period, I was never without the encouragement, the support, the feedback, the care, and the listening ear of my doctor. Often it was her concern for me and my love for her that made it possible for me to try to get through a day. There were times when I would tell myself, "Hang in there until you see your doctor because you know she cares."

Not long ago, my doctor had the flu, and she called to cancel our appointment. After a brief moment of panic, I discovered that I was more concerned about her health than my own fear that she would not come back soon. I knew that she would return when she recovered. The panic of a lost child abandoned by her mother was not there. I believe that was a significant realization since it meant that I was moving slowly toward becoming the kind of adult my doctor always said I could be. My relationship with her will not stop for awhile. My love for her will never end, but perhaps it will not be such a dependent love.

One of the statements that my doctor used a great deal was, "You must learn to look at the half full glass. The half empty glass that you always saw is not good for you."

I believe that, in a sense, I have done that in describing my recent hospitalizations. There were regressions, conflicts, disappointments, fears, aloneness, but they all dimmed as I thought about all the help I received after the disastrous experience I had during my first long-term stay. When I was admitted to my second long-term hospital my experience was different. I believe this was because the underlying attitude that governed all aspects of hospital life was respect. It was this most important quality which made me begin to feel better about myself and want to do something to help myself. I made use of every aspect of hospital life that was available to me. And now, I have, with some confidence, grasped my half-full "glass of life." I can now affirm that it is indeed half full and not half empty. Furthermore, it can become even fuller as I continue my journey, one step at a time.

CHAPTER FORTY-SIX

The Treatment of Schizophrenia: A Patient's Perspective

Esso Leete

This chapter was previously published in Hospital and Community Psychiatry, 38, *486-491. Copyright © 1987, the* American Psychiatric Association.

It has been 20 years since I first became mentally ill. As I approach 40, I find myself still struggling with the same symptoms, still crippled by the same fears and paranoia. I am haunted by an evasive picture of what my life could have been, whom I might have become, what I might have accomplished. My schizophrenia is a sad realization, a painful reality, that I live with every day. I wonder what, if anything, I could have done differently either to avoid developing schizophrenia or to lessen its severity.

After years of turmoil and lack of direction, in 1982, I made a conscious decision to put my experiences with mental illness, both positive and negative, to constructive use, educating others about mental illness and its treatment. This effort has become my mission in life, my passion. Knowing that something beneficial may eventually come from the horror of my mental illness is my consolation. My search for answers to the many questions I had about my affliction has helped me to clarify my thoughts about the needs of individuals with schizophrenia. These thoughts, which are based on my experiences, are presented here.

The Onset of Illness

Let me tell you a little about my history. I probably inherited a predisposition to mental illness; my uncle was diagnosed as having "dementia praecox," an earlier term for schizophrenia. In my senior year of high school, I began to experience personality changes. I did not realize the significance of the changes at the time, and I think others denied them, but looking back I can see that they were the earliest signs of illness. I became increasingly withdrawn and sullen. I felt alienated and lonely and hated everyone. I felt as if there were a huge gap between me and the rest of the world; everybody seemed so distant from me. I watched dispassionately as my two younger sisters matured, dated, shopped, and shaped their lives while I seemed stuck in a totally different dimension.

I reluctantly went off to college, feeling alone and totally unprepared for life away from home. I was isolative and had no close friends. As time went on, I spoke to virtually no one. Increasingly during classes I found myself drawing pictures of Van Gogh and writing poetry. I forgot to eat and began sleeping in my clothes. Performing even the most routine activities, such as taking a shower, rarely even occurred to me.

The First Break

Toward the end of my first semester, I had my first psychotic episode. I did not understand what was happening and was extremely frightened. The experience left me exhausted and confused, and I began hearing voices for the first time. Reality as others knew it had given way to the multiple realities with which I would now live.

I was admitted to a psychiatric hospital, diagnosed as having schizophrenia, treated with medications, and released after a few months. Over the next two years I was hospitalized in psychiatric facilities five times, the longest hospitalization lasting a year. During my late teens and early 20s, when my age demanded that I date and develop social skills, my illness required that I spend my adolescence on psychiatric wards. To this day I mourn the loss of those years.

When I was first hospitalized, I was young, passive, extremely dependent, and naive. I did not understand what was happening, and I was not sufficiently in touch with the world to care. I was so regressed that I hardly spoke and stayed in bed as much as possible, eagerly seizing my voices as companions. I believed I was living on Venus and, according to hospital charts, I stood on chairs and tables speaking in an incomprehensible language (presumably "Venusian").

My identity began to fragment and seemed to blend with my environment. Rather than just enjoying the wind, for instance, I thought I had merged with it. I had to stare at the sun to appreciate its warmth. Yet gradually I was able to see myself as separate from those things. As I neared discharge, I began to feel some stirring of belief in myself. It was not until much later that I made a conscious effort to develop a sense of control, realizing that I had the power to decide what form my life would take and who I would be.

After spending nearly 2 years in a series of hospitals, I began weekly outpatient therapy and medication management at the local psychiatric hospital at which I had received inpatient care. I attended a local college part-time and was married to my first husband at the end of my first semester. We moved to another state, where I continued on medication and received both individual and group psychotherapy.

My condition improved, and a few years later I discontinued outpatient therapy and requested that my medication be gradually tapered off. Throughout most of this time I was employed, first in a series of fast-food restaurants and later as a secretary at a college. For the next 10 years, I did not require hospitalization. During that time, I was divorced from my first husband and married a community mental health center psychiatrist. Although I experienced some acute flare-ups of symptomatology during that period, I had no recurrence of persistent, disabling symptoms.

EXACERBATIONS

When more serious symptoms returned about 10 years later, I denied their existence. The more people alluded to my illness, treated me negatively, and recommended I become reinvolved in therapy, the more resistant and angry I became. I had decided that I was not ill, that I did not need the medications, and that I did not wish to be involved in psychiatric treatment. I just did not want to be sick any more, an understandable desire, and I was convinced that if I got rid of the evidence of illness I would be magically cured. It didn't work.

Instead, having discontinued medications years earlier and now withdrawing from other forms of support, I experienced more symptoms. It is my belief that the actions I took were self-destructive responses to my despondency about being mentally ill. I was aided in my downhill plunge, however, by several of the psychiatric institutions at which I was treated.

DUBIOUS TREATMENT

One private psychiatric hospital in Denver was particularly destructive. I was banned from group therapy sessions, my food was monitored, my time was regulated, and my roommates were removed from my room and thus from my negative influence.

Toward the end of my hospitalization, I was placed in seclusion and restraints every day. I was forbidden to cross a red line painted on the floor, much less leave the unit. Not surprisingly, I did not improve, as such power struggles and automatic limit setting are rarely therapeutic. The more I was ostracized and punished, the angrier I became and the more

I rebelled. Slowly, however, my desperation turned to resignation and hopelessness.

To make matters worse, even my psychiatrist would not speak to me. Although he dutifully came to see me about twice a week, he stopped talking to me after the first couple of sessions, regardless of what I said, what I asked, or what I did. One day I had to actually sit on my hands to prevent myself from jumping up and strangling him out of frustration. Not only was his "silent treatment" not helpful, but it contributed substantially to my feelings of despair. Fortunately, with the help of my friends on the unit and daily one-to-one sessions with various staff, particularly two nurses who had compassion and professional integrity, I survived.

After 5 months on the unit, any therapeutic alliance that had been established was long gone. One day I announced that I would soon be escaping on the locked elevator and calmly began to collect my belongings. The staff seemed skeptical and utterly unconcerned. Within about an hour, I had successfully eloped from the unit, determined to commit suicide.

What I found on the outside, however, dissuaded me. To my real amazement, I found that people did not threaten me, did not yell at me, did not order me around, did not ignore me, and did not treat me alternately like a child or like a criminal. They were actually friendly, and for the first time in a long time I felt pleasure and power. Having felt these feelings, I fantasized that I might hold on to them and find the strength to run my own life. After two days of deliberation and real soul-searching, I decided to check out of my motel room and return to the hospital on my own, vowing to leave there cured.

THE TURNING POINT

Upon my return to the hospital I was met with silent anger. I sensed that staff were disappointed to see me again and that they had secretly wished they would no longer have to deal with me. Naively I had expected that our relationship would be better after I returned voluntarily. I assumed staff would see the evident change in my attitude and resume my treatment with the same optimism and energy I felt.

Instead, virtually all communication between staff and me ceased, and I continued to be banned from group therapy, occupational therapy, and recreational therapy. Naturally I was again restricted to the unit. Once again I experienced daily episodes of seclusion and restraint, which were precipitated by the anger and frustration I felt toward my private psychiatrist for his refusal to talk to me during our sessions.

The situation deteriorated after the staff discovered while reading my journal that I was in possession of a gun (which I had bought while contemplating suicide). I had brought the gun with me onto the unit to defend myself against the possibility of tube feeding, with which the staff had threatened me before I left the unit. I thought the sight of a gun would force them to abandon their attempt at tube feeding. I had not wanted to hurt anyone and I kept the gun unloaded and brought no bullets with me to the hospital.

Because of my "dangerous and inappropriate behavior," I was immediately placed in seclusion for 2 days. At the end of the 2 days, I learned that the head of the hospital, acting with staff input, had ordered that I remain in seclusion at least until the next visit from my doctor, who did not see me every day. I was distraught. During the 2 days I had spent in quiet seclusion, I had heard an increasing number of voices, and I was terrified they would seize this opportunity to close in on me. I did not know how I would survive even another 5 minutes in this room, let alone until I met with my doctor.

I was released from seclusion on the next day, after I saw my doctor and agreed to do everything he wished. He had threatened to send me to a maximum security unit of a state hospital for an indefinite period of time. About a week later, the hospital "released" me into the streets (actually I was kicked out), even though my psychiatrist had implied that I would need intensive on-going treatment in a locked setting.

After spending 2 days in a cheap hotel, I decided to investigate Community Care Corporation, a private psychiatric residential halfway house that one of the nurses at the hospital had told me about. I sought and gained admission to the program.

The residential program was very different from the hospital. It was structured and supervised, yet I did not feel imprisoned and at the mercy of an arbitrary staff. Unfortunately I had incorporated some of the negative messages about myself that I had learned at the hospital and had come to believe I was incapable of living successfully on the outside. At Community Care, however, I sensed that the treatment team genuinely cared about me, and therefore I did not feel an ongoing need to test limits, as I had at the hospital.

Unlike the hospital staff, the residential treatment team did not assume authoritarian, confrontative postures that result inevitably in power struggles. Instead, they encouraged and even demanded my input in treatment. They considered me a partner in my own treatment rather than a less knowledgeable inferior. The mutual fear experienced by myself and the staff at the hospital was replaced by mutual acceptance at Community Care. Medication was used in the residential program as an aid in the recovery process. In the hospital it was too often used to sedate patients into submission.

There were other differences as well. In the residential program, I was able to practice social skills in the safety of a community of peers and to learn skills by watching others practice. Psychiatric hospitals had only engendered or exacerbated feelings of dependency and low self-esteem. After several hospitalizations, I had begun to feel hopeless about the future and about my having any part in the world.

The regimentation of the hospital was missing at Community Care. The residential program expected me to take control of my life and led me to believe that I could. Staff attitudes were extremely important in building my confidence. In addition to recognizing and honestly addressing my weaknesses and problem areas, staff also pointed out my strengths and helped me make the most of them by teaching me specific problem solving techniques and daily living skills.

Each week a staff member and I independently rated my progress in specific areas. The staff did not approach my treatment with a biased view of what I could accomplish, as I felt hospital personnel had done. Staff at this facility believed in my potential, and I began to develop confidence in myself. Gradually I became aware that I was my greatest asset.

There were other benefits to the program, too. I felt that I was part of a family, which motivated me to improve my social skills and interpersonal relationships, a crucial step in the path to recovery. Group therapy showed me that other members of the program had similar symptoms and strengthened my connection to them. I also learned to do reality testing with staff and group members. The encouragement and immediate feedback I received were invaluable.

As a result of my developing confidence in myself and realistic trust in others, I was able to grow. The prejudice I had encountered was supplanted by an emerging understanding of me as a person, and pity became respect. The flexibility of the program to meet my individual needs enabled me to work forward, with the knowledge that a predictable, consistent, and caring support system was available for me should I need it.

I was now ready to take control of my life. My estranged second husband and I moved into an apartment together, and I threw myself into the task of finding employment. With encouragement from Community Care and my husband, I was successful. None of these steps were accomplished easily, but the pieces of my periodically disrupted life were coming back together.

REFLECTIONS

So that I may continue to progress, I have looked closely at what has helped me and what has not, and I have tried to understand why my condition has improved. I have come to the following conclusions.

Community-Based Treatment

Hospitals have their place in the treatment and stabilization of acute psychiatric problems. However, it is my opinion that long-term gains in functioning are made most readily and most successfully through treatment in the community. Although some community facilities are better than others, a good community support program can provide vital services for its clients, perhaps the most important of which are a familiar structured environment and close interpersonal relationships.

Living in the community allows individuals with a psychiatric illness to gain understanding and acceptance from members of a treatment program. Peers, family, and friends can also provide recognition of and respect for clients' individuality and special needs.

A community support program can help residents develop a predictable daily schedule to offset their chaotic inner existence and thus make life easier. Any number of structured activities could satisfy this need, but I have found work—a paying job—to be the most helpful. My job gives me something to look forward to every day, a skill to learn and improve, and an earned income. It is my motivation for getting up each morning, not always an easy task for psychiatric patients. My hours at work are passed therapeutically as well as productively, for through steady employment I have learned to value myself and trust in my ability to overcome my disease.

Education and Support

Education about mental illness is crucial for everyone, but particularly for patients. I resent the fact that I was not given information about my illness and the methods used to treat it, some of which I feel were harmful. For example, alternating electroshock with insulin coma therapy in 1966 only served to virtually eradicate my memories while probably adversely affecting my ability to learn new information as well. Doing so without my consent or even my awareness was criminal.

Patients and family members are entitled to education about mental illness, including its symptoms, course, and treatment; more important, perhaps, they also need to know that the disease can be managed and that there is reason to hope that the patient will live a satisfying and productive life.

Peer-run support groups can be extremely valuable to clients by offering support, friendship, hope for the future, and peer-group modeling. We as consumers of psychiatric services should meet socially with others who have had similar experiences to exchange information about coping skills and to take responsibility for ourselves. We must meet with others like ourselves to see firsthand what we have accomplished and what we can achieve.

Support groups and educational groups can help patients and their friends and family members to accept and deal with mental illness. Community mental health centers should be required to hold classes on a regular basis for both families and consumers in which various major mental illnesses can be openly discussed and information about mental illnesses shared by both professionals and clients. In fact, these classes are already taking place. Each week at the Mental Health Center of Boulder County, both consumers and family members pack a room to hear the facts about mental illnesses, hoping to gain a better understanding of these perplexing and frustrating diseases.

Medications

I believe there is also a place for medications in the treatment of major mental illnesses. Unfortunately the side effects of antipsychotic medications can often be more disabling than the illnesses themselves, and I have even experienced side effects from the pills I took to control the side effects of antipsychotic drugs. For years I fought against taking medications before I found one that worked while causing a minimum of side effects. Now I would resist discontinuing it. I now know how terrible I feel when I do not take my medication, and I realize how much better I am able to function with it.

Before I reached this important realization, I was caught in a vicious circle. When I was off the medication I couldn't remember how much better I had felt on it, and when I was taking the medication I felt so good that I was convinced I did not need it. Finally, however, I was able to make the connection between taking the medication and feeling better and to realize how very helpful the medication is to me.

I am not advocating that everyone with a mental illness take medication or that we now have medications that will work for everyone, but the use of medication is an option worth exploring by anyone with a mental illness. Letting a doctor "adjust" your brain chemistry may be frightening, and drug therapy is certainly an art when competently done. However, if psychopharmacotherapy is to be successful, the patient cannot be a passive observer; arriving at the proper type and dosage of medication requires a true partnership between doctor and patient.

Dealing with Relapse

Relapses are inevitable. Although they can be triggered by a number of different mechanisms and may have a biochemical or neurophysiological basis, their effects can often be mediated by a strong, positive relationship with one's family or other significant individuals. Above all else, it is important to deal intelligently with relapses when they occur and make the effort to begin again. Those of us with mental illnesses must try to learn what we can from the unfortunate experience of relapse and remember what helped us to recover and what did not. In that way the next relapse may be softened.

Being Realistic

Like those with other chronic illnesses, I know to expect good and bad times and to make the most of the good. I take my life very seriously and do as much as I can when I am feeling well, because I know that there will be bad times when I am likely to lose some of the ground I have gained. Professionals and family members must help the ill person set realistic goals. I would entreat them not to be devastated by our illnesses and transmit this hopeless attitude to us. I would urge them never to lose hope, for we will not strive if we believe the effort is futile.

STRATEGIES FOR PREVENTING RELAPSE

I find that my vulnerability to stress and anxiety decreases the more I feel in control of my life. My coping strategies largely consist of four steps: recognizing when I am feeling stressed; identifying the stressor; remembering from past experience what action helped in the same situation or a similar one; and taking that action.

Generally speaking, I have also learned to have a more positive outlook. I accept myself and my shortcomings (although

I try to minimize them), and I have also become more accepting of others, realizing that we cannot all be alike. I attempt to keep in touch with my feelings and to attend immediately to difficulties, including symptoms. For example, rather than letting my paranoia grow, I will take action to satisfy the paranoid feelings. If I feel uncomfortable in a public place because I am convinced someone is after me, I will make it a point to sit facing the door. Having done so, I am able to forget the paranoid feeling and go on about my life rather than letting the paranoia control me.

Because new experiences and environments create enormous pressures, I need the security of a predictable environment. I also know I must go slow when confronted with anything new, avoiding stressful situations if necessary. I have learned my particular limitations and my own sources of stress, and I mentally prepare myself to cope with situations that test my limits or cause stress by anticipating the problems that might occur.

I now know that at times I may need to spend some time alone, and I take "time out." But not too much. I also try to recognize my personal warning signs of relapse (though not always successfully). To successfully avert or diminish relapses, I have been forced to be persistent and to consistently utilize these coping behaviors.

My illness is a sobering reality, yet I am not as vulnerable to it as I once was because of my regular use of coping strategies as well as my new philosophy about my life. I have come to understand that life may be more difficult for me than it is for others and that I must preside over it more attentively for this reason. Yet every individual, regardless of whether he or she has a mental illness, must develop skills in general coping, interpersonal relations, and management of work and leisure time. It is these skills that will allow us to lead successful and happy lives.

CONCLUSIONS

There is no magic answer that will eliminate the tragedy of mental illnesses, but we need not be at their mercy. Appropriate treatment can help those of us with a mental illness to understand our disease and to learn to function in spite of it. After multiple hospitalizations, I found that any gains I had made were consolidated in community treatment, where mentally ill individuals are treated as people with strengths and weaknesses instead of mental patients who can never improve. Those with mental illnesses must try not to be disheartened, admittedly a difficult task, for having some hope is crucial.

Despite my lack of formal credentials, I have become somewhat of an expert about my psychosis; having lived with it these many years, I feel I have a personal understanding of it that could not be learned from books. I have tried to use this knowledge to live the best life my disease will allow. We consumers of psychiatric services have much to contribute in the effort to educate the public about mental illness and eradicate its stigma.

More important, however, those of us who are afflicted with a mental illness must work to understand our disabilities so we can conquer them. We must study our illness, appraise our lives, identify our strengths and weaknesses, and build on our assets while minimizing our vulnerabilities. Only then will we realize and fully use our potential and begin to overcome the stigma, discrimination, and rejection we have experienced. Only then will we reclaim our dignity and our autonomy. To achieve these goals we must change the perception of who we are and who we can become, first for ourselves and then for the public.

Although it takes time, those of us with a mental illness can overcome the disease by compensating for our handicaps. I did not choose to be ill, but I can choose to deal with schizophrenia and learn to live with it. I know I must confront my disorder with courage and struggle with my symptoms persistently, never viewing relapse as a permanent defeat and always acknowledging remission as a hard-earned victory.

CHAPTER FORTY-SEVEN

Patients' Accounts of Stress and Coping in Schizophrenia

Agnes B. Hatfield

This chapter was previously published in Hospital and Community Psychology, 40, *1141-1145. Copyright © 1989, the American Psychiatric Association.*

The concepts "stress" and "coping" are often used by clinicians to explain the behaviors of people with schizophrenia and to develop strategies for working with patients and their families.[1-6] The general assumption of these clinicians is that people with schizophrenia have a special vulnerability, probably of biological origin, to internal and external stress.[7]

Anderson[8] used the term "core psychological deficit" to explain this vulnerability, which she felt could be exacerbated in the home, work place, or treatment setting. Anderson and colleagues,[1] who elected to focus on the family as a potential source of stress, developed and tested a method of psychoeducational treatment that reduced patients' rate of relapse. The treatment involved training families in new ways of communicating and relating that, along with optimum uses of medication, reduced the stresses that led to decompensation. Kopeikin and others,[5] who also considered life events as precipitants of patients' decompensation, directed their efforts toward helping families identify, prevent, and cope with situations that were stressful to the patient.

These studies focused on stressors that are external to the patient. Patients' accounts of their experiences, however, reveal that many sources of stress are internal to the person. There is a growing interest among researchers and clinicians in learning more about the personal side of mental illness to better understand patient behaviors and to establish better rapport with patients.[9-13] As Carpenter[9] pointed out, "It is in the subjective and inner world of volition, perception, cognition, and affect that schizophrenia is manifest" (p. 534). The challenge is to find a valid way to learn about this inner world of schizophrenia.

A potentially valuable, but little consulted, source of information about the personal side of mental illness is patients' accounts that have appeared in numerous small publications, consumer newsletters, and small collections of personal stories, as well as in professional journals and, occasionally, in published books. Although several such accounts were published in the 1960s and 1970s,[14-17] more recent materials also offer valuable insights.

The purposes of this study were to learn from first-person accounts how the inner experiences of people with schizophrenia become sources of stress for them and how patients strive to cope with these stressors. First-person accounts from a wide range of sources were selected with the assumption that they supply valid and useful data for understanding and helping people with schizophrenia. The research was also guided by Estroff's suggestion,[18] based on studies of patients in their natural environments in the community, that patients' perceptions, beliefs, feelings, experiences, and behaviors are the most important units of analysis. Stress theory,[19-23] which is briefly explained below, served as a general framework for interpretation of patients' statements.

STRESS THEORY

Stress occurs when a person's resources are inadequate to meet the demands of the environment. This definition may be interpreted to include both the inner and outer environment. Stress is a painful state of disequilibrium accompanied by feelings of great tension, high anxiety, and fatigue. When individuals are stressed, they struggle to find ways of coping that will reduce their great discomfort.

This chapter is not concerned with ordinary levels of stress but rather with stress severe enough to tax an individual's capacity to cope with or adapt to it. Wrubel and associates[24] have identified some characteristics of situations that are likely to produce overwhelming levels of stress. Such situations may be unique in the individual's experience, and the individual may not be prepared to deal with them. On the other hand, stress is also produced by events that occur frequently or that have a long duration. Such situations lead to fatigue and burnout. Also stressful are situations that affect all aspects of one's existence or that are highly ambiguous. Patient accounts indicate that the experience of schizophrenia commonly has these characteristics.

Some theoreticians assume that all human beings have an innate drive toward competence.[25-27] In this view, human beings are always striving to survive physically and psychologically. They either attempt to adapt to their environment or change it. Patient accounts usually reveal an active process of coping and adapting in spite of the tremendous difficulties that schizophrenia presents.

SOURCES OF STRESS IN SCHIZOPHRENIA

Sources of stress identified in patients' accounts of mental illness include altered perceptions, cognitive confusion, attentional deficit, and impaired identity.

Altered Perceptions

Alteration of senses may involve either enhancement or blunting of perceptions, but enhancement or increased acuteness is probably most common. Visual stimuli appear sharper and brighter, and auditory stimuli seem louder. In addition, these sensations appear to change unpredictably. Since everything that we know about the world must come through our senses, people with schizophrenia experience a grossly distorted reality. They suffer high levels of stress and anxiety as they struggle to negotiate between the world as others know it and the world of their inner reality.

Sculptor and writer Mary McGrath[28] provided this account of her experience:

"I know all of the negatives. Schizophrenia is painful, and it is craziness when I hear voices, when I believe that people are following me, wanting to snatch my very soul. I am frightened too when every whisper, every laugh is about me; when newspapers suddenly contain curses, four-letter words shouting at me; when sparkles of light are demon eyes. Schizophrenia is frightening when I can't hold onto thoughts." (p. 38)

McGrath says her illness is a " journey of fear" that is "often paralyzing" and "mostly painful." Still she is hopeful because new research may help ease the burden of the illness and because of the help and caring of mental health professionals. She expresses the difficulty of living between two worlds, as does Nona Borgeson:[29]

"Where weighing the odds of probability ends, schizophrenia begins, and paranoia runs rampant. The schizophrenic doesn't think: he/she knows, false knowledge though it be, and his/her world becomes one of polarities—black or white, love or hate, ecstasy or suicidal inclinations, mortal fear or indestructibility." (p. 7)

It is instructive to review patients' descriptions of their inner world in light of what Antonovsky[30] says about human health or the state of well-being. He suggests that a sense of coherence, an "enduring though dynamic feeling of confidence that one's internal and external environments are predictable and that things will work out as well as can be expected," is crucial to well-being (p. 123). The lack of coherence and predictability that plagues the lives of men and women with schizophrenia, who have a "terrific sense of unreality" and who often feel like they are "waking up in a strange room,"[17] is certainly striking.

Cognitive Confusion

Patients in Freedman's study[15] of perceptual and cognitive disturbances in schizophrenia described themselves as "confused," "hazy," "bewildered," and "disoriented."[15] They reported that they suffered thought blocking and sometimes felt their minds going blank, and that they were unable to maintain cognitive control over their ideas. Torrey[13] reported the following example:

"My thoughts get all jumbled up. I start thinking or talking about something, but I never get there. Instead I wander off in the wrong direction and get caught up all sorts of different things that may be connected with the things I want to say but in a way I can't explain. People listening to me get more lost than I do." (p. 18)

Freedman[15] found a variety of disturbances in memory, language, and speech in the 50 autobiographical accounts she studied. Patients reported experiencing a lag between hearing a word, recalling its meaning, and formulating an answer. Speech required great concentration and conscious effort. Freedman provides the following example from a patient:

"Sometimes when people speak to me, my head is overloaded. It's too much to hold at once. It goes out as quick as it goes in. It makes you forget what you just heard because you can't get hearing it long enough. It's just words in the air unless you can figure it out from their faces." (p. 338)

The patient accounts reported by Freedman revealed that the sense of time was often distorted during acute stages of illness. Some patients said they lost all sense of time and with it, all notions of logic, order, and sequence:

"My time sense was disturbed. This was the result of intense cerebral activity in which inner experiences took place at greatly increased speed, so that much more than usual happened per minute of external time. The result was to give an effect of slow motion. The speeding up of my inner experiences provided in this way an apparent slowing down of the external world." (p. 338)

Attentional Deficit

The difficulties of meeting the ordinary demands of the environment due to cognitive confusion are compounded by problems of attention and concentration. More than half of the sample in Freedman's study specifically noted such problems and reported that their minds wandered a good deal. One patient said, "It is not that he [the patient] cannot keep to the point, but there are so many points and all equally and insistently insignificant" (p. 336).

Anscombe[31] suggested that attentional deficit is central to the problem of coping with schizophrenia. The patient often has the sensation of being captured by a stimulus rather than being able to choose what to attend. Objects seem to jump out of the environment and command attention. Patients have a sense of lack of volition and are unable to shift their attention flexibly. McGhie and Chapman[32] provided this account:

> "If I am reading I may suddenly get bogged down at a word. It may be any word, even a simple word that I know well. When this happens I can't get past it. It is as if I am being hypnotized by it. It's as if I am seeing the word for the first time and in a different way from anyone else. It's not so much that I am absorbed in it, it's more like it is absorbing me." (p. 109)

Finding themselves riveted to a particular stimulus, people with schizophrenia conclude that what they are attracted to has unusual significance.[31] David Zelt,[33] telling his story in third person, describes his fascination with colors, each of which came to have its own significance:

> "Ordinarily unimportant information from external reality took on new dimensions for him. For example, colors powerfully influenced him. At any given moment wherever David went, colors were used to express judgements about his spirituality. People used the colors of their clothes or cars to express positive or negative views of him. Green meant that David was like Christ; white stood for spiritual purity; orange indicated he was attuned to the cosmos." (p. 530)

The patient experiences enormous difficulties in achieving levels of competence adequate to meet ordinary environmental demands. Since the source of these difficulties is invisible, the world generally does not understand the patient's problems and expects more than the patient can produce. As a result, the patient often feels inadequate, anxious, and discouraged.

Impaired Identity

Alterations in the sense of self are common in schizophrenia. McGrath[28] describes her strange feelings: "If I want to reach out to touch me, I feel nothing but slippery coldness, yet I sense it is me." Later she says, "My existence seems undefined—mere image that I keep reaching for, but never can touch" (p. 638). Normally individuals have a clear sense of where their bodies end and the rest of the world begins. Without this capacity, orienting oneself in the world is extremely difficult.

With treatment, the more acute phases of mental illness tend to abate and more energy is available to attend to the external world. But Harris and Bergman[34] observed that getting better can be a mixed blessing for many clients. They are caught between the familiar patient role and the nonpatient role, which is not clearly defined. They are frightened about the future but cannot return to the past. These men and women have the awesome task of learning to accept that life is irrevocably different, and because of this difference, new meaning in life and a new way of living must be found.

Godschalx[35] studied the personal perspective of patients with schizophrenia and found that many of them struggle with issues of identity. They had great difficulty deciding how to characterize what was wrong with them. They stated variously that they had "a nervous breakdown," "spells," "anxiety," or "mental problems." Godschalx found no relationship between acknowledgment of a mental illness and either happiness or level of functioning.

COPING STRATEGIES

The many creative ways that patients use to cope with these distressing symptoms are truly remarkable. Esso Leete[36] has stated that, contrary to popular thinking that people with schizophrenia are withdrawn and passive, they are actively fighting "internal terrors and external realities" to keep their emotional balance and social composure in a world they cannot always translate.

People with schizophrenia may appear rigid and unable to change directions without difficulty. This inflexibility is one way of maintaining stability when the ground keeps shifting beneath them. Structure and predictability in the external world help compensate for the unpredictability of the inner world. Daily routines give pattern and a sense of order to life. By knowing what to expect, the person with schizophrenia can prepare [him- or herself] and thus exert a degree of control over events. Stress and anxiety lessen when events lose their sense of arbitrariness and an appearance of consistency emerges.

Stephen Weiner[37] likened his condition to that of Sisyphus, who was condemned to roll a rock up a hill only to have it slide down again: "So strategy becomes a necessity—learn to anticipate. No caffeine before a predictably stressful situation... A conscious effort to combat the automatic ideas of reference... Remind myself that coincidences do appear" (p. 9).

Jeannette Keil[38] found that she could learn to control her words and actions even if she was unable to control her racing thoughts. She worked diligently to keep her life in balance, and she pressured herself to appear appropriate. Jerry Pearson[39] said he used relationships with people to stay centered in reality: "When I am alone for too long, my thinking and emotions can produce a semi-hallucinatory state. As long as I know that I have access to other people, I think I will be all right. Living in isolation would be the worst thing that could happen to me" (p. 2). Cara Lawerance[40] found that "having too much time is like living one's life in a cave... One of the first things we should do to help recovery is to schedule our days" (p. 2).

Godschalx[35] found that her subjects were anxious about the terrors of hallucinations, the sense of being different, possible loss of control, and the likelihood of being victimized. The patients tried to deal with these insecurities by monitoring internal tensions, structuring their thinking, and taking psychotropic medication. Esso Leete[41] found it important to recognize her own warning signs of potential relapse, including decreased sleep, trouble with concentration, forgetfulness, increased paranoia, more frequent voices, irritability, and being overwhelmed by her environment.

A number of men and women with mental illnesses find an acceptable role in life by helping others. Cathy King[42] found her identity in a "fellowship of others of her own kind." In a patient self-help organization, she experienced for the first time what it means to be a part of a group. Esso Leete[41], after a long struggle with schizophrenia, is now a full-time employee at a hospital to which she was once committed. She started the Denver Social Support Group to help others cope with their mental illnesses.

Patients related many philosophical ways that they came to terms with their dilemma. Stephen Weiner[37] dealt with the unfairness of having mental illness by accepting the fact that life is not fair, although it is unfair in different ways to different people. He has chosen to accept his condition "without completely giving in to it" (p. 10).

But in accepting his condition he eschews bravado as a means of coping. "Bravado is an almost inevitable reaction to pain and humiliation," he has written. "It is easier to pretend to oneself that the pain and humiliation never existed."[43] But this tactic is a form of denial of the "almost-heroic reality that the strength to endure and overcome had to arise as a strategic reaction to an unchosen, unforeseen misfortune" (p. 6).

Zan Boches[44] has suggested that life puts various limitations on people. However, freedom to make choices always exists within these limitations. For him, life was worthwhile in spite of the limitations imposed by serious illness. Barbara Pilvin[45] came to terms with the way mental illness compromised her goals. She stated that her illness "made me understand that there are no guarantees in life, that the outcome of my plans may be beyond my control" (p. 23).

CONCLUSIONS

Clinicians now generally recognize environmental stress as a factor in aggravating the symptoms of schizophrenia. They less often acknowledge the role that internal stressors may play in creating anxiety and suffering. To more accurately explain and interpret patient behavior and to respond empathetically to patients, clinicians must learn much more about the inner world of schizophrenia. A rich source for learning about this experience is the body of widely available first-person accounts of patients.

REFERENCES

1. Anderson, C. M., Reiss, D. J., & Hogarty, G. E. (1986). *Schizophrenia and the family*. New York, NY: Guilford.

2. Beels, C. C., & McFarlane, W. R. (1982). Family treatments of schizophrenia: Background and state of the art. *Hospital and Community Psychiatry, 33*, 541-550.

3. Bernheim, K., & Lehman, A. (1985). *Working with families of the mentally ill*. New York, NY: Norton.

4. Clarkin, J. F., & Glick, I. D. (1982). Recent developments in family therapy: A review. *Hospital and Community Psychiatry, 33*, 550-556.

5. Kopeikin, H. S., Marshall, V., & Goldstein, M. J. (1983). Stages and impact of crisis-oriented family therapy in the aftercare of acute schizophrenia. In W. R. McFarlane (Ed.), *Family Therapy in Schizophrenia*. New York, NY: Guilford.

6. Left, J., & Vaughn, C. (1985). *Expressed emotion in families*. New York, NY: Guilford.

7. Zubin, J., & Spring, G. (1977). Vulnerability: a new view of schizophrenia. *Journal of Abnormal Psychology, 86*, 103-126.

8. Anderson, C. M. (1983). A psychoeducational program for families of patients with schizophrenia. In W. R. McFarlane (Ed.), *Family Therapy in Schizophrenia*. New York, NY: Guilford.

9. Carpenter, W. T. (1986). Thoughts on the treatment of schizophrenia. *Schizophrenia Bulletin, 12*, 527-539.

10. Minkoff, W. M., & Stern, R. (1985). Paradoxes faced by residents being trained in the psychosocial treatment of people with chronic schizophrenia. *Hospital and Community Psychiatry, 36*, 859-864.

11. Reiser, M. (1988). Are psychiatric educators losing the mind? *American Journal of Psychiatry, 145*, 148-153.

12. Strauss, J. S. (1986). Discussion: What does rehabilitation accomplish? *Schizophrenia Bulletin, 12*, 720-723.

13. Torrey, E. F. (1983). *Surviving schizophrenia: A family perspective*. New York, NY: Harper & Row.

14. Alverez, W. C. (1961). *Minds that came back*. New York, NY: Lppincott.

15. Freedman, M. A. (1974). Subjective experiences of perceptual and cognitive disturbances in schizophrenia. *Archives of General Psychiatry, 30*, 333-340.

16. Kaplan, B. (1964). *The inner world of mental illness*. New York, NY: Harper & Row.

17. Landis, D., & Mettler, F. A. (1964). *Varieties of psychopathological experiences*. New York, NY: Holt, Rinehart, Winston.

18. Estroff, S. (1981). *Making it crazy*. Berkeley, CA: University of California Press.

19. Coehlo, G. V., Hamburg, D. A., & Adams, J. E. (Eds.). (1974). *Coping and adaptation*. New York, NY: Basic Books.

20. Figley, C. R., & McCubbin, H. I. (Eds.). (1983). *Coping with catastrophe*. New York, NY: Brunner/Mazel.

21. Hansell, H. (1976). *The person-in-distress: On the biosocial dynamics of adaptation*. New York, NY: Human Sciences.

22. Monat, A., & Lazarus, R. (1977). *Stress and coping*. New York, NY: Columbia University Press.

23. Parad, H. (Ed.). (1965). *Crisis intervention: Selected readings*. New York, NY: Family Services Association of America.

24. Wrubel, J., Benner, F., & Lazarus, R. (1981). Social competence from the perspective of stress and coping. In J. O. Wine, & M. D. Smye (Eds.), *Social competence*. New York, NY: Guilford.

25. White, R. W. (1976). Strategies of adaptation. In R. H. Moos. (Ed.) *Human adaptation: Coping with life crisis.* Lexington, MA: Heath.

26. Mechanic, D. (1974). Social structure and adaptation: Some neglected dimensions. In G. V. Coelho, D. A. Hamburg, & J. E. Adams. (Eds.) *Coping and adaptation.* New York, NY: Basic Books.

27. Adler, P. (1982). An analysis of the concept of competence in individual and social systems. *Community Mental Health Journal, 18,* 34-39.

28. McGrath, M. E. (1984). First person accounts: Where did I go? *Schizophrenia Bulletin, 10,* 638-40.

29. Borgenson, N. (undated). Schizophrenia from the inside. In H. Shetler, & P. Straw. *A new day: Voices from across the land.* Arlington, VA: National Alliance for the Mentally Ill.

30. Antonovsky, A. (1979). *Health, stress, and coping.* San Francisco, CA: Jossey-Bass.

31. Anscombe, R. (1987). The disorder of consciousness in schizophrenia. *Schizophrenia Bulletin, 13,* 241-260.

32. McGhie, A., & Chapman, J. (1961). Disorders of attention and perception in early schizophrenia. *British Journal of Medical Psychology, 34,* 103-116.

33. Zelt, D. (1981). First person account: The messiah quest. *Schizophrenia Bulletin, 7,* 527-531.

34. Harris, M., & Bergman, H. (1984). The young adult chronic patient: Affective responses to treatment. *New Directions in Mental Health Services, 21,* 29-35.

35. Godschalx, S. M. (1986). *Experiences and coping strategies of people with schizophrenia.* Unpublished doctoral dissertation, College of Nursing, University of Utah.

36. Leete, E. (undated). Mental illness: An insider's view. In H. Shetler, & P. Straw. *A new day: Voices from across the land.* Arlington, VA: National Alliance for the Mentally Ill.

37. Weiner, S. (undated). Exhaustion and fairness. In H. Shetler, & P. Straw. *A new day: Voices from across the land.* Arlington, VA: National Alliance for the Mentally Ill.

38. Keil, J. (1984). *Overcoming the recurring nightmare of schizophrenia.* San Diego, CA: K & A.

39. Pearson, J. (1988). Need for friendship. *Alliance for the Mentally Ill of Tucson and Southern Arizona Newsletter, 5*(1), 5.

40. Lawerance, C. (1988). Having too much time, too little to do. *Alliance for the Mentally ill of Tucson and Southern Arizona Newsletter, 5*(1), 5.

41. Leete, E. (1987). A patient's perspective on schizophrenia. *New Directions for Mental Health Services, 34,* 81-90. (see Chapter 46).

42. King, C. (1987). Dissolving the barriers: reflections on coming out of the closet. *Hang Tough (newsletter of the Marin Network of Mental Health Clients), 2*(2), 8-9.

43. Weiner, S. (1987). Bravado and the mental health clients' self-help movement. *Hang Tough (newsletter of the Marin Network of Mental Health Clients), 2*(2), 4-5.

44. Boches, Z. (1989). "Freedom" means knowing you have a choice. In *Schizophrenia: The experiences of patients and families* (pp. 4-42). Arlington, VA: National Alliance for the Mentally Ill.

45. Pilvin, B. (undated). And wisdom to know the difference. In H. Shetler, & P. Straw. *A new day: Voices from across the land.* Arlington, VA: National Alliance for the Mentally Ill.

CHAPTER FORTY-EIGHT

Patient Self-Regulation and Functioning In Schizophrenia

Edna K. Hamera, Kathryn A. Peterson, Sandra M. Handley,
Ardyce A. Plumlee, and Elaine Frank-Ragan

This chapter was previously published in Hospital and Community Psychiatry, 42, 630-631. Copyright © 1991, the *American Psychiatric Association.*

Although clinicians have often been skeptical that individuals with schizophrenia can identify symptoms of their disease process, research findings dispute such skepticism. Patients appear to be aware of early indicators of exacerbation of their illness. Findings from retrospective investigations show that many patients identify nonpsychotic indicators as early warning signs and symptoms.[1,2] Examples are tenseness and nervousness or symptoms of dysphoria, such as trouble sleeping.

Prospective studies have sought to determine if early indicators predict relapse.[3-6] In most of these studies, early indicators were measured by clinicians' ratings, although Birchwood and colleagues[6] used ratings by patients and significant others. The findings from these studies suggest that although patients may experience early indicators, the presence of the indicators does not always predict relapse. Thus early indicators appear to be sensitive but not specific to relapse. However, definitions and measures of relapse differ among investigators, so the findings are tentative.

These prospective studies assume that although patients may identify early indicators of exacerbation of illness, clinicians still need to intervene to prevent relapse. Our previous findings[2] suggested that patients did not react passively to early indicators but took actions in response to them. Our work is based on a self-regulation model adapted from a model of illness representation[7] and control theory[8]. The model posits that individuals monitor symptoms that signal exacerbation of their illness and take actions to manage their illness.

Using our model and the findings from Docherty and associates[9], which showed that patients experience a progression from nonpsychotic to psychotic symptoms before relapse, we hypothesized that patients who identified symptoms of depression and anxiety as early indicators would function at a higher level than patients who identified psychotic symptoms. In addition, we explored the relationship between the type of actions patients took in response to indicators and their level of functioning.

METHODS

Study participants were selected from among patients enrolled in Community Support Services (CSS) of Johnson County Mental Health Center in Merriam, Kansas. A convenience sample of 51 subjects who had received a DSM-III diagnosis of schizophrenia at least two years previously were interviewed... Patients with secondary diagnoses of substance abuse, mental retardation, or organicity were excluded.

Two-thirds of the patients in the sample were male, and 90% were Caucasian. Their mean age was 33.5 years, and they had a mean of 12.6 years of education. Thirty-five percent were employed either full-time or part-time, and 71% resided in unsupervised living situations. The majority of subjects (63%) had a diagnosis of a paranoid subtype of schizophrenia, all were on antipsychotic medications, and all were being closely monitored by a case manager. In addition, some attended group activities at CSS.

The interviews were conducted using the Self-Regulation Interview for Schizophrenia adapted from our previous work.[2] In the open-ended interview, administered by two of the investigators, subjects were asked if they knew when they were becoming ill; if they said yes, they were asked how they knew. From the list of indicators reported, subjects were asked to select one that they particularly noticed. This primary indicator was then coded into one of three categories—anxiety, depression, or psychosis—based on the stages of decompensation described by Docherty and associates.[9]

In the interview, subjects were also asked what they did, if anything, when they experienced their primary indicator. The actions reported were coded two ways. First, they were grouped by whether or not they involved contacting health care professionals or taking prescribed medications (medical versus non-medical actions). Second, the actions were grouped into self-defeating behaviors (use of drugs or alcohol or acting out) and other actions.

Inter-rater reliability for the responses to the self-regulation interview, assessed independently by two of the investigators, ranged from 89 to 100 percent. Likewise, interceder reliability for primary indicators and action categories ranged from 96 to 100 percent.

Within a week of the interview, the subjects' case managers rated their level of functioning using the Global Assessment Scale (GAS) (10). The relationship between the type of indicator (anxiety, depression, or psychosis) and the GAS was examined using an analysis of variance with Duncan's post-hoc test. Tests were used to determine if level of functioning differed among subjects who took different kinds of actions to regulate their primary indicator.

RESULTS

All 51 subjects identified illness indicators. Forty-one percent of the subjects' primary indicators were categorized as anxiety, 285% as depression, and 31% as psychosis.

Forty-nine of the 51 subjects reported taking more than one action to regulate their primary indicator; the mean number of actions was 3.1. The most frequent action was to add new activities or focus on existing ones; for example, "get busy" or "concentrate on usual activities." Other frequently reported actions were cognitive strategies such as self-talk and behaviors such as resting or withdrawing. Of the total number of actions (N=132), only 20 were medical actions; that is, taking prescribed medication or contacting health care professionals. Fifteen self-defeating actions, involving behaviors such as using drugs or alcohol or acting out, were reported.

Subjects were asked if the primary indicator of exacerbation of their illness got better, stayed the same, or got worse in response to their most frequent action. Most subjects (N=36) reported that the primary indicator of illness improved as a result of the action. Ten subjects stated the action had no effect, and three said it made the indicator worse.

Subjects with psychotic indicators had significantly lower GAS scores (a mean of 51.17, with a range of 30 to 70) than subjects reporting indicators involving anxiety or depression (F=5.67, df=2.50, p=.01). Subjects taking medical actions did not have higher levels of functioning as indicated by GAS scores than subjects taking non-medical actions. Likewise, subjects who regulated the indicators of illness with actions that were not self-defeating were not rated as functioning better than subjects who reported regulating behaviors that were self-defeating.

DISCUSSION

The study was undertaken to evaluate the relationship between symptom self-regulation and level of functioning in patients with schizophrenia. Patients who identified nonpsy-

chotic indicators of exacerbation of illness functioned at a higher level than patients who identified psychotic indicators. The GAS, which measures level of functioning, includes symptomatology as an index of functioning but also includes job performance and relationships with family members and other people as well as use of leisure time.

The types of actions taken to regulate primary indicators were not related to level of functioning. It may be that actions are not encouraged by health care professionals, so patients have not systematically assessed what they can do to manage primary indicators of illness. Research on specificactions for specific symptom groups is needed.

The relationship between type of indicator and level of functioning found in this study may be supported in other samples and settings with different demographic and treatment characteristics. However, in our previous work,[2] the majority of nonhospitalized patients from mental health centers serving lower socioeconomic populations reported monitoring indicator symptoms and taking actions in response to indicators; implicit self-regulatory processes were present.

The findings suggest that individuals with schizophrenia could be taught to monitor early nonpsychotic indicators more effectively, which may improve their functioning and prevent hospitalization. A prospective study is needed to determine if enhancing existing self-regulatory processes is beneficial.

ACKNOWLEDGMENT

This study was funded by research grant SRG 5R21NRO1507-02 from the National Center for Nursing Research of the National Institutes of Health. Roma Lee Taunton, RN, PhD, was principal investigator and Kathryn Peterson, RN, MS, was project director. The authors thank Leslie Young, MSW, and the case managers at the community support program of Johnson County Mental Health Center for their assistance in data collection and Ronald L. Martin, MD, for comments on previous drafts.

REFERENCES

1. Herz, M. & Melville, C. (1980). Relapse in schizophrenia. *American Journal of Psychiatry, 137*, 801-905.

2. McCandless-Glimcher L., McKnight S., & Hamera E., et al. (1986). Use of symptoms by schizophrenics to monitor and regulate their illness. *Hospital and Community Psychiatry, 37*, 929-933.

3. Heinrichs, D. W., & Carpenter, W. T. (1985). Prospective study of prodromal symptoms in schizophrenic relapse. *American Journal of Psychiatry*, 142, 371-373.

4. Marder, S. R., Mintz, J., & Van Patten T., et al. (1986). Prodromal symptoms as predictors of schizophrenic relapse. In J. A. Lieberman & J. M. Kane. (Eds.), *Predictors of Relapse in Schizophrenia*. Washington, DC: American Psychiatric Press.

5. Subotnik, K. L., & Nuechterlein, E. (1988). Prodromal signs and symptoms of schizophrenia. *Journal of Abnormal Psychology, 97,* 405-412.

6. Birchwood, M., Smith, J., & Macmillan, F., et al. (1989). Predicting relapse in schizophrenia: The development and implementation of an early sign monitoring system using patients and families as observers: A preliminary investigation. *Psychological Medicine, 19,* 649-656.

7. Leventhal, H., Norenz, D., & Strauss, A. (1982). Self-regulation and the mechanism for symptom appraisal. In D. Mechanic. (Ed.) *Psychological Epidemiology.* New York, NY: Neale Watson Academic Press.

8. Carver, C., & Sheier, M. (1982). Control theory: A useful conceptual framework for personality, social, clinical, and health psychology. *Psychology Bulletin, 92,* 111-135.

9. Docherty, J., Van Kammen, D., & Siris, S., et al. (1978). Stages of onset of schizophrenic psychosis. *American Journal of Psychiatry, 35,* 420-426.

10. Endicott, H. J., Spitzer, R., & Fleiss, J., et al. (1976). The Global Assessment Scale: a procedure for measuring overall severity of psychiatric disturbance. *Archives of General Psychiatry, 137,* 766-771.

CHAPTER FORTY-NINE

Resilience and Human Adaptability: Who Rises Above Adversity?

Susan B. Fine

This Eleanor Clarke Slagle Lecture (1990) is a study of outcome—outcome that often defies the odds. It is a study of lives characterized by extraordinary hardships and remarkable abilities to move beyond them. It poses a core question: Who rises above adversity? It ventures beyond traditional concerns for pathology and vulnerability, beyond theoretical and statistical methods. In fact, its most valuable data come directly from the personal experiences of those confronted with chronic or terminal illness, physical and mental disabilities, abuse, impoverishment, the Holocaust, and other disasters. I have pursued many life narratives, not as a test of endurance in the face of human suffering (although it made for a more tearful year than most), not in search of heros and heroines (although there were many), but in an effort to more fully understand factors that influence resilient responses. The voices of the resilient send a powerful message: Personal perceptions and responses to stressful life events are crucial elements of survival, recovery, and rehabilitation, often transcending the reality of the situation or the intentions of others. The inner life (affective and cognitive processes and content) holds the potential for transforming traumas into varying degrees of triumph. Ironically, these same phenomena are often ignored in the clinical reasoning and practice of many health professions, including our own.

Consequently, this chapter is intended to heighten the reader's appreciation of the powerful interaction among a person's inner psychological life, his or her relationship to the surrounding world, and his or her emerging functional capacities. It pursues these themes by first providing an overview of theoretical constructs about the human response to adversity. Second, it focuses on extreme life events and the personal and social meaning ascribed to them. Third, it addresses the phenomenon of resilience and the means by which persons in extreme situations have coped. Implications for occupational therapy practice are then considered.

OVERCOMING ADVERSITY: A HUMAN CONDITION

The experience of adversity and the drive to rise above it are themes that characterize the human condition. The inevitability of life's trials and tribulations and the struggles between good and evil are evident in religious traditions, myths, the arts, and everyday conversation. Although adversity is ultimately a personal experience, in the bigger scheme of things it is faceless and timeless. We have grown up with both the ascendance of Cinderella and the failure of Icarus. We share such maxims as "It's always something" (Radner, 1989) or "You have to take the bad with the good." These universal themes attempt to guide us in matters of social order and disorder.

The Law of Disruption and Reintegration

There is also a professional literature devoted to understanding the human response to disruptions, the search for order and balance, and the consequences of prolonged imbalance. Although taxonomies and belief systems vary, a central theme, linked to Cannon's (1939) work in biology and physics, identifies a recurring cycle of disruption and reintegration as a natural and necessary part of one's growing capacities to adapt to internal and external change (Flach, 1988). In today's lexicon we speak of risk, stress, coping, competency, crisis theory, and biopsychosocial models. The past has been marked by a more disparate arrray of assumptions.

The relationship of stress to disease has been the highest priority among clinicians since Hippocratic times. Attempts at developing broader, systematic constructs have emerged from a number of disciplines. Psychoanalysis has given us ego mechanisms of defense as a metaphor for mental processes that handle crisis and threats. Freudian views emphasize a hierarchy of defenses that transform conflict-ridden impulses into more acceptable thoughts and actions. Ego psychology promotes reality-oriented, purposeful, conflict-free capacities (i.e., attention, perception, and memory) that are future-oriented and that render one capable of transforming situations rather than being transformed by them. In this formulation, adaptive functioning is seen as the relative use of coping capacities over defense mechanisms (Anthony & Colher, 1987). The growth and cumulative effects of coping resources and skills over the life span are reflected in Erikson's (1963) classic developmental theories.

A behaviorist tradition also emerged with an early emphasis on the consequences of concrete problem solving. Today, as cognitive behaviorism, it is concerned with the cognitive components of coping skills and the Eriksonian belief that "successful coping promotes a sense of self-efficacy, which in turn, inspires more efforts at mastering difficult situations" (Moos & Schaefer, 1984, p. 6).

Endocrinologist Hans Selye (1978) assumed importance in the disruption-reintegration debate. Half a decade of work on stress and its hormonal and neurochemical correlates has had a great impact on professional and popular views of prevention and disease management. Selye's original emphasis on the singular importance of the stressful event itself has been mediated by a growing belief that the physical or psychological impact of any demand will vary depending on how we interpret the situation and how able we are to do something about it (Lazarus & Folkman, 1984).

Moos and Billings (1982) elaborated by organizing coping skills into three areas: appraisal-focused coping (i.e., efforts to understand and find meaning in a crisis), problem-focused coping (i.e., attempts to deal with the reality and consequences of the crisis and create a better situation), and emotion-focused coping (i.e., handling the feelings provoked by the crisis).

The cognitive appraisal process (how we interpret personal experiences) is central to a great deal of contemporary thought on coping. Stress itself has been defined as a "relationship between person and environment that is appraised by the person as taxing or exceeding his or her resources and endangering his or her well being" (Lazarus & Folkman, 1984, p. 19). Although social psychology traditionally emphasizes the role of external stressors and cognitive strategies (i.e., logical analysis, mental preparation, cognitive redefinition, and avoidance or denial), internal phenomena must not be ignored. Personal theories of reality about oneself and one's world, developed over time and generally outside of awareness, serve as a filter through which we perceive, interpret, and respond to experiences (Janoff-Bulman & Timko, 1987). Disturbing thoughts and memories can also heavily influence the appraisal process (Houston, 1987).

The credibility of the cognitive appraisal paradigm is enhanced by the newly integrated discipline of psychoneuroimmunology, which is "the study of the intricate interaction of consciousness (psycho), brain and central nervous system (neuro) and the body's defense against external infection and aberrant cell division (immunology)" (Pelletier & Herzing, 1988, p. 29). The impact of personal mood and attitudes on the immune system has opened new doors for researchers and clinicians. Studies have found that one's immune system benefits from confronting traumatic memories, looking at life optimistically, and living at a mildly hectic pace (Goleman, 1989). This line of thought will no doubt continue to provide us with newer and different hypotheses about the laws of disruption and reintegration.

For now, contemporary biopsychosocial formulations represent a robust model. Capacities to meet challenging demands and stand up to disruptions depend on inborn and acquired skills, the material and interpersonal resources in the environment, and the psychosocial capacities to handle anxieties that arise when one is performing various life tasks. Successful adaptation is dependent on the degree of fit among these factors. Although mastery is both developed and sustained by manageable challenges, challenges that are too demanding or too dangerous defeat resources for coping and reintegration (White, 1976).

And dangers there are! The law of disruption and reintegration does not promise, or always deliver, a rose garden. Life events continually test the durability of the balance we try to maintain.

Ordeals Beyond Our Control

There are life events that are experienced as traumatic because they are severe ordeals beyond our control. Under circumstances of predictable, moderate stress, persons call on conventional patterns and solve problems with characteristic resources and adaptive styles. But extreme situations and the stress accompanying them are not conventional. By their nature they are beyond the range of the predictable; previous experiences have not prepared us for them. How does one prepare for a spinal tumor, a brain injury, a schizophrenic episode, or a devastating earthquake? How does one comprehend Auschwitz or Dachau, where

> *Dreams used to come in the brutal nights,*
> *Dreams crowding and violent*
> *Dreamt with body and soul,*
> *Of going home, of eating, of telling our story.*
> *Until quickly and quietly, came*
> *The dawn reveille;*
> *Wstawàch*
> *And the heart cracked in the breast.*
>   (Levi, 1965, p. xi)

Extreme experiences such as these are characterized by a lack of conventional social structure, a loss of anchor, in reality, and a lack of ability to predict or anticipate outcomes (Torrance, 1965). Although we associate such phenomena with the high drama of hostage situations, prolonged combat, or concentration camps, they may so define the experience of persons whose lives are linked with ours on a daily basis, that is, our patients. Perhaps we ourselves have endured trauma or the sudden onset of a life-threatening illness.

Being full of strength and vigor one moment and virtually helpless the next... with all one's powers and faculties one moment and without them the next . . . such a change, such a suddenness, is difficult to comprehend and the mind casts about for explanations. (Sacks, 1984, p. 21)

There are those, like Lifton (1988), who view man "as perpetual survivor... of 'holocausts' large and small, personal and collective, that define much of existence" (p. 12). Although the Holocaust was a horrifying reality, as metaphor it illuminates many other ordeals, helping to understand and negotiate them. The vivid words and images of those with illness and disability also reveal a deeper meaning of their experiences—meaning that defines the nature of their adaptive task and shapes the reality of their reintegration.

THE PERSONAL AND SOCIAL MEANING OF TRAUMA

There are many reasons to perceive extreme life events as threatening. The most stressful dimensions appear to be those that challenge personal assumptions about oneself and the structure of the world one lives in. Much of this is linked with the phenomenon of control: the ability (or perceived ability) to change, predict, understand, or accept environmental transactions within a meaningful context (Potocki & Everly, 1989). The sense of being in control and the desire for such control are believed to be crucial aspects of personality affecting physical and mental health as well as recovery potential.

The perception of self, with its elements of body image, identity, and self-worth, were dominant themes in every narrative I encountered, whether the trauma occurred in Vietnam, Theresienstadt, a hospital in London, or a city in Arizona. The pervasive threat to, or loss of, identity was as potent a force—and sometimes more significant than—any real threat to life and limb. The tattooed number on the arm of a concentration camp inmate had its counterpart in the history number on a hospital ID bracelet. As startling as this analogy may seem, in the eyes of the "number" it may well mean humiliation, a lack of personal validation, and varying degrees of dehumanization. Just as prisoners of war are stripped of rank, role, and place in their reference group, victims of fires suffer losses of important nonhuman anchors for personal identity (Rosenfield, 1989). Stroke victims, made captive by their disease and an impersonal hospital environment, lose the ability and opportunity to act on their own behalf.

In losing one's identity, one must replace it with another. How one chooses the new altered self is no small task. "Feelings of fear, vulnerability ... sadness over losses and weakness about not being able to control one's life or one's emotional reactions, contribute to feelings of defectiveness" (Marmar & Horowitz, 1988, p. 95). The impact of confinement, isolation, and perceptual distortions are described by neurologist Oliver Sacks following a near-death accident,

serious leg injury, disturbing hospitalization, and role change from doctor to patient.

> I was physiologically, in imagination, and feeling... a pygmy, a prisoner, a patient... without the faintest awareness. How could one know one had shrunk, if one's frame of reference itself shrunk? (1984, p. 157)

Experiences that reflect a loss of self-control are often a central issue in psychiatric disorders as well. It is evident in schizophrenia, for example, when unpredictable symptoms "sparkles of light into demon eyes" (McGrath, 1984) or when a partially observing ego is "aware enough to recognize the dangers of not being able to control what I'm doing or thinking" (A patient, personal communication, October 1989).

Psychological stress, induced by threats of loss of self or failure, is also highly dependent on social values and the person's acceptance of the culture's definitions of what is valuable. Finding a new self or coming to terms with the only self one has ever known is reflected in the mirror others place before us. There is humiliation and pain generated

> ...by a gait to embarrass, to make children laugh, a clumsy countering locomotion... from only the most exacting, determined efforts to control. Inside my rolling head, behind my shocked, magnified eyeballs, my brain orders, with utmost precision, each awkward jerk of thigh, leg, foot. (Weaver, 1985, p. 43)

Jean Amery provides us with a powerful metaphor for thinking about a person's sense of his or her own body and place in the world when mastery and control of that body is violated through intentional political torture, abuse, or from the pain of illness and medical procedures.

> He who has suffered torture can no longer feel at ease in the world. Faith in humanity—cracked by the first slap across the face then demolished by torture, can never be recovered. (Amery 1986, p. xiii)

There are, of course, many forms of torture. The torture that physical illness may bestow need not be limited to bodily discomfort or pain, but "visits upon [people] a disease of social relations no less real than the paralysis of the body" (Murphy, 1987, p. 4). Anthropologist John Murphy viewed his spinal tumor, growing paralysis, and confinement as an assault on his identity and a disruption of ties with others. In depicting his illness as an extended field visit to an unfamiliar culture, he identified a primal scene of sociology—the social confrontation of persons with significant flaws, where someone looks or acts differently and we are uncertain as to what to say or where to look. This robs the encounter of cultural guidelines, leaving those involved uncertain about what to expect and what to do. For Murphy, "it has the potential for social calamity" (p. 87).

This calamity is also experienced as being in limbo. Sacks (1984) viewed this as a by-product of his body agnosia and the empathic agnosia of his surgeon, who insisted that nothing was wrong. His disease and lack of a human foothold (i.e., adequate communication and validation) left Sacks with a sense of double nothingness. "Now doubly, I had no leg to stand on; unsupported, doubly" (p. 108). Kleinman (1988), in turn, characterized limbo, for those with chronic illness, as "the dangerous crossing of borders, the interminable waiting to exit and reenter normal everyday life . . . the perpetual uncertainty of whether one can return at all" (p. 181).

I heard this again and again: a common thread, a theme that plagued Holocaust survivors and Vietnam veterans as well as the physically and mentally disabled—the gulf between the self and others (family, friends, caregivers, society). Who will listen? Who will understand what we are experiencing? Who will believe where we have been and what we have endured? Who will validate us as we continue to deal with adversity and its imprints?

RESILIENCE

For some, the imprints are so deeply etched that they succumb. Others endure under conditions that seem unsupportable to health. Redl's (1969) work with adolescents who have beat the odds inspired the concept of ego resilience, that is, the capacity to withstand pathogenic pressure, the ability to recover rapidly from a temporary collapse even without outside help, and the strength to bounce back to normal or even supernormal levels of functioning. Demos (1989) suggested that, in its most developed state, such buoyancy requires "an active stance, persistence, the application of a variety of skills and strategies over a wide range of situations and problems. . . [and] flexibility . . . to know when to use what" (p. 5).

The formal study of resilience emerged in epidemiological studies on susceptibility to heart disease over 25 years ago. It is only within the past 15 years, however, that more rigorous efforts have been made to extricate it from a disease model and focus instead on "good psychosocial capacities such as competence, coping, creativity, and confidence" (Anthony & Cohler, 1987, p. x). Although healthfulness remains a less-than-perfect body of knowledge, a variety of popular and scientific resources provide direction for the reader's ongoing investigation, including descriptions of personal experiences (Brown, 1990; Browne, Connors, & Stern, 1985; Cousins, 1979; Egendorf, 1986; Gill, 1988; Heller & Vogel, 1986; Miller, 1985; Minear, 1990; Nolan, 1987; Sheehan, 1982; Trillin, 1984), situational studies of combat (Elder & Clipp, 1988; Rahe & Genender, 1983), studies of disasters (Bolin & Trainer, 1978; Lifton & Olson, 1976) and illness (Cleveland, 1984; Cohen & Lazarus, 1973), studies of the invulnerable child (Anthony & Cohler, 1987; Dugan & Coles, 1989; Garmezy & Masten, 1986; Murphy & Moriarty, 1976), and longitudinal investigations of adaptation (Chess & Thomas, 1984; Vaillant, 1977; Werner & Smith, 1982).

Resilience has been chronicled in studies of famous men and women who were highly stressed and traumatized as children, among them George Orwell, Charles Dickens, Anton Chekov, Kathe Kollowitz, Pablo Picasso, and Buster Keaton (Goertzel & Goertzel, 1962; Miller, 1990; Shengold, 1989). Resilience, however, is evident in all walks of life. What is less clear is how persons manage to marshal the necessary resources. What enabled young Ryan White, confronted with two life-threatening illnesses, humiliation, and rejection, to become so articulate a spokesman for AIDS? What contributed to the brutalized Central Park jogger's remarkable recovery and promotion in her highly competitive investment banking firm? These are questions whose answers have as many nuances as there are people and ordeals, for resilience is not all of one piece.

Resilience is made operational by cognitive and behavioral coping skills and the recruitment of social support. Lazarus and Folkman (1984) suggested that such skills do not come all at once. Rather, they are acquired through a developmental process—a process of selecting from available alternatives and having persons reinforce; the skills that are necessary to make coping possible. Studies of vulnerability and competence in children and adolescents have provided valuable insight into some aspects of this multifaceted and shifting phenomenon. Theoretical models of stress resistance view the relationship between stress and personal attributes from several perspectives: as compensation (personal attributes help to improve adjustment when stress diminishes competence), as protection (personal traits interact with stress in predicting adjustment), or as to challenge (stressors enhance competence) (Garmezy, 1983). Dispositional attributes of the child, family cohesion and warmth, and the use of external support systems by parents and children are mechanisms that buffer stress and promote resilient responses. Temperament, sex, intellectual ability, humor, empathy, social problem-solving skills, social expressiveness, and an inner locus of control have been found to influence adaptation under adverse conditions (Garmezy, 1985). These phenomena, however, show variability over time and at different developmental periods (Werner & Smith, 1982) and are influenced by changing demands of the environment. Coping, for children and adults alike, reflect traitlike and situation-specific elements (Kahana, Kahana, Harel, & Rosner, 1988).

Resilience is often measured behaviorally on the basis of the person's competence and success in meeting society's expectations despite great obstacles. Internal indexes (thoughts and feelings) are often ignored, despite evidence that impressive social competence may well be heavily correlated with depression and anxiety (Miller, 1990; Peck, 1987). Clinicians and researchers are alerted to attend to the distinctions and interactions between adaptive behavior and emotional status. Resilience needs to be examined and understood from both perspectives.

RESILIENT PERSPECTIVES

Truly functional coping behavior has been characterized as not only lessening the immediate impact of stress, but also as maintaining a sense of self-worth and unity with the past and an anticipated future (Dimsdale, 1974). It involves two distinct tasks: a response to the requirements of the situation and a response to the feelings about the situation. Author

Nancy Mairs (1986), struggling with multiple sclerosis, chronic depression, and agoraphobia, explained the process:

> Each gesture... carries a weight of uncertainty, demands significant attention: buttoning my shirt, changing a light bulb, walking down stairs. The minutiae of my life have had to assume dramatic proportions. If I could not... delight in them, they would likely drown me in age and self-pity.
>
> Yet I am unwilling to forgo the adventurous life; the difficulty of it, even the pain, the... fear, and the sudden brief lift of spirit that graces... the pilgrimage. If I am to have it... I must change the terms by which it is lived.... I refine adventure, make it smaller and smaller... whether I am feeding fish flakes to my bettas... lying wide eyed in the dark battling yet another bout of depression, cooking a chicken... [or] meeting a friend for lunch... I am always having the adventures that are mine to have. (pp. 6-7)

Mairs accepted the challenge and altered her lifestyle in the face of unpredictable capacity while maintaining some semblance of control over her life through a commitment to scaled-down adventures. Even in the presence of many serious problems she demonstrated what Kobasa (1979) and colleagues have called *hardiness*. Hardiness is characterized by challenge, commitment, and control attributes. Challenge is expressed as a belief that change, rather than stability, is normal in life and is an incentive for growth rather than a threat to security. Control is expressed by feeling and acting as if one is influential rather then helpless. Influence is operationalized through the use of imagination, knowledge, skill and choice. Commitment is a tendency to involve oneself rather then feel alienated from situations; it involves a generalized sense of purpose that allows one to find events, things, and people meaningful and to approach situations rather than avoid them.

In extraordinarily stressful situations (the ones that diminish social structure, connections with reality, and a sense of predictability), opportunities to operationalize commitment, control, and challenge orientations are greatly compromised. Nonetheless, cognitive and behavioral coping mechanisms and efforts to recruit social support emerge and find expression in the most remarkable ways. The personal perspectives of the persons whose anecdotes follow are a tribute to the resourcefulness of the human mind and spirit. Their thoughts, feelings, and actions reflect the true character of resilience.

Hope and the Will to Overcome

Hope and the will to overcome are evident in the poignant poetry of children who found comfort and inspiration in the resilience of nature while confined in a Czechoslovakian camp in 1944:

> The sun has made a veil of gold
> So lovely that my body aches.
> Above, the heavens shriek with blue
> Convinced I've smiled by some mistake.

> The world's abloom and seems to smile.
> I want to fly but where, how high?
> If in barbed wire, things can bloom
> Why couldn't I? I will not die!
> (Anonymous, In I Never Saw Another Butterfly, 1978, p. 52)

Hope and the will to overcome emerge in others as a fierce, sometimes raging will to live, that is, "the burning desire to tell, to bear witness" (Gill, 1988, p. 59), "to testifying on behalf of all those whose shadows will be bound to mine forever" (Wiesel, 1990, p. 15), "to live not for oneself, but to lament those who died [in Hiroshima]" (Tamiki, 1990, p. 30).

Affiliation and the Recruitment of Social Support

Acquiring a sense of belonging to a social group or, for that matter, to all of life, is a powerful way to sustain oneself in the face of death or other extremes. It may manifest itself by turning one's attention inward to memories and images of loved ones, by participating in an organized underground movement, or by devising a tap code to communicate through cell walls to other Vietnam prisoners of war. It also emerges through the collaboration of a therapist and a severely mentally ill woman who is struggling against great odds to restore a semblance of autonomy and self-respect:

> You believed in me... were willing to take a chance on my being able to handle an apartment when my family felt it would be a waste of money. We had hopes, I didn't want to let you down... and I haven't." (A patient, personal communication, 1989)

Finding Meaning and Purpose

The identification of purpose, or finding meaning in an ordeal, was described by Viktor Frankl (1984) as "the last of human freedoms"—choosing one's attitude in any given set of circumstances, having at least the power and the control over how you interpret and explain what happens to you. Individuals find meaning and purpose in many different ways. Some find it in an increased commitment to religion, a political ideal, or a social cause. Others find it by using intellect and creativity to combat devastating fear. Many concentration camp victims and prisoners of war played chess and built houses, nail by nail, in their mind's eye; one man prepared a full German-English dictionary on scraps of paper during his incarceration and published it after his release. Others claimed that even forced labor was sustaining.

Interestingly, despite confining, constraining situations with extremely limited resources, many sought to find meaning and retain interests, values and skills through focused, self-regulating activity. "The prisoners who fared the best in the long run were those who ...could retain their personality system largely intact ...where previous interests, values and skills could to some extent be carried on" (Hamburg, Coelho,

& Adams, 1974, p. 413). In situational studies of combat, illness, and the anticipated death of family members, Gal and Lazarus (1975) reported reductions in anxiety and feelings of helplessness even when activities did not provide actual control over the situation. In contrast, the vulnerable were described by Eitinger as those who "felt completely helpless and passive, and had lost their ability to retain some sort of self-activity" (Hamburg et al., 1974, p. 413). Our continuing efforts to understand the complex role of occupation in remediating illness and maintaining health may be greatly enhanced through studies of the spontaneous behavior of those in stressful situations.

The Capacity to Step Back

Frankl's (1984) disgust with his own trivial preoccupations with survival found him, in fantasy, lecturing on the psychology of concentration camps. Both he and his troubles became the object of a psychoscientific study undertaken by himself that later contributed to the development of a school of psychotherapy. Frankl demonstrated the capacity to step back and, in so doing, preserved a part of himself from extraordinary degradation, pain, and loss. Functioning somewhat like a solution to a figure-ground problem, this process provides one with the option of ignoring aspects of the situation that are out of one's control. It may appear as a differential focus on the good, or it may be marked by a heightened capacity for observation, that is, a period of exalted receptivity when details of events, faces, words, or sensations are retained (Levi, 1987). This is evident in the writings of Diesel (1990), Cousins (1979), Heller and Vogel (1986), Brown (1990), and Nolan (1987). None perceived themselves to be victims or survivors, but rather, witnesses to their own experience.

There is More to Oneself than Current Circumstance Suggests

The discovery of the new or real self is artfully reflected in nk's (1988) study of embodiment—the experience and aning of disability in American culture. She described a ung woman born with quadrilateral limb deficiencies who stressed her assets instead of her deficits— her womanly figure (like Venus de Milo's) and her ability to write better with her stumps than with her artificial arms. Increasingly, her rehabilitation team viewed her refusal to use prosthetics as poor adaptation.

Dugan and Coles (1989), in turn, described a 6-year-old black girl who was initiating school desegregation in New Orleans in the face of mobs, violence, and threats to her life. She hoped she would "get through one day and then another," and if she did, "it will be because there is more to me than I ever realized" (p. xiv).

Novel Applications of Problem-Solving Strategies

Coping involves creative and reflective behavior (White, 1976). Resilience is manifest in the ability to turn a familiar way of solving problems into a novel application, one that may save a life. When Sacks (1984) sustained his injury while mountain climbing alone, he was at great risk for dying of exposure. He reported that there came to his aid a kinetic melody, rhythm, and motor music. "Now, so to speak, I was musicked along" (p. 30). Remembrances of the Volga Boatmen's Song gave him the strength and rhythm to "row" himself along the ground for many hours until he found help.

Transforming Dross Into Gold

Vaillant's (1977) longitudinal study of the life and coping strategies of a group of Harvard graduates documented the way in which the mature ego mechanisms of altruism, humor, suppression, and sublimation function to transform disturbances into adaptive behavior, thus turning "dross into gold" (p. 16). This is, in part, the way the speechless, palsied Irish poet Christopher Nolan (1987) found his mellifluous voice:

> Fossilized for so long now, he was going to speak to anyone interested enough to listen.... Now he shared the same world as everyone else; he could choose how much to tell and crazily decide how much to hold back. His voice would be his written word. (p. 98)

The same mechanisms allowed comedian Buster Keaton to devote his life to making others laugh, while unable to laugh spontaneously himself (Miller, 1990). Long before Norman Cousins found health and fame in laughter and neuroscience linked it to our immune systems, humor was acknowledged to be one of the truly elegant defenses in the human repertoire (Lefcourt & Martin, 1986). "Like hope, humor permits one to bear and yet to focus upon what may be too terrible to be borne" (Vaillant, 1977, p. 386). This is precisely what ailing critic Anatole Broyard (1990) did when he quipped, "that a critically ill person needs above all is to be understood. Dying is a misunderstanding you have to get straightened out before you go" (p. 29).

Resilience is not a miraculous rescue. It can be a mere thread that wrestles itself to the surface of an otherwise despairing existence. It is reflected in the struggle of a 50-year-old chronically mentally ill woman who sustains an inner sense of altruism despite unrelenting suspiciousness, fear, and rigid thought processes. She is an ardent giver of small gifts, of greeting cards weeks before the actual event, and of postage stamps she hopes will acquire great value for the recipient's future grandchildren. The dignity and control she experiences in giving to others when she herself is in such great need allows her more comfort than she might otherwise have. It buffers her from the painful realization of how isolated and vulnerable she really is.

Hamburg et al. (1974) summarized the essence of survival under extreme duress by underscoring the importance of the maintenance of self-esteem, a sense of human dignity, a sense of group belonging, and a feeling of being useful to others.

How Durable is Resilience?

Resilient responses to ordeals have phase-specific attributes.In the acute phase, energy is directed at minimizing the impact of the stress and stressor. In the reorganization phase, a new reality is faced and accepted in part or in whole. And then there is the rest of one's life. How durable is resilience? We know it is neither a single act nor constant state. How and under what circumstances does it emerge, shift, or fail the person? Camus (as cited by Kluet, 1958) described its emergence: "In the depth of winter I finally learned that within me there lay an invincible summer." In contrast, Monette (1988) experienced its decline: "I used up all my optimism keeping my friend alive. Now that he's gone, the cup of my health is neither half full nor half empty. Just half." (p 2).

The suicides of Primo Levi and Bruno Bettelheim prompt similar questions. Why did Levi, successful chemist and award-winning author who recorded his Holocaust experiences because there "were things that imperiously demanded to be told" (1987, p.9), choose to die? Did cancer and the ill health of his mother chip away at the mission he had set for himself? Did a history of exemplary behavioral competence distract from the depression and anxiety that often accompanies it? Did a major depression go untreated? What about Bettelheim? His essays bore witness to Nazi atrocities; his provocative style challenged a world he saw as too passive and naive. He enacted solutions to some of humanity's problems by developing therapeutic environments for severely disturbed children. Did retirement, physical ailments, or the loss of a familiar social network limit his ability to play out a meaningful life story? Did his resilience run out? Or was this last sorrowful act a measure of his need to be in control, exercising his own will, his way, while he could? He spoke prospectively of these issues in the introduction to *The Uses of Enchantment: The Meaning and Importance of Fairy Tales* (1977):

> If we hope to live not just from moment to moment, but in true consciousness of our existence, then our greatest need and most difficult achievement is to find meaning in our lives... Many have lost the will to live, and have stopped trying, because such meaning has evaded them. An understanding of the meaning of one's life is not suddenly acquired at a particular age, not even when one has reached chronological maturity. (p. 3)

These anecdotes demonstrate the changing and highly personal nature of resilience, often attained at the cost of some degree of spontaneity and flexibility. This and the interplay among such factors as age, general health status, and changing roles and relationships may conspire to diminish the once raging will to live in some, while allowing others to continue to find meaning and commitment in changing life circumstances. Resilience appears to be less an enduring characteristic and more a process determined by the impact of particular life experiences on particular conceptions of one's own life history (Cohler, 1987), leading one, once again, to conclude that it is not so much what happens to people but how they interpret and explain it that makes a difference.

INTEGRATING PERSONAL MEANING, BEHAVIOR, AND REALITY: IMPLICATIONS FOR PRACTICE

Who rises above adversity? Perhaps it is sufficient to say that human capacities can shrink, hibernate, and flourish under circumstances of extreme stress; influence of personal perspective; and people, places, and things in the environment. The lives I sampled in the course of this study heightened my appreciation for the richness of the coping process and the difficulties many face with the unrelenting demands of their illness and the oft-times unresponsive health care system. Even a resilient outcome does not represent a similar linear trajectory. It often requires the empathic attention and skillful assistance of those, like us, who are empowered by training and, I hope, by inclination.

Ordeals Provide a Window of Opportunity

Physical and emotional disruptions, the circumstances that bring us and our consumers together, provide a window of opportunity. Timely and meaningful interventions can have a significant impact on the reintegration process. These interventions may involve us in multiple tasks, such as helping persons find meaning in their crises, helping them handle feelings provoked by their situation, helping them with the reality and consequences of their condition, and fostering the functional skills and behaviors that they will need to fulfill their potential. Unfortunately, individual needs and capacities do not necessarily run on the same time standard as that of third-party payers. Potential for resilience may be noted and nurtured, but not necessarily birthed in 6 inpatient days or 12 annual reimbursed outpatient visits. Illness, and certainly disability, is an ongoing process in which personal problems may constantly emerge to undermine technical control, social order, and individual mastery (Kleinman, 1988). The conflicts that arise among individual needs, professional values, and the system's priorities pose real challenges to those who need access before the window of opportunity is shut. We must examine our own role in perpetuating this dilemma. We must reevaluate and, in some instances, reframe, short- and long-term practice models. Additionally, we must educate colleagues, administrators, and insurers to the personal and financial impact of psychosocial factors on recovery and rehabilitation outcome in all areas of specialization.

Many Factors Influence Individual Response to Ordeals

Many intervening variables affect pateint's major life changes on the one hand and illness outcome on the other.

The good news is that those who rise above adversity do not belong to an exclusive club. It is not a closed system. However, some people are their own best facilitators, while others need help. Neither group should face its ordeals at the hands of caregivers and environments that induce more stress by diminishing humanistic contacts and links with reality, by neglecting the person's need to predict or anticipate outcomes, or by ignoring the inner elements of coping and competency behaviors. It is troubling to note how well many of our treatment centers fulfill the criteria for extremely stressful, negative life events.

The variability of resilience may come as bad news for some, because it does not permit a simple recipe for treatment. Instead, we must commit ourselves to understanding the complexities of personality, coping capacities, and environmental influences and use them to identify goals, interventions, and environments that are meaningful to a given person under a given set of circumstances.

Transforming Adversity Into Possibilities

Murphy (1987) reminded us that "there is a need for order in all humans that impels us to search for systematic coherence in both nature and society, and when we can find none, to invent it" (p. 33). Thoughts, feelings, and actions, influenced by neurobiology and environments are the means by which our patients attempt to invent coherence and order that is acceptable to themselves and the outside world (White, 1976). The experiences documented in the present chapter are testimony to how innovative and powerful human thoughts, feelings, and actions can be.

These capacities are also our most elegant professional tools for transforming adversity into possibilities, when we take the tame to conceive of them as such. As always, Sacks (1984) captured the essence of this phenomenon best:

Rehabilitation involves action, acts . . . [and] must be centered on the character of acts—and how to call them forth, when they have come apart, disintegrated, been "lost"—or "forgotten." (p. 182)

Calling forth the character of acts involves the therapist's understanding and using the patient's thoughts and feelings, collaborating with him or her, establishing trust, and reaching for the personal context that is partner to external reality and individual potentials for functional behavior.

Professional Entreaties

How well do we call forth the character of acts? I believe that as a group we are far more effective at defining reality and assessing and promoting performance than we are at assessing and making use of patient's views of themselves and their situation. Although our clinical prowess has grown greatly, we are too often committed only to present manifest performance. These snapshot approaches to capacity fail to reflect the unique adaptive style and potential of each person. If we are to enhance outcome, we must integrate the patients' experience of their condition and their preexisting patterns of self-regulating activity with our concerns and strategies for functional mobilization.

Kleinman (1988) proposed the use of clinical mini-ethnographic methods for acquiring a better picture, much like an anthropologist does in assessing a different culture. The ethnographer draws on knowledge of the context to make sense of behavior, allowing herself to sample the subject's experience. Occupational therapists are demographers of sorts. We have unique access to information about activities of everyday living and what it's like to live with an illness or disability. We need only to acknowledge and actualize it. But do we? Do we draw out the patient's perception of his or her situation? Or do we focus only on those aspects of function we can see, palpate, or measure?

Practice has changed dramatically over the past 30 years, as much a product of our growth and development as it is a measure of new knowledge and shifts in the health care system. We certainly have not been idle. It is therefore no surprise that we find ourselves pursuing the future with such vigor that we sometimes fail to look back to see if we have left something of value behind. I believe we are at great risk of leaving in our wake some of the most central and precious components of our practice— how people think and feel about themselves and the world in which they live. Evidence suggests that we may have already reframed the rehabilitation process to fit today's economy rather than to fit today's patients.

Our connections to the deeper personal experiences of our patients seem to be unduly mediated by professional objectivity, our personal reluctance to hear, and a narrow view of what belongs to a given area of specialization. Fleming (1989) identified the presence of practice dichotomies concerning the relative importance of the patient's personal phenomenological status and how best to relate to him or her. Although some therapists appear to use such information and their relationship in treatment, their ambivalence about acknowledging it relegates it to an underground practice and reflects troublesome conflicts in values. We must remind ourselves that psychosocial phenomena belong to everyone, irrespective of their diagnosis and health status. Practice that separates feelings from function and psychosocial from physical perpetuates disorder rather than fostering reintegration.

The profession's efforts to examine the actuality of clinical reasoning shows great promise for rescuing the person inside our patients and for allowing us to acknowledge the credibility of this element of clinical activity. Similarly, the study of resilient persons provides us with important opportunities to share their experience, rethink our beliefs about occupational therapy's domain of concern, and enrich the emerging science of occupation. Like the subjects of this chapter, "each of us maintains a personal theory of reality, a coherent set of assumptions developed over time about ourselves and our world that organizes our experiences and understanding and directs our behavior" (Janoff-Bulman & Timko 1987, p. 130). I believe that our responsiveness to the inner lives of others can add perspective to our professional assumptions and enhance our understanding of human performance capacity. In so doing, we will find ourselves far better able to help our patients refine their ventures, find meaning and purpose in their ordeals, discover there is more to themselves than current circumstance suggests, and transform the dross of their adversity into the gold of their accomplishments.

EPILOGUE

This is a work in progress. My purpose has been to examine the relevance of resilience to our practice. However, one person's efforts to orchestrate the chorus of resilient voices cannot do them justice. I urge the reader to explore this literature as well. It is likely to stimulate extraordinary personal and professional awakening. Moreover, it merits our collective thought and action, because the efforts of many are needed to give meaning to the hardships our patients endure and the difference occupational therapy can make.

ACKNOWLEDGEMENTS

I dedicate this lecture to three resilient women whose adaptive style and commitment to challenge have greatly enriched my personal and professional life: my mother, Elsie Babbitt; my mentor and friend, Gail Fidler; and my daughter, Deborah Fine. All three not only see the cup as half full, but strive to keep it overflowing for themselves and others.

REFERENCES

Amery, J. (1986). *At the mind's limits: Contemplations by a survivor on Auschwitz and its realities*. New York, NY: Schocken.

Anthony, E. J., & Cohler, B. J. (Eds.). (1987). *The invulnerable child*. New York, NY: Guilford.

Bettelheim, B. (1977). *The uses of enchantment: The meaning and importance of fairy tales*. New York, NY: Knopf.

Bolin, R., & Trainer, P. (1978). Modes of family recovery following disaster: A cross national study. In E. L. Quarantelli (Ed.), *Disaster theory and research* (pp. 233-247). London, England: Sage.

Brown, C. (1990). *Down all the days*. London, England: Mandarin.

Browne, S. E., Connors, D., & Stern, N. (1985). *With the power of each breath: A disabled women's anthology*. San Francisco, CA: Cleis.

Broyard, A. (1990, April 1). *Good books about being sick*. New York Times Book Review, pp. 1, 28-30.

Cannon, W. (1939). *The wisdom of the body*. New York, NY: Norton.

Chess, S., & Thomas, A. (1984). *Origins and evolution of behavior disorders: From infancy to early adult life*. New York, NY: Brunner/Mazel.

Cleveland, M. (1984). Family adaptation to traumatic spinal cord injury. Response to crisis. In R. H. Moos (Ed.), *Coping with physical illness* (pp. 159-171). New York, NY: Plenum.

Cohen, F., & Lazarus, R. S. (1973). Active coping processes, coping dispositions and recovery from surgery. *Psychosomatic Medicine, 35*, 375-389.

Cohler, B. J. (1987). Adversity resilience and the study of lives. In P. J. Anthony & B. J. Cohler (Eds.), *The invulnerable child* (pp. 363-424). New York, NY: Guilford.

Cousins, N. (1979). *Anatomy of an illness*. New York, NY: Bantam.

Demos, E. V. (1989). Resiliency in infancy. In T. F. Dugan & R. Coles (Eds.), *The child in our times: Studies in the development of resilient* (pp. 3-22). New York, NY: Brunner/Mazel

Dimsdale, J. E. (1974). The coping behavior of Nazi concentration camp survivors. *American Journal of Psychiatry, 131*, 792-797.

Dugan, T. F., & Coles, R. (1989). *The child in our times: Studies in the development of resiliency*. New York, NY: Brunner/Mazel.

Egendorf, A. (1986). *Healing from the war: Trauma and transformation after Vietnam*. Boston, MA: Shambhala.

Elder, G. H. Jr., & Clipp, E. C. (1988). Combat experience, comradeship and psychological health. In J. P. Wilson, Z. Harel, & Kahana (Eds.), *Human adaptation to extreme stress from the Holocaust to Vietnam* (pp. 131-154). New York, NY: Plenum.

Erikson, E. (1963). *Childhood and society*. New York, NY: Norton.

Flach, F. (1988). *Resilience: Discovering a new strength at times of stress*. New York, NY: Fawcett Columbine.

Fleming, M. (1989). The therapist with the three-track mind. In *The AOTA Practice Symposium guide 1989* (pp. 70-73). Rockville, MD: American Occupational Therapy Association.

Frank, C. (1988). On embodiment: A case study of congenital limb deficiency in American culture. In M. Fine & A. Asch (Eds.), *Women with disabilities* (pp 41-71). Philadelphia, PA: Temple University Press.

Frankl, V. E. (1984). *Man's search for meaning*. New York, NY: Washington Square Press.

Gal, R. & Lazarus, R. S. (1975, December). The role of activity in anticipating and confronting stressful situations. *Journal of Human Stress, 1*, 4-20.

Garmezy, N. (1983). Stressors of childhood. In N. Garmezy & M. Rutter (Eds.), *Stress, coping, and development in children* (pp. 43-84). New York: McGraw-Hill.

Garmezy, N. (1985). Stress-resistant children: The search for protective factors. In J. E. Stevenson (Ed.), *Recent research in developmental psychopathologies* (pp. 213-233). Elmsford, NY: Pergamon.

Garmezy, N., & Masten, S. (1986). Stress, competence and resilience: Common frontiers for therapist and psychopathologist. *Behavior Therapy J, 7*, 500-521.

Gill, A. (1988). *The journey back from hell: An oral history—Conversations with concentration camp survivors*. New York, NY: Morrow.

Goertzel, V., & Goertzel, M. G. (1962). *Cradles of eminence*. Boston, MA: Little, Brown.

Goleman, D. (1989, April 20). *Researchers find optimism helps body's defense system*. New York Times, p B15.

Hamburg, D. A., Coelho, G. V., & Adams, J. E. (1974). Coping and adaptation: Steps toward a synthesis of biological and social perspectives. In G. V. Coelho, D. A. Hamburg, & J. E. Adams (Eds.), *Coping and adaptation* (pp. 403-440). New York, NY: Basic.

Heller, J., & Vogel, S. (1986). *No laughing matter*. New York, NY: Avon.

Houston, B. K. (1987). Stress and coping. In C. R Snyder & C. E. Ford (Eds.), *Coping with negative life events* (pp. 37 399). New York, NY: Plenum.

I never saw another butterfly: Children's drawings and poems from Terezin Concentration Camp, 1942-1944 (1978). New York, NY: Schocken Books.

Janoff-Bulman, R., & Timko, C. (1987). Coping with traumatic events: The role of denial in light of people's assumptive worlds. In C. R. Snyder & S. E. Ford (Eds.), *Coping with negative life events* (pp. 135-155). New York, NY: Plenum.

Kahana, E., Kahana, B., Harel, Z., & Rosner, T. (1988). Coping with extreme trauma. In J. P. Wilson, Z. Harel, & B. Kahana (Eds.), *Human adaptation to extreme stress from the Holocaust to Vietnam* (pp. 55-76). New York, NY: Plenum.

Kleinman, A (1988). *The illness narratives: Suffering, healing, and the human condition*. New York, NY: Basic.

Kobasa, S. C. (1979). Stressful life events, personality, and health: An inquiry into hardiness. *Journal of Personality and Social Psychology, 37,* 1-11.

Lazarus, R S., & Folkman, S. (1984). *Stress, appraisal, and coping*. New York, NY: Springer.

Lefcourt, H. M., & Martin, R. A. (1986). *Humor and life stress: Antidote to adversity*. New York, NY: Springer-Verlag.

Levi, P. (1965). *The reawakening*. New York, NY: Collier.

Levi, P. (1987). *Moments of reprieve*. New York, NY: Penguin.

Lifton, R. J. (1988). Understanding the traumatized self imagery, symbolization and transformation. In J. P. Wilson, Z. Harel, & B. Kahana (Eds.), *Human adaptation to extreme stress from the Holocaust to Vietnam* (pp. 7-31), New York, NY: Plenum.

Lifton, R. J., & Olson, J. E. (1976). The human meaning of total disaster. *Psychiatry, 39,* 1-17.

Mairs, N. (1986). *Plaintext: Deciphering a woman's life*. New York, NY: Perennial Library.

Maquet, A. (1958). *Albert Camus: The invincible summer*. New York, NY: Braziller.

Marmar, E. R., & Horowitz, M. J. (1988). Post-traumatic stress disorder. In J. P. Wilson, Z. Hard, & D. Kahana (Eds.), *Human adaption to extreme stress from the Holocaust to Vietnam* (pp. 81-103). New York, NY: Plenum.

McGrath, M. (1984). First-person accounts: Where did I go? *Schizophrenia Bulletin, 10,* 638 640.

Miller, A. (1990). *The untouched key: Tracing childhood trauma in creativity and destructiveness*. New York, NY: Doubleday.

Miller, V. (Ed.). (1985). *Despite this flesh: The disabled in stories and poems*. Austin, TX: University of Texas Press.

Minear, R. H. (Ed.). (1990). *Hiroshima: Three witnesses*. Princeton, NJ: Princeton University Press.

Monette, P. (1988). *Borrowed time: An AIDS memoir*. New York, NY: Avon.

Moos, R., & Billings, A. (1982). Conceptualizing and measuring coping resources and processes. In L. Goldberger & S. Breznicz (Eds.), *Handbook of stress: Theoretical and clinical aspects* (pp. 212-220). New York, NY: Macmillan.

Moos, R. H., & Schaefer, J. A. (1984). The crisis of physical illness: An overview and conceptual approach. In R. H. Moos (Ed.), *Coping with physical illness* (pp. 25). New York, NY: Plenum.

Murphy, L B., & Moriarty, A. (1976). *Vulnerability, coping and growth: From infancy to adolescence*. New Haven, CT: Yale University Press.

Murphy, R. F. (1987). *The body silent*. New York, NY: Henry Halt.

Nolan, C. (1987). *Under the eye of the clock*. New York, NY: Dell.

Peck, E. C. (1987). The traits of true invulnerability and posttraumatic stress in psychoanalyzed men of action. In E. J. Anthony & B. J. Kohler (Eds.), *The invulnerable child* (pp. 315-360). New York, NY: Guilford.

Pelletier, K. R. Herzing, D. L. (1988). Psychoneuroimmunology: Toward a mind body model: A critical review. *Advances, 5,* 27-56.

Potocki, E. R., & Everly, G. S. J. (1989). Control and the human stress response. In G. S. Everly, Jr. (Ed.), *A clinical guide to the treatment of the human stress response* (pp. 119-136). New York, NY: Plenum.

Radner, G. (1989). *It's always something*. New York, NY: Simon & Schuster.

Rahe, R H., & Genender, E. (1983). Adaptation to and recovery from captivity stress. *Military Medicine, 148,* 577-585.

Redl, F. (1969). Adolescents—Just how do they react? In G. Caplan & S. Lebovici. (Eds.) *Adolescence: Psychosocial perspectives* (pp. 79-90). New York, NY: Basic.

Rosenfeld, M. S. (1989). Occupational disruption and adaption: A study of house fire victims. *American Journal of Occupational Therapy, 43,* 89-96.

Sacks, O. (1984). *A leg to stand on*. New York, NY: Harper & Row.

Selye, H. (1978). *The stress of life* (2nd ed.). New York, NY: McGraw-Hill.

Sheehan, S. (1982). *Is there no place on earth for me?* New York, NY: Vintage.

Shengold, L. (1989). *The effects of childhood abuse and deprivation*. New Haven, CT: Yale University Press.

Tamiki, H. (1990). Summer flowers. In R. H. Minear (Ed.). *Hiroshima* (pp. 19-114). Princeton, NJ: Princeton University Press.

Torrance, E. P. (1965). *Constructive behavior: Stress, personality, and mental health*. Belmont, CA: Wadsworth.

Trillin, A. S. (1984). Of dragons and garden peas: A cancer patient talks to doctors. In R. H. Moos (Ed.), *Coping with physical illness* (pp. 131-138). New York, NY: Plenum.

Vaillant, G. E. (1977). *Adaptation to life*. Boston, MA: Little, Brown.

Weaver, G. (1985). Finch the spastic speaks. In V. Miller (Ed.), *Despite this flesh: The disabled in stories and poems* (pp. 3-45). Austin, TX: University of Texas Press.

Werner, E. E., & Smith, R. S. (1982). *Vulnerable but invincible: A study of resilient children*. New York, NY: McGraw-Hill.

White, R. W. (1976). Strategies of adaptation: An attempt at systematic description. In R. H. Moos (Ed.), *Human adaptation: Coping with life crises* (pp. 17-32). Lexington, MA: Heath.

Wiesel, E. (1990). *From the kingdom of memory: Reminiscences.* New York, NY: Summit.

CHAPTER FIFTY

Holism in Mental Health Practice

Barbara J. Hemphill-Pearson and Margaret Hunter

This chapter was previously published in Occupational Therapy in Mental Health, 13(2), 35-49. Copyright ©1997, *Haworth Press.*

Holistic care in the United States has expanded dramatically in recent years. Many professionals, including occupational therapists, claim to be practitioners of holistic health in one form or another. Holistic health originates from orientations that reflect a close tie with traditional medical and theological systems, to orientations that use a philosophy taken from Eastern medicine and religion (DeSobe, 1981).

A growing body of evidence supports the view that health professionals should be preoccupied, not only with illness, but also with the more basic and essential human issues such as their spiritual, emotional, and educational values (Ginsburg, 1982). One of the main premises of holistic care is that the patient's mind and body are inseparable (Pownall, 1986), that the individual must be viewed as a total being. "... holistic health is an approach to treating illness, emphasizing self-responsibility, the whole person, and the process of care-giving" (Ardell, 1979, p. 393).

Human health is biopsychosocial, a combination of physical, mental, and social elements. For example, a major physical health problem will impact the person's mental and social functioning (Reed, 1983).

The purpose of this chapter is to define holism and to suggest how it can be applied in occupational therapy practice. The authors will discuss holism's historical roots, its definitions, and the fundamental theories of holism and holistic care. Holistic care as a model of practice in occupational therapy also will be presented, as well as implications for occupational practice. The authors' goal is to develop a working definition of holism and generate discussion that will offer new options for the practice of holism by occupational therapists in mental health.

HISTORICAL PERSPECTIVE

The word "holistic" comes from the Greek "bolos," or whole, meaning a way of comprehending and describing whole organisms and systems as entities greater than and different from the sum of their parts (Gordon, 1980). The term appears in the writings of Plato and Aristotle. Plato implied that attention to the person as a whole, a mind-body complex, was the best approach a physician could adopt in treating patients (Lipowski, 1984). Hippocrates emphasized the environmental impact and treatment of illness; the etiologic and therapeutic importance of psychological factors, nutrition and lifestyle; the interdependence of mind, body and spirit; and the need for harmony between the individual, the social milieu, and the natural environment (Gordon, 1982).

Many medical writers from the Roman times onward have explicitly or implicitly advocated such an approach. Benjamin Rush taught medical students the importance of viewing the patient as a whole and was concerned with psychosomatic relations (Lipowski, 1984). Later, Sir William provides the necessary framework, for example, to understand and manage stress. The holistic health approach to stress management is based on training, rather than on therapy, and on prevention rather than on cure. It focuses on the entire person—body, mind, and spirit, when dealing with psychosomatic disease.

Holistic health also includes several subsystems (Gross, 1980). These subsystems are holistic healing, self-care, and holistic medicine. Holistic healing refers to practitioner-centered activities that are adjuncts or alternatives to traditional medicine. Self-care refers to the training of consumers to aid in their own treatment, e.g., apple cider vinegar, and honey potions, earth therapy, ionization, sex therapy, and tantric medicine (LaPatra, 1978).

Holistic Medicine

Holistic medicine is a subsystem in which humanistic options for health professionals exist. Benson (1979) states that "holistic medicine is an interdisciplinary approach to health care which incorporates the principles of medicine, physiology, psychiatry..." (p. 39). It embraces a collection of therapies, including nontraditional, sometimes gimmicky therapies. There is little hard data on their effectiveness, however. According to holistic physicians, such therapies based on psychic or occult powers are psychic tools, not holistic medicine (Walton, 1979).

Gordon (1982) offers seven characteristics of holistic medicine:

1. Its insistence that each patient be understood and treated as a unique individual made up of body, mind, and spirit, and that any health care must also take into account a person's environment.
2. It emphasizes the responsibility each person should assume for his/her health.
3. It includes the promotion of health and the prevention of disease, and emphasizes the role of education in the process.
4. Practitioners use a variety of diagnostic and therapeutic measures that lie outside the canon of traditional western medical practice.
5. It emphasizes the potential therapeutic value of the setting in which health care takes place and of the psychosocial supports it makes available.
6. It stresses an understanding of and a commitment to change those social and economic conditions that perpetuate ill health.
7. It is concerned with changing the attitudes of the physicians who practice medicine and with broadening and enriching medical practice (p. 547-550).

Holistic medicine attempts to include all the techniques that modem science and empirical use have revealed to be helpful. These include biofeedback (Renshaw, 1984), meditation, psychotherapy, behavior modification, modern fluid replacement, ancient acupuncture, diet, drugs, surgery, massage (Aston, 1984), visualization (Pownal, 1986), personal responsibility, and public health. Such remedies are called "unconventional therapies" (Eisenberg, Kessler, Foster, Norlock, Calkins, and Delbanco, 1993). The authors estimate that in 1990 Americans made an estimated 425 million visits to providers of unconventional therapy. The number of primary care visits was estimated to be 388 million.

Humanistic medicine, which is considered part of the holistic medicine approach (Gordon, 1980), emphasizes the relationship between physicians and patients, and the psychological and spiritual development of both the patient and the physician. Humanistic therapies, such as gestalt, client-centered, prima, rational-emotive, and Adlerian, are used (Cole, 1982; Corey, 1986; Udchic, 1984).

Pelletier (1977) summarizes holistic medicine by offering four philosophical assumptions that underlie traditional healing practices that are the basis of a holistic perspective. First, all states of health and all disorders are considered to be psychosomatic. Psychosomatic orientation requires treating the whole person through an integrated approach. Second, each individual is unique and represents a complex interaction of body, mind, and spirit. Third, the patient and the health practitioner share responsibility for the healing process. The patient is an active participant. Fourth, diag-

nosis and treatment of pathology is obviously a medical concern, but the creation of a lifestyle conducive to health maintenance and personal fulfillment is beyond the limited scope of corrective pathology.

HOLISM AS A PHILOSOPHY

Some authors believe that today, when the term holistic is used to refer to health, it represents a philosophy or a concept based on the simple definition of the term.

Bamberg (1982) views holism as a philosophy of living. The author states that it is a "philosophy for better living through awareness of all things which touch or affect us combined with a private regimen for self-improvement which incorporates all the germane and usable information we have in a harmonic way, with others and the world in which we live" (p. 1). Newbeck (1986) states that holism is a philosophy which recognizes the individual's ability to self-heal. It is a systems-based philosophy which says that no part of us, no matter how small, functions in original isolation; no part of us works-or fails to work-without affecting the whole.

Instead of being physician-centered it should be activity-centered. The whole team's primary goal is to prevent illness,not just to overcome it. It is with the latter philosophy that the occupational therapist is most concerned. Hemphill (unpublished research) demonstrated that therapists practice holistic occupational therapy. One hundred and eleven (90%) graduates of baccalaureate programs who responded to a questionnaire, practiced holistic methods.

Occupational therapy literature's emphasis on the importance of viewing individuals as integrated organisms is consistent with the philosophy of holistic practice. Such a belief was one of the early premises on which the occupational therapy profession was founded (Johnson, 1986).

HOLISM— A PRACTICE MODEL

Holistic health can take two forms. One emphasizes holistic therapy, the other wellness. The therapy model of holistic health approaches the treatment of illness by focusing on self-responsibility, the whole person, and the process of caregiving (Payne, 1983). For example, a California health center that endorsed the practice of holistic health brought together under one roof an interdisciplinary team and provided medicine, spiritual/emotional care, and mental health care. Each discipline had to be open and aware of other disciplines. Each health professional had to interact with the other disciplines and their clients in the context of each client's own environment and personal perceptions of his/her disease (Ropp, 1982).

The holistic therapy model is also a basic frame of reference that is based on a partnership between provider and patient—one that ensures the understanding of diagnoses, initial causes, and treatment of illness—and one that is predicated on active patient participation.

Psychosocial factors that influence patients' health and disease (Abroms, 1983) are identified. Mental illness, for example, must be viewed from multiple perspectives—biological, psychosocial, and existential-moral (Abroms, 1983). There is agreement that the mind and body should be considered and treated in an integrated fashion (Brown and Zinberg, 1982). The health provider integrates family members and significant others into the patient's treatment process, recuperation, and rehabilitation.

In discussing occupational therapy practice, White (1986) defined holism in the context of wellness as a "belief in the interactive effects of the mind, body, spirit, and environment; the existence of functional interdependence among parts and wholes; . . . and the idea of individual responsibility" (p. 745). The wellness model advances prevention, rather than cure, and health enhancement, diet, exercise, meditation, positive mental attitudes, and religious faith, rather than medical treatment (Pasnau, 1982).

This second form of holistic health has led to the development of holistic centers. Each holistic center's health care process reflects nature's healing force. Thus, traditional clinical, laboratory, and diagnostic procedures are often supplemented by unconventional methods, such as exercise, visualization, role playing, acupuncture, shiatsu, meditation, and yoga. Many holistic health centers use standardized tests to help patients understand the relationship between their behaviors and their health. The centers' structure and function reinforce mutual participation and self-help. Clients are encouraged to see the center as a place for education and socialization, as well as for health and wellness (Gordon, 1980).

HOLISM IN OCCUPATIONAL THERAPY

Throughout the history of occupational therapy, holism has been an integral concept in the philosophy of treatment and health of patients. The literature mentions holism as a valuable and important concept in the philosophy of occupational therapy education and practice (Meyer, 1922; Dunning, 1973; Reed, 1984). In 1922 (Pattison), the first explicit mention of holism is made in the application of occupational therapy in the treatment of tuberculosis. It emphasized the need for holistic principles to be used if the patient was to be restored to health. In 1932 (Stevenson) holism was first mentioned in the occupational therapy literature for the treatment of the mentally ill. In an article by Taylor (1944) the therapist is reminded to "treat the whole person according to his/her individual needs" (p. 209). Trider (1970) stated that occupational therapy was the only health profession that used a holistic approach in patient treatment. In 1977 (Engelhardt) another author concluded that occupational therapy has a holistic and humanistic view of therapy and health, which was absent from other medical approaches. Bing (1981) concluded in his Eleanor Clark Slagle Lectureship that there is a "belief in the wholeness of the human—that the mind and body are inextricably conjoined" (p. 499). A research article by Ben-Shlomo (1983) suggested that thera-

pists should be concerned with the mind-body link when using physical exercise to improve self-attitudes. The occupational therapy literature does not explicitly define holism. Instead, the concepts of holism are couched within the descriptions of occupational therapy principles, methods, and techniques. Holism appears to pervade the entire profession through case studies, treatment plans and assessments. There are some central tenets that occupational therapists would agree upon, but there are other equally valid tenets of holism that are based on the individual's educational background and clinical experience. The occupational therapy treatment principles that reflect the concepts of holism range from client evaluation and treatment planning, to the coordination of services secured from other health disciplines.

In practice, holism principles would be integrated into the occupational therapy treatment plan and shared with the patient or family, giving adequate attention to biological, psychological, social, and environment factors. The client would be viewed as autonomous and as a coparticipant in health care delivery. The patient's values would be considered, and the principle of patient participation in the decision-making process encouraged (Slaymaker, 1986). These principles are consistent with current trends in managed care. Their application will prepare the occupational therapy profession to meet the coming health care reform challenges.

IMPLICATIONS FOR OCCUPATIONAL THERAPY

Occupational therapists who specialize still can remain true to their holistic training. A therapist can be specialized and treat the whole patient by integrating knowledge and care that will be attentive to all patient needs. For example, a therapist practicing in the field of mental health still examines all of the areas, including physical-motor and cognitive function, the central core of developmentally appropriate activities, and all the environmental factors that affect patients (Slaymaker, 1986);

In 1982, Hemphill proposed the integrative approach to selecting test instruments. The integrative approach encourages the therapist to view the client from a holistic view during the assessment process. The author proposed that the client be assessed from four areas of human function: psychological, behavioral, learning, and biological. These areas of human function represent frames of references that relate to their corresponding theoretical bases. By assessing the client in these four areas of human function, the therapist could apply the treatment principles that represent each frame of reference. Therefore, the therapist could be using more than one frame of reference to test a client. Using more than one frame of reference offers a holistic approach because it addresses the client biologically, emotionally, physically, and socially (Hemphill, 1982, 1989).

More recently, Kielhofner (1992) included the concept of holism as an emerging paradigm in occupational therapy.

The author views holism as an important "focal viewpoint" (p. 61) in the model of human occupation. The model proposes that the mind and brain are interrelated. Holism is seen as a physical, emotional, cognitive, social, and cultural concept that is strongly influenced by the general systems theory. The general systems theory, in turn, promotes understanding of the interconnectedness between phenomena within the body. As Kielhofner states, it provides a view of the world as a vast, integrated network of components in which parts are incorporated into wholes" (p. 63).

Bruce and Borg (1993) address holism as a frame of reference for the treatment of organic brain syndrome. In their chapter summary of theoretical principles, the authors state "the individual is understood as an integrated biopsychosocial 'whole' whose health care needs must be addressed accordingly" (p. 316).

The concept of holism is evolving in occupational therapy, and an attempt is made to show where it is now in that evolution. The following case illustration takes what is known now and applies holistic concepts to occupational therapy practice in mental health:

CASE ILLUSTRATION

Client: M.K. Caucasian Female

Primary Diagnosis: Paranoid Schizophrenia, DSM IV-Axis I

M.K. was referred for occupational therapy evaluation and treatment after being discharged from a state psychiatric hospital. She was put on a psychotropic medication and placed in a semi-independent living apartment, where she was visited by a case manager once a week to receive assistance with shopping, health care needs, and financial responsibilities. M.K. had been hospitalized three times prior to this admission. She had, however, been able to care for her 3-year-old son and hold a part-time job with supported employment for the last 6 years. At the time of the recent admission, she was neglecting her son's basic needs and, therefore, temporarily lost custody of him.

Evaluation Process

Evaluations were completed at M.K's apartment, on the bus, at the grocery story (where she worked as cashier and a bagger), and at her mother's home (where her son was living). Before evaluating her formally, time was spent developing rapport, establishing a friendship, and developing trust and equality. This was done by taking her out for coffee, by avoiding intrusive questions, and by listening and validating her concerns.

At her apartment, she was given the Bender-Gestalt. Her score of 12 showed mild organic problems. During observation of her motivation level and initiative to socially connect with others, it became apparent that she was isolated and bored. A leisure inventory showed she spent most of her free time watching television and drinking coffee. She chronically felt suspicious of other people's motives and as a result, she

spent most of her time alone. Ironically, she was less suspicious when she interacted and had a purposeful activity to engage in.

Throughout the evaluation process, M.K was asked questions related to her spiritual beliefs. She grew up as a Protestant, with little spiritual guidance. She became more religious after being diagnosed with schizophrenia and has since become afraid of the messages she hears from God, including messages about people knowing her thoughts. Otherwise, she felt little sense of universal purpose and had no desire to join a church or spiritual group.

At her apartment she was given the Motor Free Visual Perceptual Test and an unstandardized cognitive screening tool. Scores revealed she had normal visual perception, but that her short-term memory was impaired and her long-term memory was intact. Mild deficits were identified in following complex directions and in performing tasks requiring abstract thinking and problem solving. In addition, she was given the Allen Test of Cognitive Functioning and scored a level 5.

We took the bus and grocery shopped at the store where she worked, as part of the evaluation process. Observations of M.K. during these activities revealed she was remarkably strong and in good physical condition. Her range of motion, muscle tone and strength were within functional limits. She demonstrated a mild decrease in both fine and gross motor coordination. She was later evaluated using the Jepson-Taylor Hand Function Test and scored slightly below norms bilaterally. In addition, the "Imitation of Postures" was given, which indicated a mild proprioceptive deficit.

In the area of self-care, M.K. required minimal prompts for hair, teeth, skin, and nail care. Weekly visits from her case manager helped her remember to do her laundry, clean her apartment and take her medication. In addition, M.K. needed assistance in achieving a balanced diet. Her son was removed from her care partly because of poor nutrition, and M.K wanted to learn to take better care of him. All of the self-care tasks deteriorated when M.K. was under stress.

M.K. worked at the grocery store as a bagger/cashier twenty hours a week and required frequent absences due to her fluctuating stress level and hallucinations. She received support and flexibility from her supervisor, who had received training from M.K's case manager.

M.K. visited her son two times/month and wanted to regain custody of him. She had never married and was without a relationship. She wanted to develop an intimate relationship with someone new. Her parents were supportive of her as were her two siblings. She had little contact with friends or with her community and was isolated at the time of evaluation.

Treatment Summary

The treatment was designed by M.K. and the occupational therapist as a team, and was based on her desires and values. M.K.'s first priority was to develop a social support system. She wanted to meet a companion and have a hobby. To meet this goal, the occupational therapist helped her contact a local church that held ceramics classes two times a month—a hobby she was interested in pursuing. In addition, the church was looking for a volunteer to help with its coffee hour, and M.K. thought she might meet new people through helping.

Her next priority was to manage the stress that lead to symptom exacerbation. The occupational therapist suggested learning stress management and joining an aerobics class. M.K. was willing to do both and was taught stress-reduction techniques through breathing and muscle control. A portable biofeedback machine was used to accomplish this goal.

M.K.'s next priority was to receive more assistance with her activities of daily living so that she could feel attractive and present a better image to those deciding how much time she could spend with her son. A local church was found where M.K. could assist in filing and answering the phone in exchange for feedback and self-care support from the church secretary. M.K. kept toiletries and make-up at the church. In addition, M.K. could participate in the senior lunch program and receive a free, well-balanced meal.

M.K. did not find her memory to be a high priority for treatment. She was willing to carry a pocket calendar and a spiral notebook to keep track of her appointments and to write down her concerns as they occurred. She had trouble acknowledging her cognitive limitations and was not forced to accept them by the occupational therapist. The pocket calendar was attached to her purse by a cord and covered with florescent tape to remind her to use it. She was willing to participate in a weekly occupational therapy support group, which met twice a week to assist participants in problem-solving, advocacy, medication management, and health care needs.

M.K.'s other priorities included getting her sexual and intimacy needs met, getting to spend more time with her son, developing a better relationship with her family, and eventually earning more money. These areas were not dealt with initially due to time constraints and helping M.K learn to build on her strengths and recover from her hospitalization.

Over a period of time, the occupational therapist and M.K. developed a therapeutic relationship based on equal partnership. They would spend sessions either in the community, at her apartment, or at her job (meeting with her employer). All areas of her life were addressed in occupational therapy treatment, including spiritual, cognitive/perceptual, vocational, physical, sexual, and familial concerns. In addition, her family was involved in her treatment by meeting at her parent's home for some sessions. The traditional form of treatment—seeing her in the clinic-was not appropriate. The occupational therapist provided education in the areas of stress management and biofeedback, spiritual support when appropriate, sexual guidance, and diet. Addressing her as a whole, complex, person encouraged long-term stability and self-control.

SUMMARY

The authors' goal is to encourage the occupational therapy profession to develop a universally acceptable definition of holism that clearly indicates the holistic tenets involved, and that professionals can adopt and visibly translate into practice. Perhaps, a position paper on the subject is in order.

The philosophy of occupational therapy is similar to that of holism, as described by the Greeks and earlier ancient writings. Sir William Osler's prediction that medicine of the future would embrace the concept of holism has come true. Holism is an integral part of the practice of occupational therapy in mental health. M.K.'s evaluation and treatment exemplify this holistic approach to intervention in a case of paranoid schizophrenia. Physical, cognitive/perceptual, spiritual, and environmental aspects must be important components of mental health practice. In the past, paranoid schizophrenia was generally treated from a medical reductionistic model. Use of the holistic approach suggested in this chapter will ensure that, today, the person is viewed as the whole being described by Hemphill (1989), Kielhofner (1992), and Bruce and Borg (1993).

REFERENCES

Abroms, E., (1983). Beyond eclecticism. *American Journal of Psychiatry, 40*(6), 740.

Ardell, D., (1979). *High level wellness: An alternative to doctors, drugs, and disease.* New York, NY: Bantam Books.

Aston, J. (May, 1984). The power of the will. *Nursing Times, 80*(2).

Bamberg, D. (1982). Holistic health, human ecology, and you. *Occupational Health Nursing, 30*(1).

Ben-Shlomo, L. (1983). The effect of physical exercise on self-attitudes. *Occupational Therapy in Mental Health, 3,* 11-28.

Benson, H. (1979). *The mind/body effect.* New York, NY: Simon and Shuster.

Bing, R. (1981). Occupational therapy revisited: A paraphrasic journey. *American Journal of Occupational Therapy, 35,* 499-518.

Bruce, A., & Borg, B. (1993). *Psychosocial occupational therapy: Frames of reference for intervention* (2nd Edition). Thorofare, NJ: SLACK Incorporated.

Cmich, D. (1984). Theoretical perspectives of holistic health. *Journal of School Health, 54*(1), 30-32.

Cole, D. (1982). *Helping: Origins and development of the major psychotherapies.* Toronto, Canada: Butterworths.

Corey, C. (1991). *Theory and practice of counseling and psychotherapy.* Monterey: Brooks/Cole Publishing Co.

Desobe, G. J. (1981). Standards for holistic health care. *American Protestant Hospital Association Bulletin, 45*(3), 48-49.

Dunning, R. E. (1973). Philosophy and occupational therapy. *American Journal of Occupational Therapy, 27,* 18.

Eisenberg, D., Kessler, R., Foster, C., Norlock, F., Calkins, D., & Delbanco, T. (1993). Unconventional medicine in the United States. *The New England Journal of Medicine, 328*(4), 246-252.

Engelhardt, H. (1977). Defining occupational therapy: The meaning of therapy and the virtues of occupation. *American Journal of Occupational Therapy, 31,* 666-672.

Ferguson, M. (1980). *The Aquarian Conspiracy: Person and social transformation in the 1980s.* Los Angeles, CA: J. P. Tarcher, Inc.

Garai, J. E. (1979). New horizons of the humanistic approach to expressive therapies and creativity development. *Art Psychotherapy, 6,* 177- 183.

Garai, J. (1984). New horizons of holistic healing through creative expression. *Art Therapy, 1*(2), 77.

Ginsburg, I. (1982) Is a holistic model salutary? *Nursing Homes, 31*(5), 39.

Gross, S. (1980). The holistic health movement. *Personnel and Guidance Journal, 59*(2), 96.

Gordon, J. (1980). Holistic health care: its promise, its problems. *The New Physician, 29*(6), 20.

Hemphill, B. (1982). *The evaluative process in psychiatric occupational therapy.* Thorofare, NJ: SLACK Incorporated.

Hemphill, B. (1989). *Mental health assessment: An integrative approach to the evaluative process.* Thorofare, NJ: SLACK Incorporated.

Johnson, J. (1986). Wellness and occupational therapy. *American Journal of Occupational Therapy, 40*(11), 753.

Kielhofner, G. (1992). *Conceptual foundations of occupational therapy.* Philadelphia, PA: F.A. Davis Company.

LaPatra, J. (1978). *Healing: The coming revolution in holistic medicine.* New York, NY: McGraw-Hill Book Company, 94-120.

Lipowski, Z. (1984). What does the word psychosomatic really mean: a historical and semantic inquiry. *Psychosomatic Medicine, 46*(2), 159.

Lipowski, Z. (1986). Psychosomatic medicine: past and present part 1: Historical background. *Canadian Journal of Psychiatry, 31,*2.

Meyer, A. (1922). Philosophy of occupation therapy. *Archives of Ocupational Therapy,* 1.

Newback, I. (1986). The whole works. *Nursing Times, 82*(30), 48.

Nuernberger, P. (1978). *Freedom From Stress.* Himalayan International Institute of Yoga Science and Philosophy Publishers, 6.

Pasnau, R. (1982). Consultation-liason psychiatry at the crossroads: In search of a definition for the 1980s. *Hospital and Community Psychiatry, 33*(12), 992.

Pattison, H. (1922). The trend of occupational therapy for the tuberculous. *Archives of Occupational Therapy, 1* 19-24.

Pelletier, K. (1977). *Mind As Healer, Mind As Slayer.* New York, NY: Delta Publishing Company, 318.

Pownal, M. (February, 1986). All in the mind's eye. *Nursing Times, 82*(8), 26.

Reed, K. (1984). *Models of Practice in Occupational Therapy.* Baltimore, MD: Williams and Wilkins, 65.

Renshaw, J. (April, 1984). The power of the will. *Nursing Times, 80*(1), 38.

Ropp, R. (1982) A model for wholistic care. *American Protestant Hospital Association Bulletin, 45*(1), 26.

Slaymaker, J. (1986). A holistic approach to specialization. *The American Journal of Occupational Therapy, 40*(2), 117.

Stevenson, G. (1932). The healing influence fo work and play ina mental hospital. *Occupational Therapy and Rehabilitation, 11,* 85-89.

Taylor, M. (1944). Dynamic rehabilitiation. *Occupational Therapy and Rehabilitation, 23,* 310-315.

Trider, M. (1972). The future of occupational therapy. *Canadian Journal of Occupational Therapy, 39,* 3-8.

Udchic, H. (1984). Adlerian holism and holistic health. *Individual Psychology: Journal of Adlerian Theory, Research, and Practice, 40*(4), 364.

Walton, S. (1979). Holistic medicine, *Science News, 116,* 410.

White, V. (1986). Promoting health and wellness: a theme for the eighties. *The American Journal of Occupational Therapy, 40*(11), 745.

SECTION FIVE

Familial and Social Supports: Promoting Adaptation and Quality of Life

EDITOR'S NOTE

There are more than 36 million people in the United States who have physical and/or mental disabilities that are severe enough to limit their ability to perform daily activities. However, only 5% of all disabled Americans reside in institutions; the remaining 95% live in the community, residing alone or living with their family, friends, and/or professional caregivers (National Institute on Disability and Rehabilitation Research, 1999). The number of Americans with significant disabilities who reside in the community is expected to increase as a result of the continued deinstitutionalization movement and the growth of managed care (Malloy, 1995; Schreter, Schreter & Sharfstein, 1997). In addition, the consumer advocacy movement and the implementation of the Americans with Disabilities Act (ADA) has resulted in an increased demand for community integration for all persons with disabilities (AOTA, 1991; Crist, 1996; Frese, 1998; Grady, 1996; Javernick, 1991).

However, residing in one's community does not automatically ensure successful adaptation to disability or full integration into the life of the community (Dunn, Brown, & McGuigan, 1996; Grady, 1996). Persons with disabilities are often discharged into the community with inadequate skills for community living and with limited resources for adaptation (Carpentier et al., 1992; Frese, 1998; Schreter, Schreter & Sharfstein, 1997). Economic barriers, limited accessibility, and social stigma may all contribute to increased social isolation and decreased adaptive functioning (Christiansen, 1991; Fahl, 1996). The very nature of a disability and the presence of performance component deficits may also contribute to increased stress and a diminished ability to cope with the demands of one's living environment (Christiansen, 1991; Macias & Rodican, 1997). The families of persons with disabilities are also challenged by changes in the families' lifestyles, role expectations, and daily tasks (Clark & Standard, 1996; Fahl, 1996).

Underlying all of these challenges to the adaptive abilities of the individual and the family are the emotional responses to the illness itself. Shock, anger, grief, and denial may be expressed as the individual and family struggle to accept and adjust to the realities of the disability (Christiansen, 1991; Clark & Standard, 1996; Fahl, 1996; Macias & Rodican, 1997).

Successful adjustment to community living and effective adaptation to disability have been strongly linked to the provision of a supportive social network. Self-help groups, clubhouse communities, stress management, psychoeducation, and social skills training have all been found to improve significantly the patient's prognosis and to enhance the quality of life for both the person with the disability and for his or her family (Ascher-Svanum & Krause, 1991; Christiansen, 1991; Clark & Standard, 1996; Grady, 1996; Yerxa, 1996). Therefore, it is vital for occupational therapists to become adept at evaluating clients' and their families' social support needs and at providing appropriate intervention and prevention strategies to enable clients and their families to cope with the daily stresses of physical and/or psychosocial disability. It is insufficient for the occupational therapist to teach functional skills without considering the social context of these skills (Dunn, et al, 1996; Frese, 1998; Grady, 1996; Javernick, 1991).

The chapters in this section provide an overview of the collaborative processes needed to build social support networks with clients and their families. A number of social support programs for community treatment centers and for institutional, residential settings are described. These programs have successfully assisted clients and their families in functionally adapting to the challenges of living with disabilities.

However, before a practitioner begins developing family and social support programs, he or she must understand the individual family's unique context. Therefore, this section begins with a comprehensive discussion of the diverse needs of families from different ethnic and cultural backgrounds who have a family member with a serious mental illness. Frequently, these families are viewed through a western cultural, medical perspective which seriously neglects the multicultural society in which they live. Laurene Y. Finley argues in Chapter 51 that to effectively support individuals with mental illness and their families, mental health practitioners must recognize and support their diverse sociocultural contexts. She examines cultural variations in family structure, communication and presentation styles, problem solving, decision-making and conflict resolution, role expectations and help-seeking attitudes. Potential barriers to the participation of ethnic, culturally diverse families in mainstream support groups are analyzed. A multidimensional approach to bridge these cultural gaps is described in a clear, concrete manner. Finley outlines eight separate dimensions that should be considered for each family and provides relevant questions to use in assessing each of these dimensions. Practical family and provider self-assessment guidelines and approaches for applying a multicultural lens to facilitate mutual understanding of value differences and similarities are provided. Finley concludes with a list of strategies for the development of a culturally specific family support group. Throughout this chapter, examples of alternative, innovative, culturally sensitive approaches are presented to enhance collaboration with, and support of, the families of persons with mental illness.

To truly work in partnership with a family, we must strive to understand the complexity of feelings experienced by the relatives of a person with a serious illness (Fahl, 1996; Clark & Standard, 1996). One of the major emotional reactions that characterizes a family's response to their subjective experience of chronic illness is a severe sense of loss. Spouses, parents, siblings and children often have tremendous longing for the quality of their former relationship with the family member who is now chronically ill. Besides this current loss, family members experience significant grief over the loss of shared future goals, hopes and dreams. However, these losses are often not dealt with in traditional support groups which focus on the more tangible issues of family problem solving and communication.

The need for therapeutic interventions to specifically focus on family grief and coping with loss is discussed in this section's next chapter by Frederick E. Miller. He describes a format for grief therapy for relatives of persons with serious mental illness. The two main phases of his approach (which include reminiscence and readjustment) are applicable to all families who are experiencing the loss of a family member due to chronic illness, regardless of its source (i.e., physical or mental). Although, without the attainment of advanced training, grief therapy and bereavement counseling are beyond the scope of occupational therapy practice; many of Miller's suggestions on how to help a family cope with grief provide appropriate guidelines for occupational therapists to use during family interactions and in family education programs. As Miller states, understanding the realities of a family's grief and using bereavement counseling guidelines can assist in engaging them (even when they are labeled as "resistant") in more traditional family support intervention programs.

Strategies for engaging families in treatment are further explored in Chapter 53 by Kayla F. Bernheim. In her presentation, Bernheim outlines eight generic principles for developing a comprehensive, collaborative approach for involving families in the care of persons with chronic mental illness. She provides clear, practice-oriented examples to substanti-

ate each principle. She also gives constructive ideas to empower families to become part of the collaborative treatment process and to be advocates for improved quality of care. Although Bernheim's presentation focuses on the families of the chronic mentally ill, readers will find her principles applicable to families of persons with many types of chronic disabilities. These principles provide essential guidelines for the occupational therapist working with families, and their application is vital for development of effective family intervention programs.

Bernheim expands upon these collaborative principles in Chapter 54, in which she describes a support program whose aim is to develop close working relationships between the families of persons with chronic mental illness and the staff of a community residence where these patients live. She identifies the elements of an effective family support program and provides descriptive examples of methods utilized to engage families and to maintain positive collaborative relationships. Bernheim also addresses staff concerns regarding working with families and provides constructive suggestions for dealing with these issues. Bernheim again focuses on the families of persons with chronic mental illness, but readers will find her family support program description highly relevant to most residential settings in which positive professional and family collaboration is desired (i.e., nursing homes, developmental centers).

In Chapter 55, the authors also emphasize a collaborative approach among patients, families, and the interdisciplinary treatment team; however, their focus is on the acute care, inpatient psychiatric unit. They describe a short-term psychoeducational program that utilizes a holistic team approach to meet the needs of patients and their families. Psychiatrists, nurses, occupational therapists, social workers, and an administrator all work together to educate patients and their families about the nature of mental illness and to develop the skills and resources needed for effective coping. The chapter identifies the separate components of the psychoeducational program and describes the roles and responsibilities of each professional member within the program. Of particular interest to readers will be the description of the Life Skills Curriculum provided by the occupational therapy department. The utilization of individual, family, and group methods and the empathetic individuation of treatment provide patients and their families with invaluable support to develop the functional skills essential for community living.

The need for professionals to support families as they strive to cope with mental illness is further explored in this section's next chapter by Barbara Jacobs. Her touching discussion is based on her personal experience as an occupational therapist who is the parent of a child with the dual diagnosis of schizoaffective disorder and substance abuse. Jacobs explores the complexities of this diagnosis and the impact of stigma and fear on the entire family. The resulting resolution and "dual denial" that develops from this lack of understanding is realistically described. The intervention implications of this dual disability and the troubling limitations of many treatment programs are explored with personal experiences provided to substantiate the need for all practitioners to be aware of the needs of a person with a dual diagnosis and their family. Jacobs describes how her family copes with their family member's dual disability through the use of support groups and "carving out" and maintaining time for family fun. Her personal experience offers helpful guidance which she supplements with a list of concrete tips for practitioners to use when working with families who have a member with a mental illness.

The familial experience of mental illness can become very complicated when the family member with the illness is also a parent, for parenting involves a number of vital skills that may be lacking in persons with mental illnesses. The necessity to recognize the significance of parental mental illness and its impact on the family cannot be underestimated and intervention programs must be developed to address and prevent familial dysfunction. Chapter 57 addresses this complex issue by exploring the needs of mothers with mental illness and their children between birth and age five who are considered "at risk" for the development of multiple problems. The chapter's author, Mary Ann Zeitz, describes an innovative intervention and primary prevention program that provides comprehensive services to these multi-risk families. This center-based program includes a therapeutic nursery that provides a safe and predictable environment that is also stimulating and flexible to enhance children's development. This supportive environment also serves as a learning laboratory in which mothers with mental illness can model and practice effective parenting. Individualized rehabilitation programs are provided to the parents while the children are cared for in the nursery.

Intervention programs provided include educational and vocational services, stress management groups, independent living skills training and parenting education. The on-site programs for the mothers and children are supplemented with a holistic case management system, outreach services, primary and extended family support groups and substance abuse treatment. While occupational therapy is not discussed in this chapter, a number of services described by Zeitz are clearly within occupational therapy's domain of concern. These include: developmental assessments of children to determine strengths and deficits, parenting skills training to foster the successful use of child rearing practices that are developmentally appropriate, and independent living skills training to maintain the family within the community.

The development of programming which supports successful adaptation to disability and community integration is also addressed in Chapter 58 by Susan Delaney McConchie. This chapter outlines the process utilized to develop a support group for persons with physical and psychosocial disabilities. The questions posed by the author in developing this program provide relevant guidelines for the development of support groups in a diversity of treatment settings. The goals, format, and structure of the program are described. Issues regarding coleadership and logistical concerns are realistically discussed. The description of the positive effect of the support group on members' personal growth and community advocacy efforts validates the rele-

vance of support groups for persons with physical and/or psychosocial disabilities.

In Chapter 59, Sharon Mueller and Melinda Suto present stress management principles and techniques that are also applicable to a variety of patient populations and a diversity of treatment settings. Evaluation methods, intervention techniques, and group procedures utilized in their stress management program are discussed. A psychoeducational approach is used to increase members' knowledge of stress and to acquire effective coping skills.

The development of a supportive social network also provides the basis for Chapter 60. In her presentation, Harriet Woodside describes a community day treatment program for persons with chronic mental illness that developed into a "surrogate extended family" for its members. Patient population characteristics, program philosophy, and the developmental process of the program are presented. Mutual trust, respect, dignity, and friendship are emphasized throughout the presentation.

The benefits of establishing trusting, collaborative relationships with individuals and their families have been strongly supported by this section's authors. I hope readers will utilize the information presented in this section to evaluate clients' and their families' social support resources and needs and to model their interventions in the collaborative manner presented by each chapter's authors. More importantly, I hope readers will model the positive examples set by several chapter authors to design and develop innovative programs that fill the current gaps in family support services.

To assist the reader in further developing his/her skills in working with families, questions for further consideration are provided below. In addition, a number of resources for family and social support are provided at the end of this text's preface to assist readers in their evaluation, intervention, and referral process. Consumer groups and professional organizations (e.g., Alzheimer's Disease and Related Disorders Association, Alliance for the Mentally Ill) have a wealth of knowledge and experience to share; readers are urged to contact relevant organizations for further information about available services.

QUESTIONS TO CONSIDER

1. What are the major concerns and potential reactions a family may have when a family member has a physical and/or psychosocial disability? What are the unique issues a family must deal with if the disabled family member is a parent? A child? A spouse? A sibling?

2. How may the social stigma associated with a number of illnesses (e.g., substance abuse, schizophrenia) affect the patient's and family's adjustment to an illness? How may individual personal reactions to disability affect the adjustment process? What are ways occupational therapists can help individual family members cope with their family's loss?

3. What is your sociocultural background and how does this influence your view of chronic physical and mental ill-

ness? What are your sociocultural values and beliefs that may influence your ability to give and receive support? How does your family typically respond to distressful situations? To loss?

4. How can occupational therapists build collaborative relationships with clients and their families? What are relevant occupational therapy intervention goals and methods for building family and social supports?

5. What are the essential situational coping skills for community living? How can an occupational therapist facilitate the development of adaptive coping skills in patients and their families?

6. How are maladaptive signs of stress exhibited in patients' and families' behaviors? How can stress management techniques be integrated into an occupational therapy program?

7. What are the potential concerns of families who have a member of their family in a residential, institutional treatment setting? What steps can be taken by staff to maintain positive family involvement in institutional settings?

8. What are the special needs of parents who have mental illness? How may the effects of mental illness impact on one's ability to effectively parent? What are the occupational therapy assessment tools that can be used to determine an individual's parenting skills and their child's developmental level? How can occupational therapy interventions be provided to enhance successful parenting and to facilitate healthy child development?

9. What are the unique social support needs of persons with chronic mental illness? How can occupational therapists structure a treatment program that maintains a balance between goal-directed treatment and the provision of social support?

10. What resources do patients and/or their families need to maximize adaptive adjustment to disability? What are the social support options available to patients and their families? How can occupational therapists network with these resources to facilitate their use?

REFERENCES

American Occupational Therapy Association. (1991, December 5). Occupational therapy and the Americans with Disabilities Act. *OT Week,* pp. II, III.

Ascher-Svanum, H., & Krause, A. (1991). *Psychoeducational groups for patients with schizophrenia: A guide for practitioners.* Rockville, MD: Aspen Publishers.

Carpentier, N., Lesage, A., Goulet, J., Lalonde, P., & Renaud, M. (1992). Burden of care of families not living with young schizophrenic relatives. *Hospital and Community Psychiatry, 43,* 38-43.

Christiansen, C. (1991). Performance deficits as sources of stress: Coping theory and occupational therapy. In C. Christiansen & C. Baum (Eds.), *Occupational therapy: Overcoming human performance deficits* (pp. 69-96). Thorofare, NJ: SLACK Incorporated.

Clark, M., & Standard, P. L. (1996). Caregiver burden and the structural family model. *Family Community Health, 18*(4), 58-66.

Crist, P. A., & Stoffel, V. C. (1996). The Americans with Disabilities Act of 1990 and employees with mental impairments: Personal efficacy and the environment. In R. P. Cottrell (Ed.), *Perspectives on purposeful activity: Foundations and future of occupational therapy.* Bethesda, MD: American Journal of Occupational Therapy.

Dunn, W., Brown, C., & McGuigan, A. (1996). The ecology of human performance: A framework for considering the effect of context. In R. P. Cottrell (Ed.). *Perspectives on purposeful activity: Foundation and future of occupational therapy* (pp. 131-144). Bethesda, MD: American Occupational Therapy Association.

Fahl, M. A. (1996). Mental illness and family involvement. *Mental Health Special Interest Section Quarterly, 19*(3), 1-2.

Frese, F. J. (1998). Occupational therapy and mental illness: A personal view. *Mental Health Special Interest Section Quarterly, 21*(3), 1-3.

Grady, A. (1996). Building inclusive community: A challenge for occupational therapy. In R. P. Cottrell (Ed.). *Perspectives on purposeful activity: Foundation and future of occupational therapy* (pp. 229-240). Bethesda, MD: American Occupational Therapy Association.

Javernick. (1991, November 28). Moving toward therapist/consumer partnerships. *OT Week,* 15.

Macias, C., & Rodican, C. (1997). Coping with recurrent loss in mental illness: Unique aspects of club house communities. *Journal of Personal and Interpersonal Loss, 2,* 205-221.

Malloy, M. (1995). *Mental illness and managed care: A primer for families and consumers.* Arlington, VA: National Alliance for Mental Illness.

National Institute on Disability and Rehabilitation Research (1999) *www.ncddr.org.*

Schreter, Schreter, and Sharfstein (Eds.) (1997). *Managing care, not dollars: The continuum of mental health services.* Washington, DC: American Psychiatric Press.

Yerxa, E. J. (1996). The social and psychological experience of have a disability: Implications for occupational therapists. In L. W. Pedretti (Ed.), *Occupational therapy: Practice skills for physical dysfunction* (3rd Edition) (pp. 253-275). St. Louis, MO: Mosby.

CHAPTER FIFTY-ONE

The Cultural Context: Families Coping with Severe Mental Illness

Laurene Y. Finley

This chapter is reprinted from the Psychosocial Rehabilitation Journal, 21, *230-240, by permission of the author.* *Copyright © 1998.*

Families throughout the world must adjust to the onset of a psychiatric disability and its resulting complications and challenges (Lefley, 1985). In over two thirds of the world's countries, families are an essential resource to members who have either a physical or a mental illness, providing general social and psychological support in ways perceived as alien in western service delivery (Bell, 1982; Lefley, 1985). Family members may be perceived as allies and integral to the treatment process. They may travel long distances and live in close proximity to the hospital in order to "wait out" the hospitalization of a family member. They may also participate in the feeding, nursing, and medication monitoring of the mentally ill family member (Bell, 1982). In the Philippines, persons who stay with their relatives while in the hospital are called "watchers" (Higginbotham, 1979). The "watcher" family role has been emulated in more traditional psychiatric systems as a model for conducting discussion and education with families.

- Help-seeking attitudes and behavior: Strong religious and spiritual beliefs may affect conceptions about illness and health. Mental illnesses may be perceived as the "devil's work," possession by evil spirits, caused by witchcraft, or punishment for disobeying God. Ethnic family members may not make clear demarcations between physical illness, emotional illness, and spiritual complaints.

"Si Dios quiere" (If God wishes) or "Que dies nos bendiga (May God bless us) are common responses heard among Latino families, for example, caring for a member with persistent mental illness (Guarnaccia, Parra, Deschamps, Milstein, & Argiles, 1992). These refrains reflect the hopes, frustrations, and religious beliefs that may be experienced in dealing with a deeply troubling illness that frequently defies explanation.

Home remedies, folk medicine and/or folk healers, dependence on religious leaders, and prayer are different types of approaches ethnic family members may utilize either singly or collectively alongside biomedicine.

The following basic assumptions underscore our learning about ethnic families (Alston & Turner, 1994; Szapocznik & Kurtines, 1993):

- Families are embedded in a systemic context
- Ethnicity and culture are powerful determinants of family norms and patterns;
- Embedded within cultures are potential sources of strength, which can be used by families as resources for recovery and a sense of well-being (Finley, 1997);
- Engagement and involvement of ethnic families requires the successful acknowledgement and utilization of these strengths;
- Every family has a cultural context to be valued, understood, and explored.

UNDERSTANDING FAMILIES IN A MULTICULTURAL CONTEXT

Group membership for many ethnic families may be a source of pride, cohesion, safety, and a buffer against psychological stressors in times of crisis, loss, stress, or disability. Families will rely upon these strengths, coping skills, and solutions learned from the familial, cultural context (Devore & Schlesinger, 1981). On the other hand, the family's interaction with the broader, pluralistic, societal context may, at timess, contribute to tension and confusion.

At least five struggles, either singly or in combination, may be faced by these families: 1) economic survival; 2) overcoming negative societal, group stereotypes; 3) development of a clear sense of ethnic identity and heritage; 4) reconciliation of tensions stemming from acculturation of the values and behaviors of the mainstream culture; and 5) continual adaptations and responses to a circular feedback process, that is, the "victim-system" (Boyd-Franklin, 1989; Chestang, 1972; Pierce, 1970; Pinderhughes, 1982).

A by-product of racism, poverty, and oppression, the victim-system strongly limits access to the opportunity structure, which in turn limits achievement and skill attainment by members of the ethnic group. These limitations in turn produce poverty. Poverty places undue stress on familial relationships such that, over time, the family's capacity to perform social roles adequately and to support their communities may become restricted. Families may be challenged by the multiplicative effects of stigma, resulting from one or more cooccurring illnesses of a family member and a devalued "minority" status within the broader society.

All families that come for mental health services bring their unique sociocultural histories. Though not all ethnic families are trapped in the victim-system, those that are may also bring with them an additional world view in which the surrounding environment and its institutions are perceived as hostile, dangerous, and unpredictable. This "cultural paranoia" (Mirowsky, 1985), which is a protective, survival mechanism, may present itself as a family being overly sensitive, too racially or ethnically conscious or sensitive, or unduly suspicious of providers and the systems which they represent. These families are frequently wary of receiving help from outsiders. Perceiving these outsiders as intrusive or fearing that providers may perceive them as weak may explain the reluctance of many ethnic families to work with persons outside the nuclear and extended family. Neighbors & Jackson (1984), for example, found that a majority of African American respondents were more likely to make contact with their informal social network than with more formal mainstream institutions.

ETHNIC CAREGIVERS AND COPING MASTERY

Ethnic groups in the United States vary widely in cultural heritage. Values in these groups, however, seem to be closer to those of the more traditional cultures found in developing countries. These cultures tend to be more group and family oriented, interdependent, and less individualistic than members of the American mainstream (Lefley, 1990).

There is supportive evidence that the prognosis for severe and persistent mental illness may be better in more traditional cultures with extensive kinship systems as compared to cultures with more nuclear family structures (Kleinman & Good, 1985; Sartorius, Jablensky, & Korten, 1986; Waxler, 1979). A critical factor contributing to the intercultural differences could well be the view extended family members have towards the caretaking role. Caretaking is often per-

ceived as a valued involvement providing psychological, emotional, and economic buffers that differ from the Western, nuclear family experience (Lefley, 1987; 1990).

Over the last 15 to 20 years, the family therapy literature has promulgated the importance of applying a "multicultural lens" to the study of all families (Ho, 1987; McGoldrick, Pearce, & Giordano, 1982; McGoldrick, Giordano, & Pearce, 1996). Within a contextualist theoretical framework we understand that behavior cannot be understood outside of the context in which it occurs (Szapocznik & Kurtines, 1993). Consumers, therefore, are best understood within the context of their families; families are understood within their cultural context; the culture within the broader, diverse, complex, pluralistic society (Szapocznik, & Kurtines, 1993). Cultural forces are always impacting on the way in which family members interact with one another and with other systems at large.

The definition of "family support" and the design of innovative support models, therefore, must occur within the context of the family's culture (Alston & Turner, 1994) and are specifically mediated by factors such as family background, ethnicity, ethnic identity, cultural affiliation, socioeconomic status, and acculturation. Views towards mental health, attitudes about mental health services, preferences concerning interventions, types of medications, and providers may all be culturally determined. Examples of variations in world view that may influence not only family perception of formal and informal support but provide perceptions of families are:

- *Family structure.* Who is considered family? Family structures differ cross-culturally. Extended family and kinship networks may include a variety of persons both related and non-related. "Play aunts," "play uncles," godparents, neighbors, boyfriends, and members of the church family may all be part of an ethnic family's kinship system. Members of this system may be available for support of the family coping with a member with severe and persistent mental illness.

- *Communication and presentation styles.* Culturally determined presentation styles often affect the manner in which family issues and psychological distress may be presented. Some families may be more verbally expressive, open and self-disclosing; others more closed. Cultures also dictate different norms about nonverbal behaviors, such as eye contact and distances in personal space. Often incorrect motives and behavioral assessments are attributed to presentation styles which differ from those of the provider.

Studies have examined the significance of expressed emotion (EE) in the communication among family members, to relapse prevention and rehospitalization of the person with severe mental illness (Brown, Birley, & Wing, 1972; Leff & Vaughn, 1985; Vaughn & Leff, 1976; Lefley, 1992). Family members have been particularly critical of these studies, feeling that they are being held responsible for the relapse of their family member and that other powerful, environmental factors, not accounted for by these studies, may contribute to a consumer's relapse. Additional caution must be exercised in applying these outcome studies to ethnic families because they do not seem to reflect the cultural and communication styles which exist in many family structures (Lefley, 1992).

- *Problem-solving, decision-making and conflict resolution.* Some ethnic groups, such as African Americans, Italian Americans, and Latinos, tend to emphasize cooperation among the family and community group in times of distress (Randall-David, 1989). Family members may be highly involved in the decision-making process, conferring with other members and sanctioning or not sanctioning recommended forms of treatment. Learning more about the family's processes and identifying these lay members who are most involved are critical to any development of a family-professional partnership.

- *Role expectations.* Functions and responsibilities of family members may or may not be traditionally ascribed according to gender and/or age of family members. In less acculturated Latinos, for example, the male may be the key decision maker in matters outside of the home. Females may be primarily responsible for child-rearing and education, functioning as mediators between fathers and children (Guarnaccia, et al, 1992). In African American families, one might expect to find flexibility of roles within the family. Decision-making may rest with either the male or female head of household. In families in which several generations often reside in the same household, the seniors or elders may hold great influence in family decision-making.

Research on the role of family involvement in mental health is emerging in the United States, though few studies have examined the specific needs of ethnic families, the ways in which they cope with a member who has a severe mental illness, differential perceptions of caregiving duties and caregiving burden, and the patterns or differences in use of informal supports (Adebimpe, 1994; Cook, Pickett, & Cohler, 1997; Pickett, Damian, Vraniak, Cook, & Cohler, 1993). The research that exists focuses on families caring for relatives with longstanding illnesses such as severe and persistent mental illness and dementia among older adults.

The limited research has also included comparisons between African American and white caregivers. In a couple of instances, attempts have been made to include Latino families; either sample size limitations or no significant differences were found in the perceived burden between Latino and White caregivers in these studies (Stueve, Vine, & Struening, 1997).

Investigations of the differential self-perceptions of Blacks and Whites caring for a relative with severe and persistent mental illness found that Black parents challenged the stereotype that they were more likely to cope poorly and have lower self-esteem (Pickett et al 1993; Ulbrich, Warheit, & Zimmerman, 1989). Generally, Black parents, in comparison with White parents, seemed to have an ability to cope and feel better about themselves; this seemed to correlate with the

number of resources and amount of experience they had in dealing with their child's mental illness. Though Black families may live with greater life strains than Whites, in general a more pragmatic attitude seemed to allow them to maintain an outlook whereby mental illness may be seen as just another life challenge to which they must adjust.

There has been some support for ethnically-bound differences in the prevalence of depression among caregivers, though research participants were caregivers of elderly persons with dementia (Mintzer & Macera, 1992). It does appear, however, that different kinds of attributions and expectations may be made by ethnic caregivers regarding care of relatives with long-term illnesses.

Ethnic differences have also been noted in systematic studies of what caretakers do and how burdensome the family members may find their roles. White and African American parents report equivalent caregiving obligations and responsibilities. The basically equivalent duties, however, are perceived as a generally less stressful burden for Blacks than for Whites (Horwitz & Reinhard, 1995; Stueve et al., 1997). Perhaps the greater involvement of African Americans in their extended kinship system may make caring for an adult child with severe mental illness more normative and less stressful (Angel & Angel, 1993).

In a study that also considered differences in caregiving among siblings of persons with severe mental illness, important differences between Blacks and Whites were also noted. Blacks reported more caregiving duties and yet also viewed these responsibilities as less burdensome (Horwitz & Reinhard, 1995). The higher levels of perceived stigma regarding mental illness existing among White parents could have exacerbated their experience of stress and sense of burden (Horwitz & Reinhard, 1995).

These findings are perplexing in light of the systemic and institutional sociocultural conditions that daily impinge upon caregivers of non-majority groups (e. g., discrimination, a greater degree of poverty). The following is a summary of several explanations that might account for these differential results (Horwitz & Reinhard, 1985; Lefley, 1985, 1990; Pickett et al., 1993; Stueve et al., 1997):

- Attributions about illness, religious involvement, and social support may provide protective mechanisms;
- Members of some ethnic groups may be more practiced in attending to the needs of the extended family network, such that helping kin is highly valued. This normative context may help to diminish the emotional costs of caregiving;
- Ethnic caregivers may have greater access to their social support networks;
- Reliance on strong religious or spiritual beliefs such as prayer, the minister, folk healers, or the congregation may provide familial supports in a context which is more culturally congruent (Delgado & Humm-Delgado, 1982; Griffith, Young, & Smith, 1984). Pickett and colleagues (1993) point out, however, that simply having more numbers in one's familial and church network may not always mitigate against stress

for some ethnic group members. The reciprocal nature of the relationships may sometimes create additional problems contributing to a reluctance to utilize these informal supports;

- Members of different ethnic subgroups may offer alternative interpretations of psychiatric symptoms that are less stigmatizing and emphasize more normal social roles, demonstrating a capacity to integrate the person with the disability into family life (Lefley, 1990).

In summary, caregiving is shaped by multiple factors, with different groups experiencing different consequences or differences in how distress is handled. Ethnic families who are caregivers do have a story to tell that fairly consistently differs from families from the majority culture. Application of innovative methods to explore the unique strengths of ethnic families should provide a greater understanding of how culturally adaptive styles might be used effectively in working with different ethnic groups (Pickett et al., 1993). It should not be inferred, however, that members of different ethnic groups are necessarily more resilient or less distressed with caregiving demands (Stueve et al., 1997). There may be multiple ways in which a family caregiver's psychological well-being may be affected. Finding differences between any set of ethnic groups on one outcome does not assure that similar differences will be found on other measures (Stueve et al., 1997).

BARRIERS TO THE PARTICIPATION OF ETHNIC FAMILIES IN MAINSTREAM SUPPORT GROUPS

It is likely that if families from the dominant culture experience difficulties with the mental health system, ethnic and culturally diverse family needs are neglected as well (Solomon, 1988; Spaniol & Zipple, 1988)! Though family support programs have been increasing, many mutual support or self-help groups have been less successful in the recruitment of families who are not middle class, Anglo-American, or not just female participants (Borkman, 1990; Guarnaccia, et al., 1992). It is possible that underutilization of these programs stems from their incompatibility with the values and characteristics of various ethnic families. Pernell-Arnold and Finley (1992) suggest potential barriers to those programs wanting to incorporate ethnic group membership.

1. The expectation that some ethnic family members may want or feel that they need currently existing family support models may be incorrect. It is possible that these families may be quite content with the level of support derived from their kinship system. Research suggests that contact with the informal social network is more likely and that some families may utilize the network either first or in combination with professional supports (Neighbors &Jackson, 1984). We need to find out more about how the social network functions

as a referral system, the types of problems taken to the network, and how informal helpers attempt to resolve these problems (Neighbors & Jackson, 1984).

2. Current family support models may not adequately simulate the cultural patterns of support with which ethnic families may be familiar. Programs may be held in settings outside of ethnic neighborhoods or communities in places where people either feel uncomfortable and therefore either avoid attending or attend infrequently. For example, holding meetings in a mental health agency setting may be stigmatizing for some families.

3. Organizational structure and leadership styles may not be compatible with those experienced in more community settings. For example, some groups may be accustomed to formal structures; others with a more informal, relational style. If Arab family members attended a family support group, for example, in which a woman presided, where children were excluded, food was not served, or prayer not initiated either at the start of or close of the meeting, cultural dissonance might be experienced by these family members. Club Sociales, as another example, are home town clubs in Puerto Rican communities where the organizational structure fulfills multiple functions such as recreation, orientation for individuals new to the community, social services, and employment (Delgado & Humm-Delgado1982). The extent to which the family group is perceived as compatible or incompatible with these functions and needs may affect Latino participation.

4. The content of meetings may not address the needs of ethnic members. Perceived lack of practicality, type of presentation styles, and a business focus rather than a relationship orientation may all be impediments to members from different ethnic communities.

5. Social activities sponsored by a mainstream support group may not always be appreciated by members of a different class or cultural background. For example, a support group fund-raising event featuring cocktails and a night out at the symphony may not appeal to some African American participants with different food and music preferences.

6. Member composition at meetings in which only one or two ethnic family members may be present may contribute to feelings of alienation, intimidation, and isolation. Environments may not be perceived as safe or welcoming to the sharing of the family member's experiences. Perceptions of any incompatibility based on socioeconomic status, lifestyle, or family organization may result in decreased comfortability.

7. Not unlike numerous other institutions within the mainstream culture (e.g., churches, schools, mental health programs, country clubs, and corporations) family support group leaders and members are frequently uncertain and uncomfortable with diversity. They may not have the knowledge or information required to address issues of cultural competence in their group sessions and programs. Training in these areas has been

infrequent, if occurring at all. Programs desirous of change, with little preparation, are often faced with the task, perceived as insurmountable, of creating a milieu supportive of diversity with few existing prototypes or internal/external supports.

8. Ethnic group members may, indeed, be interested in family supports but find themselves in situations with competing survival demands, such as child care, transportation needs, and/or working two or more jobs. Any or all of these may present potential obstacles not addressed by many family support program models.

9. Some ethnic group members may be sensitive to either direct or indirect forms of perceived oppression and discrimination, that is, acts or institutional procedures that may help to create or perpetuate continued advantages of the majority group. There may be a level of mistrust that emanates from prior negative experiences with social systems that is easily projected onto new situations where either intentional or unintentional slights may occur.

10. Mainstream groups may fail to reach out aggressively and innovatively reach out to ethnic families. Many programs do not really know how to access ethnic communities and sometimes are without the time and resources to do so.

BRIDGING CULTURAL GAPS WITH ETHNIC FAMILIES: A MULTIDIMENSIONAL APPROACH

Normative transactions in ethnic families are frequently subject to negative misinterpretation by providers from different cultures (Lefley, 1985). A multidimensional approach to culture is required, which outlines the various contexts that can influence value formation and that can provide a framework for assessment of both shared and different worldviews between the provider and family members. Such an approach can assist providers in synthesizing family value orientations into a "cultural snapshots of each family that can then be contrasted with the provider's own snapshot" (Karrer, 1993). Clarified commonalities can be used as "bridge builders"; differences can be used as opportunities to challenge and help expand views and ways in which to conceptualize cross-cultural impact.

The following multidimensional approach outlines eight separate dimensions. Though each one is important, it may or may not be salient for a given ethnic family (Karrer, 1993). For example, for some families religious values may be more salient; for others, acculturation issues may be predominant. Variations may exist not only across these dimensions but also within each.

Socioenvironmental context. This dimension includes identification of the family's nationality; appraisal of external socioeconomic stressors, barriers, and obstacles to achievement; and the family's relationship and familiarity with mainstream cultural norms useful for accessing required goods and resources.

Kinship network. Identification of both biologically related kin as well as "fictive" kinship relationships (i .e., close friends, babysitters, neighbors, boarding home operators, stepfathers, boyfriends, and grandparents, in addition to members of the "church family," such as ministers and deacons) begins to answer the question, "who is family?" Essentially these kin relationships are potentially each family member's social network system, which can be relied upon for mutual aid or support in times of need or crisis. These persons may live either within the household, the neighborhood, the country of origin, or throughout the United States.

Gathering information on the family's perceptions of their problems, and assessing how decisions are made and problems solved facilitates the engagement process. Randall-David (1989) recommends asking the following questions in order to learn more about family perceptions: "What do you think is your problem?" "What do you think caused your problem?" "What do you think that your sickness does to your body?" "What type of treatment do you think you should receive?"

Perceived gender role responsibilities and expectations must be understood. It should be determined if the gender roles are more traditional or contemporary.

Cultural values and beliefs. The provider attempts to gather information about the attitudes, values, norms, and beliefs which guide the family. Examples are beliefs about illness and wellness; help-seeking values and behaviors (i. e., who the family seeks out when there is an illness); gender roles; attitudes towards caregiving roles and responsibilities; communication styles; and problem-solving and decision-making styles. Interdependence as a family value (i.e., the extent the family holds allegiance to one another and the group) is weighed against the value of individual, personal liberties (Karrer, 1993). Description of religious beliefs, and rites or rituals that may affect family attitudes should also be identified.

Cultural transitions and acculturation. It is important to understand the history of the family and its key transitions from one culture to the next (Jacobsen 1988; Karrer, 1993). Determining factors precipitating these transitions, length of time in this country, and past and present socioeconomic status are all critical in learning more about the family's adaptational and survival styles in adjusting to the mainstream culture.

Language. Linguistic patterns are closely related to ethnicity and culture. Language provides not only a means of communication but also a cognitive structuring of the world which is linked to one's world view, identity, self-concept, and self-esteem. What language does the family utilize in formal and informal situations? Families may be proficient in using a language for less formal, interpersonal encounters, for example, but not in formal family conferences with multiple service providers present. Do family members "conveniently" code switch, that is, possess differential skills in two languages but alternate between them, even within a single sentence? Code switching might occur when family members are under emotional stress and easily revert back to their native language.

Ethnic identity development. How do family members see themselves as members of their own ethnic group? What attitudes about their group membership are manifested? What are the attitudes about self, members from other ethnic groups, as well as members of the mainstream culture? What behaviors are exhibited as a result of how family members define themselves? Do these behaviors allow the family to interact comfortably in different cultural settings? Ethnic identity attitudes may influence the extent to which family members may be comfortable with providers from either the mainstream or other cultures (Helms, 1990). These attitudes may also affect the extent to which members may be able to incorporate themselves into family support groups in which they may be the only representitives of their cultural group.

Mistrust and discriminatory experiences. What has been the family's history and experience with discriminatory events? What are their coping styles? How do they handle their interface with institutions both within and outside of their community? Racism, for example, is a daily social stressor and unless the provider can acknowledge these experiences, he or she may be perceived as a part of just another abusive societal institution.

Regional background. Within cultures, there are wide variations based on geographical regions, living environments, and climate. These variations often affect family lifestyle patterns and values.

For example, in comparison with urban environments, rural settings may tend to be slow-paced and sanction more interpersonal proximity (Karrer, 1993).

APPLYING A MULTICULTURAL LENS: GUIDELINES AND APPROACHES

1. Apply a "cultural lens" to each family. Assume that each family is a unique representation of its culture and be able to describe each family's world view and perceptions.
2. Partner with families. Demonstrate comfort with differences by raising racial or ethnic differences, when appropriate. Ask family members directly how they may feel about working with providers from another cultural background.
3. Demonstrate genuineness and concrete support. Genuine interest in and support of one or more family members will garner respect from other family members.
4. Identify and describe one's own world view and values. Own and share them respectfully and directly with the family, when applicable.
5. Identify the family group's perception of mental illness and help seeking/coping traditions. Attend to the cultural explanations which the family may provide about the mental illness and their experiences in managing the illness. Use the family members' explanations as the framework for engaging them.
6. Use the multidimensional approach previously described to assess points of similarity and differences between one's own world view and that of the family. Use points of contact and similarities to bridge the differences.
7. Assess and support the extended family and social network. Determine the degree to which external provider or agency support may be required or acceptable to the family.
8. Develop a support model for the family that is consistent with its ethnic/cultural style and strengths (Lefley, 1990). An educational, problem-solving model, for example, may be congruent for some Latino families because it does not override the Latino family's authority or undermine the intricate pattern of Hispanic interpersonal relationships (Rivera, 1988). Members of the family system are mobilized to meet their own, self defined needs (Rivera, 1988). At the same time, using egalitarian problem-solving models, not attending to spiritual and religious needs, misinterpreting spiritual beliefs, and assessing the family as "over-involved" with one of its members with mental illness would be culturally incompatible.
9. One of the most widely studied family intervention models, that is, Behavioral Family Therapy (BFT), may be particularly applicable to ethnic families (Falloon, Boyd, & McGill, 1984; Penn & Mueser, 1996). Originally provided on an individual basis, directly in the home, it can easily involve the kinship system, that is, parents, siblings, spouses, other relatives, neighbors, or close friends and the consumer (Mueser, 1996). Family strengths are assessed and the members' understanding of the psychiatric illness is evaluated.

   A combination of home-based and clinic-based sessions have also been found to be successful. The home-based sessions, particularly when offered at the beginning of the intervention sequence may be optimal in facilitating the engagement of ethnic families who might otherwise be labeled as "resistant" (Mueser, 1996). Some ethnic families may view the family home as the appropriate place to care for their member (Guarnaccia et al., 1992).

   BFT is both family and individually goal oriented, with goals tailored to each family and each member. Family members are cast as experts, which could help to reduce potential provider threat. Communication skills training and problem solving methods are concrete, structured approaches taught to families using didactic, experiential, participatory, and/or discussion formats (Mueser, 1996). Disenfranchised, often disempowered families are empowered by the ability to attain goals and solve problems on their own through problem-solving meetings, which might be chaired by a family member with another member playing the role of the secretary.
10. It is frequently assumed that families coping with mental illness are isolated from their support networks so that a new network of families must be created.

Building upon the strengths of the social and cultural matrix within the ethnic community by developing supportive family networks within the family kinship system is another viable alternative.

Family network approaches (Speck & Attneave, 1973), as opposed to building a group of unrelated individuals, builds upon larger family networks which share kinship ties or membership in key community institutions. These networks may serve as innovative strategies for collective problem solving and conflict resolution for rural, Italian American, African American, Latino, Native American as well as numerous other ethnocultural extended family systems (Speck & Attneave, 1973). Families with more ruptured networks could be integrated with other kinship systems and community institutions with more resources for providing support (Guarnaccia et al., 1992). Alternative settings for these meetings would be needed, such as the home, the church, or a well-regarded, neighborhood community center or facility.

DEVELOPING A CULTURALLY SPECIFIC FAMILY SUPPORT GROUP

Providing family support to ethnic families may require different models and approaches, ranging from the offer of no support based on lack of need or family preference to enhancement of an already existing kinship network, outreach and incorporation of ethnic family members into already existing, mainstream programs; or culturally specific homogeneous, multiple family groups where ethnic family members are recruited and assisted in the development of mutual self-help and support. There has been some anecdotal support for the efficacy of such ethnically or culturally specific psychoeducational consumer groups, where members are all from the same cultural group, that is, gender, race, or sexual orientation (Finley, 1978; Merta, 1995; Primm, 1990; Simoni & Perez, 1995). Culturally specific groups may offer participants several advantages: 1) perception of having less conflict; 2) the use of positive cultural identification as the means for facilitating cohesion; 3) providing more support; 4) being better attended; 5) the creation of an environment of safety and protection as a buffer to a perceived hostile environment; and 6) providing more rapid symptom relief than heterogeneous groups (Finley, 1978; Merta, 1995; Simoni & Perez, 1995).

Strategies to be considered in the formation of a "same culture" or culturally specific family support group model, for African Americans or Latino families, for example, might include the following:

- Develop a clear strategy. An example might be to form a partnership with one or more ethnic family members either from an agency or from a mainstream family support group. These persons may be cultural guides or "cultural brokers" to assist in the same-culture group formation.

- Be patient and persist in your efforts. Building trust between provider, institutional systems, and ethnic family members may take time to develop. Structured, active, and directive interventions and greater self-disclosure can assist in the creation of more reciprocal relationships with family members (Simon & Perez, 1995).

- Identify and assess the ethnic/neighborhood network system (e .g. ethnic organizations, botanicas, churches, Club Sociales, sororities, fraternities). Be knowledgeable about the language abilities, acculturation levels, and adherence to traditional ethnic values. Support from community leaders can be instrumental in the successful development of a culturally specific support group model.

- Give talks on mental illness and the needs of persons with severe and persistent mental illness at churches and local community groups. Continue this process for a period of time and then try to establish a long-term relationship with the organization (Pernell-Arnold & Finley, 1992).

- Have a festive open house. Invite members of the community. Integrate culturally relevant celebratory activities, food, and music. Provide games and activities for the entire family.

- Begin a group designed to help families relate to and help their family member in the neighborhood, the church, or the family home (Pernell-Arnold & Finley, 1992). The group focus should be very pragmatic, that is, helping to solve immediate problems of behavior involving the consumer. Off-site consultation would be invaluable. Demonstrate usefulness to the family group, first and foremost. Groups should meet at times most conducive to their members. Language considerations must also be incorporated.

- Be aggressive in outreach to ethnic families. Personally contact family members of consumers served in the agency. Outreach is welcoming. Personal contacts should be made using multiple methods: 1) written contact using official letterhead; 2) culturally sensitive and "catchy" flyers; 3) by phone; and 4) by personal invitation from persons who have rapport with the family (for example, a case manager). Personal invitations should be extended to fathers, mothers, or other adults in the extended kinship system (Boyd-Franklin, 1989; Pernell-Arnold & Finley, 1992; Simoni & Perez, 1995).

- Contact or a friendly "check-in" may be required between each and every meeting. Such contact conveys personal interest and concern, and provides helpfulness with ongoing stressors while also serving as meeting reminders. Engagement of ethnic families may be intensive in its initial stages. Do not be discouraged if initial groups have a lower attendance than desired. If participants enjoy their experiences, if they find the outcomes useful, they will become the nucleus that promotes further development of the group.

- Family needs and obstacles should be anticipated. Tangible assistance may be required, for example, transportation, child care arrangements, clothing for recent immigrants.
- Give out certificates for almost everything (Pernell-Arnold & Finley, 1992), for example, attendance, volunteer activities, and participation in meetings. Family support programs for ethnic members may require built-in achievement mechanisms and recognition opportunities in order to facilitate empowerment. Provide ancillary supports and opportunities for further achievement such as adult basic education or G.E.D. classes, assistance in attending a community college and job training or placement.
- Eventually, ask for volunteers to help staff members lead other groups, speak to other groups, and/or speak with professionals (Pernell-Arnold & Finley, 1992).
- Ask participants if staff member may speak at their church or community organizations (Pernell-Arnold & Finley, 1992).
- Attempt to get a church or community organization to adopt a program, for example, a family day picnic; a talent show; an art show; or a trip to a play, museum, ball game, or park. The organization may either send volunteers or provide financial assistance (Pernell-Arnold & Finley, 1992).
- Train some of the group participants to be group leaders; conduct leadership training sessions. Consider different leadership structures, for example, rotating leadership or election of officers. Be prepared to maintain a coaching or mentoring relationship with the newly emerging leadership.
- Initially, expect greater discretion in disclosure than what might be expected in support groups of middle-class Anglo-Americans (Simon & Perez, 1995). Shame and issues of confidentiality may be major concerns for ethnic participants. Also expect differential participation by members. Persons who do not prefer to engage in discussion should be allowed this option.
- Stress harmonious social relationships. It is advisable to warn family group members that differences of opinion are inevitable and encourage the participants to devise ways to manage them (Simoni & Perez, 1995).
- Survey families. Find out what questions and concerns they may have. Expert guest speakers may come and discuss these topics of interest. The preference for outside "experts," among Latinos, for example, is consistent with cultural emphasis on power differential and value of lineality (Delgado, 1981). Consideration should be given to the cultural diversity of invited speakers.
- Provide information to families regarding how to handle not only situations of discrimination as they interface with the mental health system, but other forms of ethnic or cultural discrimination as well. What have been their experiences? What strategies or advocacy are needed to combat this additional factor?

REFERENCES

Adebimpe, Y. R. (1994). Race, racism and epidemiological surveys. *Hospital and Community Psychiatry, 45,* 27-31.

Alston, R., & Turner,W. (1994). A family strengths model of adjustment to disability for African-American clients. *Journal of Counseling and Development, 72,* 37~382.

Angel, R. J., & Angel, J. (1993). *Painful inheritance: Health and the new generation of fatherless families.* Madison, W1: The University of Wisconsin Press.

Bell, J. (1982). The family in the hospital: Experiences in other countries. In H. Harbin (Ed.), *The psychiatric hospital and the family* (pp. 120-129). New York, NY: Spectrum.

Borkman, T. (1990). Self-help groups at the turning point: Emerging egalitarian alliances with the formal health care system. *American Journal of Community Psychology, 18,* 332.

Boyd-Franklin, N. (1989). *Black families in therapy: A multidisciplinary approach.* New York, NY: Guilford Press.

Brown, G., Birley, J. L. T., & Wing, J. K. (1972). Influence of family life on the course of schizophrenic disorders: A replication. *British Journal of Psychiatry, 121,* 241-258.

Chestang, L. (1972). *Character development in a hostile environment (occasional paper No. 3).* Chicago, Ill: University of Chicago School of Social Administration.

Cook, J., Pickett, S., & Cohler, B. (1997). Families of adults with severe mental illness—The next generation of research: Introduction. *American Journal of Orthopsychiatry, 67*(2), 172-176.

Delgado, M. (1981). Hispanic cultural values: Implications for groups. *Small Group Behavior, 12,* 69-80.

Delgado, M., & Humm-Delgado, D. (1982). Natural support systems: Sourcing strength in Hispanic communities. *Social Work* 83-89.

Devore, W., & Schlesinger, E. (1981). *Ethnic sensitive social work and practice.* St. Louis, MO: C.W. Mosby Company.

Falloon, I. R. H., Boyd, J. L., & McGill, C. W. (1984). *Family care of schizophrenia: A problem-solving approach to the treatment of mental illness.* New York, NY: Guilford Press.

Finley, L. (1978). The black experience group: A therapeutic activity model for the black schizophrenic. In American Personnel & Guidance Association (Ed.), *Innovations in counseling services* (pp165-171), Washington, DC: American Personnel and Guidance Association.

Finley, L. (1997). The multiple effects of culture and ethnicity on psychiatric disability. In L. Spaniol, C. Gagne, & M. Koehler (Eds.), *Psychological and social aspects of psychiatric disability* (pp. 497-510). Boston, MA: Center for Psychiatric Rehabilitation, Sargent College of Health and Rehabilitation Sciences.

Griffith, E. E. H., Young, J. L., & Smith, D. L. (1984). An analyses of the therapeutic elements in a black church service. *Hospital and Community Psychiatry, 35,* 46-469.

Guarnaccia, P., Parra, P., Deschamps, A., Milstein, G., & Argiles, N. (1992). Si Dios queiere: Hispanic families' experiences of caring for a seriously mentally ill family member. *Culture Medicine and Psychiatry, 16,* 187-215.

Helms, J. E. (1990). *Black and white racial identity: Theory, research and practice.* Westport, CT: Greenwood Press.

Higginbotham, H. N. (1979). *Delivery of mental health services in three developing Asian nations: Feasibility and cultural sensitivity of "modern psychiatry."* Unpublished doctoral dissertation, University of Hawaii.

Ho, M. K (1987). *Family Therapy with Ethnic Minorities.* Beverly Hills, CA: SAGE Publications.

Horwitz A., & Reinhard, S. (1995). Ethnic differences in caregiving duties and burdens among parents and siblings of persons with severe mental illnesses. *Journal of Health and Social Behavior, 36,* 138-150.

Jacobson, F. M. (1988). Ethnocultural assessment. In L. Comas-Diaz, & E. E. H. Griffith, (Eds.), *Clinical guidelines in cross cultural mental health* (pp. 135-147). New York, NY: John Fey.

Karrer, B.M. (1993). The importance of understanding the cultural dimensions when treating adolescents and their families. In W. Snyder & T. Osmond (Eds.), *Empowering families: Helping adolescents* (pp. 59-70). Publication developed by contract from the Office of Treatment Improvement of the Alcohol, Drug Abuse and Mental Health Administration, Rochelle, Minn.

Kleinman, A., & Good, B. (Eds.) (1985). *Culture and depression.* Berkley, CA: University of California Press.

Leff, J., & Vaughn, C. (1985). *Expressed emotion in families: Its significance for mental illness.* New York, NY: Guilford Press.

Lefley, H. P (1985). Families of the mentally ill in cross cultural perspective. *Psychosocial Rehabilitation Journal, 8,* 57-75.

Lefley, H. P. (1987). Culture and mental illness: The family role. In A. B. Hatfield and H. P Lefley (Eds.), *Families of the mentally ill: Coping and adaptation* (pp. 30-59). New York, NY: Guilford Press.

Lefley, H. P (1990). Culture and chronic mental illness. *Hospital and Community Psychiatry, 41*(3), 277-286.

Lefley, H. P. (1992) Expressed emotion; conceptual, clinical and social policy issues. *Hospital and Community Psychiatry, 43*(6), 591-598.

McGoldrick, M., Pearce, J., & Giordano, J. (Eds.) (1982). *Ethnicity and family therapy.* New York, NY: Guilford Press.

McGoldrick, M., Giordano, J., & Pearce, J. (Eds.) (1996). *Ethnicity and family therapy* (2nd Edition). New York, NY: Guilford Press.

Merta, R. (1995). Groupwork. In J. Ponterotto, J. Casas, L. Suzuki, & C. Alexander, (Eds.), *Handbook of multicultural counseling* (pp. 567-585). Thousand Oaks, CA: SAGE.

Mintzer, J. E., & Macera, C. A. (1992). Prevalence of depressive symptoms among white and African-American caregivers of demented patients. *American Journal of Psychiatry, 149*(4), 575-576.

Mirowsky, J. (1985). Disorder and its context: Paranoid beliefs as thematic elements of thought problems, hallucinations and delusions under threatening social conditions. *Research in Community and Mental Health, 5,* 185-204.

Mueser, K. (1996). Helping families manage severe mental illness. *Psychiatric Rehabilitation Skills, 1*(2), 21-42.

Neighbors, H., & Jackson, J. (1984). The use of informal and formal help: Four patterns of illness behavior in the black community. *American Journal of Community Psychology, 12*(6), 629-644.

Penn, D. L. & Mueser, K. T. (1996). Research update on the psychosocial treatment of schizophrenia. *American Journal of Psychiatry, 15,* 607-617.

Pernell-Arnold, A. & Finley, L. (1992). *Psychosocial rehabilitation services in action: Principles and strategies that result in rehabilitation* (Contract Bid # P09-07-09-92-DP). Columbia, S.C.: South Carolina Department of Mental Health.

Pickett, S., Damian, A., Vraniak, D., Cook, J., & Cohler J. (1993). Strength in adversity: Blacks bear burden better than whites. *Professional Psychology: Research and Practice, 24*(4), 460~67.

Pierce, C. (1970). Offensive mechanisms. In F. Barbour (Ed.), *The black seventies* (pp. 265-282). Boston, MA: Sargent.

Pinderhughes, E. (1982). Afro-American families and the victim system. In M. McGoldrick, J. Pearce, & J. Giordano (Eds.), *Ethnicity and family therapy* (pp. 108-122). New York: Guilford Press.

Primm, A. M. (1990, February). Group psychotherapy can raise self-esteem in mentally ill black men. *The Psychiatric Times: Medicine and Behavior,* 24-25.

Randall-David, E. (1989). *Strategies for working with culturally diverse communities and clients* (Report No. MCH 113793). Washington, DC: The Association for the Case of Children's Health.

Rivera, C. (1988). Culturally sensitive aftercare services for chronically mentally ill. Hispanics: the case of the psychoeducational treatment model. *Fordham University Hispanic Research Center Research Bulletin, 11,* 16-25.

Sartorius, N., Jablensky, I., & Korten, A. (1986). Early manifestations and first contact incidence of schizophrenia in different cultures. *Psychological Medicine, 16,* 909-928.

Simoni, J., & Perez, L. (1995). Latinos and mutual support groups: A case for considering culture. *American Journal of Ortbopsychiatry, 65*(3), 440-445.

Solomon, P. (1988). Racial factors in mental health service utilization. *Psychosocial Rehabilitation Journal, 11,* 3-12.

Spaniol, L., & Zipple, A. (1988). Family and professional perceptions of family needs and coping strengths. *Rehabilitation Psychology, 33,* 37-45.

Speck, R., & Attneave, C. (1973). *Family networks.* New York, NY: Vintage Books.

Stevenson, H., & Renard, G. (1993). Toasting ole' wise owls: Therapeutic use of cultural strengths in African-American families. *Professional Psychology: Research and Practice, 24*(4), 433-442.

Stueve, A., Vine, P., & Struening, E. (1997). Perceived burden among caregivers of adults with serious mental illness: Comparison of black, Hispanic and white families. *American Journal of Orthopsychiatry, 67*(2), 199-209.

Szapocznik J., & Kurtines, W. (1993). Family psychology and cultural diversity: Opportunities for theory, research and application. *Journal of the American Psychological Association, 48*(4), 400-407.

Ulbrich, P., Warheit, G., & Zimmerman, R. (1989). Race, socio-economic status and psychological distress: An examination of differential vulnerability. *Journal of Heath and Social Behavior, 30,* 131-146.

Vaughn, C., & Leff, J. (1976). The measurement of expressed emotion in families of psychiatric patients. *British Journal of Social Clinical Psychology, 15,* 157-165.

Waxler N. E. (1979). Is outcome for schizophrenia better in non-industrial societies? The case of Sri Lanka. *Journal of Nervous and Mental Diseases, 167,* 144-158.

CHAPTER FIFTY-TWO

Grief Therapy for Relatives of Persons With Serious Mental Illness

Frederick E. Miller

This chapter was previously published in Psychiatric Services, 47, 633-637. Copyright © 1996, the American Psychiatric Association.

The stress experienced by relatives of persons with serious mental illness is often attributed to objective burdens such as demands on relatives' time or financial resources, and to subjective burdens encompassing a range of emotional responses to the occurrence of mental illness. Frequently noted among the latter is a powerful sense of loss and grief.

As McElroy[1] has stated, "Tremendous psychological loss and grief are experienced by families of the seriously mentally ill. The cyclical nature of some of the psychiatric illnesses and the periodic reappearance of the 'former self' creates prolonged periods of grieving...families of the mentally ill cope with this unsanctioned form of grief daily." Anthony[2] has commented on the chronic sense of loss and alienation among children of severely mentally ill parents. The child may experience "a sense of abandonment associated at times with strong separation anxiety. The parent has become withdrawn, remote, inaccessible, and unresponsive." The principal component of this sense of loss is unutterable feelings of grief for the parent "who is there but not there."

In a study of grief and bereavement among relatives of persons with serious mental illness, results obtained using the Mental Illness Version of the Texas Inventory of Grief suggested that fairly profound levels of grief may persist in relatives of patients with schizophrenia or bipolar illness years after the diagnosis was first made.[3] Among the reasons speculated for such protracted grief was the difficulty some relatives had in identifying and openly talking about their loss either because of the stigma of mental illness or because of the abstract nature of "psychic loss" in which the person lives on but the relationship changes profoundly.

It appears also that contemporary approaches to working with families of persons with serious mental illness have stressed instrumental learning such as improved communication and problem-solving skills.[4-10] Although the sharing that takes place in formats such as multiple family groups may provide some avenues for dealing with relatives' grief, specific interventions focusing on grief and bereavement have been lacking.

This chapter describes a family intervention centering on the issue of grief. The intervention is based on an adaptation of Worden's four tasks[11] of grief therapy: making the loss real, facilitating the expression of overt and latent affect, helping survivors live without the deceased, and facilitating emotional withdrawal from the deceased. The grief addressed in the intervention for relatives of persons with serious mental illness results from the loss of specific hopes and aspirations rather than loss through death. In this intervention, Worden's latter two tasks are transformed into "accommodations to the loss via relationships outside that with the mentally ill relative" and "accommodations to the loss via the relationship with the mentally ill relative."

In practice, the therapy is divided into two phases. Phase 1 focuses on the process of reminiscence, and phase 2 focuses of the process of readjustment to the loss. Specific tasks to be targeted in each phase are outlined below and illustrated with case vignettes. As has been amply noted, the process of grieving often does not conform to a neat succession of discontinuous phases. Thus the clinician must consider what follows as guidelines rather than a rigidly structured sequence.

Consistent with other forms of dynamically based grief therapy, treatment is usually short term, often consisting of about ten weekly sessions, each lasting an hour to an hour and a half. Therapy may take place in an individual format or in small groups with no more than four members.

GRIEF THERAPY TECHNIQUE

Phase 1: Reminiscence

In this phase, relatives are encouraged to "tell the story" of their relationship with the mentally ill person. The therapist acts as a guide in this process, helping the client focus on the history of the relationship rather than on current problems such as securing housing for the patient or finding the right doctor. Addressing current problems is deferred with statements such as, "Perhaps once we've gone through this process you will have a new frame within which to decide the best course of action for you." To encourage the retrospective nature of the story, the therapist may suggest that the client bring in photographs or other memorabilia associated with the early years of his or her relationship with the mentally ill person. While listening to the client, the therapist endeavors to facilitate the two tasks encompassed by this phase making the loss real and encouraging the expression of overt and latent affect.

Task 1: making the loss real. In cases of acute grief in reaction to the death of another, the need to make the loss real pertains to the catastrophic, overwhelming nature of death and the client's need for denial until he or she is ready to begin to take it all in. However, in instances of "psychic loss" —that is, situations in which the individual remains alive but the relationship is profoundly altered as in cases of divorce, separation, or illness—the sense that the loss is unreal is fostered by its insidious and often cyclical nature.[12] Relatives of persons with severe mental illness often perceive glimmers of the ill person's former self, which renews hopes for a cure and denial of the illness.

The abstract or elusive nature of the loss is described by Terkelsen[13] in his reference to the loss of the "idealized internal image" of the mentally ill person. With this image, the relative loses hopes and aspirations, which are mourned. As Terkelsen wrote, "Quite naturally, as in any family, parents, siblings, grandparents dream of the future that is implied by these future projections. Then, as the illness and its effect on the future that is realistically attainable becomes evident, some of these dreams of the affected person's future, these future part-images, come under siege."

This abstract quality may relate to the specific condition of grieving for someone who is alive but afflicted by a disease that drastically alters the person's selfhood.[1] In addition, in cases of mental illness, relationships are often cut short. Children may become ill before developing adult personalities, and parents may become ill before their children grow up and can relate to them as adults. Thus the client's mourning is mainly in the conscious or not-so-conscious realm of "If only she and I had..." and "What if we had...?"

As in other forms of dynamic grief therapy, the therapist must listen intently as the client relates his or her story for specific meanings of the loss.[14] We all have private hopes or fantasies of what specific relationships may provide. For example, a child may offer parents the hope of working through their own childhood disappointments. A child or sibling may remind the client of some other relative whom the client loves and misses.

The therapist should attempt to achieve a dynamic understanding of the loss and avoid nonspecific statements, such as "You must really miss the way your son used to be," which often derail the flow of reminiscence. It is important that the reminiscence phase is not restricted, because it not only encourages catharsis but also allows the therapist and client to specify the "problem" of loss, as illustrated in the following case vignette, so that possible solutions will be much more forthcoming in phase 2, which involves adjusting to the loss.

Mrs. Z is a 54-year-old woman whose 27-year-old son, Tony, has been ill with schizophrenia and compulsive water intoxication. For Mrs. Z. the loss associated with her son's illness is doubly tragic given that her mother was also seriously mentally ill and frequently absent throughout her youth during periods of hospitalization. As Mrs. Z recounted her early relationship with Tony, she spoke with great pride about how well she had taken care of him, remembering, for example, sewing his costumes each Halloween.

As time passed, the therapist felt secure in suggesting to Mrs. Z that as Tony became ill, it became less and less possible for her to see herself as an accomplished caregiver, despite the reality of her many efforts. In taking care of Tony, Mrs. Z herself felt taken care of and in the presence of a mother. Thus her sense of loss entailed again finding herself with no one to take care of her.

Mrs. Z responded affirmatively to this interpretation, stating that she wished that there was some way for her to feel the way she had during the "good years." By identifying this specific aspect of her loss—a diminished sense of competency as a caregiver— Mrs. Z was able to participate readily in phase 2, in which striving to find accommodations to her loss was the focus.

Task 2: encouraging expression of overt and latent affect, Many affects, including sadness, anger, guilt, anxiety, loneliness, helplessness, and relief, occur as part of a normal acute grieving process.[15] Many such emotions are manifest also in instances of psychic loss, including the sense of alienation felt by some children of psychotically ill parents or the chronic sorrow experienced by parents of developmentally disabled children.[16]

A key task in grief therapy is helping the client to emote and to begin to feel comfortable with emotions that he or she may initially find unacceptable. Although I have noticed a wide range of affects among clients who are relatives of persons with serious mental illness, I have been particularly impressed by recurring themes of anger associated with feeling abandoned and of survivor guilt, particularly among siblings of mentally ill person, examples of which are included in the following case vignette.

Mr. D is a 35-year-old man whose 37-year-old brother has been continuously ill with symptoms of schizophrenia since early adolescence. As therapy began, he focused on his anger over how he felt his parents had mismanaged his brother's care. Mr. D related that he had distanced himself greatly from his parents because of this anger, holding his parents responsible for his brother's illness and the lack of a close-knit family.

The therapist listened patiently to Mr. D's expression of disappointment and anger for the first two sessions. As Mr. D began to feel comfortable with the therapist, however, the therapist opened the door for a later discussion of latent affects by gently questioning whether or not the anger might serve to obscure other buried emotions.

Later, as Mr. D became engaged in the reminiscence phase, he began to reflect on an almost forgotten time during early childhood in which he and his brother were extremely close "almost like twins."

The therapist, continuing to explore the hypothesis that Mr. D was experiencing strong latent affect, encouraged him to spend some time talking about how losing this close relationship had affected his life. He responded with a torrent of emotion: "I've felt all alone, somehow incomplete."

With the emergence of these feelings of loneliness and his engagement in the mourning process, Mr. D's anger appeared to recede. With this change, his attitude toward his parents softened, and he realized that his sense of disconnectedness derived more from the tragic loss of his expected relationship with his brother than from any specific negligence on the part of his parents.

Phase 2: Readjustment to Loss

In this phase, the goals are to help the client find ways of accommodating to the loss that was articulated in phase 1. Thus this phase is greatly facilitated by the specificity with which unmet needs have been identified. A problem-solving approach is used to engage clients and to encourage them to consider all possible ways of meeting the unmet needs that derive from the losses that relate to the profound changes in their relationship with their mentally ill relative. In this process, the therapist helps the client to avoid premature closure or editorializing before generating a thorough list of solutions.

Task 3: accommodating to the loss through relationships with others. The heart of this task is to use the blueprint created in phase 1, which details the specific nature of the loss and the affects connected with it, to build a plan for beginning to fill the void through relationships other than that with the mentally ill relative. Relatives of persons with severe mental illness tend to seal over the loss by denying their emotional needs in many relationships, not just in the relationship with the mentally ill person. Anthony[2] noted that children of a mentally ill parent may feel not just distant from that parent but generally alienated from people. Others have noted that siblings of persons with serious mental illness may feel survivor guilt not just in the presence of their ill relative but among other people as well.[17]

The therapist and client may begin this task by examining whether the loss has somehow been generalized to other relationships. For example, the therapist may ask, "Given that you have missed the closeness you once had with your son, I'm wondering whether you have gotten all the closeness that you could in other relationships and, if not, whether you have thoughts about how to get more of this feeling with other people." The following case vignette shows how the therapist and client can work on this task.

Ms. O is a 45 year-old divorced woman whose son, Tom, in his early twenties, has been ill with a complex disorder including attention deficit disorder with hyperactivity, atypical psychosis, and polysubstance abuse that first manifested when he was ten years old. Before coming for grief therapy, Ms. O had participated in a psychoeducation group. She came to grief therapy feeling that she was somehow "stuck" in her relationship with her son.

Life for Ms. O revolved around her son's problems and treatment, and she described a pattern in which she engaged, seemingly indefatigably, in activity directed toward finding him the right program or medication, all while he remained demanding of her and yet indifferent toward being active in treatment. In the reminiscence phase, Ms. O began to work through initial feelings of hostility toward her son and then her expressions of guilt. It appeared as if her son indeed fostered this sense of guilt through his expressions of neediness. However, the guilt seemed largely rooted in her sense of tragedy about her son's life, and it also contributed to the whirlwind of activity. As Ms. O reminisced, she was able to describe another side of her son—a charismatic and gregarious side that she dearly missed.

The therapist validated Ms. O's need for intensity and liveliness in her life. He explored with her alternative ways of meeting these needs, which were not fully met by the activity related to Tom's illness. True to her assertive nature, Ms. O replied, "How about a cruise? I've never taken one."

By the next session, Ms. O had booked herself on a cruise. On her return she announced that she had met a man and went on to describe with delight rekindled emotions and optimism for her future.

Task 4: accommodating to the loss through the relationship with the mentally ill person. This task diverges most from Worden's fourth task for persons who are mourning the death of someone close to them. Worden's fourth task involves detaching from the deceased and may include actually saying "goodbye" to the deceased. In contrast, in grief therapy for relatives of persons with severe mental illness, clients are assisted in detaching from an old form of relationship with their ill relative, which is often based on the relative's being regressed, passive, or oppositional, and in embracing a new way of relating. Rather than saying "goodbye," the client is helped to say "hello" to the healthy partial self that exists in all mentally ill persons.

Many relatives entering grief therapy appear to be resigned to the idea that they can never expect much emotional sustenance from their ill relative. Many believe that the relationship will necessarily be lopsided and that they will be required to make an enormous emotional investment and get little in return from the ill person. Parents of seriously mentally ill adult children often lament feelings of being stuck in a role of perpetually caring for a young child.[18] Siblings often relate feelings of resentment that they have no one with whom to share their life experiences. Clients report that they rarely share with their mentally ill relative their own worries or hopes, apart from those directly relating to the care of the ill relative.

A primary goal in this task is to help the client embrace the idea that all mentally ill persons still have a healthy aspect, or partial self. For some clients, particularly those with frequent contact with their ill relative, this task involves helping them make an alliance with their relative's healthy partial self, with the goal of achieving a greater degree of reciprocity or complementarity.[15] Other clients simply may need a readjustment in the way they think of their ill relative, as the following vignette illustrates.

Mr. B. a 35-year-old graduate student, had lost almost all contact with his older brother, who was ill with paranoid schizophrenia and was homeless somewhere in New York City. Like Mr. D, whose case was described above, Mr. B remembered with great fondness the early years with his brother, sharing a room, at times staying up late together and listening to the radio. Mr. B's father was an alcoholic with a volatile temper who left the family when Mr. B was five years old. However, in the presence of his older brother, Mr. B felt safe and cared for. With the onset of the illness, however, Mr. B's brother began to reject him, and over time they became estranged and bitter toward one another.

Mr. B described early on in grief therapy the pain of this separation, saying, "It's like I lost two parents." He felt that he had been meandering through life, perpetually pursuing his degree while working odd jobs. He seemed resigned to his loss. "That's the painful part of grief," he said. "You can't replace what's lost." But as therapy progressed through task 3, he began to feel that it was possible to fill at least some of that void, and he seemed challenged by the prospect of finding a mentor to guide him in finishing his thesis.

About a year before beginning therapy, Mr. B had learned from a family friend the whereabouts of his brother. During task 2 of grief therapy, the therapist wondered aloud about a parallel between Mr. B's feeling lost and adrift and his brothers being hard to locate or lost. This suggestion occasioned a rich discussion in which Mr. B was able to begin to work through his feelings about somehow needing a "presence" of his brother in his life. Mr. B began to feel that if eventually he was able to be of assistance to his brother even if from a great distance it would help Mr. B himself to rekindle the sense that one person could play a role in guiding another person's life.

Mr. B was enormously hesitant to risk rejection by his brother, feeling that direct contact at this point was premature. He did feel ready to have the friend deliver a note to let his brother know that he still cared about him and was available to meet sometime in the future.

DISCUSSION AND CONCLUSIONS

The case materials presented here suggest that grief therapy may be effective for some relatives of persons with serious mental illness. It is noteworthy that most of the clients in these cases previously participated in other interventions for relatives of mentally ill persons including psychoeducation and support groups. Each client felt that the opportunity to specifically address feelings of loss complemented the gains made in the other therapies. For many clients grief therapy appeared to enrich their relationship with their mentally ill relative perhaps by helping them to overcome the defenses of denial and intellectualization that had buffered the acute pain of loss.

Other investigators have commented on family members resistance to participating in interventions designed to address their relationship with their mentally ill relative.[19] Most such interventions use a coping or rehabilitative model in which clients must accept the limitations imposed by their relative's illness and find optimal modes of adaptation. However, such acceptance would he hampered if not impossible for family members who have not been given the opportunity to truly mourn the losses associated with having a mentally ill relative. Indeed, rather than facilitating the reminiscence inherent in the grieving process, mental health professionals often become frustrated with patients' relatives, feeling that they are living in the past and need to make the best of the present. Perhaps the guidelines presented here will suggest more productive ways for mental health professionals to engage such "resistant" families.

Given the lack of a control group and the small number of subjects included in the cases, conclusions about the overall efficacy of grief therapy for relatives of persons with serious mental illness cannot be made. Future large-scale, randomized studies that will use the Mental Illness Version of the Texas Inventory of Grief to evaluate the efficacy of this grief therapy approach are planned. The possibility that grief therapy may complement or augment the gains from a psychoeducational approach will also be investigated.

Individual grief therapy appears to afford clients a greater opportunity to tell their own stories and to engage the therapist directly, and group grief therapy allows clients to associate their losses with those experienced by the other group members. Further comparisons of the individual and group formats are needed.

REFERENCES

1. McElroy, E. (1987). The beat of a different drummer. In A. B. Hatfield & H. P. Lefley (Eds.), *Families of the mentally Ill: Coping and adaptation*. New York, NY: Guilford.

2. Anthony, E. (1973). Mourning and psychic loss of the parent. In E. Anthony (Ed.), *The child and his family*. New York, NY: Wiley.

3. Miller, F. E., Dworkin, J., Ward, M., et al. (1990). A preliminary study of unresolved grief in families of seriously mentally ill patients. *Hospital and Community Psychiatry, 41,* 1321-1325.

4. Canive, J. M., Sanz-Fuentenebro, J., Tuason, V. B., et al. (1993). Psychoeducation in Spain. *Hospital and Community Psychiatry, 44,* 679-681.

5. McFarlane, W. R., Dunne, E., Lukens, E., et al. (1993). From research to clinical practice: Disseminition of New York State's family psychoeducation project. *Hospital and Community Psychiatry, 44,* 265-270.

6. Goldstein, M. J. (1992). Psychosocial strategies for maximizing the effects of psychotropic medication for schizophrenia and mood disorders. *Psychopharmacology Bulletin, 28,* 237-240.

7. Ranz, J. M., Horen, B. T., McFarlane, W. T., et al. (1991). Creating a supportive environment using staff psychoeducation in a supervised residence. *Hospital and Community Psychiatry, 42,* 1154-1159.

8. Hogarty, G. E., Anderson, C. M., Reiss, D. J., et al. (1991). Family psychoeducation, social skills training, and maintenance chemotherapy in the after-care treatment of schizophrenia: II. two-year effects of a controlled study on relapse and adjustment: Environmental-Personal Indicators in the Course of Schizophrenia (EPICS) research group. *Archives of General Psychiatry, 48,* 340-347.

9. Spencer, J. H., Glick, I. D., Haas, G. L., et al. (1988). A randomized clinical trial of in-patient family intervention, III: effects at six-month and 18-month follow-ups. *American Journal of Psychiatry, 143,* 1115-1121.

10. Greenberg, L., Fine, S. B., Cohen, C., et al. (1988/2000). An interdisciplinary psychoeducation program for schizophrenic patients and their families in an acute care setting. *Hospital and Community Psychiatry, 39,* 277-282.

11. Worden, J. W. (1982). *Grief counseling and grief therapy: A handbook for the mental health practitioner.* New York, NY: Springer.

12. Burke, M. L., Hainsworth, M. A., Eakes, G. G., et al. (1992). Current knowledge and research on chronic sorrow: A foundation for inquiry. *Death Studies, 16,* 231-245.

13. Terkelsen, K. G. (1987). The evolution of families' responses to mental illness through time. In A. B. Hatfield & H. P. Lefley (Eds.), *Families of the mentally ill: Coping and adaptation.* New York, NY: Guilford.

14. Piper, W. E., McCallum, M., & Azim, H. F. A. (1992). *Adaptation to loss through short-term group psychotherapy.* New York, NY: Guilford.

15. Raphael, B. (1983). *The anatomy of bereavement.* New York, NY: Basic Books.

16. Olshansky, S. (1962). Chronic sorrow: A response to having a mentally defective child. *Social Casework 43,* 191-193.

17. Moorman, M. (1992). *My sister's keeper. Learning to cope with a sibling's mental illness.* New York, NY: Norton.

18. Pickett, S., Cook, J., & Cohler, B. (1994). Caregiving burden experienced by parents of offspring with severe mental illness: the impact of off-timedness. *Journal of Applied Social Sciences 18,* 199 207.

19. Anderson, C. M. (1977). Family intervention with severely disturbed in-patients. *Archives of General Psychiatry 34,* 697-702.

CHAPTER FIFTY-THREE

Principles of Professional and Family Collaboration

Kayla F. Bernheim

This chapter was previously published in Hospital and Community Psychiatry, 41, *1353-1355. Copyright © 1990, the American Psychiatric Association.*

The past decade has witnessed a tremendous resurgence of interest in working with families of chronically mentally ill persons. This interest has been spurred by several factors, including deinstitutionalization; documentation of the enormous emotional, financial, and interpersonal impact of an individual's serious mental illness on family life;[1-3] and the demonstrated effectiveness of psychoeducational interventions in reducing relapsed recidivism rates of some (most schizophrenic) patients.[4-6] Widespread critical reevaluation of theories about the family's role in the etiology of major psychiatric disorders has resulted in the suggestion that the conceptual framework of "coping and adaptation" should replace that of "family pathogenesis" as the basis for clinicians' approach to families.[7]

While, on the whole, the professional community is moving toward greater empathy for and cooperation with patients' relatives, there are still pitfalls ahead. Consider, for example, the frequently exhibited "we-do-that" syndrome. When asked whether an agency works with patients' relatives, the director answers, "Of course, we do that! We provide six sessions of psychoeducation." Are family members invited to treatment planning sessions? "Well, no." Do you have a family advisory committee?. "No." A mechanism for relatives to communicate grievances? "No." Do your psychiatrists regularly check with relatives before changing patients' medications? "I don't know." Have staff members been trained to understand family burden and family coping? "Not formally, no."

Genuine collaboration with families is widely advocated in principle, but elusive in practice. Each of the following eight generic principles is a necessary component of a comprehensive approach to family involvement in the care of chronic mentally ill patients.

Principle 1: View relatives who desire to participate as empowered members of the caregiving network. The experiences of relatives and, indeed, of consumers themselves have long been discounted and are only now being taken seriously by mental health professionals. However, family members may have expertise in identifying behavioral signs of impending decompensation, specifying situations that are likely to prove stressful to their ill relative, remembering which medications have been most or least helpful, and describing the likely impact of various behavioral and social interventions.

Family members have knowledge that may be otherwise inaccessible to clinicians about who the patient is as a person and what his (or her) temperamental style, needs, aspirations, values, and interests are. A coherent history of the patient's illness and treatment can rarely be obtained from a stack of discharge summaries. Rather than begin treatment de novo at each decompensation, good care requires continuity that can be immeasurably enhanced by adding families' expertise to that of clinicians'.

Principle 1 also implies mutual decision making. Here again, both patients and families have, until recently, been disenfranchised. Assuming that the patient consents, both formal and informal strategies for involving relatives in planning can be used. While some relatives may wish to be present at formal treatment planning sessions, others may prefer meeting with a single staff member before or after such sessions. Some may wish to be involved only at points of transition or trouble, while others may prefer regular contact.

A prerequisite for implementation of principle I is mutual respect. Insofar as clinicians' thinking about families is still framed in pejorative language that includes such concepts as dysfunctional family systems, overprotective mothers, double binds, communication deviance, sabotage, denial, infantilizing, and high expressed-emotion family, we will be unable to engage in genuine collaboration.

Principle 2: Provide adequate orientation. The mental health system, which is often complex, arcane, and jargon filled, presents a formidable barrier to (a family's) successful adaptation to the mental illness of a relative. Family members are likely to interact with multiple providers from many different agencies simultaneously. Inadequate orientation often causes or contributes to friction between staff, patient, and family members.

Each agency or service provider has the obligation to help the patient and family understand its own particular functions, roles, and rules. They should be explained both face to face and in writing (for reference at a later time). After orientation, family members should understand how the agency fits into the overall rehabilitation plan, should know the names and roles of each of the relevant staff members, and should be aware of the conditions under which the patient would be terminated or transferred from the agency's care. In addition, relatives should recognize ways they can be involved in the patient's rehabilitation plan and should be able to identify the mechanisms available for ongoing information exchange between staff and family.

Principle 3: Provide multiple channels for communication. Both formal and informal mechanisms for exchanging information are desirable. Such mechanisms include regular phone calls inviting relatives to treatment or rehabilitation planning sessions, a newsletter, a family grievance procedure. a family advisory group, and social gatherings for patients, relatives, and staff.

Principle 4: Aim services towards reducing family burden. Psychoeducational programs described in the literature have generally been based on the theoretical construct of "expressed emotion" as a presumed causal factor in psychotic relapse. This construct has come under significant criticism.[8]

Within the alternative framework of coping and adaptation, it is common sense to provide services designed to reduce family burden. Doing so would be expected to decrease the level of stress and tension within the family, to the benefit of all members. Such services include a combination of emotional support, information, education, advice, skills training, crisis intervention, respite care, and case management. In addition, family members' sense of isolation could be decreased by bringing them together with others in a similar situation through referral to local Alliance for the Mentally Ill support and advocacy groups.

Principle 5: Develop individualized service plans. Numerous intra- and interfamilial differences contribute to the need for an individualized approach to families. Cultural background, educational level, density of social networks, preference for group versus individual services, previous experience with mental illness, and each relative's own typical responses to hardship and grief are just a few of the variables that must be considered in designing services.[9] Patients' parents are likely to require different services than patients' siblings or children.

Clearly, a variety of services must be provided in each locality. However, agencies within a given region can cooperate to provide a range of services rather than duplicating services within each agency. The service plan for each family should be developed in the context of an initial consultation phase in which relatives and staff can make a joint assessment of the family's needs and wishes.[10]

Principle 6: Respond flexibly to changing needs over time. Just as treatment plans are reviewed regularly, plans for family involvement should also be updated. This activity requires mechanisms for obtaining feedback about the family's perceptions and wishes. With respect to individual cases, informal mechanisms can be used. They include regularly reviewing relatives' goals and objectives and asking participants at the end of an hour's consultation or a psychoeducational session whether the time seemed well spent. Other, more formal consumer satisfaction measures, such as surveys and questionnaires, can also be used.

Principle 7: Involve family representatives in systemic planning and oversight. Family advocacy constitutes a healthy redirection of (the) relatives' wish to be useful and provides the professional community with a rich source of energy and insight. Only from consumers and their families can clinicians learn how the system meets, or fails to meet, the subjective needs of those it is meant to serve.

Mental health professionals who are also consumers or relatives of consumers can be particularly valuable in bridging the gap between principles of autonomy and consumerism and those of professional care and treatment. Efforts to recruit and train these professionals should be a priority systemic family involvement, and like individual family involvement, should be reevaluated regularly and modified as needed.

Principle 8. Make an ongoing commitment to staff training, consultation, and support. Collaboration with families of patients is a relatively new concept. Many staff have been trained in models of family pathogenesis that are antithetical to these new ways of working. Their professional identities and skills are tied to those models. They may feel threatened, frightened, and angry about families' newfound assertiveness and (be) unable or unwilling to develop a working alliance with patients' relatives.

Collaboration raises some new issues for staff, including concerns about how confidentiality principles should be interpreted, particularly when relatives function as caregivers. Other issues include shifting of priorities to accommodate family work when time and money are limited and management of loyalty conflicts when families are active participants in treatment.

Clearly, staff who feel inadequately skilled and anxious cannot be instructed successfully to work with families. Staff will initially require sensitization to the needs of families, updates on new theoretical models, and skills training, followed by regular supervision and case consultation in responding to families' needs. The period of transition to greater cooperation with families can be expected to last a year or more. Procedures for orienting new staff should be revised to include a module on family-professional collaboration as it is enacted in the particular agency or system the new staff are entering.

CONCLUSIONS

Family-professional collaboration is currently in vogue. Clinicians are struggling to bring down old barriers to collaboration and experimenting with new ways of relating to patients' relatives. To prevent a return to business as usual when initial enthusiasm has passed and to avert hesitation at the threshold of real partnership, a thoughtful systemic approach to change is needed. It is hoped that the principles offered here will encourage such an approach.

REFERENCES

1. Hatfield, A. B. (1978). Psychological costs of schizophrenia to the family. *Social Work, 23,* 355-359.

2. Lefley, H. P. (1987). Aging parents as caregivers of mortally ill adult children: an emerging social problem. *Hospital and Community Psychiatry, 38,* 1083-1089.

3. Francell, C. G., Conn, V. S., & Gray, D. P. (1988). Families' perceptions of burden of care for chronic mentally ill relatives. *Hospital and Community Psychiatry, 39,* 1298-1300.

4. Leff, J., Kuipers, L., Berkowitz, R., et al. (1982). A controlled trial of social intervention in the families of schizophrenic patients. *British Journal of Psychiatry 1*(41), 121-134.

5. Falloon, I. R. H., Boyd, J. L., McGill, C. W., et al. (1985). Family management in the prevention of morbidity of schizophrenia: Clinical outcome of a two-year longitudinal study. *Archives of General Psychiatry, 42,* 887-896.

6. Anderson, C. M., Reiss, D. J., & Hogarty, G. E. (1988). *Schizophrenia and the family.* New York, NY: Guilford.

7. Hatfield, A. B. & Lefley, H. P. (1987). *Families of the mentally ill: Coping and adaptation.* New York, NY: Guilford.

8. Kanter, J., Lamb, H. R., & Loeper, C. (1987). Expressed emotion in families: A critical review. *Hospital and Community Psychiatry, 38,* 374-380.

9. Terkelsen, K. G. (1987). The meaning of mental illness to the family. In A. B. Hatfield & H. P. Lefley (Eds.), *Families of the mentally ill: Coping and adaptation.* New York, NY: Guilford.

10. Wynne, L. C., Bernheim, K. F., & Wynne, A. R. (1988). *Key issues for training in family therapy with the long-term seriously mentally ill and their families.* Presented at the National Forum for Educating Mental Health Professionals to Work With the Long-Term Seriously Mentally Ill and their Families, Chevy Chase, MD.

CHAPTER FIFTY-FOUR

Promoting Family Involvement in Community Residences for Chronic Mentally Ill Persons

Kayla F. Bernheim

This chapter was previously published in Hospital and Community Psychiatry, 41, *668-670. Copyright © 1990, the American Psychiatric Association.*

During the past decade, several factors have combined to highlight the importance of mental health professionals supporting, educating, and collaborating with families of chronic mentally ill patients. First, families have been more outspoken about their experiences in caring for ill relatives.[1,2] They have clearly expressed their views of professional services[2,3] and of what they want from service providers.[4,5]

Second, a model that focuses on family coping rather than on family pathology and that supports families as partners in rehabilitation is now available.[6] Third, family-based interventions have been shown to reduce relapse and recidivism.[7-9] As a result of these developments, many agencies, representing a variety of inpatient and outpatient settings, have established programs of family support or education.

Families of chronic mentally ill patients and the staff of community residences where patients live have much in common and potentially much to offer each other in managing the day-to-day problems in living posed by chronic mental illness. However, they have historically had little contact. In this chapter, we describe an attempt to develop closer working relationships between families of chronic patients and staff of a community residence, with particular emphasis on managing staff anxieties about increased involvement of families in patients' rehabilitation.

PROGRAM DESCRIPTION

East House Corporation, based in Rochester, New York, serves both seriously mentally ill patients and recovering alcoholics. Its mental health program, which will be the focus of this report, includes a quarterway house with 18 beds, four supervised group homes with a total of 54 beds, and scatter-site apartments that provide a total of 46 beds with various levels of supervision. Some of the agency's residential components had informally involved patients' families in various ways for several years. However, since the fall of 1987, the agency has trained staff and developed a multifaceted, formal family support program. The program is currently in place within the mental health component and is being developed within the alcoholism component.

The elements of the family support program include orientation, family consultation, group activities, and ongoing communication with families.

Orientation

Relatives appear to find careful orientation to the agency's services, policies, rules, and procedures very valuable. When a prospective resident is initially interviewed, the intake worker explores the person's family situation and identifies the family members who constitute the immediate support network. The agency's philosophy about including families in the rehabilitation effort is explained to the prospective resident. This discussion provides the opportunity to work through any resistance the patient may have about staff working with relatives.

In our experience, the overwhelming majority of residents and families respond positively, often enthusiastically, to staff's attempts to involve family members. Situations in which prospective residents are initially completely unwilling to allow family involvement are handled on a case-by-case basis and are generally resolved through negotiation and compromise.

Before admission, family members are offered a tour of the house and are oriented to the agency's intention to involve and support relatives. After the resident's acceptance for admission, relatives are invited to meet with staff to share information. An initial plan for family involvement and services is developed and placed in the resident's record. If the family is unable or unwilling to attend a meeting, staff contact the family by telephone to discuss the plan. Program staff adopt a welcoming attitude that relatives and staff can capitalize on later if either chooses. An orientation packet containing East House materials and information about community resources is provided to relatives during this initial phase.

Individual Family Consultation

Since the needs of each family and resident are unique, individualized plans for contact are made whenever possible. For some families, an occasional phone call may be all that is required, while for others, weekly telephone contacts that follow patients' home visits may be instituted. Other families may prefer face-to-face meetings to coordinate approaches to various problems.

Flexibility is the cornerstone of individual family consultation. As needs change, so do the frequency and format of contacts. For example, transitions, particularly those in which residents move to a more independent living situation, are as difficult for relatives as for residents, Program staff increase contact with family members as they work through their concerns about the move and become oriented to the prospective setting.

Group Activities

Family members participate in organizing support groups, educational and social events. Some of these events are agency-wide, and others are limited to individual residences. The educational and social activities include residents as well as relatives and staff.

Communication Channels

The agency's annual report, agency-wide newsletter, orientation brochures, and bimonthly newsletter for families are available to residents and family members.

To ensure ongoing feedback from family members, all interested relatives are invited to join an advisory group that meets with administrative staff four times a year. This group has participated in the development of a survey of family attitudes, has suggested topics for educational offerings, and has reviewed anticipated changes in agency policies and services. The group is open to families of prospective residents and past residents as well as families of current residents. In addition, about one-quarter of the members of the agency's board of directors have experienced mental illness, alcoholism, or substance abuse in their families.

TRAINING ISSUES

Staff members were understandably skeptical about the agency's plans to develop family services. Most had been heavily influenced in their previous training by theories that implicate the family in pathogenesis. Staff members' implicit orientation had been that the therapeutic community is a benign substitute for a dysfunctional family of origin. The majority had little, if any, experience interacting with residents' relatives.

Training has focused on helping staff develop empathy for relatives. Issues such as family burden, stages of adaptation, responses to stigma, variability in coping styles, cultural background, availability of other supports, and attitudes toward mental illness have been addressed. Listening to family members tell their own stories has been an essential element in this sensitization process.

Staff were particularly concerned about confidentiality issues. A problem-solving, case-specific approach to issues of confidentiality is needed in family support program that rely in part on sharing of information among staff, patients, and family members. New staff members, particularly those who had come from agencies or institutions with rigid confidentiality policies, needed to learn to approach each situation that required a judgment about confidentiality thoughtfully and creatively.

During their orientation, new staff receive four hours of training about working with families. This training includes, but is not limited to, the confidentiality issue. Even experienced staff needed both formal training and informal support and consultation to develop a more flexible approach to this complex, anxiety-producing area.

Staff were also fearful about conducting family therapy. They were uncertain about their skills and felt that if they opened the door to family work, they would be unable to set limits appropriate to their role. In addition, they wondered if they would find themselves overwhelmed by a double caseload when they tried to respond to the needs of family members as well as to residents' needs. They were also concerned that if they developed empathy for the relatives, they would be unable to fulfill their role as advocates for residents.

To address these concerns, the agency promoted an atmosphere of experimentation within which the staff could feel comfortable trying out new behaviors, working though their feelings with colleagues and supervisors, and gradually developing greater ability to identify the needs they could reasonably expect to fill. A recent 50-item survey of attitudes about families and family services completed by all program staff indicated that staff have overwhelmingly favorable attitudes toward family work and have found the positive response of both residents and relatives surprising and gratifying.

Family members' responses to a 43-item survey on satisfaction with services provide an indication of the success of staff training. The survey was conducted by mail in late 1988. Eighty-three surveys were returned, for an overall rate of 63% (79% of families whose relatives were served by the agency's mental health component and 18% of families whose relatives were served by the alcoholism component in which family services had not yet been extensively developed). Eighty-five percent of respondents felt that staff were doing a good job with families, and 78% felt staff were adequately trained to work with families.

DISCUSSIONS

Rather than hiring specialty staff to work with families, East House chose to integrate family work into the jobs of all counseling staff. Clearly, this approach requires extensive staff training and preparation. However, as has been argued elsewhere,[10] we feel this approach results in a higher level of satisfaction for residents, relatives, and staff.

It can be argued that family support and education should be provided by community mental health center staff than by community residence staff. However, our experience shows that brief family psychoeducation, which is frequently provided by mental health centers, is no substitute for ongoing, open communication that facilitates rehabilitation planning and reduces family members anxiety. Furthermore, even if community mental health centers consistently were to support families involvement in rehabilitation, communication between community residence staff and families, who share both interest and experience in the management of day-to-day problems in living with chronic mentally ill people, would still be important. All agencies that serve this population should reach out to families, each from their own unique perspective. The content of the contacts is less important than establishing a process of collaboration in which families who wish to be engaged as partners in rehabilitation have the opportunity to do so.

To summarize, keys to family support at an agency or institutional level include an attitude of welcome and cooperation, individualization of services, and multiple mechanisms for communication. Flexibility in planning, continuous evaluation and change to meet consumers' needs, and ongoing commitment to staff training, consultation, and support are also necessary. Ideally, these elements should be available in all settings in which the chronic mentally ill are served.

ACKNOWLEDGMENT

The author thanks Jim Sorrentino for his helpful suggestions for revision of this paper.

REFERENCES

1. Doll, W. (1976). Family coping with the mentally ill: an unanticipated problem of deinstitutionalization. *Hospital and Community Psychiatry, 27,* 183-185.

2. Hatfield, A. B. (1978). Psychological costs of schizophrenia to the family. *Social Work, 23,* 355-359.

3. Holden, O. F., & Lewine, R. R. J. (1982). How families evaluate mental health professionals, resources, and the effects of illness. *Schizophrenia Bulletin, 8,* 628-633.

4. Hatfield, A. B. (1979). Help-seeking behavior in families of schizophrenics. *American Journal of Community Psychology, 7,* 563-569.

5. Yeas, J. P. What families of the mentally ill want. *Community Support Service Journal 2*:1-3, 1981

6. Hatfield, A. B. & Lefley, H. P. (1986). *Families of the mentally ill: Coping and adaptation.* New York, NY: Guilford.

7. Anderson, C. M., Reiss, D. J., & Hogarty, G. E. (1986). *Schizophrenia and the family.* New York, NY: Guilford.

8. Goldstein, M. J. & Kopeikin, H. S. (1981). Short- and long-term effects of combining drug and family therapy. In M. J. Goldstein (Ed.), *New developments in interventions with families of schizophrenics.* San Francisco, CA: Jossey-Bass.

9. Leff, J., Kuipers, L., Berkowitz, R., et al. (1982). A controlled trial of social intervention in the families of schizophrenic patients. *British Journal of Psychiatry, 141,* 121-134.

10. Bernheim, K. F., & Switalski, T. (1988). The Buffalo family support project: promoting institutional change to meet families' needs. *Hospital and Community Psychiatry, 39,* 663-665.

CHAPTER FIFTY-FIVE

An Interdisciplinary Psychoeducation Program for Schizophrenic Patients and their Families in an Acute Care Setting

Linda Greenberg, Susan B. Fine, Cynthia Cohen, Kenneth Larson, Arlene Michaelson-Baily, Phyllis Rubinton, and Ira D. Glick

This chapter was previously published in Hospital and Community Psychiatry, 39, *277-282. Copyright ©1988, the American Psychiatric Association.*

Clinical efforts to provide "state of the art" treatment of schizophrenia in acute settings are influenced by several factors, including biomedical advances, the patient's special vulnerabilities, family relationships, and staff expertise. The limited availability of community-based resources, constraints on reimbursement and length of hospital stay, and high relapse and rehospitalization rates, further confound the picture.

Medication, structure, a protective environment, and family intervention are considered important components of treatment of acute schizophrenic episodes,[1,2] but there are few substantive data and little agreement about the specific elements that make up an effective "brief-treatment package" during acute episodes of the illness.[3,4]

The crisis intervention and symptom reduction models that currently prevail in the treatment of schizophrenia do not adequately address primary deficit symptoms, social adjustment, and community tenure. Mobilization for discharge is often perfunctory and influenced by factors external to the differential needs of the schizophrenic patients. Patients frequently return to the community poorly prepared to deal with environmental stressors.

The time is long overdue for reordering and clarifying the goals and content of the time-limited inpatient phase of schizophrenia treatment. This chapter describes a psychoeducational treatment program at the Payne Whitney Psychiatric Clinic in New York that we believe is responsive to the needs of acutely ill schizophrenic patients and their families as well as to the constraints imposed by the larger health care system. The chapter delineates the program's goals and techniques and describes the multidisciplinary staff's role in achieving the program's objectives. A rationale is provided for implementing the program in other acute care facilities with comparable populations and lengths of stay.

PSYCHOEDUCATION: A MODEL

While education has been a component of the treatment repertoires of many mental health disciplines,[5-11] it has often taken a backseat to psychodynamic, interpersonal, and biological methods. During the past decade, however, psychoeducation has gained considerable visibility as an important treatment for schizophrenia. The psychoeducational model is a systematic, goal-directed psychosocial technique that uses a collaborative approach in which clinicians, patients, and their families learn from each other. The goals of the process are to impart information and enhance understanding of the illness needed treatment resources and supportive services; increase daily living skills and adaptive capacities; acknowledge patients' and families' capacities and their right to know about the illness; and create a more productive alliance between patients, families, and mental health professionals.[12,13]

The rationale and efficacy of these efforts in long-term in situational and community-based settings have been well documented in the past decade by the pioneers of the psychoeducation movement.[14-21] A few clinicians within acute care settings have also reported their efforts to provide psychoeducation to patients or families.[2, 22-25] However, to the best of our knowledge, there have been no reports of a comprehensive interdisciplinary treatment program designed to meet the needs of schizophrenic patients and their families during hospitalizations.

PROGRAM SETTING

The setting for the psychoeducation program is the 104-bed inpatient service at the Payne Whitney Psychiatric Clinic of the New York Hospital—Cornell Medical Center. The inpatient service is made up of five units, each staffed by an interdisciplinary team of mental health professionals, trainees, and support personnel.

While inpatient programs, such as the psychoeducation program, are developed and initiated at all levels, guidelines for clinical practice are formulated by the director of inpatient services, as well as by unit and discipline chiefs. Administrative staff support policy and programs.

The distribution of leadership and the ongoing collaboration among the disciplines involved in the psychoeducation program have served to diminish staff burnout and sustain the staff's interest and expertise throughout the four years in which the program has operated. In addition, inservice training and supervision of staff are considered necessary to update practice, introduce educational techniques to new personnel, overcome existing biases, and enhance efficacy.

Although numerous questions about schizophrenia remain unanswered, the psychoeducation team adheres to the stress-vulnerability view of schizophrenia.[26] According to this position, symptoms are exacerbated when "...biological vulnerability increases, stressful life events overwhelm individual's coping resources, the individual's social supports diminish."[27]

The clinic's patients and their families are representative of the socioeconomic and educational mix of our urban setting. Patients range in age from 18 to 65 and include some experiencing their first episode of schizophrenia as well as those with more chronic conditions.

The 30-day average length of stay at the clinic requires rapid diagnostic assessment, treatment, and discharge planning. The majority of discharge referrals are made to outside agencies and practitioners. Continuity of care and utilization of community-based resources, therefore, are influenced by many factors arising after the patient has left our facility.

PROGRAM DESCRIPTION AND OBJECTIVES

The program consists of several components, each administered by one or more members of various mental health disciplines. Separate components are conducted by psychiatrists, nurses, occupational therapists, and social workers; a program administrator participates in family workshops. Each component has been designed to meet the distinct needs of patients and family members. However, all components work toward enhancing participants' cognitive and interpersonal strengths and adaptive capacities and decreasing their feelings of guilt and hopelessness.

The program's objectives are fostered by:

- Providing participants with an overview of current information about schizophrenia, which emphasize the relationship between a "biological vulnerability of unknown origin"[20] and a susceptibility to stress and overstimulation.
- Teaching participants about symptoms and the effects of medication to encourage compliance and prepare patients and family for early warning signs of relapse and side effects of medication.
- Increasing participants' awareness of environmental stress and its relationship to relapse.
- Creating a working alliance between the patients, their families, and staff to diminish resentment and blame, identify and implement short-term goals, and establish a foundation for ongoing treatment during the fluctuating course of the disease.
- Identifying individual strengths of the patients and the families and teaching them strategies for managing activities of daily living, positive and negative symptoms, and other distressing behaviors.
- Providing the patients with opportunities for practice, repetition, and reinforcement of adaptive skills to encourage their generalization and durability after discharge.
- Encouraging networking among families to lessen isolation and stigma.
- Supporting realistic hope by informing the patients and their families of the most current research information.
- Establishing contacts for the patients and their families with mental health professionals who support these goals in the community.

These services are thought to complement rather than replace medication and other needed treatment; therefore, the patients have an opportunity to benefit from the additive effects of combined biopsychosocial therapies.

Referrals to each of the program's components are coordinated through each unit's chief psychiatrist and multidisciplinary team. This forum deals with such issues as when and how to inform the patient and the family of the diagnosis, their readiness for information and involvement in the program, and their responses to the educational content and techniques. All patients and families are assessed for their need for psychoeducation, and if they are admitted to the program, for their level of progress.

Psychoeducation is not suitable for some individuals, but most patients on the inpatient service are treated in one or more psychoeducational components. Monitoring and maintaining the balance between individual capacities and program content and techniques are particularly high priorities; it is this balance that facilitates the application of psychoeducation to an acute population.

COMPONENTS OF THE PROGRAM

The Psychiatrist as Coordinator

The psychiatrist has a dual role that involves coordinating and consulting with the unit-based team and directly introducing psychoeducation into the patient's treatment package.

The psychiatrist's use of educational techniques during individual sessions with patients represents an expansion of the psychiatrist's traditional armamentarium.

To the degree that the patient's acute symptoms and cognitive difficulties allow, the psychiatrist spends at least two sessions reviewing the patient's symptoms and diagnosis in a simple and empathic manner. Whenever possible, these sessions precede the psychiatrist's discussions with the family. This information, as well as material about the patient's treatment and prognosis, is repeated and expanded on throughout the hospitalization until the patient manifests changes in behavior and compliance indicating he [or she] has adequately comprehended the material.

Depending on the sophistication of the patient and the family and the nature of the patient's recovery process, the psychiatrist may discuss the patient's vulnerability to stress and problems in information processing, offer information about medications and their side effects, introduce the subject of etiology, and present schizophrenia as a fluctuating but chronic illness that can be managed.

Within this model, the relationship between the patient and the psychiatrist becomes more collaborative, as the patient is encouraged to actively contribute his or her experience with symptoms and medication to the treatment process. If the patient is too cognitively impaired throughout the hospitalization, the collaborative exchange described above occurs only with his [or her] family.

Nursing Education Sessions

All of the nurses on the inpatient service teach patients about schizophrenia and its treatment. They also recommend strategies for minimizing stress based on their daily observations and information obtained from admission assessments. The nurses use a specific teaching assessment instrument developed for schizophrenia that outlines instructional techniques and incorporates questions about the patients' understanding of the illness and its treatment. Mental health workers reinforce information provided by the nurses and encourage more positive behaviors under the direction of the head nurse.

The nurses present information in individual sessions as soon as the patient's diagnosis and treatment plans have been established and the patient appears able to understand the material. Teaching is not initiated for the patients who appear overwhelmed or extremely fearful or who need to deny the illness until staff establish a stronger alliance with them and they become more accessible. The patients may be given reading material before they attend a teaching session if it appears that they would be less threatened by a written introduction. Modifications in the patients' diagnoses or treatment plans may require additional educational contacts.

The nurses also provide informal instruction about the patients day-to-day experiences and expectations as a way of augmenting more formal contacts and providing the patients with greater understanding of their illnesses and a better opportunity to actively participate in the management of their treatment.

Life Skills Curriculum

The Life Skills Curriculum, offered by members of the occupational therapy staff, addresses basic aspects of community adjustment through the use of formal instruction and task-oriented techniques. The principal objective of the curriculum is to maximize the patient's potential to function in the community, a goal as relevant for the patient hospitalized for 30 days as it is for one with a lengthier institutional tenure.[28]

The curriculum is offered during five weekly classes and in a flexible number of one-on-one tutorials, a format that aims to be both manageable for the patient and relevant to his [or her] needs. The lessons address such issue as personal goal setting, stress management, social skills, self-care, time management, home management, leisure-time planning, and use of community resources.

All of the curriculum's modules emphasize problem-solving and communication skills that can be generalized to a variety of life situations and establish an expectation that problems can be solved. Patients identify their problems, strengths, learning needs, and progress through self-assessments completed before and after they take the course.

The curriculum uses group discussions, lectures by staff and patients, role-playing, simulated tasks, video and audio tapes, computerized and paper and pencil exercises, reading assignments, and other resources to facilitate individual and group goals. Patients have opportunities to practice skills through "homework" assignments, which they complete on the inpatient units, in the program's mental health library, while attending other clinic-based rehabilitation programs, or during visits to the community.

While formal data on the outcomes of the curriculum aren't available, patient self-assessments, an important element of the psychoeducational process, indicate that they have gained a sense of satisfaction from mastering biosocial elements of independent living and from playing an active part in improving their own functioning.

Family Sessions

Because schizophrenic patients are discharged in increasing numbers to the care of family members,[29] a social worker leads family sessions, with a psychiatric resident present during the early meetings to offer psychiatric diagnoses. The sessions are geared toward helping the family develop cognitive and behavioral skills with which to deal with both the acute and the ongoing manifestations of the patient's illness.

Four to ten family sessions take place during the course of the patient's hospitalization. The first meetings focus on establishing an alliance between the family members and the clinicians.[15] These early contacts, which do not include the patient, provide an opportunity for the family to express anger, frustration, guilt, and anxiety about the patient, about the mental health system, and about the future. The clinicians focus on current issues rather than on lengthy family histories, which tend to reinforce the family's feelings of blame and guilt.[17]

Once the diagnosis of schizophrenia has been discussed, that social worker meets alone with the family to help them process information about the patient's diagnosis, treatment, and discharge planning. These sessions address the family's ongoing concerns about the future, strategies for coping with the patient's bizarre behaviors, the relationship between stress and symptoms, the patient's continued compliance with effective treatments, and the importance of a predictable, nonintrusive home environment that supports the patient's assets and a gradual increase in his [or her] responsibilities.[22]

Giving information and advice in a timely fashion and using forthright and empathic responses to the family's questions are characteristic of this problem-solving and collaborative technique. The family members are encouraged to offer their ideas about management strategies, for they are viewed as experts in their own right. Siblings and children of the patient are encouraged to attend family sessions or to meet separately with the therapists. Patients are generally included in the sessions after they have discussed their diagnosis with their psychiatrist or their nurse.

The contacts with the staff provide families with support in dealing with the stigma of having a schizophrenic family member and the burden of assuming a caretaking role. Family members of all ages often need permission to fulfill personal needs that have long been ignored.

Because continued support in the community is so critical to the family, the social worker actively cultivates and makes referrals to clinicians who use a family-focused treatment model. Unfortunately such referrals are not always feasible, as more traditional interventions for families of schizophrenic patients sometimes prevail.

Mental Health Library

As the psychoeducational program developed, it became apparent that patients and their families had a need for suitable literature about schizophrenia, other mental illness, human development, and daily living skills. The Phyllis Rubinton Mental Health Resource Library,[30] paid for through private funds, began as a joint venture of the clinic's psychiatric library and occupational therapy department.

Occupational therapy staff oversee the collection and disseminate information about the library, as well as current ideas and developments in patient and family education, to other staff through formal presentations, distribution of materials, and a bimonthly mailing of selected articles suitable for patients and families.

Patient access to the library is monitored by an occupational therapist. The therapist guides patients to resources relevant to their interests, stress tolerance, and cognitive abilities; deals with their immediate emotional reactions to materials; leads a discussion group that provides support and reinforces intellectual mastery of the material; and communicates with staff about the patients' selections and responses. The multidisciplinary team, in turn, uses the readings in individual and family sessions to facilitate treatment goals.

Patients with good functional histories seem the most motivated to use the library. Selections focusing on symptoms and medication, vignettes about people who have adapted to their illness, and guidance in managing time are of particular interest. Families are drawn to literature dealing with diagnosis, prognosis, the natural course of the disease, treatment approaches used by leading experts, and ways of coping with specific stressors.

Family Workshop

A workshop taught by a team of professionals provides another arena for helping the families to understand and manage the patients' illness. The workshop is modeled on the Survival Skills Workshop on Schizophrenia at the University of Pittsburgh,[18] but has been modified to meet the intramural and family needs that rise within a short-term setting.

The three-to-six-hour workshop takes place on Sundays or in the evenings in order to maximize attendance. An interdisciplinary team consisting of a psychiatrist, a social worker, an occupational therapist, and an administrator present a historical perspective on schizophrenia and review symptoms, somatic treatments, rehabilitation, and family coping strategies. The administrator provides an overview of methods for dealing with the mental health delivery system, reviewing such topics as obtaining insurance for the chronic mentally ill, negotiating bureaucracies, expediting referrals to agencies, and registering complaints within the institution, as well as information about the rights of the mentally ill.

The more didactic components of the workshop are balanced by informal discussions, in which team members work to clarify information, answer questions within the limits of available knowledge, and stimulate problem solving by the families. The staff collaborate in a cohesive but open and nondogmatic manner to provide the families with needed respect and empathy as well as clarification and guidance.

Coordination and referrals to the workshops are managed by a social worker. Referrals may be made any time after the patient has been on the unit for a week until a week after his [or her] discharge, provided there are at least two other families available to participate; the maximum number of families that can attend a workshop is six. Children under 12, family members who are actively psychotic, and the patients themselves are not included in workshops.

A controlled study indicated that six months after completing the workshops, participants demonstrated a statistically significant increase in knowledge about schizophrenia and a trend toward improved attitudes about the patients.

CONCLUSIONS

Limiting the objectives of brief hospitalization to symptom reduction and crisis intervention in the face of limited healthcare services may undermine the tenuous gains patients have made by the time of their discharge and contribute to the high human and economic costs of schizophrenia. On the other hand, a brief, focused, interdisciplinary psychoeducational program, designed to respond to the strengths and special vulnerabilities of schizophrenic patients and their families, can provide a foundation for posthospital adjustment and longer-term management of this disorder.

This treatment model involves the active participation of both patients and families in a range of structured, gradually more complex learning experiences that emphasize the here-and-now, stimulate cognitive and social-interpersonal capacities, and offer information and guidelines that contribute to greater understanding of the illness and its ramifications. When introduced in a timely, individualized, and empathic manner, this model promotes greater responsiveness among patients and their families to other important biological and psychological treatment approaches during both the inpatient and the after-care phases of treatment.

Controlled research studies will more accurately evaluate the impact of this effort, but the need for new models for brief inpatient treatment of schizophrenia is already clear—sufficiently clear, at least, to stimulate other practitioners to address the problem.

ACKNOWLEDGMENT

We dedicate this article to the late Phyllis Rubinton, MLS, in recognition of her innovative ideas and dedication to psychoeducation.

REFERENCES

1. Drake, R. E. & Sederet, L. I. (1986). In-patient psychosocial treatment of chronic schizophrenia: negative effects and current guidelines. *Hospital and Community Psychiatry, 37,* 897-901.

2. Glick, I. D., Clarkin, J. F., Spencer, J. H., et al. (1965). In-patient family intervention: A controlled evaluation of practice: preliminary results of the six-month follow-up. *Archives of General Psychiatry, 42,* 882-886.

3. Collins, J. F., Ellsworth, R. B., Casey, N. A., et al. (1984). Treatment characteristics of effective psychiatric programs. *Hospital and Community Psychiatry, 35,* 601-605.

4. Maves, P. A. & Schulz, J. W. (1985). In-patient group treatment on short-treatment care units. *Hospital and Community Psychiatry, 36,* 69-73.

5. Heinrichs, D. W. (1984). Recent developments in the psychosocial treatment of chronic psychotic illnesses. In J. A. Talbott (Ed.), *The chronic mental patients.* Orlando, FL: Grune & Stratton.

6. Narrow, B. W. (1984). *Patient teaching in nursing practice.* New York, NY: Wiley.

7. Falvol, D. R. (1985). *Effective patient education.* Rockville, MD: Aspen.

8. Haas, L. D. (1946). *Practical Occupational Therapy* (2nd Edition). Milwaukee, WI: Bruce.

9. Goldstein, A. P., Gershaw, N. J., & Sprafkin, R. P. (1979). Structured learning therapy. *American Journal of Occupational Therapy, 33,* 635-639.

10. Hollis, F. (1964). *Casework: A psychosocial therapy.* New York, NY: Random House.

11. Crow, M. S. (1967). Preventive intervention through parent group education. *Social Casework, 48,* 161-165.

12. Anderson, C. M. (1977). Family intervention with severely disturbed patients. *Archives of General Psychiatry, 34,* 697-702.

13. Hatfield, A. (1983). What families want of psychotherapists. In W. R. McFarlane (Ed.), *Family therapy in schizophrenia.* New York, NY: Guilford.

14. Paul, G. L. & Lentz, R. J. (1977). *Psychosocial treatment of chronic mental patients.* Cambridge, MA: Harvard University Press.

15. Lamb, H. R. (1976). An educational model for teaching living skills to long-term patients. *Hospital and Community Psychiatry, 27,* 875-877.

16. Liberman, R. P., Massel, H. K., Mosk, M.D., et al. (1985/1993). Social skills training for chronic mental patients. *Hospital and Community Psychiatry, 36,* 396 403. (Reprinted in Cottrell, R. P. (Ed.). (1993). *Psychosocial occupational therapy: Proactive approaches.* Bethesda, MD: AOTA.)

17. Anderson, C. M. (1983). A psychoeducational program for families of patients with schizophrenia. In W. R. McFarlane (Ed.), *Family therapy in schizophrenia.* New York, NY: Guilford.

18. Anderson, C. M., Reiss, D. J., Hogarty, G. E. (1986). *Schizophrenia and the family.* New York, NY: Guilford.

19. Falloon, I. R. H., Boyd, J. L., McGill, C .W., et al. (1982). Family management in the prevention of exacerbations of schizophrenia: A controlled study. *New England Journal of Medicine, 306,* 1437-1440.

20. Snyder, K. D. & Liberman, R. P. (1981). Family assessment and intervention with schizophrenics at risk for relapse. *New Directions for Mental Health Services, 12,* 49-60.

21. Left, J., Kuipers, L., Berkowitz, R., et al. (1982). A controlled trial of social intervention in the families of schizophrenic patients. *British Journal of Psychiatry, 141,* 121-134.

22. Anderson, C. M. & Reiss, D. J. (1982). Family treatment of patients with chronic schizophrenia: The in-patient phase. In H. T. Harbin (Ed.), *The psychiatric hospital and the family.* Jamaica, NY: SP Medica & Scientific Books.

23. Themes, L. O., Bajema, S. L. (1983). The life skills development program: history overview and update. *Occupational Therapy in Mental Health, 3,* 35-48.

24. Ogren, K. (1983/2000). A living skills program in an acute psychiatry setting. *Mental Health Special Interest Section Newsletter American Occupational Therapy Association, 6,* 1-2.

25. Fine, S. B., & Schwimmer, P. (1986). The effects of occupational therapy on independent living skills. *Mental Health Special Interest Section Newsletter (American Occupational Therapy Association) 9,* 1-3.

26. Main, J. (1980). Chronic schizophrenia from the standpoint of vulnerability. In C. Baxter & T. Melnechuk (Eds.), *Perspectives in schizophrenia research.* New York, NY: Raven.

27. Faloon, I. R. H. & Liberman, R. P. (1983). Interactions between drug and psychosocial therapy in schizophrenia. *Schizophrenia Bulletin, 9,* 543-552.

28. Fine, S. B. (1980). Psychiatric treatment and rehabilitation: What's in a name? *Psychiatric Hospital, 11*(Fall), 8-13.

29. Godman, H. H. (1982). Mental illness and family burden: A public health perspective. *Hospital and Community Psychiatry, 33,* 557-560.

30. Michaelson, A., Nitzberg, L., & Rubinton, P. (1984). Mental health resources library: A consumer guide to the literature. *Psychiatric Hospital, 15,* 133-139.

CHAPTER FIFTY-SIX

Dual Diagnosis: A Parent's Perspective

Barbara Jacobs

My name is Barb, and my son has both schizoaffective disorder and an addiction to street drugs. It took me a long time to be able to say that in one sentence. This is my story.

We first recognized that something was terribly wrong with our eldest son in 1986 when he was 16 years of age and a sophomore in high school. At that time, I worked as an occupational therapist at a free-standing substance abuse treatment facility. We thought that he was probably chemically dependent, and it was my hope and prayer that 30 days with my experienced and esteemed colleagues would "fix" him, and we would have our son back. It was while he was in alcohol and other drug abuse (AODA) treatment that someone suggested that he had probably been experiencing some psychiatric symptoms for several years and was using marijuana and other street drugs to "self-medicate." As a result, I told myself that he was really mentally ill, and all he needed was the appropriate combination of psychotropic medications to make him feel "normal"; then he would not need street drugs.

The road from denial to acceptance is long and bumpy, even for the experienced mental health care professional. What he has, of course, is a dual diagnosis.

DEFINITION AND IMPLICATIONS

In some psychiatric circles, dual diagnosis is a term used to describe a person with both a psychiatric disorder and a developmental disability (Torrey, 1988, p. 89). For the purposes of this chapter, however, dual diagnosis means the coexistence of substance abuse or dependence and a mental illness (Evans & Sullivan, 1990, p. ix). With a dual diagnosis, each disorder seems to exacerbate the other. In our son, it appears that the confused, concrete thinking of his schizoaffective disorder interferes with his ability to understand and internalize a 12-step program. Poor problem-solving skills make it difficult for him to recognize a relapse in progress and to take the neces-

sary steps to avoid a full-blown relapse. The power of his addiction, his impulsiveness, and his quest for immediate gratification reinforce his need for a "quick fix" when he experiences stress. Stress often exacerbates his psychiatric symptoms, which in turn leads to drug-seeking behavior.

The dual nature of the disability makes treatment difficult. The confrontational approach of many AODA programs is at odds with the warm, supportive care usually offered to persons with mental illnesses. Professionals trained in either discipline find it difficult to accommodate the needs of both illnesses in one person. Through our son's experiences in several different treatment programs, I have learned that dual diagnosis programs, from an AODA perspective, tend to believe that as long as the psychiatric symptoms are medicated, the program can proceed as it would with any other patient. This approach discounts the so-called "negative" symptoms of schizophrenia, for example, "apathy, social withdrawal, poverty of thoughts, blunting of emotions, slowness of movement, [and] lack of drive." (Torrey, 1988, p. 79), which do not respond to most medications but can severely affect functioning. The tendency toward confrontation immobilizes many persons with mental illnesses, which makes treatment ineffective. Psychiatric programs frequently do not address some of the issues facing dual diagnosis, such as coping with urges to use drugs and identifying triggers to those urges. Often psychiatric professionals who are accustomed to being supportive and nurturing have difficulty treating substance abusers whose coping skills include manipulating, lying, stealing, and other antisocial behaviors (Woolis, 1992, p. 111). Persons with a dual diagnosis, although exhibiting these using behaviors to some extent themselves, have difficulty recognizing them in others and are vulnerable and suggestible when interacting with chronic drug users because often persons with a dual diagnosis do not have the appropriate social and assertiveness skills to cope effectively.

The social stigma attached to both mental illness and addiction means that persons with a dual diagnosis experience a triple dose of rejection Not only are they not accepted by society as a whole, but also they are not well accepted by either the drug-using community or other persons with mental illnesses. Our son has frequently encountered persons at Narcotics Anonymous or Alcoholics Anonymous meetings who view psychotropic medications as mood-altering chemicals. These persons interpret his need for medications as drug-seeking behavior and urge him to stop taking them. They often tire of the "weird" behaviors associated with his mental illness. Persons with mental illnesses view drug addiction as a moral weakness and an inability to "just say no." The net result of this is that it is almost impossible for a person with a dual diagnosis to develop the positive peer support system that we all know is so important to recovery. If there are supportive family members, the person becomes increasingly dependent on parents, siblings, and extended family members to meet his or her social, emotional, and financial needs. As a result, family members "often find themselves depleted emotionally and financially" (Evans & Sullivan, 1990, p. 10) and sometimes simply give up and withdraw.

MEDICATION COMPLIANCE

Can you remember a time when a physician prescribed an antibiotic for you, and you stopped taking it before the recommended 10 day course because you were better and wanted to save the rest for another time when you are really sick again? Persons with mental illnesses are no different. They do not want to put chemicals in their body that they do not really need, so when they feel better, they frequently experiment with whether they need them at all. Of course, the result is that symptoms return. When a dual diagnosis exists, this usually means a return to the street drugs initially used to self-medicate.

Part of the reason that persons with mental illness do not want to take psychotropic medications is that they have uncomfortable side effects as well as some serious consequences (e.g., tardive dyskinesia). Our son learned about the side effects of the medications he was taking early in his illness while in a psychology class at our local junior college. The instructor was unaware of our son's dual diagnosis and was therefore unable to reassure him or instruct him as to how to proceed if he noticed the side effects in himself. As a result, he stopped taking his medications and experienced a return of his psychiatric symptoms, which in turn triggered a relapse of his drug abuse. Perhaps he was just looking for an excuse to return to his drugs of choice, but maybe more thorough information from treatment professionals could have prevented this particular relapse.

Taking medications for an extended period of time requires a level of acceptance of the need to do so. Because of the stigma attached to both mental illnesses and addiction, persons with a dual diagnosis often have "dual denial.' If they can get by without the medications, their thinking goes, maybe they are not really mentally ill. In our son's case, it was more socially acceptable to be an addict than to be 'crazy.' It

took a lot of trial and error and several relapses for our son to accept the need for medications. Currently, he seems to appreciate that the medications can help him to feel better, but I am not sure that he understands the limits of what they can do for him. A couple of weeks ago, he was complaining that they were not helping him sleep the way he wanted them to. And the last time I talked to him, he said that some people in a new Narcotics Anonymous group he attended were suggesting that he cannot be truly clean and sober as long as he takes his medications.

We all know that prescribing medications is not an exact science and that finding the optimal combination of chemicals for each person often involves a long course of trial and error. Changing drugs, however, can be tricky for anyone with a mental illness but especially for someone with a history of self-medication with street drugs. It does not take much for a person with a dual diagnosis to turn to the drugs that initially helped take care of the problem. Our son's last relapse seems to have been contributed to accidentally by a change from fluoxetine (Prozac) to risperidone (Risperdal). He had been discharged from an in-patient treatment program where he was taking Prozac because of an exacerbation of depressive symptoms. After-care was provided by a community support program. The psychiatrist with the community support program took him off the Prozac and prescribed Risperdal because he had been using the Risperdal successfully before the in-patient treatment. When the Risperdal did not relieve the depression the way he wanted it to, our son again turned to his drug of choice. He may have been in the relapse process anyway, but changes in medications must be carefully supervised.

HOW A DUAL DIAGNOSIS AFFECTS FAMILY MEMBERS

Living with someone with a dual diagnosis, even if he or she is not actually under the same roof, is much like riding a roller coaster. Plummeting downhill into a crisis has the same out-of-control sensation, and the upward climb is just as agonizingly slow. Even sitting on top of the summit has the uneasy expectation of the next downhill rush. This illness can take a tremendous toll.

Imagine that your son, 17 years of age, home from in-patient treatment for only 3 days, has just run away from home 10 days before Christmas. How do you respond? You are feeling angry, scared, sad, and hurt. What do you do with all those feelings? Do you argue with you spouse, trying to assign blame? Do you yell at the other children out of frustration and fear that someday they too will run away? Do you withdraw to your bedroom so that no one sees you cry? Do you make dinner and try to carry on a "normal" routine so that other family members can experience a little stability?

What do you do when this kind of thing happens again and again, and nothing you do seems to make a difference? How do you respond when your friends tell their children not to play with yours? What do you say when your sister asks you whether you have any idea what you did wrong in raising your son so that she can avoid doing the same thing with her children? Where do you get the energy to cope?

I call dual diagnosis a "no casserole" disease. If your son were hospitalized with cancer, neighbors would band together to form a network of support for you, possibly bringing dinner to your home each night, picking up your other children after school, or just calling to chat. Because of the fear attached to both mental illnesses and substance abuse, families often are isolated in facing their devastating consequences.

Because of fear and lack of understanding, family members sometimes isolate themselves from each other. The last crisis in our family resulted in each of our other children going to their own rooms alone while we sat at the dining room table with the police officer answering questions for his report. What is normal when the situation clearly is not?

Claudia Black, Melodie Beattie, and Janet Woltitz have written extensively about the effects of substance abuse on family members, and I suspect that most of us are familiar with the three rules that seem to govern dysfunctional families: "don't talk, don't trust, don't feel" (Evans & Sullivan, 1990, pp. 132-133). I suggest that these three behaviors can be effective as temporary coping skills in allowing family members to function appropriately through a crisis. It is when these short-term coping strategies become long-term behaviors that the family becomes dysfunctional.

The concept of "enabling" becomes confusing for me when the disabilities associated with mental illness are added to the substance abuse It is clearly enabling to call a spouse's employer to excuse him from work when he has a hangover. But is it enabling or compassionate understanding of a person's limited social skills to give a son food when he's spent his grocery money on drugs because a drug-using "friend" has persuaded him to get high? Early in our son's treatment efforts, when he was bouncing back and forth from substance abuse to psychiatric programs, we had drug counselors and 12-step family support groups espousing "tough love" and psychiatrists suggesting more compassion.

HOW ONE FAMILY COPES

Our son is the eldest of five children, so when he became ill at 16 years of age, his siblings were quite young. There were three boys: 14, 13, and 10 years of age, and a girl 7 years of age. It was important to me that they understand as much as possible what was happening to their brother and family and that their needs be met along with the needs of their ill brother. All of them participated in age-appropriate "concerned others" groups at a local psychiatric facility that had a 12-step drug treatment program. The children's program was developed primarily for children of substance abusers, which did not accurately address the feelings and experiences of our children and did not really help them to feel less alone as siblings of someone using drugs. However, they were able to come to an understanding that they did not cause their brother's behavior, they could not control it, and they could not cure it. The groups gave them permission to talk about what was happening in their family in a safe and nurturing environment. Because they had difficulty identifying with the physical and emotional abuse described by other group members, I think that they tended to minimize their own distress. I talked to professionals at each of their schools to let their teachers know to look for signs of stress.

My husband and I attended Families Anonymous meetings, a 12-step support group for parents and adult family members of substance abusers. There we learned about enabling, tough love, and letting go. We had an opportunity to share our experiences with others in similar situations. Periodic therapy sessions kept the lines of communication open and helped us to be comfortable with each other as we struggled with our individual reactions and emotions.

During the first 6 months of our roller coaster ride, we recognized the need to continue having fun as a family, at least as much as possible. Toward that end, we planned a trip to Florida for Easter week, optimistically assuming that our son would have completed treatment by then. As it turned out, he was hospitalized at an in-patient psychiatric program in another city. We went to Florida anyway and had a wonderful, relaxing, and healing family vacation, forgetting at least for a while the turmoil in our lives. Although I returned home feeling refreshed, I had a nagging memory of sitting around a conference table with the adolescent treatment team talking about the negligent parents who had "dumped" their child with us and skipped town.

Since then we have taken several family vacations and had many family celebrations. When our son is available, he joins us. We miss him when he is not there, but we still have fun.

Despite our efforts to have fun together, there is often a feeling of overwhelming sadness and grief. As with any chronic illness, grief is an ongoing process. Not only do we grieve the loss of the son and brother we once had, we grieve his lost potential. In an address to the student body about drug abuse, one of our sons began by saying, "Two years ago, my brother died," referring to the onset of symptoms. Another brother once lamented, "I wish he would act like a real big brother." As each of his younger siblings move on to a different life stage, our grief is renewed by the realization that our firstborn may never accomplish that stage. Often the accomplishments of his siblings coincide with a relapse of his drug use, perhaps his way of coping with his own negative feelings about himself. The illnesses affects extended family members as well. My son's grandparents, cousins, aunts, and uncles all experience loss to varying degrees.

It was fairly easy to be involved in our son's treatment while he was an adolescent. As soon as he reached his 18th birthday, however, contact with counselors and psychiatrists had to be initiated by us, and information was not always readily shared. It puzzled us that treatment professionals often expected us to provide a home for him upon discharge but could not help us to understand how to handle his baffling behaviors or provide the appropriate supportive environment. It was discouraging when counselors made assumptions and drew conclusions about our son's behavior without consulting us. After all, had not we lived with him all his life, where a professional may have only known him days? I question my own involvement; perhaps I have not really learned how to let go. Despite all the problems he causes, he is still my son.

I still participate in an ongoing support group, though I now prefer groups focusing on mental illness rather than on substance abuse. I found two educational programs sponsored by the National Alliance for the Mentally Ill to be helpful. They are listed in Appendix A, along with other books and support services available to families. Recovery for our family members is a continuous process, and we move in and out of supportive activities as the family members' needs dictate.

IMPLICATIONS FOR THE HEALTH CARE PROFESSIONAL

My purpose in telling this story is twofold. I want to help heathcare professionals understand the experience of family members faced with a long-term disability. The occupational therapy literature on families focuses on children or older adults, yet everyone has a family. In today's health care environment, we need more than ever to depend on family members to support our treatment efforts. It is essential that our treatment efforts likewise support the family's needs. If we can recognize and treat family members as "lay practitioners" on our treatment team, I believe that more positive outcomes will occur for everyone. I have included a list of "Tips for Dealing With Families" (see Appendix B) as well as a list of readings related to family members facing chronic illnesses. I hope that they are helpful in determining your future roles with families.

Additionally, I want to help health care professionals understand how difficult life must be for a person who has both a mental illness and a drug or alcohol addiction. This is not only a difficult population to treat, but also it is truly a terrible way to live. I want to challenge us to discard our biases about "counseling the mentally ill substance abuser" or treating the substance abusing mentally ill, and treat the person behind the dual diagnosis. Let us use our unique skills as occupational therapy practitioners to focus on their abilities to function in valued occupational roles by considering the personal skill development and the environmental supports needed to function.

APPENDIX A

Resources for Families

National Alliance for the Mentally Ill (NAMI)
2101 Wilson Boulevard
Suite 302 Arlington

VA 22201 703-S23-7600
1-800-950-NAMI

Most states have a NAMI chapter. Contact the above for local information. I accessed both "The Journey of Hope Family Education" and "How to Enter the World of Schizophrenia." Through my local NAMI chapter. Our local chapter has a lending library, monthly educational programs, various support groups for both consumers and family members, and a monthly newsletter. There is a nominal annual membership fee.

Families Anonymous, Inc.
PO Box S2a
Van Nuys, CA 91408

Local chapters will often be listed in the yellow pages of your telephone book. Our local chapter sponsors several support groups and provides educational pamphlets for a small fee. Families Anonymous uses the 12-step philosophy of Alcoholics Anonymous.

Alcoholics Anonymous
940 Rockefeller Building
614 Superior Avenue, NW
Cleveland, OH 44113
216-241-7387

Local chapters will be listed in the yellow pages of the telephone book as will information about local meetings of Alanon and Alateen. Information about Narcotics Anonymous, Cocaine Anonymous, and Naranon may likewise be found in the yellow pages of your telephone book.

Department of Health and Human Services
Social Security Administration
Baltimore, MD 21235
1-800 234-5772

This agency can provide helpful information about the availability of Social Security Income for persons with disabilities. For information about the location of your nearest office, call 1-800-772-1213.

APPENDIX B

Tips for Dealing with Families

1. When a patient is discharged from a hospital or rehabilitation center, family members ultimately become responsible for his or her care, whether aftercare is planned or not. It is important to recognize the important role in patient care and to help family members understand their role and its potential as well as its limitations.

2. Do not make the assumption that family members will ask for what they need. Offer help. Most persons will be overwhelmed and intimidated by the health care system.

3. Do not assume that someone else has already provided information or that once is enough. Use every opportunity you can to help family members understand what is happening to their loved one.

4. Family members should be treated with the same respect as any member of the treatment team or aftercare team. They can provide information that may be useful to professionals, and they need information as well as to facilitate appropriate care in the community.

5. Children and siblings are affected, too. Parents should be encouraged to include children in discussions and to respond as honestly as possible to their questions and fears. Do not assume, however, that parents will be able to meet all of their children's need for information and reassurance during this stressful time. They may need assistance and suggestions in accessing appropriate supports for their children.

6. Adult siblings and children can be an important source of support for both the patient and the primary caregiver. They need to be included In the education and treatment process so that they have all the information they need.

7. Involve the patient in as much of the family member education process as possible. It is important for family members to have a common knowledge base.

8. Common goals (including family members as well as the patient) will facilitate the treatment process. Motivation is a crucial factor in goal attainment.

9. Engage family members as soon as possible in the treatment process. The longer family members are separate from the process, the more foreign it becomes.

10. Provide both written and verbal information. Handouts are great, but persons learn in various ways. It is important to use as many channels as possible to convey information, especially during this stressful time. Verbal interaction can serve to comfort as well as teach.

REFERENCES

Evans, K, & Sullivan, L M. (1990). *Dual diagnosis: Counseling the mentally ill substance abuser.* New York, NY: Guilford.

Torrey, E. F. (1988). *Surviving Schizophrenia. A family manual* (2nd Edition). New York, NY: Harper & Row.

Woolis, R. (1992). *When someone you love has a mental illness.* New York, NY: Putnam.

RELATED READING

Clark, C. A., Corcoran, M., & Gitlin, L. (1995). An exploratory study of how occupational therapists develop therapeutic relationships with family caregivers. *American Journal of Occupational Therapy, 49,* 587-594.

Gitlin, L. N., Corcoran, M., & Leinmiller-Eckhardt, S. (1995). Understanding the family perspective: An ethnographic framework for providing occupational therapy in the home. *American Journal of Occupational Therapy, 49,* 802-809.

Hatfield, A. (1982). *Coping with mental illness in the family: A family guide* (Available from the Nation Alliance of the Mentally Ill, 2101 Wilson Boulevard; Suite 302, Arlington, VA 22201)

Hatfield, A. (1993). *Dual diagnosis: Substance abuse and mental illness* (Available from the Nation Alliance of the Mentally Ill, 2101 Wilson Boulevard; Suite 302, Arlington, VA 22201)

Hatfield, A., & Lefley, H. (Eds.). (1987). *Families of the mentally Coping and adaptation.* New York, NY: Guilford.

Hyde, A. (1987). *Living with schizophrenia: A guide for patients and their families.* Chicago, Ill: Contemporary Books.

Johnson, C. B., & Deltz, J. C. (1985). Activity patterns of mothers of handicapped and non-handicapped children. *Physical and Occupational Therapy in Pediatrics, 5,* 17-25.

Johnson, J. T. (1988). *Hidden victims: An eight-stage healing process for families and friends of the mentally ill.* New York, NY: Doubleday.

Mueser, K., & Gingerich, S. (1994). *Coping with schizophrenia. A guide for families.* Oakland, CA: New Harbinger.

Torrey, E. F. (1995). *Surviving Schizophrenia. A manual for families, consumers and providers* (3rd Edition). New York, NY: Harper Collins.

Woolis, R. (1992). *When someone you love has a mental illness: A handbook for family, friends, and caregivers.* New York, NY: Putnam.

CHAPTER FIFTY-SEVEN

The Mothers' Project: A Clinical Case Management System

Mary Ann Zeitz

This chapter is reprinted from the Psychosocial Rehabilitation Journal, 19(1), 55-62, by permission of the author. *Copyright © 1995.*

In a recent survey analysis of state policies and programs that affect "at-risk" children and their mothers with mental illness, the authors concluded that "the full extent of these high-risk groups of significantly mentally ill women and their children, and the most effective means of intervention, remain unknown" (Nicholson, Geller, Fisher, & Dion, 1993). Services to stabilize the family may be provided either by state child welfare workers or subcontracted to community agencies who may have little or no familiarity as to the serious mental health issues involved. Families become known to them when the parent is in psychiatric crisis and their children are at risk for out of home placement. While services are largely unfunded and ignored by mental health officials at the state level, comprehensive and effective intervention services are offered in Chicago by the Thresholds psychosocial rehabilitation program through one of its efforts to deliver specialized services to particular populations, in this case to mothers and children, through a program known as The Mothers' Project. This program offers an intensive case management system for the families, primary intervention services to the children through a therapeutic nursery program, as well as comprehensive array of services through the larger agency.

In the state of Illinois there has been recent ongoing media attention to the matter of parents with mental illness owing to the failure of the child welfare system to deal effectively with particular cases resulting in tragic outcomes. The result has been an initiative for the Department of Mental Health and the Department of Children and Family Services (IDCFS) to work in collaboration "in the best interest of the child." Interestingly enough, children are more often removed from their family of origin and this is due to lack of understanding of the issues involved. A recent study of state records conducted for The Report of the.Mental Health Task Force (Astrachan et al, 1994) found that of 15,000 open cases with IDCFS in Cook County alone, 5% have a head of household who has been hospitalized in a state operated facility. A full 6% of all children in substitute care have one or both parents who have serious mental illness. While there are those individuals who are screened and whose children are in immediate danger, there are many families who are not in imminent danger so that a more thorough evaluation could be conducted and intervention services can be offered. To these families, the Thresholds Mothers' Project offers treatment for the mother and child aimed at stabilization in the community and reduction of risk factors.

In those cases in which questions persist about the suitability or advisability of return of a child to a parent with serious mental illness, and in those cases in which children are returned to such a parent, there is a need for a clinical case management system with well-trained case managers. A major problem in child protection is the need to link multiple resources to better serve children and parents. A well-supervised, focused case management program can accomplish this goal.

PROGRAM DESCRIPTION

The essential features of such a treatment program are a holistic case management model that treats the family while focusing on the mother and child; comprehensive services that are agency-(or center) based as well as community and home-based; and a recognition of the central importance of parental mental illness and its impact on the family. The Thresholds Mothers' Project was the first intervention program developed for psychiatrically ill mothers and their young children offering comprehensive services to both mother and child. The necessity of individualized services for all participants at one site has been increasingly highlighted because of the disorganized, chaotic, isolated nature of these multirisk families, the difficulties encountered in engaging them, and their staggering rates of program attrition. In order to overcome the many obstacles they face, this program has developed the flexibility to meet these families "where they're at" and the persistence to achieve trust, to weather setbacks, and to accommodate developmental changes. The program takes a child advocacy stance while recognizing that the child is best cared for by his own family. Parents are actively encouraged to adopt this conviction not only for their own children, but for the children of this community. Efforts need to be placed in helping the family live independently and successfully in the community by recognizing and addressing their needs. At any given time, 30 families participate for varying lengths of time ranging from 1 to 2 or more years of program involvement. Enrollment is either voluntary or court mandated and referrals are from professionals in the community who feel that the child's development is at risk because of parental psychopathology. This program works in collaboration with a number of inpatient and outpatient facilities including the University of Illinois Pregnancy and Postpartum Treatment Program, which cited the Mothers' Project as intensive treatment of choice on an outpatient basis in a recent article (Miller, 1992).

The center-based program seeks to address the need for primary intervention for the children of parents with mental illness. Clinical data on these children indicates that they often display problems in interpersonal relationships, verbal-conceptual functioning, attentional skills, and mood or affect. They have been long identified as being at risk for the development of cognitive, psychiatric, and emotional deficits. The center-based program also provides a milieu that fosters the development of a supportive peer group for parent participants who are often isolated from the community by nature of, and as a result of, their mental illness. This peer group reinforces the need for management of the symptoms of mental illness and the implementation of child rearing practices that are cognizant of developmental level. The supportive network continues on into the community as families seek to help one another. The center-based program also seeks to teach parents the skills they need to manage their mental illness in order to avoid repeated rehospitalization, as well as the skills necessary to successfully parent their children. The specific program components available to all participants in the center-based program include the Psychosocial Program; Therapeutic Nursery; Family Support Service; Treatment of Substance Abuse Issues; and Ongoing Assessment.

Psychosocial Program

The Thresholds Psychosocial Program offers each participant a comprehensive program to enable her to seek better employment, housing, social life, education, and physical health, while seeking to reduce unnecessary psychiatric hospitalizations. The advantage of a psychosocial rehabilitation approach is that it seeks to build on the strengths of the participants while acknowledging and treating deficits. The program is unique because of the comprehensive nature of the services that is especially important to women with young children. The mothers participate in the nursery according to individual plans and are then able to pursue their personal rehabilitation programs on the same site. They can have lunch with their children and check on them frequently. It

has been found through the years that the psychosocial program offers women with young children a special path to rehabilitation not available elsewhere. Vocational services can be especially tailored for each mother so that she can move at her own pace, beginning with an on-site situational assessment and continuing with work adjustment services and job development services that are sensitive to her role as a mother. These services are offered as a transition back into the community when treatment issues for mother and child are resolved and the child is ready to be referred to local day care or kindergarten. The mothers are asked to focus on improvement of parenting capacity during the child's preschool years. The mothers, in particular, make use of a self-contained education program, working toward a GED and learning basic literacy skills. These skills are increasingly important for the mothers as they help their children with the learning fundamentals. In addition, these basic literacy skills are critical in basic independent living survival skills. A number of current participants have been able to enroll in local community college-level courses that are offered in the evening or that are self-paced, and then use their education time to study and complete assignments. Social programming in groups—including Mothers' Therapy Group, Child Development Class, Infant Group, Medication Attitudes, Parenting Skills, Life Skills, Family Milieu Group, Stress Management, and Goals Group—is not only based on knowledge of these subjects and how to present them to mentally ill parents, but also on issues raised in each program area as being problematic to the specific families involved. The self-esteem enhancing opportunities found in both the social and vocational programs have positive effects on the mother-child dyadic relationship. The thrust of all groups is to aid in the formation of a safe, secure, non-judgmental peer group in which the mothers may operate. Mothers are actively encouraged to interact with each other outside of program hours so that they can develop an ongoing social support system that is so often absent for persons with severe and persistent mental illness.

Case Management Services

As a part of case management services, planning consists of the case manager identifying services to meet the needs of the child and family. This brokerage approach (Portland State University, 1993) links the family to services in a delivery system that is neither well-coordinated nor flexible. The program can be involved as representative payee to pay rent and utilities, to manage funds, to attest to the fact that mother and child are involved in rehabilitative programming, and to teach budgeting skills. The mother is helped in obtaining all appropriate state and federal funding (WIC, SSI, SSDI, Public Aid, etc.) to which she might be entitled. All medical services necessary to mother and child are arranged by the program. This includes prenatal through postnatal services including contraceptive information and materials. Counseling, marital therapy, and psychotherapy are available either directly or through referral by the case manager.

Psychiatric services are provided by the agency's consulting psychiatrists and medication compliance is stressed and reported regularly. The advantage to provision of those services on site is the ability to give clear, concrete feedback as to the mother's functioning in the program rather than reliance on subjective reporting by the patient who may or may not be medication compliant. This consultation is particularly sensitive to the need for mothers to be appropriately medicated so that they may attend to the needs of their growing child while having adequate symptom control.

Therapeutic Nursery

The therapeutic nursery, including infant, toddler, and preschool rooms, has as its purpose the provision of primary intervention services in a safe, stimulating, caring environment that will facilitate cognitive and emotional development. Assessments of the children include both standardized tests and situational assessments to determine the child's initial deficits and strengths and to monitor whether deficiencies are mediated through the provision of therapeutic services. In general, studies comparing children of well mothers and mothers with mental illness suggest that maternal psychopathology influences social-emotional development and social maladjustment during the school years, and cognitive functions such as attention and problem-solving abilities (Stott et al., 1983). Because of the remarkable progress that the children make once intervention is provided, it is felt that many deficits can be attributed to deficits in the mother-child relationship. Some children are affectively deprived over long periods of time. The child is not able to regulate the tension that he feels and becomes either more irritable or withdraws into a shell-like appearance. The child does not reach out to other adults in his environment because he has not been effective with his mother. The child may actually look depressed. He may not cry even when it is appropriate to do so. He may form loose, defensive relationships. Some mothers are deficient in the ability to provide contingent responsivity. The child needs to know that the world is an orderly, predictable place in order to learn. This may be as simple as knowing that when he smiles, someone will smile back at him. In order for language to develop, the sounds an infant makes must be reinforced and assigned logical, consistent meaning by the mother. A strong bond to an adult is crucial for development. Unfortunately as the child begins to show more delays, the mother feels more incompetent and may respond even less to the child.

The primary goal in the therapeutic nursery is to advance the child's ability to both use language functionally and to systematize experience through mastery of conceptual/cognitive processes while simultaneously helping the child to develop a solid sense of self. The successful implementation of this program depends on the teacher's ability to form warm relationships with the children and mothers who choose to identify with her and her modeled behaviors; a knowledge of child development so that her expectations of the children and limit setting are age-appropriate; her recognition that activities should be verbally accompanied to encourage children to observe, compare, and contrast experiences at a symbolic level; and the ability to make a safe, predictable environment. The mothers are asked to work in the nursery one half morning per week as teaching assistants. The staff also has the opportunity to model alternative strategies and to give direct intervention. The primary teacher pays particular attention to promoting bonding and stimulating interaction between mother and child. She teaches the mother good child care routines, observational skills, and knowledge of the stages of normal child development through her own child. The staff models good interactive behavior such as holding eye contact, talking with children, repeating their sounds, describing their behavior, and interpreting that behavior so that the mother can become a partner in these activities and continue them on her own.

The therapeutic nursery is child-centered. The environment is designed to meet the needs of children from birth to 5 years of age and is stimulating and flexible. The atmosphere is one of warmth, nurturance, and safety for both mothers and children. Family activities like birthday parties and holiday celebrations take place in the nursery. It is a place to share, play, have fun, and learn. There are behavioral expectations and limits. The major tool of intervention is that the program recapitulates good child development practices and good parenting skills as a model for mothering and appropriate dyadic interaction. The mothers are nurtured and educated by staff in the same manner that the staff wishes them to deal with their children. There are some general strategies used by the teaching staff in the nursery. One is to build a working relationship with each mother. It is essential for staff to know the mother well and for mothers to understand the role of the teacher so that appropriate boundaries are established. The teacher is the person responsible for the child's development while they attend the Therapeutic Nursery Program. It is differentiated that mothers must get nurturing from their own caseworker who is available to nursery staff any time during the day. Teachers start by acknowledging that mothers know their own children better than the staff does, that they can help staff make the children comfortable in the nursery, and that this partnership will help their children grow. The bonus of establishing such a positive supportive relationship is that the mother is more likely to stay in the program longer and be better able to allow her child to form a strong attachment with the child's primary teacher, which in turn will benefit the child's development.

Family Support Services

Family support services are offered to fathers, husbands, and parents of participants. When a father is actively involved with the mother or child, a weekly fathers' group is held. The purpose of that meeting is to educate him regarding the nature of mental illness and medication as well as to provide support in dealing with a partner with a mental illness. In addition, problems regarding effective parenting are discussed. Family members are routinely referred to appropriate community services, and if the father also has mental illness, he is referred to psychiatric services. In families that have two parents with mental illness, the Mothers' Project has offered flexible programming that allows for both or either to participate with the child on a scheduled basis. Compliance with referrals to outside services is also monitored.

A weekly parents group is offered to the parents of mothers involved in the program when they are a part of the extended family support system available to help both mother and child. The purpose of this whole agency-based group is to help parents understand the nature of mental illness, to offer support, and to help with planning for provision for their daughter and grandchild. These siblings and grandparents are recognized as important stabilizing influences for the family and the child so that relationships are nurtured between the family, the extended family, and the project staff. Treatment planning often entails identifying family members who are or would be available to assume care of the child during periods when the parent is unable to do so due to psychiatric or other situational crisis. These family members may attend staffings or program functions, but the program goal is ongoing engagement to ensure stability for the child. During periods of psychiatric instability, their involvement with the child may be critical in avoiding substitute foster placement.

Substance Abuse Treatment

Substance abuse treatment is also offered because, besides mental illness, women in the Mothers' Project may also be confronting these issues. Use of mood altering substances takes on special significance for this population because persons with mental illness often have more extreme reactions to substances, both because of their idiosyncratic brain chemistry and because they may be combining illicit substances with prescribed medications. Symptoms also may become exacerbated resulting in inappropriate medication dosage. These women often demonstrate deficits in judgement with regard to child rearing. Use of substances can further weaken reasoning ability, impair judgement, and increase emotional liability. All incoming members are screened using an agency formulated Mentally Ill Substance Abuse Checklist (MISA). Mothers are offered on-site education and support groups several times per week. Off-site treatment compliance is monitored. In addition, the agency has on-site testing equipment to detect alcohol, cocaine, marijuana and derivatives, and PCP. The Mothers' Project facilitates inpatient detoxification and treatment if the mother cannot be maintained in the community.

Ongoing Assessment

To evaluate the effects of this program on both mothers and children, ongoing assessment is administered at regular intervals. This enables the program to gauge the degree of positive change that results from program services and provides valuable feedback regarding services that need to be altered. Daily individual case notes are kept on participation as well as weekly team notes for planning. Children are assessed at program intake using the Revised Denver Developmental Screening Test

(Frankenberg, Goldstein, & Camp, 1971) suitable for children age 5 and under. This test provides gross assessments of developmental delays in four major areas: gross motor coordination, fine motor coordination, language development, and social/personal growth. These measures are also administered every 6 months. In addition project staff measure the mother s parenting capacity through the use of the H.O.M.E. protocol (Caldwell & Bradley, 1984). The Global Assessment Scale (Endicott, Spitzer, Fleiss, & Cohen,-1976) is used to measure level of psychiatric impairment.

The Thresholds' client tracking system monitors changes in the mothers' residence, physical health and well-being, substance abuse issues, employment status, and hospitalization occurrences on a monthly basis throughout their participation in the Mothers' Project. The program relies strongly on functional assessment that reflects actual behaviors of mothers and children. The most important area examined is that of attitude toward, and management of, symptoms of mental illness, including: denial/acceptance, medication compliance as well as level of symptom relief, and an understanding of the impact of symptomatology and rehospitalization on the developing child. Of equal importance is the ability of the mother to manage her child appropriately using developmentally relevant skills. The mother needs to provide for the child's physical safety and well-being as well as provide emotional and cognitive stimulation for the growth of her child. The child's development is also assessed noting whether he or she is a difficult child to manage. The affective connection from mother to child is examined as well as any disparate attachment toward siblings. Finally, the mother's social support system is assessed including the relationships that she has made in the program. The mother's ability to form relationships with staff and other participants usually parallels her ability to form a relationship with her child or children.

Ongoing assessment is primarily used for treatment planning and for monitoring the effects of the program on the family. Both strengths and weaknesses are documented. Assessments have been used to help parents regain and retain custody of children who are involved in the child welfare system. The program provides written documentation to the juvenile court and may videotape interaction between mother and child. Sometimes assessment is used to document the mother's inability to parent her child. The program is a mandated reporter and is required to report to appropriate authorities instances of risk, abuse, neglect, environment injurious for harm, and dependency. Participants are aware of this but choose to continue in the program because of the strong, non-judgmental support available to them.

Outreach Services

The home-based program seeks to address the needs for continuity of services into the place where mothers and children live. Individual work with the family is accomplished by all involved staff through this home-based program. While home visits are made on a monthly basis to all families, younger participants receive weekly visits as a part of the

Therapeutic Nursery Program. Child care workers teach mothers appropriate ways to stimulate cognitive development. They help mothers to establish regular reasonable child care routines and schedules, aiding the mother in creating a home that is safe, pleasant, and organized to facilitate optimal development. Staff visit in the evening, particularly when there is a health care crisis with the child. This further helps to create relationships and a caring community in which the families can function.

Outreach staff are also able to receive and distribute the donations of household furnishings, clothing, and other needed equipment more effectively and efficiently. Outreach services range from crisis intervention, to finding an apartment, to helping to organize the home, to obtaining necessary entitlement program funding. Outreach staff can be used to teach activities of daily living including nutrition planning, grocery shopping, and the skills necessary to clean and maintain an orderly apartment.

Although many of the participants of the Mothers' Project live independently in the community, the program has developed an independent living program based on three levels of functioning. Initially families begin in structured agency apartments with 24-hour staff, including personnel certified to deal with issues of substance abuse. After successful stabilization in this setting, families are placed in a residence that has a live-in house manager, and requiring a weekly community meal and house meeting. Families that have succeeded at this level are offered housing in a building within one mile of the agency-based program. These apartments have leases held by Thresholds. Families are able to remain long-term in these apartments and receive home visits at least once weekly. It is essential that the mother receives guidance in developing independent living skills such as paying rent and other bills in a timely manner; negotiating for the regard and the services of the landlord; providing a safe living environment for her family; and providing, through adequate budgeting and organizational skills, a healthy home environment with food, adequate health and hygiene practices, and proper furnishings, clothing, and toys.

The community-based program seeks to address the need for linkage to services necessary for independent functioning and advocacy for participants. At the agency-based program, children and families are regularly screened through well-baby clinics, vision screening, dental screening, and staff child development specialists. When further evaluation or immediate service are indicated, participants are referred to medical, dental, and psychological services through liaisons that have been made with local area hospitals and clinics (including Planned Parenthood). Those programs are chosen specifically because of their willingness to serve low income families and to work with project staff. Casework child care, and/or outreach staff regularly attend these visits with parents and act as spokespersons for the family, helping them to understand information presented to them and aiding in the implementation of recommendations made. Each staff person in the Mothers' Project is responsible for advocacy for all families at a variety of levels. This may range from advocating

for a change in treatment plan to better serve the mother or child, to the completion of written assessments and reports to involved agencies so that services can be obtained. When participants are involved in the child welfare system, staff regularly accompany families to juvenile court to report on the progress—or lack of progress—that they have made in regaining or retaining custody of their children.

Some women seen by the Mothers' Project lose custody of their children to the foster care system because of a dramatic and rapid onset of symptoms. During that period mothers are unable to give minimal care to them. They often reintegrate rapidly. If there is no extended family available or willing to care for the child, the mother may opt for an alternative to placement of the child. The Mothers' Project has located a licensed foster family who is paid a per diem rate to provide respite care for the child to allow for minimal disruption of the family. This allows continued contact between mother and child. Some parents have up to 28 respite days available to them. The program has discovered that often parents choose to have other participants provide such care for their children. The staff offers outreach support for the respite-providing family including home visits, help with shopping and help with transportation to and from the agency-based program.

CONCLUSION

While the study conducted by Nicholson et al. (1993) reflects the lack of services available to families who are trying to parent young children and have at the same time, a serious mental illness, there are programs such as the Mothers' Project that offer services to this population effectively (Dincin et al., 1993). The clinical case management model developed by this program offers a comprehensive array of service options for the family and particularly for the "at risk" child. It should be noted that the program assumes a child advocacy stance that recognizes that the child is best cared for in the context of the child's own family. Mothers are actively challenged to identify with values that demand attention to, and safety of, children. The most salient feature of the program is its psychosocial treatment model that is supportive, non-judgmental, and encourages problem solving and skill building. Nurturance combined with adequate supportive services provides a milieu in which gains can and have been made. These services are cost-effective when compared to the cost of hospitalization. Mothers come in to the program with as many as 50 psychiatric hospitalizations and may have no further rehospitalization during 3 years of participation. For the whole agency, the average number of hospitalizations prior to coming into Thresholds is 6.9, but the rehospitalization rate of members active in the program is 15%, as compared to a national average of 35%. If the Mental Health Task Force survey is correct, the cost to the state of Illinois would be well over $8,000,000 for specialized substitute care for each year that these children remain in foster care in Cook County alone. These children historically remain in long-term foster care in the state of Illinois with little hope of returning home.

The cost to the family and the child cannot be calculated in terms of repeated separations that may be unwarranted and could be avoided with adequate supportive services.

REFERENCES

Astrachan, B., Bell, C., Budd, K., Feys, N., Geraghty, T., Heyrman, M., Kane, D., Kruesi, M., Lelio, D., Leventhal, B., Miller, L., Williams-McCargo, C., & Zeitz, M. (1994). *Report of the mental health taskforce special Wallace case investigation team.* Unpublished report to the State of Illinois Legislature, p. 3, March 8.

Dincin J., & Zeitz, M. (1993) Helping mentally ill mothers. *Hospital & Community Psychiatry, 44*(11), 1106-1107.

Endicott, J., Spitzer, R. L., & Fleiss, J. L. (1976). The global assessment scale for measuring overall severity of psychiatric disturbance. *Archives of General Psychiatry, 33,* 766-771.

Focal Point. (Winter/Spring, 1993). Case management for families and children. The Bulletin of the Research and Training Center on Family Support and Children's Mental Health. Research and Training Center, Portland State University.

Miller, L. (1992). Comprehensive care of pregnant mentally ill women. *The Journal of Mental Health Administration, 19*(2), 170-177.

Nicholson, J., Geller, J., Fisher, W., & Dion, G. (1993). State policies and programs that address the needs of mentally ill mothers in the public sector. *Hospital and Community Psychiatry, 44,* 484-489.

Stott, F., Musick, J., Clark R., & Cohler, B. (1983). Developmental patterns in the infants and young children of mentally ill mothers. *Infant Mental Health Journal, 4*(3), 217-235.

CHAPTER FIFTY-EIGHT

Establishing Support and Advocacy Groups

Susan Delaney McConchie

This chapter was previous published in Mental Health Special Interest Section Newsletter, 5-6, 8. *Copyright* © *1989, The American Occupational Therapy Association, Inc.*

Establishing community-based support groups can be a new challenge for occupational therapists. Do you have a yen to explore new directions or to develop new roles for yourself? You have the skills and the background to be of tremendous help to persons in your community, agency, or hospital. Your local newspaper will list support groups or self-help groups that are already operating. Reviewing these listings may give you the impetus to start a group to help meet an identified need in your practice or program.

Several years ago I joined the staff of a community mental health agency. As I continued to work there, I realized that many of our clients had problems that went beyond their stated diagnoses. With the administration's approval, I developed a simple questionnaire to circulate to the staff. The results did confirm my observations: A total of 75 patients, or 8% of the outpatient caseload, carried a secondary diagnosis of such disorders as cerebrovascular accident, cerebral palsy, multiple sclerosis, heart conditions, and so on. Some of the major reasons these clients had been referred to the mental health clinic were such problems as marital conflicts, depression, and feelings of isolation. They were having problems adjusting to the physical aspects of their disabilities, and problems dealing with agencies and service providers; these needs had not been addressed. Armed with these findings, I approached the agency director and persuaded him that we could better address these people's dual needs by establishing a support group designed specifically for them. He agreed, and a very rewarding chapter in my career began. What follows is an outline of the process we used to develop our group, a description of the group, and a partial discussion of subsequent issues and developments.

GETTING STARTED

Work or Volunteer Project?

The first thing to decide is the context of the project: Do you want to establish a group as part of your regular work load or as a volunteer project within your community? In terms of productivity, payment for services, and so on, you will have to weigh the pros and cons of each option carefully—including agency policies and politics. My own opinion is that it is better to undertake the project as a staff member, because you will have more resources available to you and the group in that context. The task then becomes one of providing education and training skills to the consumers involved, thus enabling them to take over the running of the group themselves. The leaders can then become consultants, which is a less time-consuming role.

Identification of Community Needs

What are some of the needs you have identified in your work setting that are not being met by your existing program? List them first, and then brainstorm with coworkers for additional needs they have identified. You may have some community requests to consider as well; as local community members became aware of our programs, requests came in to the agency for assistance in developing a variety of other groups, such as one for family members of persons with chronic mental illness, one for persons with eating disorders, and another for pregnant teenagers

Time and Coleadership Issues

If you have decided to have a coleader, identify someone who shares your ideas and enthusiasms and is willing to assume new roles. Having a similar theoretical orientation is also important, and it is helpful to have a coleader with background in the content area you have chosen to stress—perhaps someone who works in a different agency or setting.

Coleadership takes time, and it is important to be sure that your administrator or supervisor understands this. Coleadership does not mean that the group can be twice as large. Time is needed for preparation and for postgroup processing. You will have to decide how much time you can realistically devote to this new project, because—as you will see when you begin—you are not leading a traditional occupational therapy treatment group. In the initial planning stages, 3 hours per week may be needed for planning, phone contacts, group meetings, and processing; later, 2 hours should be sufficient. It is, however, easier to schedule more time initially than to create it later on!

Establishing the Format

Early decisions might include the size of the group, how transportation will be arranged, the meeting location, and whether or not to have a coleader. Other considerations are the age range of participants and how long the group will run (will it be ongoing or time limited?).

Another variable is group content. What type of group format do you envision? Will your group be strictly educational, with films and lectures, or do you envision a self-help model in which the group members determine the agenda? Do you want to provide a purely supportive group environment, or do you want to teach members advocacy skills? To a large degree, answering these questions determines the leaders' roles. For the remainder of this chapter, it is assumed that you have decided to combine aspects of both support and self-help groups and that your ultimate goal is to see this group maintain itself in the community. Eventually, your role would be that of some kind of informal consultant.

Other Considerations

Additional questions to consider before starting a group might include these: What will your referral process be? How will you screen interested people for membership? How will in-group emergencies be handled? What about general communication with referring staff? Will the agency charge a fee, or will contributions be voluntary? Will refreshments be made available? Consulting the literature on various support and self-help systems may help you decide these questions; you may also want to attend local meetings of other groups nd talk with group members.

As with any kind of program, recordkeeping is extremely important. Because ours was a new venture, keeping detailed notes proved very helpful when we decided to expand the program into new areas. Records were also kept of any critical issues that needed to be passed on to clients' primary therapists (clients agreed to allow them access to this information). Attendance records were also maintained.

SUPPORT GROUP FOR PERSONS WITH PHYSICAL HANDICAPS: DESCRIPTION OF PILOT GROUP

A description of this group is presented to help illustrate client and staff development and growth as this agency-based support group changed to a community-based self-help and advocacy organization.

The data generated from the aforementioned questionnaire proved quite helpful in establishing our group. Appropriate clients were identified within the agency. An outpatient therapist with three such clients in his caseload expressed interest in coleading the group. He was selected as coleader, and we began our planning by discussing the kinds of needs his clients presented. The questionnaire also helped us identify other clients and their primary therapists for further referrals.

Goals and Plans

We set specific goals for the new group, including (a) facilitating a support network among the members, (b) using the group as a forum for sharing information and resources, and (c) teaching clients to become their own advocates. Transportation was determined to be the client's responsibility, although suggestions to meet this need would be available. Because the clients would retain their primary therapists, case management issues would be directed to the original therapist.

All initial members of the group had come to the agency with symptoms of depression, and in one case suicidal ideation was an issue. We suspected that the members' depressions might increase as members shared the stresses of their disabilities, so we decided to teach group members early on how to use the agency's existing emergency services and similar emergency services in the community at large.

We then interviewed prospective members, explaining the purposes of the group. This allowed us to evaluate the clients' communication skills informally, identify their primary issues, determine the main reasons they were interested in joining the group, and verify other agency contacts or connections they might already have.

Group Members

We were cautious at first, so our original group consisted of only six members (three other potential members were placed on a waiting list). Though the following thumbnail sketches are limited at best, I think they will help the reader begin to understand the group's makeup. The extraordinary variety of backgrounds in the group should be noted.

Sue was a 35-year-old widow with two pre-teenage children. She had severe multiple sclerosis and had recently begun using a wheelchair. Derek, in his early 30s, had juvenile diabetes. Blind since 19 years of age, he had recently gone through a divorce and was learning to live by himself. Greg, Derek's friend, was 55 years old and nearly blind. He was quite depressed over his increasing dependence and near isolation (he lived on a farm in a rural community). Mary, 35 years of age, had severe scoliosis as well as other physical problems. She was severely depressed and at times suicidal. Carla, a 17-year-old high school student, had moderate cerebral palsy and evidence of learning disabilities and speech impairments. She frequently threatened to act out her feelings as a means of coping with her depression. Finally, there was Bill, 35, who had sustained a severe head injury in his work as a farmer. Bill was phobic and had many residual difficulties from his injury.

The First Meeting

The group's first meeting was scheduled, and all members were in attendance. We began by asking them to share something about themselves, especially about their disabilities and needs. As coleaders, we also shared briefly about ourselves and more specifically about our interest in this group and why we felt the group could be useful. We were amazed at the outpouring of feelings that took place; clients said that it was the first time that anyone had shown interest in their disabilities. They talked about events that had been crushing to them, and about what it meant to them to be labeled. They also shared feelings of loneliness, fear, and severe isolation. All were experiencing family problems (including, in many cases, marital problems) that seemed directly related to their physical conditions. They also evidenced an astonishing lack of knowledge about their various disabilities and their resulting difficulties. They suffered from fragmentation of services, and had little idea of how to access needed benefits and services, such as transportation or social security income. Access to buildings was very limited at that time. Financial problems were evident, and members had great fears for the futures of their children. The list of unsolved issues went on and on.

The group bonded early on, and little by little started to create an additional network outside of the agency. Group members made telephone calls to one another between meetings. The leaders noted the expressions of anger in the group and supported self-advocacy efforts as they emerged. After a few months of meetings, it became clear to all of us that we needed a concrete way to focus members' feelings of outrage over a general lack of services and accommodations for people with physical disabilities. As coleaders we supported the clients' idea of writing a letter about their issues to the agency director and board. We were somewhat worried about our job security as a result, and spent some time reassessing our position and its consequences. Although we remained somewhat anxious about the agency's response, we came to the conclusion that actions needed to follow ideals. The letter was written by the group and typed by an agency secretary.

This turned out to be a critical turning point for our group and for us as coleaders. We had been the leaders, they the clients, but now that distinction was blurred to some extent. We had become activists.

In response to the letter, the agency director came to a group meeting and listened to the group's complaints. Together we came up with a plan to remedy the most essential issues. Accessible, if not glamorous, bathroom facilities were provided, as were parking lot signs, a buzzer system to open the door near the ramp, and another railing on the stairway. Group members worked with agency staff members to get these tasks completed outside of group time, while we as coleaders spent extra time on the telephone with our rather nervous consumers, supporting them, helping them decide what to say to staff involved in the renovations, and so on. We soon found that we had in effect two groups, one needing ongoing support at meetings and the other wanting to take our time to address issues in the community. This latter group wanted to get other persons with disabilities involved in advocacy.

The Next Stage

At about this time, a flyer about a leadership skills training program appeared on our agency bulletin board. We took advantage of this program and helped three of our group members enroll. They came back to group sessions full of ideas and ready to establish another group in the community to tackle additional issues. We saw that establishing this type of community group would empower these clients and could provide a mechanism where advocacy and self-help would be the norm rather than just a new service within the agency. We spent several of the next support group sessions planning the community group, deciding on a name, coming up with topics of general interest, and compiling a speaker list. We discussed when and where this new group would meet, how to secure a meeting place, and the need for publicity to reach others who could profit from such a group. We provided transportation to meetings with staff persons from other agencies, and provided guidance and suggestions on additional topics as they were raised.

The original group of six clients formed the core of the new group, Handicaps for Handicaps, that began to meet on a monthly basis in the local Salvation Army gym. For the members, choosing a name for this new group seemed to be part of the needed process of freeing themselves for this next stage of development. These early members became the officers of the new advocacy group; my coleader and I served as consultants. The initial support group continued within the agency.

As time went on, referrals began coming from other agencies to both groups. My coleader and I continued to meet regularly and learned to divide issues between the groups. We discovered that we had created a type of aftercare group that we could recommend to clients when they had graduated from the agency support group. The support group continues to meet at the agency today and continues to provide long-term support for clients. The community group, which later changed its name to The Coalition of the Handicapped, became a true advocacy group. Among this group's accomplishments were marked parking spaces for disabled people, ramps and curb cuts in downtown areas, and increased awareness of and adherence to federal, state, and local codes for all new public construction. It was instrumental in improving transportation networks for disabled people in our area. Social events and an informal telephone network sponsored by this group helped members feel less isolated.

The Coalition of the Handicapped served as a rallying point and as a forum for client-agency interaction. Representatives from a variety of health-related agencies were frequent observers, speakers, or guests at monthly meetings; interagency collaboration grew as a result of the group's efforts. Community consciousness was raised as well, because the group refused to have its concerns overlooked or ignored. Group members also became active members of their communities, and attended such local meetings as city council meetings.

In addition to The Coalition of the Handicapped, the original agency-based support group served as a stepping-off point for several other community-based self-help groups, including two groups for parents of students with special needs and an educational and support group for people with diabetes and their families. Staff training models were developed to help agency and community caregivers more fully understand the dual diagnoses represented by clients with both emotional problems and physical disabilities. Eventually, a presentation was made at a regional mental health conference about this program.

SUMMARY

I've tried to share the beginnings of one effort in advocacy. I believe that the role of occupational therapy in the development of such systems is a natural extension of community practice. I hope that this chapter provides food for thought and gives you the impetus to review the needs of your own system.

I would like to thank Richard Stayton, MSW, who served as coleader of the pilot group described in this article, and Carolyn Crane Nicholson, MEd. Both are employed at Monadnock Family Services in Keene, New Hampshire.

CHAPTER FIFTY-NINE

Starting a Stress Management Program

Sharon Mueller and Melinda Suto

Within the last few years, stress management has become the subject of numerous lectures and workshops. They are sponsored by educational institutions, health care agencies and the business community. What precisely is meant by the phrase "stress management" as it relates to (mental) health care services? For our purposes, we have defined stress management as the "coping behaviors that are learned to reduce the effects of overstress resulting from the environment, the social and cultural milieu, and specific life events." The purpose of this chapter is to convey general knowledge of stress and how it affects people, and to explore individuals' stresses and find effective ways to cope with them.

Although most people could benefit from learning skills with which to cope with life stresses, there exists a high-risk population that we will focus on in this chapter. Specifically, these people are: patients (and their families) with a psychiatric disorder, patients who are chronically ill (e.g., diabetes, rheumatoid arthritis), the elderly and the physically handicapped.

People chosen for this group had a variety of psychiatric diagnoses (except those currently psychotic or suicidal), but it was more useful to judge their degree of maladaptive coping behavior than to rely solely on medical diagnoses. Referrals were accepted from the local Community Care Teams, and for people currently in the Day Program. Those clients who attended the Day Program and the stress management group had increased opportunities to practice their new skills within a supportive setting and receive feedback on their attempts.

In developing this program, material was used from books by Hans Selye (1976; 1971) and Rosenman & Friedman (1978), and prevailing theories on subjects such as nutrition, yoga, balancing exercise, work and play, etc. The treatment program used an educational model and allowed for group discussion. This format encouraged group support, problem-solving and a sharing of personal experiences. During the two and one half hour, once-weekly meetings, homework was discussed, new information presented, and the final half hour involved application of relaxation techniques (i.e., yoga, progressive relaxation, etc.). A handout covering the day's material was also available to participants during this five-week period. Specific outlines for each stress management session are summarized below, followed by a detailed discussion of selected topics.

Session one dealt with the aims of the group, confidentiality, and participants' responsibility, and outlined the following four sessions. The topics covered in the first session were defining stress, sources of stress, psychological signs of stress, physiological signs of stress, finding one's optimum stress level, the importance of paying attention to signs of over-stress, a personal evaluation that included client goals and individual stressors, and relaxation exercises.

Session two discussed the correlation between stress and illness, reducing negative effects of stress, replacing maladaptive coping behaviors, and changing attitudes toward situations.

Session three included an examination of attitude changes, healthy lifestyles, more relaxation techniques, and analyzing individual work/play/sleep patterns.

Session four covered specific stresses inherent in the following life periods: childhood, adolescence, young adulthood, middle age, and aged. Also, we elaborated on the handling of over-stress arising from home, work and social situations.

Session five included a discussion of physical exercises to use when faced with stressful situations, listing in point form of "things to remember" in dealing with stress, role-playing difficult situations using the video, and evaluating of the program to find out whether people achieved their goals.

Defining stress is an important aspect of the program since many people are not aware that they are experiencing a physiological or psychological response to stress. Individual differences are also important. Some people thrive on being busy, whereas others have a much lower tolerance for a busy schedule. Similarly, different people have various methods for handling stress. One person relaxes by doing physical activities, whereas another person prefers to do relaxation exercises or read.

The correlation between stress and illness was also discussed. Emphasis was placed on the ability of the individual to influence his or her health in a positive manner by dealing effectively with stress and by using healthy coping behaviors such as relaxation, yoga, or physical exercise, as opposed to doing such things as overeating and oversmoking. A healthy lifestyle is an important tool in dealing with stress. Such techniques as assertiveness training can be useful, as can attitude change. For example, a person can learn to say "I would like to get this done," instead of "I must get this done."

Having a balance between work, play and sleep is also important. One exercise used in the course is a "life pie." Clients are asked to divide the pie according to how much time they spend at work, play and sleep over a 24-hour period. These are then divided further into whether these activities are physical or mental. In this way, they can look at how much time is spent in each area and can evaluate where changes are needed to achieve a balanced life style.

The course also deals with the effects of change on stress level. Although Hans Selye's stress scale is outdated, it is discussed briefly, and the importance of not having too much change at one time is emphasized. If, for instance, someone had just changed residences as well as recently married, it might not be a good time to change jobs as well. Even positive events can be stressful when they involve change, and limiting the number of changes occurring at the same time is an important factor in preventing overstress. It is also important to consider stresses specific to different aspects of life. Home, work and social situations each present certain problems. Stresses arising from home life and social situations are primarily related to skill and comfort in interpersonal relationships. Although work stresses involve these areas, they also involve pressures specific to the job. Stresses arising from any one area can affect the individual's ability to function in another.

The following procedures are used to evaluate how individuals deal with stress. In each instance, clients are asked to identify what they find stressful, and to consider how they are currently dealing with these stresses. Are they doing such things as oversmoking, overeating, or overdrinking to cope, or are they using more healthy methods? If their usual methods seem inadequate, more useful ways of dealing with stress can be pointed out. Particular attention should be paid to the individual's own stress tolerance. Is he or she a "racehorse," or a "turtle?" What is fun for one person may be stressful for another.

Skills such as diaphragmatic breathing, relaxation exercises and yoga can be taught as alternatives to unhealthy coping behavior. Other behaviors, such as assertiveness training, leading a generally healthy and balanced lifestyle, and using breaks in the day's routine for relaxation and exercise, are useful as well. Limiting change when under stress is also an important technique, as is being assertive and direct about

needs and sharing feelings. A list of specific stresses with possible solutions can then be generated, providing the client with a number of alternatives. The more alternatives the individual has available, the less likely [he or she is] to be overwhelmed by stressful situations.

It is also important to be aware that different life stages give rise to certain specific stresses. A child just starting school, for example, will experience stress as a result of the necessity to leave home, make friends, and function independently, whereas the adolescent will be more concerned with the issues needed to [be dealt] with as he or she changes from child to adult. The child or adolescent who is under stress may demonstrate it by stuttering, nail-biting, poor eating and sleeping, or rebellious behavior. If this type of behavior is apparent, it is useful to find out what specific stress is occurring and to look at more positive ways of dealing with it.

Likewise, the young adult, the middle-aged and the elderly each have their own set of problems. The young adult will have to make career choices and become emotionally and financially independent. The adult in the middle years will be likely to experience such things as the "empty nest syndrome," accepting the problems of aging and perhaps looking after aging parents. Again, it is important to evaluate the specific stress and to adapt healthy methods of dealing with it. The middle years can be used as a time to reevaluate life roles and goals and to set new goals for the next 30 years.

Perhaps no age group has more problems of stress than the elderly. Loss of physical or mental ability, loss of friends, power, independence, and role in society all contribute to the difficulties of the older citizen. Stresses can be identified and alternate solutions generated for each problem. Planning ahead of time for change of lifestyle can be particularly useful as it enables the individual approaching retirement to cushion the effects of change by developing interests away from work, building a network of friends and developing a variety of interests.

In evaluating techniques for handling stress, several things become apparent. A variety of techniques are needed because specific situations require different skills. In addition, it was evident that different methods work for different people. When clients evaluated the stress management program, no specific technique was seen by the group as being most helpful. Individual groups found different things useful. Some found relaxation exercises and yoga most helpful, whereas others found sharing feelings, being assertive and leading a more balanced lifestyle most important.

A number of stress management techniques can be adapted for use in the general hospital setting. Health care teaching needn't take a great deal of staff time and can pay off in extra dividends for the patient. First, he needs to evaluate his lifestyle. Get him to do a "life pie" to assist him in his evaluation. Is his life balanced between work, play and sleep? Does he get adequate exercise and rest? What stresses is he currently under and what is he doing about [them]? What changes are happening in his life and can some of these be postponed? Will there be any long-term effects of illness and what stress management techniques can he use in view of this illness? The person with coronary difficulties, or the patient with a permanent physical disability, who formerly used vigorous physical exercise as a form of relaxation, will need to look at alternate methods of coping with stress. Relaxation exercises and yoga can be taught, and patients could be given cassette tapes to listen to and follow. Teaching the patient to cope with the physical aspects of illness is also important. Talk to the patient and try to ascertain how he or she views that illness. Keeping the stresses of different life periods in mind and helping to evaluate the patient's lifestyle can be useful in identifying the stresses a patient may be under, and can help in planning the nursing care.

In summary then, there are certain general principles in stress management. These are as follows:

1. We need to reevaluate our life patterns and to take control over our lives.
2. Stress weakens psychological resistance as well as immunological response.
3. Be aware that your emotional and physical health affect each other.
4. Avoid excessive simultaneous life changes. Be aware of which pace of life is appropriate for you and pay attention to yourself.
5. If feeling uncomfortable, stop to consider why and make any appropriate changes.
6. Maintain a steady pace at work and play. Avoid great swings in activity levels. Pace yourself.
7. Remember to equalize stress through variety in daily activities.
8. Live at a tempo and direction best suited to yourself. Remember, "One man's work is another man's play."
9. Adopt a healthy lifestyle and a positive attitude.
10. Work on clear communication to decrease tension in interpersonal situations. Don't be afraid to make your needs known.
11. Learn a variety of coping techniques so that if one doesn't work you can use another.
12. Note those around you who cope well and try mimicking their behaviors.
13. Remember, it's not stress in itself that is harmful but rather, what you do or don't do to deal with it.

REFERENCES

Rosenman, R. & Friedman, M. (1978). *Type A behavior and your heart.* New York, NY: Fawcett Crest.

Selye, H. (1976). *The stress of life.* New York, NY: McGraw-Hill.

Selye, H. (1971). *Stress without distress.* New American Library.

Pelletier, K. (1977). *Mind as healer, mind as layer: A holistic approach to preventing stress disorders.* New York, NY: Dell Publishers.

Holmes, T. & Rahe. (1967). The social readjustment rating scale. *Journal of Psychosomatic Research, 2.*

CHAPTER SIXTY

The Day Center and its Role as a Social Network

Harriet Woodside

This chapter was previously published in Hospital and Community Psychiatry, 36, *177-180. Copyright © 1985, The American Psychiatric Association.*

When chronic mentally disabled persons move into supervised care settings in the community after living in a large mental hospital for 2, 10, or 20 years, they usually arrive without any social links to their new home or neighborhood. If they are fortunate, they may find an old friend from their ward in the residence who can introduce them to some of the other boarders and point out the local doughnut shop. If they are especially fortunate, they will attend a day program, or they may have a conscientious case manager to help them establish new roots.

However, the deinstitutionalized often move from a ward where they had some social life and involvement in occupational and recreational programs to a new home chosen because it had a vacant bed or was in the same catchment area as the hospital they were leaving. Accustomed to having all activity occur under one roof in a highly controlled way, many of the deinstitutionalized seem to hover in the community as though waiting for something to happen.

If no comprehensive social networks are organized by members of the community or staff at the residence, it becomes the concern of the mental health professional to assist the chronic mentally disabled living in the community to find and maintain social links. While the need for social contacts for the chronic mentally disabled has often been identified, concrete descriptions of programs addressing this need are not plentiful.

I will begin by discussing the chronic psychiatric patient's need for social networks, and then describe the Fennell Program Day Center that provides a social network for its clients.

THE IMPORTANCE OF FRIENDS AND FAMILY

Test and Stein[1] list the following as characteristics of the chronic psychiatric patient:
- A high vulnerability to stress

- Deficiencies in coping skills such as budgeting, using public transportation, and preparing meals
- Dependency so extreme that they perceive themselves as helpless and requiring massive support from people and/or institutions in order to survive
- Difficulty in working in competitive jobs
- Difficulty in managing interpersonal relationships, especially close ones

These characteristics may be the result of the disease process, the result of lasting incapacities that remain after an acute episode, the result of the process known as "institutionalization," or an intertwining of several factors. If we take these characteristics into account, it seems that most chronic psychiatric patients do not have the ability to seek social contact with others. Yet North American investigators have found that the social network is an important indicator of outcome,[2] even though it is very difficult for the disabled person to maintain.[3,4]

Cross-cultural studies supply evidence that the nature and form of the social network is important to the health of the chronic mentally disabled. One major cross-cultural study has shown better outcomes for individuals with schizophrenia in developing countries, compared with outcomes in developed countries.[5] In interpreting these findings, Mosher and Keith[6] point out that extended kinship networks and natural support systems protect schizophrenic patients from stress. The importance of social support systems in relieving stress for schizophrenic patients is also emphasized by other authors.[7,8]

Because the close and caring social network of communal villages like those in Nigeria or Laos does not exist in North America, our chronic mentally disabled require some substitute that will mediate their anxiety while helping them to maintain coping skills. Support for this premise comes from Linn and her associates,[9] who compared 10 day treatment centers. They found some to be more effective than others in reducing the symptomatology of schizophrenic patients, in changing some attitudes about the hospital, and in delaying relapse. Centers that focused on counseling their patients were less successful than those offering occupational therapy and recreational activities. Linn and her associates suggest that a nonthreatening environment offering activities rather than insight-oriented therapy is an effective model for management of the chronic schizophrenic patient. These findings imply that low-stress group programs that include tasks for the participants will meet the needs of the deinstitutionalized chronic population.

THE FENNELL PROGRAM DAY CENTER

In the fall of 1980 another occupational therapist and I began planning a program for deinstitutionalized clients from the two chronic care wards (known as the Fennell Program) of Hamilton Psychiatric Hospital in Hamilton, Ontario. The day center is part of the Fennell Program community team that provides case management and program planning for 100 discharged patients.

The original goals of the day center were to improve the quality of the clients' lives, to regularly monitor their behavior, and to offer structure and support to help them maintain their present status. We did not focus on the program's potential for building and maintaining a social network.

Our clients are between 26 and 77 years of age; they have been hospitalized from two to 40 years. Of the 23 people we currently see, 12 are men and 11 are women; 19 are out-patients.

Of these out-patients, 11 have a diagnosis of schizophrenia and four have a schizoaffective disorder. The remaining four have various diagnoses, each reflecting a chronic psychiatric condition. Eighteen live in supervised board-and-care residences; one lives at home.

Their relationships with other people are generally unilateral. For example, while patients receive support and encouragement from residence staff, they rarely help each other. They constantly request cigarettes from fellow out-patients, but, because their financial resources are limited, they seldom reciprocate.

All but three have very little contact with their family. Five report friendships with other ex-patients, but only one reports having regular contact with friends who are not ex-patients or residents of the board-and-care home. Some report casual relationships with storekeepers and others in the immediate community, and all see a case manager on a regular basis. For many, the day center is the only regular activity in which they engage outside of their residence.

The day center is open two days a week from 9:30 a.m. to 3:00 p.m. It is housed in the Sunday school rooms of a centrally located church. Clients come either 1 or 2 days. The program varies greatly, and much of it is planned by the entire group.

The overall objective of the program is to provide activities that will interest the participants, although we do not expect any one activity to interest everyone. Activities include five-pin and lawn bowling, maintaining a large vegetable garden in the summer, indoor gardening in the winter, collating and stapling newsletters and information packages for community groups free of charge, cooking, and participating in birthday parties, holiday events, calisthenics, folk dancing, and simple crafts sessions. (The crafts are usually sold to add to the group's funds.)

The clients also sing, watch movies rented from the local library, and take trips to places of interest in the community.

Most visitors to the day center are struck by its warm, concerned atmosphere. One client started calling the day center "the club" and thus characterized it as a place that provides a sense of belonging, interest, and friendship. There is a good deal of joking and teasing among clients and staff; unusual behavior is generally treated in an appropriate way.

This atmosphere developed slowly. It is undoubtedly strengthened by case managers who continually encourage their clients to attend. The two occupational therapists serve as role models, clearly showing concern for their clients (for example, by telephoning absent clients) and appreciation of clients' talents. As with any group, the more verbal members are helpful in stimulating and maintaining conversation and establishing a spirit of optimism. Those who have been at the day center for a while serve as role models for newcomers.

Although the church was selected for its location, facilities, and willingness to house the day center, several members of the congregation and staff have quite naturally befriended our clients. The caretaker, ministers, secretary, and some members of the congregation now chat with our clients and request their help around the church. We feel that in a small way true community integration is taking place; its natural development and reciprocity have done much to boost self-esteem of our clients.

From the start we set the goal of maintaining, rather than rehabilitating, our clients. The entire program reflects that decision. We keep pressure and stress at a level we know the clients can tolerate and rarely insist that people participate. Instead, we try to offer a variety of activities so that all of the clients will be able to complete successfully and enjoy at least one activity.

Consequently we have not seen major improvement in skills and abilities. However, we have seen dramatic changes in our clients' level of socialization and in their desire to come to the center. It is as though we have touched their innate need to form interpersonal relationships and to give and receive meaning from others.

DISCUSSION

When faced with the problem of creating programs that will take into account the characteristics of the chronic mentally disabled as well as the effects that their illness and long periods of hospitalization have had on them, health professionals may vacillate between despairing and attempting to design the most comprehensive and sophisticated program yet devised.

Even when we planned what we thought were low level, and therefore possible, goals, we underestimated our clients' degree of disability. The first thing we learned was to lower our expectations to match extremely limited skill levels, poor or erratic motivation, lack of self-esteem, difficulty in expressing ideas, and years of accumulated hurts from hospital experiences and family and community rejection.

Once we gave up grand plans and focused on understanding our clients, treating them with respect and dignity, and finding projects that they could accomplish successfully and that were familiar to them, the group began running itself. It became cohesive and positive in outlook. As though soothed by gentleness and concern, clients slowly began to try new activities and to help each other. For instance, members who feared public transportation began taking the public bus to the center. Other clients attempted a new craft or volunteered when an extra partner was needed for folk dancing. These changes occurred only after a client had developed a sense of trust and a genuine liking for the day center.

Thus it is possible for chronic mental patients to function in social networks that are open and reciprocal. Each member is capable of giving as well as of receiving. The silent, most isolated members of our center are often among the first to offer part of their lunch to someone who has forgotten to bring one. In turn, the more outgoing clients acknowledge such isolation and make a point of noticing and praising a new shirt or blouse worn by a withdrawn member.

However, while the social networks of our clients have expanded, they are still largely limited to mental health professionals and ex-patients. This finding is not necessarily negative or surprising since all individuals are generally most comfortable in the company of people with whom they share experiences and interests.

Mosher and Keith[6] note that community support systems "are intended to provide the support that has been lost because of the dissolution of extended kinship networks or discharge from hospital." It is possible to view our day center as a surrogate extended family for some clients. The staff members become parents or family leaders, and the sharing of meals and housekeeping duties adds a note of domesticity to the environment. As in a family, reciprocal roles develop that involve relating to others and carrying out activities. Some clients regularly perform chores or run errands without being asked. Others provide humor, tenderness, or advice.

As has been described, the social network at the day center is slowly extending into the church and urban community. Church members who have known some of the clients for more than 2 years often remark that they are more outgoing and that they look happier. Through our volunteer work of collating and stuffing envelopes, we have friends at the arts council, the women's center, and other local agencies, and occasionally clients will mention that they have passed a familiar face on the street.

Thus the developing social network has had a ripple effect on many areas of our clients' lives. They now have a definable role, that of group member, which encompasses volunteer, companion to others, and participant in sports or crafts. This role provides a needed stability and focus for each client. With the concomitant improvement in self-esteem, this role also enables clients to cope with stress more successfully. At the same time the protective nature of the group shields clients from stress.

CONCLUSION

From its start, the day center was led by mental health professionals backed up by a competent team of case managers.

Although the literature reflects hopes that communities will offer programs to integrate and occupy discharged chronic psychiatric patients, such programs cannot be established without professional help. Our clients are still symptomatic, and they have frequent crises requiring professional support. The development of an efficacious program demands a knowledge of the clients' disease process, the ability to assess their strengths and weaknesses, and a suitable and flexible response to their needs. It also demands reconsideration of what constitutes success; we have found that success may be best measured by voluntary attendance rather than by actual participation. We hope that as the community becomes better educated and more sensitized, it will respond to the chronic mentally ill as the church did, accepting them without making many demands. However, we cannot expect the community to provide programs for them without some informed leadership.

Turner and Shitren[10] feel that a manufactured social system will create supportive relationships for the chronic mentally disabled who live in the community. Our experience indicates that such a system initially should be a protected and protective one. Once a client participates willingly, other goals, such as improving one's quality of life or becoming involved in community activities, will be more attainable. Although the security of a safe place and people who care may not improve the behavior of some clients, it does appear to cushion life's stresses and give meaning to daily existence.

REFERENCES

1. Test, M. A., & Stein, L. L. (1978). Community treatment of the chronic patient: Research overview. *Schizophrenia Bulletin, 4,* 350-364.

2. Strauss, J. O., & Carpenter, W. T., Jr. (1977). Predictors of outcome in schizophrenia, III: Five-year outcome and Its predictors. *Archives of General Psychiatry, 34,* 159-163.

3. Lipton, F. R., Cohen, C. I., Fischer, E., et al. (1981). Schizophrenia: A network crisis. *Schizophrenia Bulletin, 7,* 144-151.

4. Pattison, E. M., & Pattison, M. L. (1981). Analysis of schizophrenic psychosocial network. *Schizophrenia Bulletin, 7,* 135-143.

5. Sartorius, N., Jablonsky, A., & Shapiro, R. (1978). Cross-cultural differences in the short-term prognosis of schizophrenic psychoses. *Schizophrenia Bulletin, 4,* 102-113.

6. Mosher, I. R., & Keith, S. J. (1980). Psychosocial treatment: Individual, group, family, and community support approaches. *Schizophrenia Bulletin, 6,* 10-41.

7. Solomon, K. (1978). Societal structure and prognosis. *Schizophrenia Bulletin, 4,* 314-315.

8. Westermeyer, J., & Pattison, E. M. (1981). Social networks and mental illness in a peasant society. *Schizophrenia Bulletin, 7,* 125-134.

9. Linn, M. W., Coffey, E. M., Klett, C. J., et al. (1979). Day treatment and psychotropic drugs in the aftercare of schizophrenic patients: A Veterans Administration cooperative study. *Archives of General Psychiatry, 36,* 1055-1066.

10. Turner, J. E., C. & Shitren, I. (1979). Community support systems: How comprehensive? *New Directions for Mental Health Services, 2,* 1-13.

Professional Development: The Attainment, Maintenance, and Promotion of Excellence

EDITOR'S NOTES

Professional development is a continual life-long process; it does not end when one receives an academic degree or professional certification. Rather, being a member of a profession requires an ongoing commitment to the attainment and maintenance of excellence. Competent occupational therapists value this pursuit of excellence and are personally responsible for their professional development. (Foto, 1998; Sabari, 1985; Welles, 1988). Our professional organization, the American Occupational Therapy Association (AOTA), recognizes this need for ongoing career development and has set the ethical standard that "the occupational therapist shall actively maintain high standards of professional competence...(and)...the individual shall recognize the need for competence and shall participate in continuing professional development" (AOTA, 1988, p 795).

The benefits of a lifelong commitment to one's professional development are numerous. Increased personal pride and satisfaction in one's work; improved health care services for consumers and their families; enhanced professional image among policy makers, reimbursers, administrators, and the multidisciplinary team; and the prevention of burnout and professional stagnation are all viable outcomes of the continual pursuit of professional excellence. (Baum & Law, 1998; Davis, 1998; Depoy, 1990; Foto, 1998; Johnson, 1996; Jones & Kirkland, 1984).

While it is evident that today's health care system is fraught with realistic constraints and significant limitations, occupational therapists can respond proactively to these challenges and continue to achieve professional mastery. (Baum & Law, 1998; Christiansen, 1996; Foto, 1998). Rather than bemoan the constraints and complexities of today's health care system, readers are challenged to emulate many of this text's authors, who have met and/or continue to meet challenges head-on throughout their professional careers.

The ongoing development of a professional career requires the individual to utilize numerous resources. Clinical supervision, peer support, professional networks, mentorships, self-study, in-services, workshops, conferences, and postprofessional education can all be employed to attain and maintain professional excellence (Davis, 1998; Depoy, 1990; Kolodner & Hischmann 1997; Wells, 1988). The chapters in this final section explore professional development issues and offer a number of effective strategies for ensuring professional mastery.

The personal responsibility of the individual to continue to pursue professional mastery is the focus of this section's first chapter by Suzanne Peloquin. The philosophical and ethical principles underlying the need for a commitment to continued professional learning are identified; however, as Peloquin emphasizes, the individual is ultimately responsible and accountable for his or her own professional development responsibilities.

In the next chapter, Deborah Yarett Slater and Ellen S. Cohn present a developmental model for professional growth, which can be utilized for staff development. Developmental concepts are discussed, and relevant clinical examples highlight pertinent points. Practical strategies and recommendations for the implementation of staff development programs are provided. The personal and professional benefits of these programs are emphasized.

A continuum for professional development is also presented in Chapter 63 by Joan C. Rogers, who explores the role of professional sponsorship in selecting and developing leaders for occupational therapy. Rogers explains the diversity of potential sponsorship relationships and defines the qualities, roles, tasks, and benefits of these supportive affiliations. Strategies and examples for implementing sponsorship relationships are provided. The value and efficacy of sponsorship for attaining and maintaining professional excellence is presented.

A frequent outcome of the pursuit of excellence in one's professional career is the assumption of a leadership position to initiate change within established systems. Competent occupational therapists can move confidently into leadership positions and be at the forefront of new and innovative health care programming. A number of excellent examples of occupational therapists fulfilling nontraditional roles have been presented in this text (e.g., Schindler, director of a forensic psychiatry program; Watanabe, supervisor of a psychiatric consultation-liaison program; Barth, director of a program serving the homeless). These model occupational therapists who have assumed leadership roles in a diversity of systems of care are just a few of the exemplary occupational therapy practitioners who have utilized their professional expertise to respond proactively to professional challenges.

However, therapists who are in the earlier stages of their professional development may question their abilities to initiate change. The "how-tos" of developing innovative programming within the constraints of many systems can often seem beyond the grasp of less experienced practitioners. This section's next chapter by Joanne Valiant Cook presents a case study of an occupational therapist's three and a half year developmental process to become a leader for innovation and change within a medical bureaucracy. The vital importance of understanding the barriers to program initiatives and the power and politics of negotiating for change is strongly emphasized. The ability of this occupational therapist to emerge as a leader to promote cultural change and succeed in bringing her program proposal to fruition provides a striking role model. Her vision, flexibility, patience, perseverance, resourcefulness, and unwavering commitment to her clients are qualities that we all must emulate to fully develop our leadership potential. Cook concludes her analysis with clear, concrete, realistic suggestions for initiating change based upon the lessons learned from this exceptional therapist's experience.

The need for leadership to initiate cultural change within an organization is also explored by Brent H. Braverman and Deborah Walens in Chapter 65. The focus of these authors' discussion is the manager's role in creating a "culture of education" that is supportive of students' fieldwork experiences. Because the challenges of today's practice environment has resulted in the troubling trend to eliminate or restrict fieldwork placements, the role of the manager in facilitating administration's and staff members' appreciation of the value of clinical education has become critical. As they explain, providing fieldwork education is a primary professional responsibility that can have many quality of care benefits in an environment characterized by cost-containment and limited resources. In addition, fieldwork education has been identified as one of the most influential factors in determining students' practice preference; therefore, it is vital that occupational therapists in mental health practice, develop and maintain their commitment to providing quality clinical education experiences to future practitioners. (Quinn, 1993). Braverman and Walens provide an overview of five realistic and concrete steps the manager can use to create an environment that welcomes fieldwork education as an opportunity to attain organizational, departmental, and practitioner goals.

Implementing new programs in environments that may resist innovations requires significant marketing skills. This section's next chapter by Karen Jacobs defines marketing concepts and describes the four components of a marketing approach. As Jacobs advocates, all practitioners must learn these marketing tools and techniques to ensure that the programs they design and develop effectively meet a market need and that the value of occupational therapy is recognized in the marketplace. She challenges occupational therapists to embed marketing into their professional and personal lives by promoting the benefits of occupational therapy for well-being and life-long health.

While the acquisition of marketing skills will assist occupational therapists in surviving and thriving in challenging practice environments, additional skills are needed to respond proactively to the dramatic changes rendered by managed care. In Chapter 67, Brent H. Braverman and Gail S. Fisher present the basics of managed care and describe major organizational approaches to implementing managed care. The implications of managed care and these organizational changes for the current and future practice of occupational therapy are explored. The authors emphasize proactive strategies for professional survival in a managed care environment and highlight the need for practitioners to increase their knowledge and understanding of public policy and fiscal realities. Gaining a perspective that is broader than one's own practice environment and advocating for occupational therapy on a personal, professional, and legislative level are viewed as critical to surviving managed care. Expanding the role of the occupational therapist from primarily a direct service provider to consultant, case manager, and/or other indirect service roles; enforcing the collaborative OT/OTA partnership; and facilitating improved interdisciplinary team functioning are also essential for success in a managed care environment. Braverman and Fisher augment their discussion of these important issues with specific practical suggestions as to how occupational therapy practitioners can acquire the skills needed to assume major roles in shaping the future of managed health care.

Peloquin continues this exploration of the implications of managed care for occupational therapy in the next chapter. She examines the incongruence between the concepts and realities of management and those of providing care, and asserts that occupational therapists must manage their practice well. However, Peloquin challenges occupational therapists to move beyond simply managing care to become more active in inspiring care. As she notes, our professional heritage and inherent functioning is one of inspiration; therefore, occupational therapists must engage in actions to shape environments that inspire care. Peloquin concludes with a list of general suggestions on how to infuse inspirational functions into established managerial functions.

While it is essential that occupational therapists work to inspire and maintain caring within a managed care environment, it is also critical that we engage in scientific inquiry to validate the efficacy of our profession. In this text's final chapter, Karen L. Rebeiro provides a strong argument for increased research on the use of occupation as a means to mental health. Her discourse is based on a comprehensive overview of occupational therapy literature which substantiates her premise that historically, occupational therapists have focused more on defining, defending, and debating the philosophical beliefs of their profession at the expense of producing research that operationalized this shared philosophy. While the theoretical literature supports occupation as a distinguishing feature of occupational therapy; and describes occupation as a basic human need that gives meaning to life, promotes physical and mental health, and organizes behavior within multiple personal, sociocultural and contextual dimensions; there are few published research studies available to back these claims. The implications of this discrepancy between established philosophy and existing research are explored by Rebeiro. She proposes that reconciling what we say with what we do in practice is essential if occupational therapy is to be recognized as a valued profession in current and future practice arenas.

Given the recent growth of professional competition in health care, Rebeiro cautions that our professional future may be dependent upon the availability of science that substantiates our philosophical beliefs. She advocates for an increase in research to scientifically validate the use of occupation as therapy and advises all occupational therapists to conduct single case studies to document the therapeutic benefits of occupation. Collectively, these single case studies can provide a body of empirical data that can support the unique role and contribution of occupational therapy in mental health practice. The value of research to professional growth and career development can not be underestimated. More important, as Wendy Wood (1998) noted, occupation is in the research literature of many professions but occupational therapy is not. Therefore, as she cautions, "occupational therapy's fate will be sealed not by—any other outside entity but by how we rise to meet the challenges that have presented themselves to us" (Woods, 1998, p 408).

Readers are challenged to integrate the information and ideas presented in this text to begin (or continue) their personal pursuit of professional excellence. Abdicating this personal responsibility for professional development will result in external forces determining our profession's destiny (Foto, 1998). I believe our profession can become a powerful force in current and evolving systems of care if all occupational therapists assume personal responsibility for attaining, maintaining and promoting excellence in occupational therapy. Therefore, Carpe Diem!

QUESTIONS TO CONSIDER

1. What is your current level of professional competence? Where are you along the continuum of professional career development?

2. What are your personal and professional values and beliefs? How do these influence your professional growth? Are you actively pursuing excellence in your professional career? If not, what is deterring you?

3. What competencies and strengths do you have to offer others to enhance their professional development? What supportive and collaborative relationships can you establish with others for your mutual professional benefit?

4. How does the attainment and maintenance of professional excellence benefit the individual occupational therapy practitioner? What are the benefits of professional mastery for the occupational therapy profession and for consumers of health care?

5. What is your style of dealing with change and possible opposition to change? What are your advocacy skills? Do you tend to be more diffident or more assertive when dealing with

conflict? Would your current advocacy style be effective in initiating a program innovation such as the one described by Cook in Chapter 64? What attitudes and/or behaviors would you need to change and/or develop to be more effective in advocating for change within entrenched systems?

6. How does clinical research relate to one's professional career development? What are research questions you may be interested in exploring? Is there a particular client you are working with whose experiences with occupational therapy would provide a meaningful case study? What are practical, realistic strategies you can utilize to implement research within a clinical setting?

7. How can you enhance your professional growth and career development? How can potential deterrents to growth be changed into professional opportunities? What are the resources and supports available from the American Occupational Therapy Foundation (AOTF), state and local occupational therapy associations, and other professional organizations that can assist occupational therapists in their career development? How can occupational therapists utilize these resources in their ongoing pursuit of excellence?

REFERENCES

American Occupational Therapy Association. (1988). Occupational therapy code of ethics. *American Journal of Occupational Therapy, 42,* 795-796.

Baum, C., & Law, M. (1998). Nationally speaking: Community health: Responsibility, an opportunity, and a fit for occupational therapy. *American Journal of Occupational Therapy, 52,* 7-10.

Christiansen, C. (1996). Nationally speaking: Managed care: Opportunities and challenges for occupational therapy in the emerging systems of the 21st century. *American Journal of Occupational Therapy, 50,* 409-412.

Davis, C. M. (1998). *Patient-practitioner interaction: An experimental manual for developing the art of health care* (3rd Edition). Thorofare, NJ: SLACK Incorporated.

DePoy, E. (1990). Mastery in clinical occupational therapy. *American Journal of Occupational Therapy, 44,* 415-422.

Foto, M. (1998). The Merlin factor: Creating our strategic intent for the future today. *American Journal of Occupational Therapy, 52,* 399-402.

Johnson, J. A. (1996). Old values: New directions: Competence, adaptation, integration. In R. P. Cottrell (Ed.), *Perspectives on purposeful activity: Foundation and future of occupational therapy* (pp. 577-582). Bethesda, MD: American Occupational Therapy Association.

Jones, J. L., & Kirkland, M. (1984). Nationally speaking: Continuing education to continuing professional education shift to life-long learning in occupational therapy. *American Journal of Occupational Therapy, 38,* 503-504.

Kolodner, E. L., & Hischmann, C. L. (1997). Mentors and proteges: Partners for professional development. *Administration and Management Special Interest Section Quarterly, 13*(3), 1-4.

Quinn, B. (1993). Community occupational therapy in Canada: A model for mental health. *Mental Health Special Interest Section Newsletter, 16*(2), 1-4.

Sabari, J. S. (1985). Professional socialization: Implications for occupational therapy education. *American Journal of Occupational Therapy, 39,* 96-102.

Wells, C. (1988). Ethics and related professional liability. In S. C. Robertson (Ed.), *Mental health focus: Skills for assessment and treatment* (pp 3-90 - 3-106). Bethesda, MD: American Occupational Therapy Association.

Wood, W. (1998). Nationally speaking: Is it jump time for occupational therapy? *American Journal of Occupational Therapy, 52,* 403-411.

CHAPTER SIXTY-ONE

Continued Learning: An Adaptive Response

Suzanne Peloquin

Current issues surrounding our professional preparation are well articulated in the occupational therapy literature. The range of controversial topics, from entry-level requirements to specialization options, reflects a wide variety of compelling themes. Credibility and competence, for example, are two recurrent themes underlying arguments for specialization and standardization of curricula (King, 1986). This [chapter] focuses on the theme of personal responsibility for continued learning as one which merits consideration in any discussion about continued education. Continued learning will be characterized here as an adaptive and accountable response that each of us can formulate.

CONTINUED LEARNING AS AN ADAPTIVE LIFE RESPONSE

As mental health practitioners, we scrutinize life experiences. As occupational therapists, we invoke principles and we structure tasks to facilitate healthy responses among our patients. We often speak of achieving a balance and of being adaptive. In advocating a holistic view, we caution our patients and our fellow professionals alike against neglecting significant portions of their lives. We encourage our patients to accept and to assume responsibility for themselves.

In light of our discussion, it seems appropriate to apply these same principles to our life experiences as professionals. If the principles are important, we should benefit from characterizing our professional lives with the principles of balance, adaptive responses, a holistic view, and responsible actions that we recommend to others. In the process of applying these principles to our professional lives, we will be highlighting the theme of personal responsibility for continued learning.

Balance is a principle important to us as therapists. Richard Bolles (1981) describes a balance phenomenon that he calls the "three boxes of life." He refers to a tendency adults have in our culture to sequentially inhabit three distinct life spaces: the world of education, the world of work, and the world of leisure. We proceed through these phases chronologically, and, within each distinct phase, there is the threat of being "boxed in." Young adults (18-22) can spend a disproportionate amount of time in the education box, sometimes to the exclusion of meaningful work or play. Mature adults inhabit the work box, often removed from education, and put off significant play until retirement. Older citizens can become trapped in a leisure box, playing until death. To get out of the boxes, Bolles recommends what he calls life/work planning. What he proposes is endorsed by occupational therapists everywhere: a balance of functions within each life phase.

The portion of Bolles' (1981) thinking that is especially relevant here is adding lifelong education as a component to be balanced within each period of life. As occupational therapists, we speak most often of a work/play balance; Bolles insists that learning must be added to all life phases. He describes lifelong learning as inseparable from work and play because the combination of all three gives life its zest, aim, and mission.

Do occupational therapists perceive education as a lifelong enterprise? Once degree and certification are in hand, do we tend to heave a sigh of relief and end our student role? Do we tend to get "boxed in" by our world of work, depriving ourselves of a vital balance?

Although there is a real probability of getting boxed into a state of imbalance, we need to recognize that we are capable of a different response. We can achieve a balance, and we can commit to learning beyond the box of education.

A second principle that occupational therapists endorse is responding in an adaptive manner. It seems incongruous for therapists who advocate change and adaptation to the environment to be unresponsive professionally to changes around them. Continued learning in our day-to-day practice is an imperative survival strategy. We need to stay current in theories and techniques. It is the rare homemaker who is unaware of the existence of the microwave. Hopefully, it is the rare occupational therapist who is unfamiliar with the contents of DSM-(IV) or the relevance of... (reimbursement standards). Continued openness to those issues relating to our practice can be seen as an adaptive professional response.

A third concept therapists value is a holistic view of man. Although we sometimes struggle with our generalist training, we acknowledge its merit in providing us with a more comprehensive understanding of our patients. How could holistic professionals ever justify in practice or in principle any disregard for growth in professional endeavors while developing other aspects of their lives?

A last therapeutic concept we might relate to our professional lives is assuming personal responsibility. Most therapists carry professional liability insurance, a concrete reminder of the responsibility we exercise each day. In the final analysis we are responsible for our professional behaviors. Only continued learning about clinical issues can secure our ability to make responsible clinical decisions in a rapidly changing world.

If we reflect about ourselves as professionals, and if we apply to our professional situation those principles we value, one conclusion is plausible. It is congruent to assume individual responsibility for learning throughout the life span and to find experiences that can facilitate professional development.

Continued Learning as a Form of Accountability

Beyond what we owe ourselves, there are others to whom we are accountable for continued learning. We have a responsibility both to our patients and to our profession. In a service profession, our patients are the reason we exist (Brunyate, 1985). We owe each of our patients the best techniques and alternatives within our means. Our code of ethics commits us to the education of the consumer of health services on matters of health that are within the scope of occupational therapy. Our consumers deserve and increasingly demand our best and most current knowledge. Only through continued learning can we remain accountable to this new breed of informed patient.

We represent a profession. We sit in rounds, report at patient conferences, and serve on committees, representing far more than ourselves. Once certified, we claim the right to be called occupational therapists or occupational therapy assistants. One consequence of this right is the responsibility to represent our titles well. To represent well includes being cognizant of the situation at hand. It requires continued learning. We mastered what was taught when we were in school, but our theoretical mastery cannot stop there.

Our profession conducts the business of occupational therapy. Some of us balk at this notion as if business were the antithesis of service. The fact is that, in our diverse settings, we engage in business endeavors. Prominent business representatives featured in the book In *Search of Excellence* (Peters & Waterman, 1984) report successful business strategies. One strategy is the fostering of creativity, innovation, and continued learning. Success in business requires a commitment to making the business matter and making the business "work." As participants in the business of occupational therapy, we have a vested interest in learning more about how to make it grow and prosper.

When we respond to our patients and our profession with continued learning, we are responding accountably. Given our responsibility to be current and authentically professional, if we do not take the initiative for continued learning and demonstrate that initiative each day, others may step in to structure, legislate, or otherwise ensure our accountability.

Cultivating Opportunities for Continued Learning

If continued learning is vital on many fronts, then commitment to the process must be developed early and rekindled at regular intervals. Throughout this chapter, use of the phrase *continued learning* in lieu of *continued education* has been deliberate. The two phrases are not necessarily synonymous. While education is a stimulus, it does not always produce a learning response. We may teach facts and skills, but we do not always teach our students to learn.

John Gardner (1963) in *Self-Renewal* reminds us that "the ultimate goal of the educational system is to return to the individual the burden of getting his own education" (p. 12). Our Slagle lecturers have spoken over the years about fostering the drive to learn. Yerxa in 1967 (1985) spoke of the *authentic* professional as that individual who recognizes his or her responsibility to be a lifelong student. Fidler in 1966 described learning as a growth process. She encouraged us to set in operation a learning process that will endure. She cited a passage from a student log illustrating the process being set in motion: "I wonder sometimes if this course is not to teach us so much as it is to make us learn—it would seem that what I am learning is how to learn and teach myself—this conviction grows stronger each week" (1985, p. 149). Once set in motion, the learning process must continue in response to practitioners' needs. And here we face a challenge.

Mental health therapists across the country have markedly different practices and needs, as reported in a survey done by the American Occupational Therapy Association (1982). Opportunities for continued education may vary considerably, but opportunities for continued learning always exist. Given the drive to learn, and the mind-set of a lifelong student, therapists can find opportunities everywhere. We have professional colleagues, journals, publications, bibliographies, special interest sections, and other opportunities available to us. If we have the desire to learn, we will find many suitable vehicles. What we may periodically need is the kind of inspiration that we once received from the best of our teachers and mentors.

Our enthusiasm for continued learning may, as it would for any other task, run in spurts. The energy required must be generated. While we must rely on ourselves to maintain the initiative, isn't it good to know that the effort makes a difference to someone? Certainly it helps to remember that the energy expenditure significantly benefits us, our patients, and our profession. But isn't it a revitalizing moment when a coworker, a colleague, a supervisor, or a former teacher notices the effort? We can help one another to want to continue learning; we can, with the smallest of gestures, make a great difference.

CONCLUSION

Several controversial premises underlie current discussions about our preparation for practice. The theme of personal responsibility is pertinent to those discussions. As our profession seeks to establish guidelines for educating its members, it is crucial to remember that in the absence of individual commitment to continued learning, structured programs may be meaningless. Therapists must want to learn. They must perceive continued learning as an adaptive and accountable response that benefits them, their patients, and their profession. The drive for and belief in continued learning needs to be carefully cultivated and nurtured as a prerequisite to our ability to grow, serve, and prosper.

REFERENCES

American Occupational Therapy Association, Division of Continuing Education. (1984). *AOTA competency based curriculum in mental health.* Rockville, MD: AOTA.

Bolles, R. N. (1981). *The three boxes of life.* California: Ten Speed Press.

Brunyate, R. W. (1985). Powerful levers in little common things. In *A professional legacy: The Eleanor Clark Slagle Lectures in occupational therapy* (p. 29). Rockville, MD: American Occupational Therapy Association.

Fidler, G. S. (1985). Learning as a growth process: A conceptual framework for professional education. In *A professional legacy: The Eleanor Clark Slagle Lectures in occupational therapy* (pp. 137-155). Rockville, MD: American Occupational Therapy Association.

Gardner, J. (1963) *Self-Renewal.* New York, NY: Harper & Row.

King, L. J. (1986). Competence and credibility: A challenge to professional self-discipline. *Occupational Therapy Forum, 1*(6), 13-14.

Peters, T. J., & Waterman, R. H. (1984). *In search of excellence.* New York, NY: Warner Books.

Yerxa, E. J. (1985). Authentic occupational therapy. In *A professional Legacy: The Eleanor Clark Slagle Lectures in occupational therapy* (pp. 155-175). Rockville, MD: American Occupational Therapy Association.

CHAPTER SIXTY-TWO

Staff Development Through Analysis of Practice

Deborah Yarett Slater and Ellen S. Cohn

This chapter was previously published in the American Journal of Occupational Therapy, 45, *1038-1044. Copyright* © *1991, The American Occupational Therapy Association, Inc.*

In an era in which our profession faces a personnel shortage in mental health practice, the retention of experienced occupational therapists is a timely and critical issue. Bailey's (1990) study of the reasons why occupational therapists have left the field documented that attrition is a serious problem for the profession and for the facilities and persons it serves. Bailey noted that "the largest group of survey respondents who have left the profession [35%] did so after 5 to 10 years in practice" (p. 37). With therapists leaving the profession so early in their careers, we are confronted with a shortage of experienced therapists to serve as role models, supervisors, and mentors for newer staff members. One way that we can increase the retention of experienced therapists is by creating incentives. Innovative staff development programs may serve as a viable, practical, and economical strategy to address attrition and retention.

Like many other health care professions occupational therapy offers little career mobility. Many staff members believe that if they are competent, they will receive recognition and benefits by promotion into managerial positions. Such promotions, however take them away from clinical practice. Thirty-one percent of the respondents in Bailey's (1990) study identified poor opportunities for career advancement as a major reason for leaving the profession. The biggest complaint was that our profession is two-tiered, that is, it consists only of clinical staff and department director positions. Despite the existence of career ladders in some facilities, differentiation by salary, title, and responsibilities is limited.

Through their years of practice, seasoned therapists have integrated knowledge and expertise but have received little recognition for their repertoire of clinical skills. The lack of experienced clinicians is particularly problematic when coupled with the complexity of today's health care environment. Cost-containment, greater pressure for productivity, shortened lengths of stay, and patients with complicated medical and social needs require the skills of experienced therapists (Brollier, 1985). In this increasingly complex environment, occupational therapists must develop the ability to critically analyze practice situations.

This need for critical thinkers has been a recurrent theme in our profession (American Occupational Therapy Association [AOTA], 1987, 1990; Cohn, 1989; Parham, 1987; Rogers, 1983/1986; West, 1990/1996). This need is reinforced by the fact that the best role models for new professionals are committed occupational therapists who use an integrated approach to practice (Christie, Joyce & Moeller, 1985). Support for the development of clinicians who can analyze their practice and who are committed to providing quality care presents a challenge to supervisors and administrators alike. Such support can be partially provided through programs that focus on meeting the developmental needs of staff. Accordingly, the purpose of this chapter is to describe an approach to staff development in which reflection on and evaluation of ideas are encouraged, rewarded, and expected as a part of everyday performance. The various developmental needs of staff members as they move from novice to expert are described, as are methods that encourage continual reflection on and evaluation of practice.

STAFF DEVELOPMENT CONCEPTS

Components for successful staff development programs are identified in the management literature. Traditional staff development programs generally consist of formal courses, workshops, conferences, or a series of in-service training events that teach isolated skills and procedures (Pecora & Austin, 1987). These programs focus on immediate gains and productivity as goals rather than on the long-range needs of participants (Kaufman, 1974). Even when supported by the organization, these approaches may not prove to be effective.

Lieberman and Miller (1979) claimed that an effective staff development program should be integrated with the organization's goals and, equally important, integrated with the professionals' goals. They suggested that we focus on the interface between the staff's needs and values and the organization's goals. One way to accomplish this is to use the work itself to stimulate and reinforce professional growth and development. Thus, if the conditions and content of staff development programs are realistic, supervisors will have a better chance of changing behaviors and attitudes. Variation of on-the-job activities to present challenges can create opportunities for self-assessment that provide a basis for ongoing learning. The department director and immediate supervisors play an important role in creating a climate that encourages such self-reflection (Kaufman, 1974).

Another component to be considered in the design of staff development programs is the use of role models, or mentors. This is one of the most powerful strategies available to us for shaping, teaching, coaching, and assisting future therapists (Cohn & Czycholl, 1991; Rogers, 1982/2000; Sabari, 1985; Schon, 1983, 1987). Gitterman and Netter (1968) advocated coupling this notion of role modeling with peer learning to design staff development programs. They suggested setting up situations where staff with varying degrees of experience brainstorm to share their perspectives and ideas.

Conferences, workshops, or other forms of continuing education help clinicians broaden their knowledge base and develop advanced skills. Problems may arise, however, when clinicians have more than adequate knowledge and information about professional issues, strategies, techniques, and skills but simply cannot operationalize such knowledge. One objective of staff development programs, therefore, may be to turn knowledge into action. Analysis of practice can help clinicians break away from procedures and practice concepts that are viewed as fixed formulations and help restore abstractions to their original state. Supervisors can help other clinicians conceptualize patterns of practice, so that learning is not bound to the specific situation in which the learning took place.

To be effective for staff development, supervisors need a thorough understanding of both adult learning and career development. Adult learners are generally "independent, self-motivated learners whose experience orients them to practical issues." (Pecora & Austin, 1987, p. 135). They prefer to apply new knowledge immediately. Thus, effective staff development should focus on skills relevant to the job environment with frequent feedback on the effect of the staff member's actions while the action is taking place (Knowles, 1980). Smith & Elbert 1986) supported this premise by stating that "learning must be integrated with action if training is to produce progress" (p. 129).

THE PROCESS USED FOR ANALYZING PRACTICE

The process for analysis of practice developed for the AOTA/American Occupational Therapy Foundation (AOTF) Clinical Reasoning Study, although not conceived as a staff development program, provided an opportunity for the application of some current staff development concepts, such as role modeling, peer learning, the provision of immediate feedback, and the creation of a climate in which the evaluation of ideas was rewarded. The study took place in the occupational therapy department at University Hospital in Boston, Massachusetts, and continued for 2 years. Initially, seven therapists, each with more than 5 years of experience and diverse backgrounds in occupational therapy specialty areas, began analyzing their practice and the reasoning that directed their choice of actions. The principal investigator, an anthropologist, was assisted by occupational therapy graduate students in a process that involved videotaping patient-therapist therapy sessions. Before and after the therapy sessions, interviews with each therapist were videotaped. In the pretherapy interviews, therapists described their work with the patient and imagined or hypothesized how the session would unfold. During the posttherapy interview, the therapists described what happened in the session and identified key points at which specific reasoning resulted in specific actions. Segments of these videotapes were then analyzed and discussed by the therapists themselves, researchers, and other area clinicians in formal study groups. During the second year of the study, an additional group of seven therapists, each with approximately 1 year of experience, joined the study. Because the researchers conducted separate groups for the novice and experienced therapists, we were able to explicate the differences between the reasoning processes of novice and expert clinicians.

NOVICE TO EXPERT

Integration of the findings from the Clinical Reasoning Study with Dreyfus and Dreyfus's (1986) Model of Skill Acquisition provides an organizing framework for a staff development program. Dreyfus and Dreyfus identified a developmental continuum for growth that involves five career stages: novice, advanced beginner, competent, proficient, and expert. The stages represent increasingly complex ways of responding to practice. Data from the Clinical Reasoning Study demonstrate how these stages apply to the development of occupational therapists.

Stage I: Novice

The novice recognizes various facts and features relevant to the acquisition of new skills and learns rules for determining actions based on those facts and features. Elements of the patient's disability to be addressed in occupational therapy are so clearly and objectively defined for the novice that they are recognized without reference to the overall situation in which they occur (Dreyfus & Dreyfus, 1986). These elements are called context-free, and rules are applied regardless of what else is happening, that is, they are applied in isolation. For example, novice occupational therapists are taught how to assess joint range of motion, muscle tone, or balance and are given rules for how to conduct these procedures. They learn to identify what is normal and what is not, but generally do not consider other aspects of a disability— for example, the effects of joint range limitations on function. Because novices have limited experience with the situation they face, they must be given rules to guide their performance. Consequently, they judge their performance by how well they followed the rules.

In the AOTA/AOTF Clinical Reasoning Study, the novice clinicians focused primarily on objective findings, observable signs, and rules by which to make decisions (Cohn & Czycholl, 1991). Their reports about patients typically included information recalled from course work. They recalled characteristics of the clinical conditions studied and matched them to their patients. For example, a therapist unfamiliar with the diagnosis of Parkinson's disease might read a reference to learn about the symptoms of this illness, yet fail to recognize that the symptoms, such as bradykinesia, will affect the patient's ability to perform routine tasks.

While reflecting on her own development, a relatively new clinician recalled her interactions with patients. She reported that she saw the medical conditions first because she believed that was what she was hired to do—treat the medical condition. She stated, "Once I get my skills down, I can then focus on the interaction." After she became comfortable with the medical focus, she felt free to focus on the patient as a person. Thus, we see that novice occupational therapists focus on context-free elements, that is, the disease processes, free from the context of the patients who have these diseases.

Stage 2: Advanced Beginner

Once novices gain more experience with patients, they learn to consider additional cues, which enable them to consider elements that relate to the patient as an individual. Dreyfus and Dreyfus called this new element situational, in which rules for skill acquisition include both situational and context-free components. For example, occupational therapists at this stage are beginning to consider patients' occupational performance in the context of their patients' expected discharge environments. Advanced beginners recognize the presence and absence of behavior but are not yet able to attach meaning to it, because they are still searching for familiar patterns to assist in problem identification. At this stage, they are still unable to determine priorities. To further clarify this point, try to visualize a patient with spatial perceptual problems performing self-care. The advanced beginner may recognize spatial perceptual impairment in a patient performing self-care but fail to realize that the patient's inability to learn compensation techniques for self-care may be due to a poor attention span as well as decreased motivation. The advanced beginner does not yet see the entire picture.

A relatively young therapist involved in one of the Clinical Reasoning Study groups explained that she structured her treatments according to a framework she learned in school, that is, she had developed a structure to organize her observations for herself. She had a limited ability to sort out significant data, however. The therapist was so focused on the patient's weak right arm that she decided "not to do anything with the other arm because it was okay." However, the patient's potential to function was based on compensatory training of the unimpaired arm. This example illustrates that the therapist was still unable to see the patient's priorities.

Stage 3: Competent

A competent practitioner, according to Dreyfus and Dreyfus (1986), still "sees the situation as a set of facts" (p. 24). Not only do competent practitioners see more facts, but they are also able to identify which facts or observations are relevant. This recognition of crucial facts allows the competent practitioner to determine which aspects of a patient's conditions are most important at a given time. Although competent therapists are able to individualize therapy based on their broader understanding of a patient's problem and are able to handle multiple patient care demands with a feeling of mastery, they lack the flexibility and creativity that characterizes more experienced therapists' work.

Elstein (1978) found that the identification of cues and the generation of multiple hypotheses were two traits demonstrated by successful clinical decision makers. He also found that persons who could gather multiple cues were also able to construct several hypotheses and hold them in abeyance in order to gather additional cues to evaluate the various hypotheses. In the Clinical Reasoning Study, the experienced therapists were able to attend to more patient cues than were novices. They also constructed many hypotheses and seemed to anticipate the need to formulate these hypotheses on a temporary basis. They understood that their initial image of their patients would change as they collected more data. As their images changed, they in turn revised their initial therapy plans.

Stage 4: Proficient

Proficient therapists perceive a situation as a whole rather than as isolated parts. They have a sense of direction and a vision of where the patient should go, and they are able to take steps toward that goal. Proficient therapists are able to recognize and deal with unfamiliar situations and consider options, because they have the experience-based ability to recognize the nuances of a clinical problem. For example, a proficient therapist was able to adapt her handling of a baby addicted to cocaine when she realized that the baby was reactive to tactile input. Consequently, her treatment approach changed dramatically. Proficient therapists are able to see the whole condition. Experience helps proficient therapists identify what typical events to expect in a given situation and how plans need to be modified in response to these events. Proficient therapists can also recognize when the expected picture does not materialize.

By simply learning the diagnosis, such as cerebellar malfunction, the proficient therapist forms a specific mental image of the patient who has this problem and selects evaluation procedures accordingly. The therapist will also hypothesize about the patient's response to therapy before meeting the patient. Once the evaluation is completed, the proficient therapist will modify the initial hypotheses based on unexpected findings.

For the proficient therapist, certain features of a situation stand out as salient and others recede into the background. Once the important elements are identified, the proficient therapist then thinks analytically by combining rules and guidelines to make decisions. As therapy progresses, the salient features, treatment plans, and expectations are modified. No deliberation occurs—it appears just to happen as the therapist draws from similar experiences that trigger plans that have worked in the past and may be reapplied to new situations. Experienced therapists have a mental library full of experiences, whereas novices or students do not (Benner, 1984; Dreyfus & Dreyfus, 1986). (*Note:* Benner's study of nurses was based on Dreyfus and Dreyfus's original work. Benner's study was published in 1984, whereas Dreyfus and Dreyfus did not formally publish their work until 1986.).

In the Clinical Reasoning Study, we observed that novice therapists felt less comfortable revising their plans than did experienced therapists. Newer therapists worked hard to develop a treatment plan and were less likely to alter it when they confronted obstacles, whereas proficient therapists seemed to revise their plans automatically.

Stage 5: Expert

Expert therapists use rules and guidelines in a manner completely different from the novice therapists. The rules shift to the background. Experienced therapists appear to have an "intuitive grasp of each situation and zero in on the accurate region of the problem" (Benner, 1984, p. 32). In this context, intuition refers to a thorough understanding of a situation based on reflections of experiences. Intuition is not irrational, unconscious, or guesswork, but rather, the product of situational involvement and recognition of similarity. The rules, then, are unhitched to the sequence in which they were learned and are applied and adapted to a new situation more easily.

In the Clinical Reasoning Study, experienced therapists intuitively knew when to push a patient toward a higher level of function and when to let go to avoid failure (Mattingly, 1988). For example, an expert therapist intuitively knew when to set limits to increase tolerance for structured therapy. This intuitive judgment is based on correct identification of relevant cues at a particular time in the patient's therapy, and a variety of medical, physical, and psychosocial factors are considered. Expert therapists recognized rules but moved beyond the rigid application of these guidelines based on an inner sense of knowing what to do next. "When things are proceeding normally, experts don't solve problems and make decisions; they do what normally works" (Dreyfus & Dreyfus, 1986, p.31) . However, when confronted with obstacles or new situations, expert therapists demonstrated the analytic abilities described above.

Summary

This continuum of a professional's career can be used as a basis for the design of an effective staff program that influences professional growth from novice to expert. Regardless of their experience, all clinicians may benefit from reflecting on their practice. Experienced staff can instruct those with less experience by example. Because experienced staff may have limited opportunities for advancement in occupational therapy, which is a two-tiered field, sharing their expertise with others in a public forum offers them some recognition. Novice staff members can benefit from observing the broad repertoire of strategies that the proficient and expert clinicians use to engage patients and to reach their collective goals. Other benefits include heightened awareness and interpretation of cues that influence clinicians' actions, identification of successful therapy strategies, and alternatives for meeting treatment goals, all of which lead to a broad approach to practice.

STAFF DEVELOPMENT USING CASE STORIES

The basic elements of the process used to analyze practice in the Clinical Reasoning Study were integrated into departmental staff meetings at University Hospital in Boston. Case stories were created around the process of therapy. Some of these stories involved reports of the constant revision of therapy over time or how the patient and the therapy changed. Textbook descriptions of patients' clinical conditions and a listing of short-term and long-term goals were avoided to make the case stories more meaningful. Clinicians selected a therapy session to videotape, then chose a brief segment of that session and identified a number of leading questions to structure the group discussion. These questions included: (a) identification of treatment strategies that were or were not successful; (b) identification of points in the therapy session in which the therapist confronted obstacles; (c) naming of the story of the session; (d) identification of choice points where changes in the therapy were made; and (e) Who is this patient and what does he or she care about? (i.e., what brings meaning to this patient's life?).

Staff with all levels of experience as well as any students present in the department met so that differing viewpoints, comments, or alternatives could be shared freely among them. As might be expected, staff responses to the process-oriented case story format generated concerns that generally correlated with their stage of professional development. Novice therapists focused on concrete skill acquisition. For example, they enjoyed seeing someone else in action; hearing others in the group discuss alternative approaches. challenges. and techniques that were used when the clinician got stuck; or seeing other specialty treatment areas. Experts, on the other hand, seemed more interested in observing how clinicians engaged their patients. Additionally, the experts were interested in how clinicians create a future with and for their patients, whether there were conflicts in the stories, and how the illness experience affects the patient. These clinicians focused on the more phenomenological aspects of occupational therapy. Although the clinicians viewed and integrated video segments on different levels, they all gained knowledge and benefited from open professional discussions, which often went beyond the specific cases to broader issues affecting the practice of occupational therapy.

Clinicians who had been videotaped articulated tangible ways in which they thought videotaping and analyzing practice in reflective study groups changed their thinking and their approach to practice. Changes noted among clinicians included increased personal insight into their response to patients, increased ability to take a reflective stance toward their practice, different approaches to analyzing and labeling observation, and improved ability to hypothesize about therapy outcomes. These enhanced skills were also observed in supervision. Clinicians became more adept at articulating their own reasoning process. In supervision sessions, the clinicians began to solve problems based on a broader perspective about what might have been happening in therapy.

Additionally, the process of analyzing videotapes vividly illuminated the complexity of practice and helped clinicians understand why fieldwork students struggle to put it all together. Supervisors were able to differentiate students' problems and restructure the learning experience to facilitate specific skills such as observation, identification of cues, generation of hypotheses, formulation of the patient's future, or engagement of the patient in a collaborative process. Acknowledging the complexity of practice helped clinicians appreciate what they were doing, stimulated their interest, and validated their professional identity. Many participants articulated that the very process of analyzing their practice renewed their interest in, enthusiasm for, and pride in the profession of occupational therapy. It was notable that during the 2 years in which the Clinical Reasoning Study took place, there was no staff turnover. A sense of departmental morale and group cohesiveness were additional outcomes of such study groups (Slater, 1989).

RECOMMENDATIONS FOR IMPLEMENTING A STAFF DEVELOPMENT PROGRAM TO FACILITATE REFLECTION ON PRACTICE

Although this staff development program evolved from a research project, other departments could easily replicate its essential components. Implementation of analysis of practice may be started with staff members who are interested in reflecting on and exploring their own practice. Participation on a voluntary basis would allow therapists to take the initiative and responsibility for planning their own professional development. Persons who volunteer could form two-member teams to interview, observe, and videotape each other. The teams could then meet in larger study groups. The study group leadership might rotate as each clinician showed his or her own videotape and structured the discussion and questions to his or her own developmental needs. Each leader might identify an interesting, difficult, exciting, challenging, or unusual therapy session to videotape and discuss. Another option would be to use an outside facilitator, such as a local occupational therapy faculty member, as a group leader. This facilitator could address potentially threatening situations that may arise as colleagues begin to share their philosophical and personal differences.

Some therapists might find this process threatening. To minimize this possibility, we recommend that supervisors serve as role models by showing that they are willing to risk making their own reasoning process explicit. That is, they must model the process and demonstrate that examination of one's practice can be a rich learning experience. We believe that newer therapists will develop an understanding of their own reasoning processes by observing experienced therapists who question their own practice and by having permission to question others in a nonthreatening manner.

Before the videotaping sessions, the clinician is interviewed. He or she is asked to describe the patient from a narrative perspective, that is, to tell his or her story of the patient (Mattingly, 1990). The clinician is then encouraged to imagine what he or she expects to happen during the therapy session, what accomplishments might occur, or what difficulties might be encountered. Such open-ended questions facilitate a broad perspective and shift the focus away from a description of techniques and a listing of long-term and short-term goals. The clinician may construct a hypothetical story as he or she imagines the session will unfold.

After the videotaping, a posttherapy interview is conducted. The interview format might include a narrative description of what actually happened in the therapy session. The team may view the video together and generate specific questions. Topics of discussion might include specific techniques, patient-clinician interaction, key decision points in the session, frames of reference that inform the clinician's thinking, challenges, surprises, and frustrations. The posttherapy interview serves to enhance clinicians' awareness of what thoughts and actions guide their practice. The teams might then present their case stories to the study group or entire department for a larger discussion.

Given the pressure for productivity and tight schedules common to most occupational therapy departments, successful implementation of this program must be sensitive to time constraints. The process could be integrated into an existing scheduled meeting time during the day. Additional time for this process would be minimal if regular treatment sessions were videotaped and existing supervisory and staff meetings were used for study groups. Ideally, management staff with reduced productivity requirements, personnel from the hospital education department, or student volunteers could be used to videotape the therapy sessions.

CONCLUSION

We propose that ongoing reflection on practice in the work environment can help experienced clinicians serve as role models and mentors for novice therapists and remain enthusiastic and proud of their profession. This approach may also have a positive effect on staff turnover as therapists develop a renewed investment in their practice. Our experience with the staff at University Hospital has demonstrated the benefits of a process-oriented approach to staff development. By videotaping therapy as well as pretherapy and post-therapy interviews with therapists, followed by group analysis, we encouraged our clinicians to link thought and action in practice. This, in turn, can enhance the quality of care for patients.

ACKNOWLEDGMENT

Parts of this paper appeared in "Facilitating a Foundation for Clinical Reasoning" by E. S. Cohn & C. Czycholl. In E. B. Crepeau & T. LaGarde (Eds.), *Self-Paced Instruction for Clinical Education and Supervision: An Instructional Guide* (pp. 159-182). Rockville, MD: American Occupational Therapy Association. Copyright © 1991 by The American Occupational Therapy Association, Inc.

REFERENCES

American Occupational Therapy Association. (1987). *Occupational therapy: Directions for the future. Occupational therapy education and practice proposals for action.* Rockville, MD: Author.

American Occupational Therapy Association. (1990). *Directions for the Future Symposium Proceedings.* Rockville, MD: Author.

Bailey, D. M. (1990). Reasons for attrition from occupational therapy. *American Journal of Occupational Therapy, 44,* 23-29.

Benner, P. (1984). *From novice to expert.* Reading, MA: Addison Wesley.

Brollier, C. (1985). Occupational therapy management and job performance of staff. *American Journal of Occupational Therapy, 39,* 649-654.

Christie, B. A., Joyce, P. C., & Moeller, P. L. (1985). Fieldwork experience, Part 1: Impact on practice preference. *American Journal of Occupational Therapy, 10,* 671-674.

Cohn, E. S. (1989). Fieldwork education: Shaping a foundation for clinical reasoning. *American Journal of Occupational Therapy, 43,* 240-244.

Cohn, E. S., & Czycholl, C. M. (1991). Facilitating a foundation for clinical reasoning. In E. B. Crepeau & T. LaGarde (Eds.), *Self-paced instruction for clinical education and supervision: An instructional guide* (pp. 159-182). Rockville, MD: American Occupational Therapy Association.

Dreyfus, H. L. & Dreyfus, S. E. (1986). *Mind over machine.* New York, NY: Free Press.

Elstein, A. L. (1978). *Medical problem solving: Analysis of critical reasoning.* Cambridge, MA: Harvard University Press.

Gitterman, A., & Netter, I. (1968). Supervisors as educators. In F. W. Kaslow & Associates (Eds.), *Supervision, consultation and staff training in the helping professions* (pp.100-114). San Francisco, CA: Jossey-Bass.

Kaufman, H. G. (1974) *Obsolescence and professional career development.* New York, NY: Amacom.

Knowles, M. (1980). *The modern practice of adult education.* New York, NY: Association Press.

Lieberman, A., & Miller, L (1979). *Staff development: New demands, new realities, new perspectives.* New York, NY: Columbia University Press.

Mattingly, C. (1988). *Educational materials: A new approach for reflecting on clinical malpractice.* Unpublished report of the AOTA/ AOTF Clinical Reasoning Study.

Mattingly, C. (1990). The narrative nature of clinical reasoning in occupational therapy. In M. H. Fleming (Ed.), *Proceedings of the Institute on clinical reasoning for occupational therapy educators* (pp. 22-24). Medford, MA: Tufts University, Conical Reasoning Institute.

Parham, D. (1987). Nationally Speaking—Toward professionalism: The reflective therapist. *American Journal of Occupational Therapy, 41,* 555-561.

Pecora, P., & Austin, M. (1987). *Managing human services personnel.* Newbury Park, CA: Sage.

Rogers, J. C. (1982/2000). Sponsorship: Developing leaders for occupational therapy. *American Journal of Occupational Therapy, 36,* 309-313. (see Chapter 63).

Rogers, J. C. (1983). Eleanor Clarke Slagle Lectureship—1983: Clinical reasoning: The ethics, science, and art. *American Journal of Occupational Therapy, 37,* 601-616. (Reprinted in Cottrell, R. P. (Ed.). (1996). *Perspectives on purposeful activity: Foundation and future of occupational therapy* (pp. 327-339). Bethesda, MD: AOTA.)

Sabari, J. S. (1985). Professional socialization: Implications for occupational therapy education. *American Journal of Occupational Therapy, 39,* 96-102.

Schon, D. (1983). *The reflective practitioner How professionals think in action.* New York, NY: Basic.

Schon, D. (1987). *Educating the reflective practitioner.* San Francisco, CA: Jossey-Bass.

Slater, D. (1989). Clinical reasoning as a staff development process. In *Proceedings of the mini-course in clinical reasoning.* Baltimore, MD: American Occupational Therapy Foundation.

Smith, H. L. & Elbert, N. F. (1986). *The health care supervisor's guide to staff development.* Rockville, MD: Aspen Systems.

West, W. L. (1990/1996). Nationally Speaking—Perspectives on the past and future, Part 2. *American Journal of Occupational Therapy, 44,* 9-10. (Reprinted in Cottrell, R. P. (Ed.). (1996). *Perspectives on puposeful activity: Foundation and future of occupational therapy* (pp. 571-576). Bethesda, MD: AOTA.)

CHAPTER SIXTY-THREE

Sponsorship: Developing Leaders for Occupational Therapy

Joan C. Rogers

Stogdell defined leadership as "the process (act) of influencing the activities of an organized group in its efforts toward goal setting and goal achievement."[1, p.10] Leaders are needed within occupational therapy to formulate and implement the goals of our professional organization, The American Occupational Therapy Association (AOTA), and to promote the missions of occupational therapy in the health care delivery system. Effective leadership is a learned process. Socialization for leadership may occur in a planned or haphazard fashion. This chapter discusses one method of selecting and developing leaders for occupational therapy professional sponsorship.

SPONSORSHIP

Definition

A sponsor is one who assumes responsibility for another. Hence, a professional sponsor is an individual who takes responsibility for the professional enhancement of another individual. Shapero, Haseltine, and Rowe[2] described the professional sponsorship system as a continuum of advisory and support persons who may be differentiated in terms of levels of influence and impact. Mentors, symbolizing an intense and hierarchical relationship, are at one end of the continuum, and "peer pals", reflecting a less influential and more egalitarian relationship, are at the other.[2] The sponsorship system, which is also called *patronage*[2] and *networking,*[3-5] is focused on the *politics of career advancement*. The emphasis is on the cultivation of relationships to get ahead professionally. For example, an occupational therapist may seek and develop contacts with those professionals, administrators, and legislators who have power and authority relevant to their career plans.

Mentors

In Greek mythology, Mentor was Odysseus' counselor. In the same spirit, the word *mentor* is used in reference to a trusted advisor or guide. Historically, mentorship represented a formal or informal relationship between a prestigious, established older person and a younger person.[6] The type of support given was often financial. Rowe captured the meaning of mentor, as intended in this [chapter], when she remarked, "A mentor is a person who comments on your work, criticizing errors and praising excellence. This person sets high standards and teaches you to set and meet high standards."[7, p 41]

Mentor Roles

The mentor serves as a supporter, educator, and advocate for the protégé. Moral support is necessary for professional as well as for personal growth. A chief function of the mentor is to *believe* in the protégé's abilities. The mentor sets up performance objectives for the protégé and conveys the expectation or message that the protégé can accomplish these. This affirmation assists the protégé in acquiring an image of competence. A self-image of competence, or of the ability to master tasks, facilitates a sense of security, which gives the protégé "growing space" and supports purposeful risk taking.[8]

Conformity or imitation is not expected of protégés. Mentors respect the integrity and autonomy of their protégés and help them to discover and explore their own potentials. They do this by directing a career clarification process that includes commenting on ambitions and difficulties, assisting in integrating new ideas and experiences, and aiding in the formulation and ordering of career objectives. Through this dialogue, protégés become more aware of their abilities and shortcomings. This enables more realistic career planning and implementation.[8] Epstein[9] viewed mentors as "creators of competence."[9, p.13] They take pleasure in the achievements of those they have nurtured and are not intimidated by their promotion and success.[8]

In the capacity of educator, the mentor provides multiple opportunities for informal or incidental learning. For example, the protégé may be invited to observe the mentor negotiating a contract for a needs assessment for occupational therapy services in a long-term care facility. Observation and discussion of a particular negotiation generally fosters a better understanding and appreciation of the negotiating process than is possible through lecture and reading. The mentor elucidates the interaction by making explicit to the protégé how he or she thought about the negotiation at each step. In a similar manner, the protégé has access to many learning situations that would be unavailable without the mentor.

Another important educational function of the mentor is that of providing insight on professional issues. Written records and reports tend to convey little of the dynamics of decision making. The AOTA Bylaws,[10] for instance, document the advent of the Specialty Sections, but the rationale for their emergence is difficult to retrieve. A mentor who served on the Bylaws Committee at the time the Specialty Sections were established would have detailed knowledge about their historical and philosophical significance and could share this with others. The expertise and positions of mentors frequently places them at the center of such decision making and makes them valuable sources of oral history.

Strategies for surviving in bureaucratic environments constitute an important facet of professional behavior. As Rowe stated, one needs to "learn the organizational chart and how the place really works."[7, p.41] The place may be a work setting, such as a hospital or school, or an organization, such as the AOTA. The major concern here revolves around power and politics. The mentor assists the protégé in sensing and understanding the political climate. Knowledge of things such as who owes whom a favor, where the informal power lies, what the unwritten rules are, and how to approach an authoritarian administrator provides an "inside" perspective on group and organizational dynamics. Such assistance is invaluable in managing a bureaucracy efficiently and successfully.

The prompt acquisition of information may be as important to survival as the mere receipt of information. Daniels[3] noted that the expeditious relay of information on issues that require fast action allows maximum preparation time and, hence, may make the difference between success and failure. As an established professional, the mentor's position generally provides access to information that is not readily available to the neophyte. This may include notice of job vacancies before public posting, the specific orientation desired in grant applications, and the types of information a particular job interviewer wants to hear. Even where speed is not critical, the mentor can provide assistance that allows tasks to be completed with greater ease. Referral to key references and resource persons reduces the time expended to locate relevant information. Clarification of guidelines for report and proposal writing lessens the anxiety associated with interpreting ambiguous regulations. Such directives constitute labor-saving devices that contribute to work efficiency and productivity.

In addition to being a supporter and educator, the mentor is also an advocate. In this capacity, the mentor introduces the protégé to those in positions of influence and power, recommends the protégé for tasks and responsibilities, and is appropriately assertive when the protégé is criticized. Through such mechanisms the protégé gains visibility and is assisted in establishing a professional communication system. Daniels[3] described the sense of mastery and self-worth that is derived from an understanding of an acceptance into informal networks.

From this discussion, it should be clear that a mentor is more than a role model. Role models exert a passive influence on another. The manner in which they enact their professional role, their personal styles, and their specific characteristics may be emulated. Learning occurs principally through observation and imitation. Role models may, but are not required to, nurture, support, or educate.[2, p.11]

Qualities of the Mentor

To serve as a supporter, educator, and advocate, certain personal qualities are desirable. The ability to relate well on a one-to-one level, together with such attributes as authenticity, openness, sensitivity, responsiveness, and availability is advantageous.[8] Another favorable quality is generativity. Erikson[12] defined generativity as concern with establishing and guiding the next generation. The mentor's motivational power emanates from this concern or caring. These humanistic dimensions are supplemented by professional competence that embodies skill, commitment, and accountability.[8] Competence constitutes the essential quality needed by a mentor.

Qualities of the Protégé

It is also advantageous for the protégé to possess certain traits. In view of the commitment of time and effort required to transform talents into competencies, those seeking an advisor need to convince prospective mentors that they are worth an investment in time and effort. Hence, it is desirable for them to display a willingness to learn, and [to] exhibit career directness and trust in the mentor.[8] The protégé may invite a mentorship by seeking and offering help. Protégés are appreciative of the help received and acknowledge this, when and as appropriate, to the mentor and others.[7]

Mentor-Protégé Relationship

The special qualities of the mentor-protégé relationship emerge from the professional competence and senior position of the mentor. The relationship is hierarchical, not democratic. The protégé with talent, and rudimentary skills, is given a chance to learn from the mentor.

Although hierarchical, the relationship is also mutualistic. Both persons give and receive in a mutually beneficial way. The mentor gives knowledge and support in exchange for the protégé service. Work with the head is traded for work with the hands, so to speak. Pilette[8] remarked about the spiritedness of the interaction. She observed that after talking with one's mentor one may feel intellectually and physically energized. The perception of mutualism resides between the two parties.

Others may well perceive the relationship to be parasitic; however, if either the mentor or the protégé senses that one party is not adequately reciprocating, the positive quality of the relationship is generally destroyed.

The mentor will generally follow the protégé through a sequence of career developments and will facilitate job entry and mobility at many points along the way.[8] The intensity and continuity of the relationship account for its restrictive and exclusionary nature. Since it is difficult for a mentor to sponsor more than a few protégés simultaneously, every learner desiring a mentor may not find one. Buber captured the essence of the mentor-protégé relationship when he said, "Without either being concerned about it they learned, without noticing they did the mystery of professional survival. They received the spirit of affirmation."[13, p.89]

Collegial Relationships

Sponsor relationships range from those that are hierarchical to those that are collegial.[2] At the opposite end of the sponsorship continuum from mentors are peer mentors,[5] "peer pals,"[14] and networks.[4,5] Like mentors, these dyads, groups, or organizations are focused on career development and job-related issues and seek to serve the same functions as mentors—psychological support, advising, information giving, and referral. Peer and network relationships may be distinguished from the mentor-protégé relationship in terms of the egalitarian quality of the former. Each participant in the collegial relationship sometimes acts as a leader and sometimes as a follower. Thus, the notion that sponsors must be more powerful and successful than those they sponsor is contradicted by the concept of peers helping each other to succeed in their careers. These collegial relationships also differ from mentorship in that they are available to more persons and are less exclusive.

Networks generally have a broader power base than peer mentorships and "peer pal" groups. According to Welch,[5] the peer mentor dyad is based on complementary talents. A clinical specialist wanting to learn research skills and a faculty member possessing such skills and seeking to renew clinical skills would constitute a viable partnership. In the *peer pal* model,[14] sharing is encouraged among a small group of people. As the term is commonly used, *networking* implies a larger group than *peer pals*. Also, in networks, there is generally less emphasis on the development of specific vocational or professional skills and more emphasis on upward career mobility. Competence in specific occupational skills is assumed. Networks operate on the principle that it is *who* you know, not *what* you know, that gets you ahead. By participating in a network, one comes in contact with people who are in positions potentially useful to one's career and who know other people who are in positions potentially useful to one's

career. Conversely, one's own position and contacts can be useful to others in the network. The interpersonal linkages formed in and through networks are used to advance one's career primarily through referrals and recommendations. Although the impact of networks may be less personal than that of a mentor or a peer pal group, the outreach contact capabilities are much greater.

THE VALUE OF SPONSORSHIP FOR OCCUPATIONAL THERAPY

Sponsorship provides an effective, appealing, and personalized strategy for developing leaders for occupational therapy. It is built on a concept of intraprofessional and interprofessional support, which has lacked wide acceptance in "female" professions such as occupational therapy. Levinson and associates[15] observed that women establish fewer mentor relationships than men do. At the same time, Sheehy[16] and Estler[17] documented the importance of a mentor in adult life. The dearth of women in mentorships has been attributed to a lack of opportunity as well as to the general failure to socialize women for leadership positions.[18] Others[8, p.14] have commented that the sense of distrust and competitiveness among women themselves discourages cooperative interaction. Duncan and Partridge[14] put forth the interesting hypothesis that women may not recognize the association between power and support networks. Whatever the reason, it has become apparent that little has been gained by neglecting sponsorship as a vehicle for leadership development. Recognizing this, women across the country have been joining to form support partnerships and networks to service their career aspirations in much the same way as the *good ole boys'* network has done for men.

Sponsorship can be used by occupational therapists in a variety of ways. The intent of the following discussion is to furnish some examples of its application, rather than an exhaustive list of possibilities.

The concept of hierarchy, as embodied in the mentor-protégé relationship, can be extended to many types of dyads—faculty member-student, instructor-professor, novice clinician-experienced clinician, clinician-administrator. The one-to-one situation is particularly conducive to sharing the subjective aspects of professional behavior. For example, personal experience has indicated that, by verbalizing how one thinks about and reacts to a particular client case, students are assisted in developing clinical reasoning skills and in coping with their reactions to the severely disabled. Similarly, peer reviews of one's articles and conference proposals may be useful in illustrating that scholarly life is usually a combination of successes and productive failures. Professional meetings and conferences afford opportunities for mentors to introduce their protégés to professional leaders through informal gatherings and spontaneous contacts.

Within occupational therapy, the peer group notion is probably best reflected in the local Special Interest Sections. Such groups may serve as a vehicle for addressing both conceptual and career advancement issues. In gerontology, for example, therapists are needed who can conceptualize practice in the aging services network, including protective services, nutritional sites, and senior citizen centers. The Special Interest Sections provide a logical forum for such exploratory thinking. After roles and functions have been projected, strategies for articulating them to persons in power and authority can be developed, tested, and evaluated. When positions for occupational therapists are created in such settings, members of the Special Interest Section can be instrumental in referring qualified therapists for the position and in preparing them for the application and interview process.

Within the AOTA, the Special Interest Sections, as well as all other organized groups, may be construed as issue-oriented networks. Assuming that the interests of gerontological occupational therapy were being neglected in AOTA policies and actions, the Gerontology Special Interest Section could be mobilized to exert pressure on the policy and decision-making bodies. Application of *networking* principles would involve identifying and patronizing those office holders sympathetic to gerontological issues, persuading and converting other elected and appointed officials, promoting the election and selection of candidates supportive of gerontological issues, and courting the assistance of other AOTA units. These activities would be carried out through person-to-person contacts and organized actions, with the keen recognition that by helping the causes of gerontological practice, gerontological therapists would be helping themselves and each other.

The power base of occupational therapists could be substantially increased if therapists joined *organized* support networks such as the Philadelphia Women's Network, or the Bay Area Professional Women's Network. Network contacts can assist in maneuvering occupational therapists into the administrative positions in occupational therapy units, health care settings, social programs, and governmental agencies. They may also be critical for eliciting support for such objectives as licensure legislation and reimbursement by health insurance plans. Networks vary in membership characteristics and degree of structure. Some are restricted to men or women, to certain occupational classifications or job levels, or to personnel in a particular facility. Others cover broad geographical regions and are open to all regardless of occupation, position, or sex. Meeting agendas range from informal career-oriented discussions to planned programs dealing with topics such as agenda planning, the negotiation process, and assertiveness. The selection of a network to join emerges from one's career development needs.

Mechanisms for gaining access to power bases, such as the good ole boys' network, also merit attention. Many of these ties are developed through associations made during the college years. In recognition of this, it may be advisable for occupational therapy students to take their courses in administration and supervision in schools of business and public or hospital administration, which have as their expressed purpose the education of administrators and executives. Such an educational strategy might not only foster a sharp appreciation of how the administrator's mind operates, it might also facilitate collegial relationships with those who will come to exert control over the delivery of occupational therapy services.

Finally, attention should be directed toward the psychological benefits of sponsorship, regardless of the particular form it takes. Professional role strain, also known as "burnout," is prevalent among professionals.

Many therapists are disillusioned with their careers. They may work alone. They may not feel like part of a team. They may realize little administrative support and may rarely receive recognition. The information-giving, psychological support, and advocacy inherent in sponsorship could help alleviate such role strain and foster the innovative visions that occupational therapists have about occupational therapy. Sponsorship creates a sense of belonging to a social network designed to help people succeed.

In conclusion, sponsorship does not require large expenditures of money and time, or large numbers of therapists to initiate. One therapist can affirm another and, from here, various kinds of social support structures can grow. For each therapist there is a double challenge— to select someone to sponsor and to acquire a sponsor.

ACKNOWLEDGMENT

This paper is based on an address given at the Annual Conference of The American Occupational Therapy Association in San Antonio, Texas, 1981.

REFERENCES

1. Stogdell, R. J. (1974). *Handbook of leadership: A survey of theory and research.* New York, NY: The Free Press.

2. Shapero, E. C., Haseltine, F. P., & Rowe, M. P. (1978). Moving up: Role models mentors, and the "patron system". *Sloan Management Rev, 19,* 51-58.

3. Daniels AK. Development of feminist networks in the health sciences. *In Proceedings of The Conference on Women's Leadership and Authority in the Health Professions,* HEW Contract #HRA 230-76-0269,1977, (pp. 25-35)

4. Kleiman, C. (1980). *Women's networks.* New York, NY: Ballantine Books.

5. Welch, M. (1980). *Networking.* New York, NY: Warner Books.

6. Kelly, L. Y. (1978). *Power guide—the mentor relationship. Nurs Outlook, 26,* 339.

7. Rowe, M. P. (1977). Go hire yourself a mentor. In *Proceedings of the Conference on Women's Leadership and Authority in the Health Professions,* HEW Contract #HRA 230-76-0269 (pp. 41-42).

8. Pilate, P. C. (1980). Mentoring: An encounter of the leadership kind. *Nurs Leadership, 3,* 22-26.

9. Epstein, O. F. (1974). Bringing women in: Rewards, punishments, and the structure of achievement. In R. B. Kuncsin (Ed.), *Woman and success* (pp. 13-21). New York, NY: William Morrow and Co. Inc.

10. Bylaws. (1978). *AOTA Member Handbook* (pp. E-1-E-9). Rockville, MD: The American Occupational Therapy Association.

11. Haseltine, F. P. (1977). Why be a role model when you can be a mentor? In *Proceedings of the Conference on Women's Leadership and Authority in the Health Professions,* HEW Contract #HRA 23-76-0269 (pp. 37-39).

12. Erikson, E. H. (1950). *Childhood and society.* New York, NY: W. W. Norton & Co.

13. Buber, M. (1965). *Between man and man,* New York, NY: Macmillan.

14. Duncan, J., & Partridge, R. (1980). Peer pals: Overcoming the obstacles to leadership development. *Nurs Leadership, 3,* 18-21.

15. Levinson, D. J., Darrow, C. M., Klein, E. D., Levinson, M. H., & McKee, B. (1974). The psychosocial development of men in early adulthood and the middle transition.. In O. R. Ricks, A. Thomas, M. Roff (Eds.), *Life history research in psychopathology* (Vol .3). Minneapolis, MN: The University of Minneapolis Press.

16. Sheehy, G. (1976). *Passages.* New York, NY: E.P. Dutton & Co., Inc.

17. Estler, S. (1977). Women in decision-making. In *Proceedings of the Conference on Women's Leadership and Authority in the Health Professions,* HEW Contract #HRA 230-76-0269 (pp. 197-208).

18. Diamond, H. Patterns of leadership. *Educ Horizons, 57,* 59-62, 78-79.

CHAPTER SIXTY-FOUR

Innovation and Leadership in a Mental Health Facility

Joanne Valiant Cook

This chapter was previously published in the American Journal of Occupational Therapy, 49, 595-606. Copyright © 1995, The American Occupational Therapy Association, Inc.

This (chapter) presents a case study description and analysis of the long negotiation process of implementing change in services and service delivery for clients with severe mental illness who were outpatients of an acute care psychiatric unit of a general hospital. The change—the formation of a multidisciplinary team to provide ongoing, coordinated care—was proposed and negotiated by an occupational therapist.

The purpose of this (chapter) is to reveal and interpret the developmental process involved in seeking to make organizational, program, or service changes in medical bureaucracies. At a time when health services are in a state of change or flux in terms of demands from the public and funders, it seems useful for providers of mental health services to be aware of and prepared for the delays and roadblocks they may encounter as they attempt change. Such understanding may support the change-makers in maintaining the perseverance that is often required to achieve successful innovations.

This case study is one component of an extended ethnographic research study, conducted by the author between 1983 and 1989 in a medium-sized Canadian city, of the evolution of an outpatient clinic for clients with schizophrenia. Although the events described in this chapter took place more than a decade ago, a current ongoing research study of an attempt at introducing a new rehabilitation service in a large provincial psychiatric hospital (analogous to state psychiatric hospitals in the United States) reveals that similar processes of development are occurring. That is, although the context of events in terms of time and place are different and thus one cannot generalize the results of the 1980s study, it does appear that the processes themselves and the analysis of those processes meet the criterion of "transferability' (Lincoln & Guba, 1985, pp. 297, 316) to situations where health care professionals are attempting to introduce new services. Case study analysis of organizational change may offer lessons that can assist those who wish to be leaders of interventions in programs and interventions in health care.

The process of innovation that is described here occurred before participant observation at the site began. The history was obtained from an analysis of all available documentation of the process and in-depth, tape-recorded and transcribed interviews with key participants including the occupational therapist; the directors of the departments of psychiatric services, social work, psychology, and day care therapy; and all the members of what became known as the Schizophrenia Clinic Team. The history of the process is, therefore, a reconstructed account based on the participants' memories as well as written reports and minutes of meetings. The sequence and description of events were consistently reported by the above named informants and supported by the written sources. The criterion of credibility for qualitative studies (Krefting, 1991; Lincoln & Guba, 1985) would thus appear to be partially met by the triangulation of sources and the later prolonged engagement and my observations at the site. In addition, this reconstruction was read and supported by three of the participant in the study, thus providing the "member checks" that Lincoln & Guba (1985, p. 314) recommended as another technique to enhance the credibility of findings.

This (chapter) is organized in two parts. Part I provides a chronological description of the process of initiating change in mental health services and an analytic understanding of difficulties in implementing new programs of care. Part II examines the role of leadership in fostering change and the contribution of professional ideology to the commitment to effecting change.

PART I: THE DEVELOPMENTAL PROCESS OF INNOVATION

The Context for Change

By the late 1970s, the neglect and seeming abandonment to the streets of deinstitutionalization persons with chronic mental illness was being described in professional journals, exposed in the popular press, and examined by commissions of inquiry (Bachrach, 1983; Cook, 1988). Some of the professional staff members in the Psychiatric Services Unit of the hospital described in this case study were increasingly concerned about the lack of programs, coordination of services, and even the availability of access to the resources that did exist, for an ever-growing population of clients requiring ongoing care. The occupational therapist described the situation in her place of employment at that time as follows:

At that point, the treatment of schizophrenia was done on an individual basis. Therapists and psychiatrists were working independently. There were no formal mechanisms for coordinating treatment. Individuals who were *really* ill could quite easily have as many four therapists. So you had multiple therapists but no mechanism for coordinating. If you had a concern or problem or you wanted to clarify something, you tried catching the psychiatrist in the breezeway or coffee lounge or in the hall. It was a very loosey-goosey system. It has a rather humorous sound to it, but in actual fact, with the nature of schizophrenia and the kinds of multiple problems that our clients* had, for myself and for other people it was very ineffective and at times dangerous. Crisis intervention was almost impossible because there was no unified approach as to how the case was going to be handled. You really didn't have the opportunity to discuss the outpatient approach with the psychiatrist or other staff, so it was really challenging.

On a more global level, Psychiatric Services had no unified concept of how we were going to treat schizophrenia. Some people used a medical approach, some people used a psychological approach, some people used a supportive centered approach, some humanistic, and there were even people who had a more layman approach. So we had a lot of problems. People were coming from different angles and there was no opportunity for collaboration. Clients were not being informed or educated about their illness. They often had very poor compliance with treatment as a result. There was a revolving door that was incredible. People would be bopping in and out—I'm sulking about the more seriously ill. We had what called the "lounge-crowd" of young schizophrenics that would hang around the hospital and smoke and drink coffee. They had no sense of direction, but it was more symptomatic of the problems that they had.

Families were blamed for the illness. A lot of families became very distressed. I received numerous calls and letters from parents wanting help. At that time people were actually being referred to Social Work to be assessed to see if family pathology was causing the illness.

The starting point, really, for us were the patients, their families, and their needs. And the needs were multiple. Several clinicians and representatives from all disciplines were really concerned about the situation and really wanted to improve our aftercare for, at that point, what we called "the chronic population." And the result of that was informal meetings.

(*The terms client and patient were used interchangeably by the clinic staff members, although client had become the preferred term by the conclusion of this study.)

By 1980, the environmental pressures for improved and more available services to deinstitutionalized clients were increasing. The members of the newly formed local chapter of the Friends of Schizophrenics (an organization similar to the National Alliance for the Mentally Ill [NAMI] in the United States) were requesting professional help for their ill relatives and for themselves. The physicians, both general practitioners and psychiatrists, at the hospital were also finding the increasing numbers of persons who were chronically ill a demanding responsibility due to the multiple social and functional problems with which these clients presented. The revolving door problem, crisis episodes, and the "lounge crowd" worried the hospital administrators.

The First Initiatives: 1979-1980

In the late months of 1979, one of the psychiatrists began to feel overwhelmed by the pressure of the large caseload of patients with schizophrenia that he was carrying:

I had reached the stage where I couldn't go any further... I couldn't handle it... there wasn't sufficient back-up... there was a steady increase year by year... So at that time I presented a seminar, at one of the Friday morning inservices [in house education series] on the problem of schizophrenia. I became convinced that we had to do something about it.

A small group of clinicians, including the occupational therapist, a social worker, and a nurse who were also concerned about the lack of coordination and follow-up of outpatients, began to meet once a week for short periods with this psychiatrist to discuss these issues in regard to his patients. In late May 1980, the occupational therapist wrote a memo to her department manager outlining in considerable detail the need for and benefits of a formally designated, multidisciplinary, outpatient team for the coordination of services for the chronically ill who required continuing care (see Appendix A). The combination of the psychiatrist's inservice, the occupational therapist's memo, and the visit of a British psychiatrist who pointed out the inadequacies of care for this specific population led the director of the Psychiatric Services to bring the issue before the Professional Advisory Committee for Psychiatric Services (PAC). This body met monthly to plan, approve, and evaluate services and programs. It was composed of department chiefs or managers from the various disciplines and hospital administration. Three months later, a Task Force on Continuing Care, chaired by the chief of Social Work, was convened to define the current needs of the chronic population, to establish their future needs for programs, and to submit a report by the end of the year.

The Initial Negotiations: August 1980-March 1982

The task force included the clinicians who had been meeting weekly with one psychiatrist and other department chiefs and representatives. The task force met regularly for 8 months and then held a 2-day workshop in an attempt to reach consensus on how to proceed with its mandate. The divisive issue was whether a program should be established to provide care for a small number of the most obviously disabled, clearly defined, chronic, users of resources (the position of the chairperson of the task force) or whether a service only for patients with schizophrenia, both newly diagnosed and chronic, should be undertaken (the psychiatrist's position).

In the minutes of the PAC meeting of May 11, 1981, the chairperson of the task force is reported as stating that "after nine months of work the task force was grinding to a halt." One month later he reported that, although some short-term goals, such as establishing a list of needy patients, had been met, the problem of defining the population to be served was at an "impasse situation" and would probably require resolution by PAC. On October 16, 1981, PAC requested recommendations from the task force for review. In December 1981, the Chairperson of the task force submitted to PAC a "majority proposal for a continuing care program for chronic psychiatric patients" which was to begin with a modest caseload of 32 patients who would be provided with the services of a multi-disciplinary team. The report was tabled for several months until the psychiatrist's minority report favoring the establishment of a program for patients diagnosed as having schizophrenia was presented to PAC on March 8, 1982.

The minority report contained indications of the problems and conditions encountered by those who had such high hopes for the policy of deinstitutionalization and to which the occupational therapist was responding in recommending a team-coordinated service. As Cameron (1978) had written, "the severely mentally ill, on the other hand, are more professionally frustrating; treating them has been largely eschewed with the reorganization of the health system" (p. 323). The minority report outlined the reality of practice, which had resulted in many persons with chronic mental illness suffering from neglect in the community:

> If we are drawing up a program covering all types of chronic mental illness, then I would see no special role for a psychiatrist in the program apart from what is happening now. We would be dealing with very much the same patients we have around the unit now and each of them is under the care of a psychiatrist. I am unclear as to how we could develop a meaningful program for those inpatients because most of them are really just being carried and there is not too much hope for therapeutic improvement. I feel it will be difficult to find a psychiatrist who would devote himself to the chronic care program as envisioned by our committee, because it would soon become a dumping ground for patients who are really untreatable. On the other hand, it might be possible to find a psychiatrist for an active and interesting schizophrenia program, which I think is much more important for this area.

After much discussion, a compromise motion was ordered to PAC: "that the various individuals from departments involved meet to establish a team to begin dealing with chronic patients—specifically schizophrenic patients—in a formalized fashion."

Planning the Schizophrenia Clinic: April 1982-December 1982

The members of what was designated as the Continuing Care Team first met in April 1982. The membership included the original members of the group who had been meeting regularly with the psychiatrist and representatives from the Day Therapy and Nursing Departments. The director of the Psychiatric Services Department asked the occupational therapist to be the chairperson of the team meetings. In June 1982, after three meetings, the chairperson submitted a report on the team's progress, which included issues of patient identification, the development of a registry system, and a preliminary model of team functioning in regard to coordination of treatment and review of patients' progress. The team continued to meet once a week for 1 hour. In a transcribed interview the therapist-chairperson described the process that led to the proposal for a Schizophrenia Clinic:

> We looked at the schizophrenic clients we were working with that had problems and we studied them all in depth and we made lists of patients and worked out what themes were emerging. The whole process was really unsatisfactory because all we were doing was studying, but in the meantime our clients were still having problems and nothing was happening. So, finally the team got frustrated and decided what we really needed was a team approach for starters and we needed good case management. That was what was emerging from the discussions. So we decided that the best approach would be to develop a schizophrenic clinic and [the psychiatrist] actually called it The Schizophrenic Clinic. That's where the beginning for that concept came from.

In December 1982, a formal proposal written by the occupational therapist-chairperson was submitted to PAC (see Appendix B). The proposal reflected all the concerns expressed in her May 1980 memo, but now they were more specifically detailed in terms of establishing a schizophrenia clinic that would meet the "combined needs of psychiatrists, other professional staff, the patients, his family and community agendas." The proposed clinic format retained the private relationship of psychiatrists to their clients but gave them each a block of time to meet with the multidisciplinary team to discuss their roster of clients and plan for the coordinated delivery of services.

Resistance to and Acceptance of the Plan: January 1983

At the January 1983 meeting of PAC, the chief of Social Work (and former chairperson of the task force) in a written memo and in person at the meeting, criticized the schizophrenia clinic proposal in terms of its scope, staffing, and program design. He argued persuasively for the development of "a quality service for a smaller number of chronic patients" [rather than] diffusing our efforts by attempting a limited service for all schizophrenic patients. He further argued that there were insufficient staff resources to mount the clinic as proposed and that more specific programs needed to be developed. The chairperson of the Continuing Care Team had recently been appointed senior occupational therapist for Psychiatric Services and in that capacity now attended PAC meetings. As she listened to the arguments against the proposal she told me that she began to "feel desperate." She was sure PAC would turn down the proposal and ask for the development of a program or programs for a population (rather than establishing a clinic format with team input to meet the needs of individuals); then the whole process would go back to the beginning and it would take another 2 years or more to reach any decision. She said, "as an [occupational therapist] I have started a lot of new programs here and I know that approach doesn't work." Her feeling of desperation was also influenced by the recent suicide of one of her clients. She believed that the death might have been prevented had the clinic concept been realized, so she argued "that if we could just start with good case management even though we didn't have a lot of resources, then at least we would be making some inroads and giving it a start." After much discussion, PAC agreed—with the proviso that the Clinic Team develop a program proposal to be submitted to the District Health Council for independent funding. The departments of social work, day therapy, and occupational therapy each agreed to give 6 hours of staff member time per week to the clinic.

The occupational therapist and the social worker on the Continuing Care Team were asked to write the proposal for additional funding, within some severe limits imposed by PAC members and particularly by the director Of Psychiatric Services. They were told to keep the proposal modest and to only request funding for a half-time social worker and half-time nurse. (The original plan from the Continuing Care Team included additional day therapy and occupational therapy staff.) PAC believed that the existing services with their 6-hour per week commitment were adequate. In addition, the director believed that there was a greater chance of securing funding if the proposal was small. (Ironically, the director explained to me in an interview that he had been mistaken. In fact, the Ministry of Health totally funded as requested all proposals ranked number 1 and 2 by the District Health Councils. The Schizophrenia Clinic proposal was ranked number 1 and thus could have received much larger funding. The lack of adequate funding was a source of many subsequent problems in the Clinic's development.)

The occupational therapist reported that she:

fought and advocated for increased occupational therapy involvements as the department's resources were stretched to the limit. Moreover, we deal with this population of clients more than any other department.

It was an uphill fight and it's typical of the problems of recognition for the contribution of occupational therapy as a professional service.

The application for funding had to be submitted only 2 weeks after PAC approved the clinic proposal. Many unpaid, overtime hours were spent in completing the forms required by the Ministry of Health guidelines. At the last moment, the director of Psychiatric Services agreed to include a request for additional occupational therapy time but not for day therapy time. With the exception of the staffing requests, the proposal submitted (see Appendix C) was, in essence, the same program proposed in the submission to PAC, which itself was very similar to the multidisciplinary team concept proposed in the original memo sent by the therapist to her department manager (see Appendices A and B).

The Implementation of the Clinic-March 1983

The psychiatrist from the Continuing Care Team was appointed as the director of the Schizophrenia Clinic, and the occupational therapist was given the informal title of team coordinator (i.e., responsibility for day-to-day administration of the clinic but without administrative authority).

The first formal case conference clinic was held in March 1983 before funding was approved. By September 1983 the occupational therapist in her role as team coordinator had, using letters and memos, convinced all the psychiatrists who had a roster of clients with schizophrenia to schedule regular clinics with the team. In October 1983, the provincial Ministry of Health granted the program funding for a trial period of 2 years, with permanent funding dependent upon two annual Ministry evaluations. It was the first schizophrenia clinic in Canada. There were various service programs (such as vocational assessment and training, social skills groups, and activities of daily living groups) throughout the country at that time but no multidisciplinary clinics offering individualized, client-centered, case management to a population with a specific condition.

This process of innovation took more than 3 years to reach fruition. In the late 1960s, when deinstitutionalization was well under way, a critical account of the problems faced by workers in mental health facilities reported that "innovative talking has been encouraged, while innovative action has been resisted" (Graziano, 1969, p. 10). Similarly, almost 20 years later Kinston pointed our that "getting new ideas into the health system and properly used is a long term effort" (1983, p. 1163). As the narrative above illustrates, the idea for a multidisciplinary team service for the persons with severe mental illness took several years and a great deal of effort to reach implementation. An understanding of the obstacles and barriers to innovation in mental health care requires an exploration of the realities of bureaucratic organization, of cultural differences in the health professions and practices, and of differences in power between interested stakeholders.

Understanding Obstacles and Barriers to Innovations in Health Care

A useful framework for summarizing the process of initiating this innovation is Tichy's (1981, 1983) conceptual scheme of problem cycles. He stated that there are three systems in mutually influencing relationships in any organizations: the technical, the political, and the cultural. Any organization has:

> three basic elements... the technical design problem... social and technical resources must be arranged so that the organization produces some desired result... the political allocation problem... allocating power and resources... who will reap benefits...[and] the ideological and cultural mix problem... to determine what values need to be held. (Tichy, 1981, p. 165).

In very simplified terms, what occurred during the departmental process described here can be conceptualized as follows: There was a technical problem—the vision of services to a new clientele, the deinstitutionalized client with chronic illness; the proposed solution to this technical problem involved cultural change in values, practices, and organizational structure; the cultural change proposal became the focus of political negotiation, challenge, and opposition. Each of these waves of activity took place within a medical bureaucracy in a time of changing social and political approaches to persons who were mentally ill. These varying cycles, contexts, historical circumstances were intertwined in the long process that eventually led to the adoption of the innovative change.

The Reality of Barriers to Innovation Within a Bureaucracy

Many of the propositions developed by Downs (1967) on problems of change in bureaucracies were borne out during the ongoing negotiations for the initiation of the Schizophrenia Clinic. For example, Downs stated that in the large bureaucracies "nearly every major structural or behavioral change is preceded by study of the need for such a change carried out by one or more committees" (1967, p. 275). The 3 years required to implement the original idea proposed by the occupational therapist can be partially explained by the barriers posed to innovation in bureaucracies. The appointing of committees, then a task force, then a workshop, then a feasibility team, and so on, each needing approval from yet another layer of the hierarchy, bogged down the decision-making process in terms of both time and competing alternative approaches. An additional problem was that this change was initiated from the bottom up in an organization accustomed to directives issued from the top down. Those with the authority to make decisions—the members of PAC —were department and administrative chiefs who were not involved in day-to-day interaction with these clients. Most of those working toward the implementation of a multidisciplinary outpatient service were lower-level staff employees in terms of the hierarchical arrangement of

decision making, until the occupational therapist became a member of PAC. The problems of change initiated from the bottom up in a bureaucracy that "can mire staff in a morass of detail and conflict" (Weissman, 1982, p. 44) were evident in this attempt to develop a new service. That is, organizations that are arranged in hierarchical form, with clearly defined departments and professional role definitions, are more likely to require longer time frames for negotiation toward decision making because of the multiplicity of interests, professional practices, and authoritative channels.

The Reality of Cultural Differences in Delaying Consensus

Morgan (1986) identified another important factor in understanding the process of change in organizations. "Traditionally the change process has been conceptualized as a problem of changing technologies, structures and [people... [but]... effective change also depends on changes in images and values that are to guide action... organizational change implies cultural change" (pp. 135-138). Some of the delays encountered in developing the Schizophrenia Clinic resulted from a dispute over values and behavioral solutions. The opposing proposals from the chairperson of the task force and the Continuing Care Team chaired by the occupational therapist illustrate the cultural diversity. One proposed defining the problem as a question of use of services and the need to establish *group* programs for the chronic users of such services. The other proposed an *individualized*, psychiatrist-team-directed, direct service delivery to a more clearly identified population in need of specialized services. These were different philosophies of intervention, evidenced different values as to the neediest population, and proposed different professional responses as a solution.

The emergent solution for a case management service took many months of cultural defining work by the Continuing Care Team. This process was not just one of innovation but one of fundamental cultural change. The focus of practice was to be on the community and the clients who lived there, rather than on inpatient care. The approach was to be individualized, coordinated services to the client and family, not the provision of group programs. The services were to be integrated, comprehensive, and coordinated by a collaborative and overlapping team, rather than fragmented, technical expertise provided by several departments. The primary goal was rehabilitation (maintaining and enhancing function), not treatment to effect cure. The new service was designed to provide continuing after-care, not short-term acute care.

Although the cultural solution among the members of the Continuing Care Team evolved through consensus, its eventual adoption depended on the ability to mobilize support for the proposal within the hospital. Both the delayed nature of this innovation process and the eventual adoption were influenced by political activity and differential access to power.

The Reality of Power and Politics in Negotiating for Change

In their classic work on psychiatric institutions, Strauss, Schatzman, Bucher, Ehrlich, and Sabshin (1964) conceived of the institution as an arena of negotiation and the eventual working structure and practices as a negotiated order. Several illustrations of the negotiating process culminating in the Schizophrenia Clinic have been provided. However, the process of negotiation was not between equals in each context. The adoption of the proposal depended on the ability to mobilize the power resources within the hospital.

As Kanter (1983) pointed out, there is a "political side to innovation... it requires campaigning, lobbying, bargaining, negotiating, caucusing, collaborating and winning votes. That is, an idea must be sold... and [there is a need] for power to turn ideas into action" (p. 216). Or as Graziano (1969) so cogently put it, "the *conception* of innovative ideas in mental health depends upon creative, humanitarian, and scientific forces, while their *implementation* depends, not on science or humanitarianism, but on a broad spectrum of professional and social politics" (p. 10).

Traditionally, in mental health facilities, decision-making power is vested in the medical profession, department heads, and top administrators. In this hospital, the decision-making body was the PAC composed of such persons. Initially, neither of the two prime movers for the innovation (the psychiatrist and the occupational therapist) was a member of this body. It was only at the end of the process, by virtue of a promotion that the occupational therapist was able to attend the meetings and lobby for the adoption of the clinic proposal. Occupational therapists as a group have traditionally held less powerful positions among medical professionals. Maxwell and Maxwell (1977) attributed this lack of power to the history of medical sponsorship and hence control of occupational therapy, to the diffuse and not-well-understood expertise of its practitioners, to its association with chronicity, and rehabilitation rather than the more dramatic acute care medical practice, and to its being a predominately female profession. This lack of power has led to a pattern of adaptation to the health care hierarchy that was characterized as "diffidence" by Maxwell and Maxwell (1977, p. 83).

Perhaps, in this case, the occupational "diffident" pattern of lobbying for support by writing memos and being part of the task forces and committees, but being unable to directly participate in the decision-making level of the hierarchy, partially accounts for the length of time it took to finally implement the original idea. In spite of being able to secure the support of the director of Psychiatric Services, the innovation was almost lost due to the skillful, persistent, and, as later events proved, prophetic opposition of the chief of Social Work who served as the chairperson of the initial task force. (The chief of Social Work's criticism of the scope and ambition of the clinic proposal proved over the years to be valid as the team struggled with inadequate human and material resources to meet the needs of an ever-increasing clientele.) As Downs (1967) pointed out, opposition to change is more likely to occur when the change will reduce the resources one has to control and decrease the importance of the functions currently fulfilled. The proposed clinic format would be under the control of the medical profession. The opposing proposal for group programs would have provided opportunities for an expansion of Social Work jurisdiction and, hence, control. The detailed critique of the clinic proposal in terms of its inadequacies in design, goals, and resources almost blocked the innovation. In the end, the proposal was approved because it met the interests of those who had control over the decision—the psychiatrists and the hospital administrators. The former would get the support services they needed and the later could be seen to be providing further community service (which, in their interest, also resolved the lounge crowd nuisance and the revolving door problem) but at a low cost because the program was to be funded by an external grant from the Ministry of Health. The power brokers had to be convinced that it was in their interests to approve the program. The length of time required for the lobbying, persuading, and stating the case that the occupational therapist pursued was prolonged by political opposition from those who had something to lose or nothing to gain if her innovative idea was adopted.

Persistence and Innovation: Professional Values and Cultural Leadership

This chronology of the process of effecting an innovation in the delivery of mental health services illustrates the lengthy negotiations, persuasion, meetings, and discouragements faced by those who would initiate change in medical bureaucracies. This chronology makes understandable those situations in which service providers give up their attempts to improve service delivery. Why, in this situation, did an occupational therapist persevere to institute this innovation? What enabled her to persevere in spite of setbacks, delays, and opposition? In part II of this case study, some possible answers to those questions are explored. The thesis to be argued is that the philosophy (values and beliefs or professional ideology) adhered to and the professional practice experience of the primary change agent were important personal resources and stimuli for leadership activities.

PART II: THE ROLE OF PROFESSIONAL IDEOLOGY IN LEADERSHIP AND CULTURAL CHANGE

Kanter (1983) described those who effect change or innovation as entrepreneurs. She wrote "entrepreneurs are above all visionaries. They are willing to continue single-minded pursuit of a clearly articulated vision, even when the line of least effort or resistance would make it easy to give up" (p. 239). What enabled the occupational therapist in this case study to continue pushing for change while others gave up the fight when consensus could not be reached? What can account for the eventual acceptance of her original proposal for an out-patient multidisciplinary team? Why did she emerge as the informal leader of a cultural change and its eventual implementation? One possible interpretation is that her professional affiliation and experience as an occupational therapist provided her with the beliefs and values (professional ideology) that were used as personal resources for initiating change.

The Nature and Function of Professional Ideologies

Wilson defined ideology as

a set of beliefs about the social world and how it operates, containing statements about the rightness of certain social arrangements and what actions would be undertaken in the light of those statements. An ideology is both a cognitive map of sets of expectations and a scale of values in which standards and imperatives are proclaimed. Ideology thus serves both as a clue to understanding and as a guide to action, developing in the mind of its adherents an image of the process by which desired changes can best be achieved (1973, pp. 91-92).

Similarly, Marx characterized the ideology of a profession as a "morally charged mandate for action" (1969, p. 81). The literature on organizational life cycles and organizational culture examines the importance of ideology as a resource in creating new meaning in innovative activity, to legitimate those activities and to develop an identity or ethos that provides direction and purpose (Abravanel, 1983; Lohdahl & Mitchell,1981; Smircich, 1983). Thus, the primary function of ideology is prescriptive.

If ideology provides the stimulus to action, one can presume that when innovative activities are proposed within an organization, there is a different ideology underpinning those proposals. Ideology

becomes a central feature of the innovative organization. The ideology summarizes the values and ideals that the founders intended the new organization to epitomize... by using the ideology as a resource, the founders... may be able to generate... commitment... and value consensus (Lohdahl & Mitchell, 1981. pp. 186-187)

The adherence to ideological values can serve to attach meaning to situations and the actions required within them. Those meanings and prescriptions for action are the resources of those who lead cultural change.

The Role of Leadership and Shared Meaning in Innovation: The Cultural Connection

In an analysis of leadership, Smircich and Morgan (1982) declared:

Leadership [is] The Management of Meaning... Leadership is realized in the process whereby one or more individuals succeed in attempting to frame and define the reality of others... they emerge as leaders because of their role in framing experiences in a way that provides a viable basis for action (pp. 257-258).

Schein (1985), in an analysis of cultural change in organizations, declared that

as I began to think through the issues of how culture changes, I again realized the centrality of leadership— the ability to see a need for change and the ability to make it happen. Much of what is mysterious about leadership becomes clearer... if we link leadership specifically to creating and changing culture (pp. x – xi).

Hall (1982) defined leadership as being "what a person does above and beyond the basic requirements of his position. It is the persuasion of individuals and innovativeness in ideas and decision making that differentiates leadership from the sheer possession of power" (p. 161). Bennis (1979) expanded this definition by stating that "leadership involves more than managing, more than just being an idea man, it involves questioning the routine" (p. 42). There are three requisite characteristics for determining leadership or change agent implied in the foregoing quotations: (a) the ability to recognize the need for change; (b) the ability to define, create, or develop meaningful realities or bases for action to meet the need; and (c) the capacity to mobilize resources to implement the change.

The occupational therapist in this case study went beyond the mere requirements of her job, questioned the routine modes of therapeutic practices with persons with chronic mental illness, and proposed an alternative reality of service. In proposing a new service, she was introducing a different ideological system of beliefs, that is, a different cultural frame for practice. Both the psychiatrist and the occupational therapist on the Continuing Care Team saw a need for change in the after-care services for clients with chronic mental illness. The psychiatrist defined it in terms of requiring support services from others:

[T]o treat patients with schizophrenia is a lifetime job... the social problems are so great. It seemed to me that the psychiatrists would be willing to treat schizophrenics if they got support. Just as I was prepared to treat them if I got support.

On the other hand, the occupational therapist had defined the need in terms of ongoing, individualized client care that required the coordination and integration of services and workers by enhancing communication through a formally structured team mechanism. Both professionals worked toward defining the situation, but from different perspectives. With the exception of his minority report to PAC, the psychiatrist did not participate as actively in the various task forces and meetings as did the occupational therapist, nor did he outline in writing the detailed proposals supported by treatment principles that the therapist continuously circulated (see Appendices A and B). These various written memos and proposals documented the therapists' vision of service (Bennis, 1979) and they began to establish a meaning structure as the basis of action.

It is the third requisite that most distinguished the occupational therapist rather than the psychiatrist as the primary change agent and emergent leader. Kanter (1983) stressed "the link between individual entrepreneurs and their coalitions or teams. Individuals initiate... and then work through teams to bring ideas to innovation. Prime movers push—by getting more and more people involved in action vehicles that express the change being promoted" (p. 35). Because of her participation in the various task forces and committees and her appointment to PAC and chairmanship of the Continuing Care Team, the therapist slowly gathered support from others who came to share her definitions and they, through interaction, began to develop shared understandings of the need for and type of change required.

It is "shared meanings that permit organized activity to emerge and assume coherence... for unless meanings are in some sense shared, there can be no alignment and coordination of action" (Morgan, 1984, p. 315). The occupational therapist described the final consensus on meaning in terms that confirm Louis's (1983, p. 50) statement that: "A key premise of a cultural view is that meaning is emergent and intersubjectively negotiated."

We decided what we needed was a team approach, for starters, and we needed good case management. That was what was emerging from the discussions. With the problems we had, we had to start with the clinic, the team, and case management. That was the only logical place to start, but interestingly enough that took a long time to evolve—that concept. It seems so obvious when you look at it, but it wasn't obvious when we were groping with the start. At one point people were looking at starting a program here in the hospital—a social program, a work program, etc.—and that would have been putting the cart before the horse. You can't rehabilitate on that basis.

The on-going consultations in weekly meetings and the written proposals on goals, objectives, and rationales prepared by the occupational therapist were instrumental in bringing the clinic to being, as Kanter (1983) stated, "prime movers push in part by repetition" (p. 296). In the midst of the ambiguity and ad hoc nature of the 3-year process of initiating the multidisciplinary clinic ideas, the therapist's written proposals provided some structured meaning even as they were being negotiated.

However, as Schein (1983) contended, "cultures do not start from scratch. Founders and group members always have prior experience to start with" (p. 221).This insight on prior experience leads to questions about content of the ideology underpinning the innovation known as the Schizophrenia Clinic.

Professional Ideology as a Resource in Promoting Innovation: The Values of Occupational Therapy

In 1986, 3 years after the clinic was established, the occupational therapist provided for some new members of the team what she termed a historical review of the clinic development in the following words:

[My] purpose is to provide some information about the clinic's development, to help us regain, or for the new people, to gain an understanding of our philosophy, central concepts and organization ... What I'm wanting to highlight through this review is that there arc certain central concepts that are important to the clinic. Number one is that we are client-centered. We are looking at the client first and administration second. Now that is why the program was established. Secondly, that we wanted to look at the development of a holistic, coordinated approach. As we all know individuals with schizophrenia have a multiplicity of problems that really require a team effort. When you look at the clinic, each member of the team has a very specific role. There is some overlap, but there are so many things to look at, that a team effort is required. Along with the team approach is the understanding that the clients are going to relate to a team, not just one individual. So if someone leaves or is sick, or on holiday, that client doesn't feel like he has no one to relate to—they have got a team. The third concept is that schizophrenia is a mental illness and that informing clients and their families about the diagnosis is important and that education is really going to facilitate community adjustment. Along with that concept is our feeling that client participation in their treatment and taking responsibility is important. The fourth is case management and the importance of good linkage between the community and the hospital resources and really helping the client to make the links and have access to that. A final point that is essential to clinic functioning is that It is a point of contact for clients, community, and staff.

Most occupational therapists reading the above quotation will recognize the description of the Schizophrenia Clinic as an embodiment of many of the fundamental beliefs, values, and principles of practice of the profession. The writings of many of those honored by their profession with the Eleanor Clarke Slagle lectureship in the United States (American Occupational Therapy Association, 1985) or the Muriel Driver Lectureship in Canada (Baptiste, 1988; Carswell-Opzoomer, 1990; Judd, 1982, Law, 1991; Polatajko, 1992) and the Canadian publication on *Guidelines for the Client Centered Practice of Occupational Therapy* (Canadian Association of Occupational Therapists, 1991), among others, espouse those central values and beliefs of occupational therapy that Yerxa has stated "speak to vital human needs and ensure that people with chronic conditions will be able to lead satisfying lives instead of being throw away people in tomorrow's world" (Yerxa, 1991, p. 9).

Smith (1984) has advised that those who would attempt organizational change must provide a new language, as the old language maintains the old ways. In contrast to the traditional language of psychiatric practice, there are different conceptions for services illustrated in this therapist's historical review and in the documents and proposal for the establishment of the multidisciplinary team clinic (see Appendices A, B, and C): *holistic,* not specific psychotherapeutic care; clients, not patient; *quality aftercare* for clients and families, not acute care for the ill patient; *case management* and *education* to promote *function,* not just medical treatment to effect cure; *participation* of clients and families in treatment planning, not passive reception of service; and *coordination* of services, not brokerage or fragmentation of expertise.

In focusing her efforts on developing comprehensive services for persons with chronic mental illness, the therapist in this case study also reflected the commitment of those persons often devalued by other professional and lay groups. Yerxa has commented on this essential value of occupational therapy practice:

> Otherwise devalued, mental patients were perceived humanistically by the pioneers in occupational therapy as people worthy of dignity... the valuing of a person's essential humanity in spite of severe and sometimes chronic disease, was central to the practice of the original therapists... The historical values of the profession have been transmitted to modern occupational therapists, as may be seen in current patient advocacy efforts as well as in occupational therapists' traditional provision of services to the most severely and chronically disabled patients. Such patients are often seen as "beyond help" by many other professionals because of extensive and irreversible pathologies. (1983, p. 151)

Perspectives differ on the need for innovation in service for the deinstitutionalized clients in this study, as enunciated by the psychiatrist and the therapist. With the institution of the Schizophrenia Clinic, the psychiatrists gained the back-up, supportive services to deal with nonmedical needs of these clients, which were often responsible for their previous neglect by many professionals (Baxter & Hopper, 1982; Cameron, 1978; Cook, 1988; Rob, 1980; 1983; Morrissey & Tessler, 1982. Although one of the premises of deinstitutionalization policy was to provide access to psychiatric care in the community, the resistance to working with this clientele by psychiatrists and some other professionals was unpredicted (Cameron, 1978). The basic needs of persons with schizophrenia are for fundamental, educational, and supportive services, not the talking therapies that many professionals prefer to offer. Further, the difficulty of working with persons with severe mental illness must not be discounted in understanding the reluctance of many professionals to accept them as clients. Often any progress they make may be small and may take place at a very slow pace. There may be setbacks and relapses and the clients themselves can sometimes be demanding, belligerent, frustrating, and uncooperative (Estroff, 1981; Pranger & Brown, 1992; Price, 1993). In this case the occupational therapist's commitment to serving the chronically ill was crucial in instigating the long process of improving the services available to them.

Professional Values, Leadership, and Change

The Schizophrenia Clinic as envisioned and, in most respects, as embodied reflected the fundamental values and practice beliefs of occupational therapy to which the therapist in this case study was dearly committed. This commitment appeared to serve as an important driving force in her consistent efforts to realize a vision of improved service. But it

has also been noted that leadership requires more than vision and ideas. Successful change masters also require "a longer time horizon, conviction in an idea, no need for immediate results or measure and a willingness to convey a vision of something that might come out a little different when finished" (Kanter, 1983, p. 239).

This process to effect organizational change began with the initiative of a professional in the middle ranks of a hierarchically structured medical bureaucracy. By most accounts such efforts from "the grass roots" (Kanter, 1983, p. 180), the "muddling" middle manager (Feldman, 1980, p. 3) or the "lower level staff change agent" Weissman, 1982, p. 4) are doomed to failure or as Kanter puts it, "withering" (1983, p. 102). Generally, this lack of success is due to the inability to mobilize resources, particularly political power and support (Graziano, 1969) and due to the general inertia and resistance to change in service bureaucracies (Downs, 1967; Golembiewski, 1985; Kanter, 1983; Kinston, 1983; Mechanic, 1980). In such contexts and circumstances, said Mechanic,

> [u]nusual leadership is often necessary... A change in direction requires a leader who can communicate to others the sense of excitement in a new venture and who has the organizational skills to bring the necessary people and organizations together. In the absence of a strong incentive—such as available funding—it is extraordinarily difficult to *build the necessary momentum* (1980, p. 179, emphasis added).

In spite of the barriers and obstacles to innovation, a leader did emerge who was able to maintain the momentum to eventually put a multidisciplinary team and the clinic together. Her leadership position came about as much by default as by appointment. It appears that by always maintaining the idea of a holistic, multidisciplinary, coordinated, education and case management service she kept the cultural vision in the foreground. The role of defining the reality, of imparting a sense of mission, of creating new cultural form led to her emergent leadership. As others came to share those understandings and see that it gave purpose and shape to their hopes and working life, her position as unofficial team coordinator solidified. The Schizophrenia Clinic as implemented was a somewhat altered creation but was based nevertheless upon the occupational therapist's original vision of a multidisciplinary team designed to coordinate services for persons with chronic mental illness.

Much of what we read in professional journals and the popular press documents the powerlessness of so called lower-level participants to effect change in organizations. In this case, one person did make a difference. A new delivery of services was established that reflected the occupational therapist's values and beliefs about the importance of client participation, the individual worth of those with chronic illness, the necessity of continuous and ongoing support, the client's potential for growth, and the recognition of the holistic nature of humans, which requires coordination and integration of services to meet their varied needs. Yerxa (1983) discussed the difficulties and challenges faced by therapists who strive to maintain those values in medically dominated settings:

Owing to [the value differences between medicine and occupational therapy], occupational therapists have sometimes had difficulty implementing their values in the traditional medical setting... Occupational therapy has been sufficiently audacious to create and sustain its own unique mode of practice while surviving within, and contributing to, health in the medical milieu. In many respects this persistence of professional values and a singular philosophy, in the midst of conflicting ideals and philosophies, has been intrepidly daring (p. 157).

When the therapist in this case was asked why she kept trying for so long to effect change when so many others might have given up, her explanation was somewhat less sophisticated than Yerxa's, but value-laden nevertheless. She said "the bottom line was improved patient care and that's what sees you through all this muck." The profession and its clients need more change making therapists who are so committed to professional values that they "intrepidly" see their way through "all the muck."

CONCLUSION:
LESSONS TO BE LEARNED

Nothing changes quickly. Those who wish to initiate new programs or services within bureaucratic organizations muse be prepared to be persistent and persuasive over a long time period.

Have a clear and consistent vision. Change agents are often required to clearly articulate the components of change to many participants in a variety of meetings.

Maintain the vision with new language. In order to change a culture (both the values and the practices) new meaning must be developed through the use of new terminology used consistently when explaining or negotiating for change.

Put it in writing. In this case study, the therapist was the one person who kept the mission in front of others by writing memos and proposals for the change. In time, those written proposals maintained the vision by reiterating new language.

Build coalitions. Change is much more likely to occur if it is supported by other professionals and administrators. This factor also adds to the time line but is necessary for success in both the initiation phase and the maintenance of the innovation once implemented.

Recognize stakeholder's interest. This follows from building coalitions. Everyone involved in institutional change has "turf" or professional concerns that can hinder or help the process of change. Being aware of such interests means that adjustments and compromises can be made to change proposals to encourage support.

Be flexible. This follows from the previous lesson. It does not mean compromising the vision for change but allows for the adjustments necessary to build strong coalitions.

Don't give up or give in. As shown in this case study, initiating change often requires a long-term commitment of energy. One's values can be resources in maintaining enthusiasm. Hold on to them.

APPENDIX A

Outpatient Multidisciplinary Team Memo (May 26, 1980), Abridged

A. team approach would provide a mechanism for:
1. Identifying patient needs, establishing treatment goals, developing and implementing treatment programs
2. Coordinating and integrating treatment programs
3. Providing a systematic review of patient progress
4. Improving quality of care
5. Improving communication among staff and facilitating consistent patient treatment
6. Promoting development of treatment programs based on clearly identified patient needs
7. Maintaining staff morale and impetus in treating this challenging group of patients

APPENDIX B

Proposal for Schizophrenia Clinic (December 13, 1982), Abridged: Objective and Goals for Clinic

The overall objective of the clinic is to promote the development of good quality treatment services for schizophrenic patients and their families in the community. More specific goals include the following:
1. Provide a formal system for organizing the delivery of treatment care to schizophrenia patients including psychiatric and psychosocial aspects
2. Develop a multidisciplinary team approach to the outpatient treatment of schizophrenic patients
3. Provide a system of mutual staff support and peer consultation
4. Provide a point of contact for the patients, their families and community agencies
5. Promote research, education and program development in the area of schizophrenia.

APPENDIX C

Summary Outline Of Program (Ministry Application: January 1983)

It is proposed to establish an aftercare clinic for schizophrenic patients and their families that will comprise several components. A system of case management involving the assignment of a prime therapist and the contributions of a multidisciplinary team will be put in place with a designated psychiatrist in charge. Members of the team will act both as direct service providers and as consultants in their particular area of expertise.

The clinic will perform a coordinating function in relation to existing programs that serve the schizophrenic patient. e.g., out-patient, day therapy social/recreation programs.

The clinic will provide a point of contact for staff, patients, their families, and community agencies. Patient and family crisis situations will receive quick and thorough response with the aim of preventing relapse and/or admission to hospital. The clinic program will offer patient and family education about the medical and psychosocial aspects of schizophrenia in the form of teaching and support groups.

Finally, the program, through focusing on one particular patient population, will develop an intimate knowledge of gaps in service for the schizophrenia patient and consequently will produce comprehensive recommendations for further program development.

ACKNOWLEDGEMENTS

I acknowledge the valuable feedback received from Betty Yerxa, EdD, LHD (Hon), OTR, FAOTA, and Helene Polatajko, PhD, OT(C), as well as the reviewers for the *American Journal of Occupational Therapy*.

This research was supported by the Social Sciences and Humanities Research Council of Canada Doctoral Fellowship.

REFERENCES

Abravanel, H. (1983). Mediatory myths in the service of organizational ideology. In L. Pondy, P. I. Frost, G. Morgan, & T. C. Dandridge (Eds.), *Organizational symbolism* (pp. 273-293). Greenwich, CT: Jail Press.

American Occupational Therapy Association (1985). A professional legacy. *The Eleanor Clarke Slagle lectures in occupational therapy, 1955-1984*. Rockville, MD: Author.

Anthony, W., Cohen, M., & Farkas, M. (1990). *Psychiatric rehabilitation*. Boston, MA: Center for Psychiatric Rehabilitation.

Bachrach, L. (Ed.) (1983). *Deinstitutionalization. New directions for mental health services series*. San Francisco, CA: Jossey-Bass.

Baptiste, S. (1988). Chronic pain, activity, and culture. *Canadian Journal of Occupational Therapy, 55*, 179-185.

Baxter, E., & Hopper, K. (1982). The new mendicancy: Homeless in New York City. *American Journal of Orthopsychiatry, 52*(3), 393-408.

Bennis, W. (1979). Why leaders can't lead. In R. Kanter & B. Stein (Eds.), *Life in organizations* (pp. 36 48). New York, NY: Basic.

Cameron, J. (1978). Ideology and policy termination. Restructuring California's mental health system. In J. Man & A. Wildavsky (Eds.), *The policy cycle* (pp. 301-328). Beverly Hills, CA: Sage.

Canadian Association of Occupational Therapists (1991). *Occupational therapy guidelines for client-centered practice*. Toronto, Ontario: COOT Publications.

Carswell-Opzoomer, A. (1990). Occupational therapy: Our time has come. *Canadian Journal of Occupational Therapy, 57*(4), 197-204.

Cook, J. V. (1988). Golfman's legacy: The elimination of the chronic mental patient's community. *Research in the Sociology of Health Care, 7*, 249-281.

Downs, A. (1967). *Inside bureaucracy*. Boston, MA: Little, Brown.

Estroff, S. E. (1981). *Making it crazy: An ethnography of psychiatric clients in an American community*. Berkeley, CA: University of California Press.

Feldman, S. (1980, Fall). The middle management muddle. *Administration Mental Health*, 3-11.

Golembiewski, R. T. (1985). *Humanizing public organizations*. Mt Airy, MD: Lomond.

Graziano, M. (1969). Clinical innovation and mental health power structure: Social case history. *American Psychologist, 24*(1), 10-18.

Grob, G. N. (1980). Abuse in American mental hospitals in historical perspective: Myth and reality. *International Journal of Law and Psychiatry, 3*, 295-310.

Grob, G. N. (1983). Historical origins of deinstitutionalization. In L. L. Bachrach (Ed.), *Deinstitutionalization* (pp. 15-30) San Francisco, CA: Jossey-Bass.

Hall, R H. (1982). *Organizations structures and process*. Englewood Cliffs, NJ: Prentice-Hall.

Judd, M. (1982). The challenge of change. *Canadian Journal of Occupational Therapy, 48*(4), 117-124.

Kanter, R. M. (1983). *The change masters*. New York, NY: Simon & Schuster.

Kinston, W. (1983). Hospital organization and structure and its effect on interprofessional behavior and the delivery of care. *Social Science and Medicine, 17*(16), 1159-1170.

Krefting, L. (1991). Rigor in qualitative research: The assessment of trustworthiness. *American Journal of Occupational Therapy. 4*(3), 214-222.

Law, M. (1991). The environment: focus for occupational therapy. *Canadian Journal of Occupational Therapy, 58*(4), 171-180.

Lincoln, L., & Guba, E. (1985). *Naturalistic inquiry*. Newbury Park, CA: Sage.

Lodahl, T. M., & Mitchell, S. M. (1981). Drift in the development of innovative organizations. In J. R. Kimberly, R. H. Miles, & Associates (Eds.), *The organizational life cycle*. (pp. 184-207). San Francisco, CA: Jossey-Bass.

Louis, M. R. (1983). Organizations as culture bearing milieu. In L Pondy, P. J. Frost, G. Morgan, & T. C. Dandridge (Eds.), *Organizational symbolism* (pp. 39-53). Greenwich, CT: JAI.

Marx, J. H. (1969). A multidimensional conception of ideologies in professional arenas: The case of the mental health field. *Pacific Sociological Review, 12*(2), 75-85.

Maxwell, J. D., & Maxwell, M. P. (1977). *Occupational therapy. The diffident profession.* Kingston, Ontario: Queen's University.

Mechanic, D. (1980). *Mental health and social policy.* Engelwood Cliffs, NJ: Pretence-Hall.

Morgan, G. (1984). Opportunities arising from paradigm diversity. *Administrative Science Quarters, 16*(3), 306-327.

Morgan, G. (1986). *Images of organization.* Beverly Hills, CA: Sage.

Morrissey, J. P., & Tessler, R. C. (1982). Selection processes in state mental hospitalization: Policy issues and research directions. *Research in Social Problems and Public Policy, 2,* 35-79.

Polatajko, H. (1992). Naming and framing occupational therapy: A lecture dedicated to the life of Nancy B. *Canadian Journal of Occupational Therapy, 59,* 189-200.

Pranger, T., & Brown, G. (1992). Burnout: An issue for psychiatric occupational therapy personnel? *Occupational Therapy in Mental Health, 12*(1), 77-92.

Price, S. (1993). New pathways for psychosocial therapists. *American Journal of Occupational Therapy, 47,* 557-559.

Schein, E. (1985). *Organizational culture and leadership.* San Francisco, CA: Jossey-Bass.

Smircich, L. (1983). Organizations as shared meanings. In L. Pondy, P. L. Frost, G. Morgan, & T. C. Dandridge (Eds.), *Organizational Symbolism* (pp. 55-56). Greenwich, CT: JAI.

Smircich, L. & Morgan, G. (1982). Leadership: The management of meaning. *The Journal of Applied Behavioral Science, 18*(3), 257-273.

Smith, K. (1984). Philosophical problems in thinking about organizational change. In P. S. Goodman & Associates (Eds.), *Change in organizations* (pp. 316-374). San Francisco, CA: Jossey-Bass.

Strass, A., Schatzman, L., Bucher, R., Ehrlich, D., & Sabshin, M. (1964). *Psychiatric ideologies and institutions.* New York, NY: Free Press of Glencoe.

Tichy, N. (1981). Problem cycles in organizations and the management of change. In J. R. Kimberly, R. H. Miles & Associates (Eds.), *The organizational life cycles* (pp. 163-183). San Francisco, CA: Jossey-Bass.

Tichy, N. (1983). *Managing strategic change. Technical, political and cultural dynamics.* New York, NY: Wiley.

Weissman, H. H. (1982). Fantasy and reality of staff involvement in organizational change. *Administration in Social Work, 6*(1), 37-45.

Wilson, J. (1973). *Introduction to social movements.* New York, NY: Basic.

Yerxa, E. J. (1983). Audacious values: The energy source for occupational therapy practice. In G. Kielhofner (Ed.), *Health through occupation: Theory and practice in occupational therapy* (pp. 149-162). Philadelphia, PA: F.A. Davis.

Year, E. J. (1991). Occupational therapy and medicine: A comparison of values. *The Link, 7,* 1-2.

CHAPTER SIXTY-FIVE

Creating a Culture of Education: The Manager's Role in Supporting Fieldwork Education

Brent H. Braveman and Deborah Walens

This chapter was previously published in Administration and Management Special Interest Quarterly, 14(3), 1-3. *Copyright © 1998, The American Occupational Therapy Association, Inc.*

The number of accredited occupational therapy programs has grown dramatically over the past few years. Although this has decreased the shortage of clinicians, it has created a new shortage—one of fieldwork education sites. Fieldwork education has and continues to be a mayor priority for the profession. According to the American Occupational Therapy Association's (AOTA, 1993) *Occupational Therapy Roles* document, the scope of the occupational therapy practitioner's role includes key performance areas at the intermediate level of "Supervises/teaches occupational therapy practitioner, students, and other staff performing supportive services and/or other aspects of service provision, and participates in the fieldwork education process. (p. 10). Managers play a critical role in defining fieldwork education as a practitioner's responsibility. In addition to supporting the fieldwork education process by contracting with academic institutions to accept students, the occupational therapy manager plays an important role in facilitating member appreciation of the educator role. The manager can be a needed advocate for staff members after they have accepted a student by ensuring support from administration and facilitating a positive experience that the staff members will want to repeat. This (chapter) is an overview of five steps to creating a "culture of education."

1. How can accepting students assist you in achieving your department and organizational mission?
2. What vision for the future can you describe to staff members and others that includes a role for students?
3. What is your own philosophy on the responsibility of occupational therapy practitioners to be involved in fieldwork education?
4. What historical experiences do staff members have that will either facilitate or hinder your efforts to develop a fieldwork program?
5. What exists in your current department and organization culture that supports or hinders the successful development of a fieldwork education program?

Answering these questions can assist you in anticipating and overcoming potential roadblocks. Your staff members and others in your organization must view fieldwork education as a positive step to achieving department and organization goals. Becoming aware of previous negative experiences with fieldwork education and capitalizing on positive experiences will assist you in developing a critical level of support. Most important, when developing support for fieldwork education, you must realistically determine that you can make the investment of personal, department, and professional resources to the process of educating students (Griswold & Strassler, 1991; Walens, 1991).

STEP ONE: EVALUATING YOUR OWN CONTEXT

The process of creating a culture of education begins by completing an evaluation of your practice environment. This evaluation includes answering five pivotal questions that will help put fieldwork education on the right foot. The five questions are:

STEP TWO: CREATING A CULTURE TO SUPPORT FIELDWORK EDUCATION

A first step in creating a culture to support fieldwork education is to examine the "psychological contract" that exists between yourself as a proxy for the organization that employs you and the employees who report to you. Schermerhorn, Hunt, and Osborn (1994) explained that a psychological contract exists between every employer and employee and that this contract "is an informal understanding that includes the set of expectations that are held by the individual that specify what the individual and the organization expect to give to and receive from each other in the course of their working relationship. (p. 51)." The expected exchange is anticipated during the recruitment phase but can be either confirmed or denied later during actual employment. Establishing an expectation that part of the role of all staff members includes ongoing participation in fieldwork education can become part of this psychological contract. That is, after it is established that taking students is simply a "part of the job," staff members will come to expect fieldwork education as part of the ongoing exchange of value between themselves and their employer. The psychological contract can be further validated by the manager who finds ways to bring real-life value to the fieldwork educator role. This can be accomplished by including statements about fieldwork education in job descriptions, performance appraisal systems, and competency evaluation systems. Additionally, because staff members seldom receive additional financial rewards for accepting fieldwork students, and because it means considerable work, you must be able to clearly articulate the benefits of involvement in fieldwork education in terms of personal and professional. These may include improved supervisory skills, impetus for the examination of one's own practice, and exposure to developing knowledge bases currently presented in academic settings.

STEP THREE:
EVALUATING YOUR
DEPARTMENT'S PREPAREDNESS

Many of the barriers that staff members identify to accepting fieldwork students are likely to center on real concerns about their own preparedness to provide a quality learning experience. It is possible to praise staff members for the professionalism and ethics that underlie these concerns while not allowing this fear to prevent you from moving forward. The concerns of staff members regarding skill development as an educator can be addressed by obtaining formal or informal education to become a fieldwork instructor. Continuing education is periodically available through academic institutions, state associations and AOTA or can be customized by bringing speakers to your department for inservice education. Most academic fieldwork coordinators are willing to assist new fieldwork sites in developing their programs and with the ongoing maintenance of a program. Generally, all you need to do is ask. State associations are another resource for identifying experienced fieldwork educators in your local area who are willing to provide inservice education or share previously developed resources so that you do not have to "reinvent the

wheel." Many publications are available from AOTA, such as the newly published *The Fieldwork Anthology: A Classic Research and Practice Collection* (Privott, 1998) and *Self-Paced Instruction for Clinical Education and Supervision (SPICES)* (Crepeau & LaGarde, 1991). AOTA regional fieldwork consultants and the AOTA fieldwork program manager are readily accessible by calling 1-800-SAY-AOTA. (The Fieldwork Educators Competency Self-Assessment Tool will be available to assist fieldwork educators in evaluating the areas where they need further knowledge or skills.) Finally, AOTA members may subscribe free of charge to AOTA's Special Interest Section listservs. A listserv is an e-mail "bulletin board" where participants may post questions or requests for assistance, and others on the listserv may respond to such requests through e-mail.

STEP FOUR:
JUSTIFYING PARTICIPATION
IN FIELDWORK EDUCATION

Whether you work in a medical facility and are experiencing the crunch of managed care or you work in a community or educational system and are faced with shrinking tax dollars, we have all been asked to do more with less and justify all that we do. All practitioners have these pressures and may ask you to justify the decision to begin a new time-intensive effort such as a fieldwork education program when they can barely keep up with current demands for delivering services. Often, the basis of this thinking is a concern for quality care, but what we need to recognize is that fieldwork education and quality care are not mutually exclusive in achieving goals.

Another concrete method of evaluating the effect of a fieldwork education program is to complete a week-by-week analysis of expected productivity to be provided by the fieldwork educator and the student. Table 65-1 gives an example formulated on the basis of a department with an expectation for 6 hours of billable service per 8-hour day per staff member. Under this progression, the fieldwork educator and the student together provide a total of 1,532 billed time units (1 time unit a 15 minutes) over a l2-week period compared with the expected 1,440 billed time units for the staff member alone without the student. Although you must evaluate the true cost-benefit relationship for your own setting, the example in Table 65-1 is a conservative model because it allows for 10 hours of supervision during Weeks 1 and 2, and it assumes that, beginning Week 6, the staff member is only carrying one half of a caseload and that the remainder of the staff members' time is devoted to supervision or to other department efforts. Of course, it is recognized that when a fieldwork educator encounters a problem student, this model will not apply. However, by using other creative models of fieldwork education (e.g., two fieldwork educators for one student, or two fieldwork students paired with one part-time fieldwork educator), the payoff can be even greater than that outlined

Table 65-1

Expected Treatment Units During a Level II Fieldwork Expedience

Week	1	2	3	4	5	6	7	8	9	10	11	12
Educator	80	80	80	80	80	60	60	60	60	60	60	60
Student	6	6	40	40	40	60	60	80	120	120	80	60

here. Staff members can likewise be freed up to work on special projects or take advantage of leave time if supervision is shared by more than one staff member. These benefits can be explicitly included in the expectations of the psychological contract regarding your fieldwork education program.

STEP FIVE: AVOIDING COMMON MISCONCEPTIONS

There are several common misconceptions that exist to dissuade a manager from developing a fieldwork education program. First, some managers have avoided accepting students because of the lead time involved in the contract process. Education programs often ask facilities to accept a reservation for a fieldwork student up to 1 year or more in advance. The fear that a reservation might have to be canceled due to staff member turnover or layoffs can enter into the decision to not take students. In fact, although no fieldwork education coordinator enjoys a last-minute cancellation, they do expect that cancellations will occur from time to time. Furthermore, most fieldwork coordinators would prefer that you cancel an educational experience that you know will be a poor one than take a student into a bad situation. Second, there has been the misconception that all fieldwork experiences must be full-time (40 hours per week) and be classified as pediatrics, physical disability, or mental health. Although this is true in some academic programs, the standards for AOTA accreditation for education programs dictate only the minimum number of hours of Level II fieldwork (940 hours for occupational therapists/440 hours for occupational therapy assistants) and that at least half of the sustained fieldwork experience is desirable on a full-time basis (AOTA, 1991a, 1991b). Most education programs have the occasional need for part-time affiliations that last longer than 12 weeks and are willing to accept a wide range of fieldwork experiences, including home health care, community based practice, and combinations of more than one practice area. Managers are encouraged to contact academic fieldwork coordinators to discuss creative options that their program may be able to offer.

CONCLUSION

Fieldwork education is a critical step in the education of occupational therapy practitioners, and occupational therapy managers play an important role in facilitating the development of fieldwork education programs within their facilities. Numerous resources exist to assist the manager in the development and ongoing support of such programs such as those cited within this (chapter). Managers interested in developing fieldwork education programs are encouraged to contact AOTA...or one of the authors for more information.

REFERENCES

American Occupational Therapy Association (1991a). *Essential guidelines for an accredited educational program for the occupational therapist*. Rockville MD: Author.

American Occupational Therapy Association. (1991b). *Essentials and guides for an accredited educational program for the occupational therapy assistant*. Rockville, MD: Author.

American Occupational Therapy Association. (1993). *Occupational therapy roles*. Rockville, MD: Author.

Crepeau, E. B. & LaGarde, T. (Eds.) (1991). *Self-paced instruction for clinical education and supervision (SPICES)*. Rockville, MD: American Occupational Therapy Association.

Griswold, L. A., & Strassler, B. (1991). Formulating a fieldwork philosophy and resources. In E. B. Crepeau & T. LaGarde (Eds.), *Self-paced instruction for clinical education and supervision (SPICES) (pp. 21-39)*. Rockville, MD: American Occupational Therapy Association.

Privott, C. R. (Ed.). (1998). *The fieldwork anthology: A classic research and practice collection*. Rockville, MD: American Occupational Therapy Association.

Schermerhorn, J. R., Hunt, J. G., & Osborn, R. N. (Eds.) (1994). *Organizational behavior in the new workplace. Managing organizational behavior*. New York, NY: Wiley.

Walens, D. (1991). A conceptual model of practice for school system therapists. In A. C. Bundy (ed.), *Making a difference. OTs and PTs in public schools*. Chicago, Ill: University of Illinois at Chicago, Department of Occupational Therapy.

CHAPTER SIXTY-SIX

Innovation to Action: Marketing Occupational Therapy

Karen Jacobs

This chapter was previously published in American Journal of Occupational Therapy, 52, 618-620. Copyright © 1998, The American Occupational Therapy Association, Inc.

Living in process is being open to insight and encounter. Creativity is becoming intensively absorbed in the process and giving it form. (Smith as quoted in Schaef, 1990)

We live in uncertain and unpredictable times. As Fradette and Michaud (1998) noted in their book, *The Power of Corporate Kinetics*, "If we can no longer depend on our ability to predict the future, we can create a dynamic business design that can capitalize on the unpredictable, to turn it to our advantage" (p. 19). One mechanism to "capitalize on the unpredictable" is to embed marketing into our daily occupations, whether it is describing the value of occupational therapy while providing direct services to a client, speaking to parents about the benefits of occupational therapy while waiting to pick up one's child from an after-school sport, or presenting on health and wellness at a local senior health fair.

Marketing the value of occupational therapy is our collective responsibility. It will take a commitment from all of us to continuously innovate, evolve, redefine, and reinvent ourselves:

- It will require that we instantly respond to new demands and seize new opportunities.
- It will require that we continuously ask ourselves, "What business are we in?"
- It will require that we challenge ourselves to ignore traditional thinking and business boundaries and be creative.
- It will require designing new products and services for smaller markets.
- It will require that we "serve a single customer and act in zero time" Fradette & Michaud, 1998, p. 117).

I believe that we should be a market leader in the promotion of lifelong health and well-being, which supports fulfilling and productive lives. To accomplish this goal, we need to ensure that we provide the following three things and be exceptional in at least one: (a) product leadership *(our products must be the best)*; (b) operational excellence, effectiveness, and efficiency *(we must always deliver on what we say)*; and (c) customer intimacy and connectedness *(we must try to delight our customers)* (Labovitz & Rosansky, 1997).

AOTA's National Awareness Campaign has been a superb beginning to reaching millions of people, but we need to continue the momentum and be even more effective in our marketing efforts. This increased effectiveness will require that we focus on occupational therapy's value—its benefits rather than its features. The features of occupational therapy are the assessments, evaluations, interventions, consultations, and so forth that we provide. Rather than explaining occupational therapy's features, we need to reframe all that we do into its benefits. We promote lifelong health and well-being, and the mechanism to achieve this benefit is through participation in meaningful occupation.

In the past decade, marketing has become more commonplace in health care organizations and, in fact, has become a necessary component to staying competitive in the American health care system.

Traditionally, occupational therapy practitioners and health care organizations have developed their products on the basis of what they thought the customer wanted relative to their own plans. Marketing reverses this process.

Because marketing is an important aspect of service delivery, it is vital that all practitioners understand it. Practitioners need to learn the tools and techniques of marketing just as they needed to learn the tools and techniques of occupational therapy. This (chapter) briefly introduces some marketing concepts, but I highly recommend that practitioners continue to acquire knowledge and develop skills in marketing by attending workshops, taking continuing education courses, or acquiring advanced degrees in business. In general, we all need to become more business savvy.

Marketing should be embraced as a dynamic that includes the successful analysis of a need, the design of a product or service to meet the need, the uniting of that product or service to a potential user, and the use of a product or service by the consumer. Ideally, a marketing approach is used before the development of any product or service.

A MARKETING APPROACH

A marketing approach requires a detailed marketing plan that should be developed yearly and updated regularly. Measurable and achievable objectives should be set, with responsible persons designated to monitor outcomes. The four components to a marketing approach are (a) analyzing market opportunities, (b) researching and selecting target markets and market strategies, (c) developing marketing strategies, and (d) executing and evaluating the marketing plan.

Analyzing Market Opportunities

Analysis of various elements in the marketplace is the first step in a marketing approach. The market itself needs to be defined and may be selected simply on the basis of geographic territory. The market consists of all actual or potential buyers of a product, service, or idea. Identification of attractive target markets includes the analysis of marketing opportunities. This analysis consists of (a) self-audit, (b) consumer analysis, (c) competitive analysis, and (d) environmental assessment (Jacobs, 1989, 1997; Jacobs & Logigian, 1994).

Self-Audit. A self-audit assesses the strengths and weaknesses of, opportunities for, and threats to the practitioner or organization. Factors to be assessed might include the following:

- *Strengths:* product leadership; operational excellence, effectiveness, and efficiency; customer intimacy and connectedness; clinical expertise (e.g., the practitioner's qualifications, such as a master's degree; specialized training; board certification, such as in pediatrics, neurorehabilitation, or board-certified professional ergonomist); and effective outcome measures
- *Weakness:* inadequate staffing, ineffective marketing, limited finances, and poor reputation (Beaton, 1995)
- *Opportunities:* demographic (e.g., aging population), expansion into industry-based practice, increased funding sources, and legislation (e.g., Reauthorization of the Individuals With Disabilities Education Act of 1990 [Public Law 105-17])
- *Threats:* competition for scarce resources, changes in funding sources (e.g., managed care), and changes in legislation (e.g., salary equivalency, Balanced Budget Act of 1997 [Public Law 105-33])

This self-audit assists in understanding how well or poorly prepared a practitioner or organization is to meet the marketplace demands. Ascertaining what one does well and maintaining one's product or service at an optimal level are critical aspects of marketing.

Consumer analysis. A consumer analysis delineates potential customers in order to understand their needs and wants for products or services.

Competitive analysis. Identifying other providers of similar services will provide a snapshot of the kinds of services being offered in a particular locale, and analyzing these services will both reduce the potential for overlap and help to identify areas that are not being served. Opportunities for collaboration or joint ventures may surface at this time (Jacobs, 1997).

Environmental assessment. An environmental assessment attempts to predict what impact present and future demographics, political and regulatory systems, cultural and economic or financial environments, psychographics, and technology have on products and services (Jacobs, 1997).

Researching and Selecting Target Markets and Market Segments

After the marketing opportunities have been analyzed, the market's needs can be determined through research, which might include observation, survey, or even experimentation to test hypotheses. After research is completed, the market is segmented, that is, divided into target markets or groups of consumers with similar needs, wants, or interests. The groups are further segmented into smaller, distinct groups that might require separate products and promotions. Ideally, we should attempt to customize our products to serve a single customer! According to Beaton (1995), there are three criteria for segmentation:

- Measurability: Whether the service provider can collect information on service utilization and the reasons underlying the pattern of use.
- Accessibility: Whether the service provider can apply marketing effort to reach a selected segment of the market.
- Substantiality: Whether the selected services are large enough to merit a different mix of marketing activities. (pp. 8-9)

After segmentation is done, it is followed by targeting, which, according to Beaton, can be carried out in different ways:

- Undifferentiated marketing: When the same mix of marketing activities is offered to the entire market, such as in marketing occupational therapy to the general public.
- Differentiated marketing: When marketing programs are designed for different market segments, such as marketing to various specialties within occupational therapy.
- Concentrated marketing: When marketing is concentrated on one segment of the market, such as care of the elderly. (p. 9)

All of these strategies help in deciding where products or services should be positioned in the market and in developing marketing strategies.

Developing Marketing Strategies

The marketing approach continues with the development of a marketing mix. The marketing mix is a particular blend of marketing variables, called "the four Ps" (product, price, place, promotion), that are used to meet the needs, wants, or interests of this well-defined target market. It is what an individual or organization can do to influence the demand for their products or services (Jacobs, 1997). The remainder of this section focuses on promotion.

Promotion is the vehicle of communicating information to the consumer about the products' or services' merits. (Occupational therapy practitioners should remember to reframe the message to primarily promote the (benefits of products and services.) The instruments of promotion are advertising, sales promotion, publicity, and personal selling, and the methods of promotion are only limited by imagination and financial resources. All promotional activities should be piloted with a small segment of the target group so that modifications can be made before full distribution. Messages should be succinct, using 15-word or less sound bites or tag lines, bullet points, or a question-and-answer format. Occupational therapy practitioners should use the AOTA tag line, "OT... skills for the job of living," whenever possible. In addition, word-of-mouth recommendations by present and past consumers are a powerful promotional tool. I encourage all practitioners to keep a log of testimonials from their consumers and use them whenever marketing products or services.

Advertising involves the use of a paid message presented in a recognized medium and by an identified sponsor with the purpose to inform, persuade, and remind. The AOTA's National Awareness Campaign has been successful in reaching millions of consumers and potential consumers through advertisements in *People Weekly, Family Circle, Better Homes and Gardens,* and *USA Today.*

Sales promotion is the use of a wide variety of short-term incentives to encourage earlier or stronger target market response to the purchase of products or services. This approach is optimized when used in conjunction with advertising (Kotler & Clarke, 1990). Some examples of consumer sales promotion tools are samples, coupons, gifts, contests, and demonstrations (Jacobs, 1997).

Publicity is free promotion; however, despite this positive feature, one has little control over its placement, and, thus, it becomes difficult to focus the message on specific target markets (Jacobs, 1997). For example, a radio spot discussing a topic such as preventing cumulative trauma injuries would be consider publicity.

Personal selling is the most effective form of promotion. It involves face-to-face communication between the practitioner and the consumer. Some examples of personal selling methods are making presentations at meetings, providing continuing education workshops, and lecturing to professional organizations.

National Occupational Therapy Month provides an excellent opportunity to promote the benefits of occupational therapy. I encourage practitioners to plan ahead and contact the AOTA Public Relations department for a promotional resource packet. The packet contains suggestions for celebrating the month, camera-ready advertisements, "skills for the job of living" logos, story ideas, public service announcements, and sample news releases, to name a few.

EXECUTING AND EVALUATING THE MARKETING PLAN

After the target market has been selected and the marketing mix developed, the marketing plan is implemented. Because marketing is a dynamic activity, the plan will require periodic and ongoing reexamination to evaluate its effectiveness. A specific time frame, such as a 12-month period, should be delineated to measure whether objectives and goals are being met. A system of regular review is essential so that modifications can be made when needed (Jacobs, 1997).

CONCLUSION

The use of a marketing approach will allow practitioners to approach the health care environment proactively and be ready to meet the changing needs and wants of the marketplace. In all times of change, there is a chance for great opportunity. I challenge all practitioners to make a commitment to marketing the value of occupational therapy.

REFERENCES

Balanced Budget Act of 1997. Pub. L. No. 105-33, 111 Stat. 251.

Beaton, J. (1995). *Marketing handbook for occupational therapists.* London, England: College of Occupational Therapists.

Fradette, M. & Michaud, S. (1998). *The power of corporate kinetics.* New York, NY: Simon & Schuster.

Jacobs, K. (1989). Work hardening in the health care system. In L. Ogden-Niemeyer & K. Jacobs (Eds.), *Work hardening: State of the art* (pp. 111-126). Thorofare, NJ: SLACK Incorporated

Jacobs, K. (1997). Marketing strategies. In J. Pratt & K. Jacobs (Eds.), *Work practice: International perspectives* (pp. 267-276). Oxford, UK: Butterworth-Heinemann.

Jacobs, K. & Logigian, M. (1994). *Functions of a manager in occupational therapy.* Thorofare, NJ: SLACK Incorporated.

Kotler, P. & Clarke, R. (1990). *Marketing health services.* London, England: Prentice Hall.

Labovitz, G., & Rosansky, V. (1997). *The power of alignment.* New York, NY: Wiley

Reauthorization of the Individuals With Disabilities Education Act of 1990. (1997). Pub. L. No. 105-17.

Schaef, A. W. (1990). *Meditations for women who do too much.* San Francisco, CA: Harper Collins.

CHAPTER SIXTY-SEVEN

Managed Care: Survival Skills for the Future

Brent H. Braveman and Gail S. Fisher

This chapter was previously published in Occupational Therapy in Health Care, 10(4), 13-31. Copyright ©1997, *Haworth Press. Reprinted by permission.*

INTRODUCTION

The 1980s and 1990s have been a time of dramatic and consistent change in the way health care is delivered. The rate of infiltration of managed care has varied from market to market; yet, its growth and impact on health care organizations and personnel have nonetheless continued. This growth and the resulting competition have forced health care providers to continue to provide quality services but at a lower cost.

To respond to the demands of changing patterns of reimbursement, many public and private health care providers have begun to utilize common strategies to lower costs, shorten lengths of stay and increase systematic efficiency. These strategies impact occupational therapy practitioners directly, yet, they are frequently ill-prepared to respond to changes constructively. With adequate preparation, occupational therapy practitioners may not only respond to organizational change, but may play a major role in helping to shape their organization's future. This preparation requires gaining an understanding of the changes occurring in the local health care market and developing new skills as clinicians, supervisors, managers and leaders.

The purpose of this (chapter) is to:

1. Present and define the most common strategies currently being utilized by health care providers to respond to managed care and the resulting implications for occupational therapy practitioners.
2. Present and define the skills and strategies which occupational therapy practitioners can utilize to effectively respond to the changing health care environment.

MANAGED CARE BASICS

Managed care systems seek to contain or reduce costs while assuring the quality of health-related services. They utilize several strategies to accomplish these goals. First, a prospective payment system is used rather than the traditional fee-for-service basis. This is usually implemented by using capitated reimbursement, where a provider of services is paid a set amount for each managed care plan enrollee, no matter what services are provided. This provides an incentive to the provider to limit costs as much as possible to maximize profits. Second, a gatekeeper, usually a primary care physician or a case manager, is responsible for managing the care of an individual patient, and must authorize services provided by others. This usually results in lower utilization of specialist physicians and other health care professions, including occupational therapists. Careful screening of the need for services is utilized to determine whether the anticipated outcome justifies the cost. When rehabilitation services are needed, it is desirable to provide services in the least costly manner, such as in outpatient and home settings. Third, managed care organizations use utilization review procedures to monitor whether services are necessary and appropriate for the individual patient's situation (Landry and Knox, 1996). They may also collect data on quality of services and patient satisfaction and publish this data for use by enrollees and providers (The American Occupational Therapy Association Managed Care Project Team, 1996).

ORGANIZATIONAL APPROACHES FOR SURVIVING MANAGED CARE

Networks

Most health care providers have realized that in order to survive into the next decade, they must be able to link together with others to become part of a "seamless" system of care. Insurers are seeking "one-stop shopping" encompassing cost-containment, quality, and convenience for their customers. A primary strategy to accomplish these goals is developing or joining a network of health care providers. The establishment of a network ranges from somewhat informal referral agreements among specialty providers to comprehensive vertically integrated health systems (The American Occupational Therapy Association Managed Care Project Team, 1996). A vertically integrated health care system is an arrangement whereby a health care organization offers either directly or through others, a broad range of patient care and support services (Conrad, 1990). The ideal managed care delivery system has been envisioned as an organized body of health services and financial mechanisms that operates in an integrated and systematic fashion to manage and provide the right prevention, wellness, medical, and related services at the right place, time, and cost (Wolford, Brown, & McCool, 1993). As we continue to see a proliferation of larger and more fully integrated health care networks, occupational therapy practitioners will experience new opportunities and new challenges. New opportunities may arise for occupational therapy practitioners to utilize their skills in the areas of quality assurance or programs that emphasize disease prevention. Occupational therapists who have advanced skills in the analysis and adaptations of environments may be naturals to assume the role of case manager, a major component of managed care (Fisher, 1996). However, fewer therapists may be able to successfully operate as private practitioners without ties to a network. The days of the entrepreneurial occupational therapist who operates his or her own professional practice are coming to a close (Landry, 1996). Therapists will likely need to reorganize their private practices to align themselves with a network to take advantage of contractual referral arrangements.

Product Line Management

Product line management is a strategy in which personnel are reorganized from traditional discipline specific departments such as occupational therapy or physical therapy to "product lines" which are organized according to the service they provide. An example might be a Cardiovascular Services Product Line in which surgeons, nurses, social workers, and occupational and physical therapists providing care are organized to report to one administrator and medical director responsible for the "line" or for a variety of cardiovascular services ranging from surgery to outpatient cardiac rehabilitation. Product line organization allows minimization of administrative overhead more accurate tracking of the costs and revenues associated with delivery of a particular "product," and increased continuity of care. In an organization arranged in product lines the level of contact which the occupational therapy personnel in one product line might have with occupational therapy personnel in other product lines in the same facility might vary from frequent to none at all! While this organizational strategy offers clear advantages in the areas of team communication and decision-making, it also provides challenges to staff who no longer necessarily report to members of the same discipline. A particular chal-

lenge is that of providing adequate supervision to new graduates who must focus on the development of basic competencies. Staff operating in this model will need to learn new methods of solving discipline-specific clinical problems and planning for their development as occupational therapy practitioners. Existing paradigms regarding the amount and type of supervision provided to entry level occupational therapy practitioners, and how this supervision is provided, may need to be reexamined by the profession.

Skill Mix Change

As more of the health care market becomes capitated, the focus of health care providers will be on delivering high-quality, low-cost care. More and more, occupational therapy practitioners will need to evaluate the benefits of their services on a "cost per unit of care basis." The cost per unit of care has begun to be utilized as a tool to benchmark organizational cost efficiency against competitors. An organization determines the cost per unit of care for occupational therapy by dividing the total of all expenses related to the provision of all occupational therapy services during a set time period by the number of billable units of service provided during that same period. Occupational therapy managers who find that their cost per care exceeds that of competitors may expect to come under pressure to find ways to lower costs. A primary approach to lowering the cost per unit of care is to utilize less expensive technical or support personnel in place of more costly professional staff. Examination of the "skill mix" (ratio of OTRs to COTAs or aides) will be a necessary step in lowering the cost per unit of care. This means that as a profession we must change our current paradigm regarding the COTA/OTR partnership and how the roles of each are utilized. With the increased use of nonprofessional staff, OTRs have had to become more proficient as supervisors and case managers. The OTR role will increasingly become one of evaluator, communicator, educator, and trainee. The COTA will provide the bulk of the hands-on-care (The American Occupational Therapy Association Managed Care Project Team, 1996). As we move away from a fee-for-service basis to a more capitated system of reimbursement, occupational therapy (and all allied health professionals) may now be viewed by organizations as an expense rather than a source of revenue. This means that we must seek ways of achieving the same outcome of treatment but at a lower cost. The Tri-alliance (The American Occupational Therapy Association, The American Physical Therapy Association, and The American Speech-Language-Hearing Association) has recognized the use of multiskilled aides who are trained across disciplinary lines as an effective means to meet this challenge. In their position paper, *Use of Multiskilled Personnel,* the Tri-alliance stated, "Assignment of tasks to aide-level personnel with requisite direction and supervision results in efficient and cost-effective use of professional-level health care practitioners. The Tri-alliance does not support the use of "multiskilling" at the technical or professional levels (OT Week, 1996). In this document, multiskilling has been differentiated from the term cross-training, although at times these words have been used interchangeably. As opposed to multiskilling (training across disciplinary lines) cross-training in this document refers to training within one's discipline in practice areas which were previously unfamiliar.

Skill mix changes, while limiting the role of OTRs in direct treatment, may provide new opportunities for providing other types of service delivery. For example, occupational therapists may be called on to act as consultants to other interdisciplinary team members regarding a patient that may not need direct care. Occupational therapists will be more reliant on family members and support staff such as aides to help carry out occupational therapy related activities when treatment time is limited. This indirect service, which is provided by training others and monitoring their activities, has a history of being provided in nonhospital settings, such as school system practice and home health care. Participation in more consultation and indirect service requires us to shift our mind-set about what "real occupational therapy" is. Occupational therapy practitioners can be encouraged to see the value and power in helping others to become knowledgeable so they can assist patients and clients in becoming more functional.

Reengineering/Operational Improvement

Reengineering or organizational improvement strategies utilized by organizations vary. They range from organized, systematic approaches intended to change the culture of an organization through continuous quality improvement (CQI) techniques, to contracting with consulting firms to reengineer systems and jobs to eliminate waste and lower expenses. Reengineering typically means reducing the workforce, tightening the scope of service, shrinking overhead, modifying processes, and redefining service delivery (Brayman, 1996). Operational Improvement is a term which has been coined to describe reengineering efforts which focus on the implementation of employee-suggested changes in work flow to reduce costs (Lumsdon, 1994). These programs provide training to middle managers and staff in techniques to analyze and redesign work flow such as "leveraging" tasks which shifts duties from high-priced professional staff to the lowest paid but appropriately skilled worker. This may then result in increased expectation for provision of billable service by professional staff. Another common operations improvement approach is the consolidation of departments or medical units. An organization which previously operated an occupational therapy and a physical therapy department with separate managers may consolidate these departments into one, allowing elimination of one expensive managerial position. While many prestigious health care systems raise the benefits of a CQI approach for long-term change, they have also implemented operational improvement programs for short-term savings. The implementation of such programs can have devastating effects on the unprepared department. Organizations often conduct these efforts by contracting with outside consulting agencies. These agencies are hired on a percentage basis so that the higher the rate of savings they find for the institution, the higher their compensation. Department managers might expect that consultants will come armed with "summary" data from other organizations on expected levels of productivity, cost per unit of care or skill mix ratios. With the implementation time line of such projects often being 6 to 9 months, there is seldom time to collect adequate data specific to your facility. Without this data you are left defenseless against the sometimes considerable arguments these consultants can make.

Critical Pathways

A critical pathway is "an optimal sequencing and timing of interventions that is developed by a multidisciplinary team for a particular diagnosis" (Sinnott, 1994). Critical pathways map out the routine elements of care which occur with the vast majority of patients with a given diagnosis. The goals of critical pathways include: (1) minimizing the delays in providing care that sometimes occur due to system inefficiencies rather than by intent, (2) maximizing the quality of care through efficient utilization of resources, (3) establishing a basis for comparison when measuring the quality of care provided and (4) to project the length and cost of treatment (Abreu, Seale, Podlesak, & Hartley, 1996). Critical pathways often incorporate standing orders for such services as occupational therapy or physical therapy. For example, they may delineate what day post-admission or surgery services are to begin. A standing order may be as simple as an order for screening by a professional with full evaluation and treatment requiring a second order. However, in institutions where roles are well defined and disciplines have established professional credibility, standing orders may be more comprehensive, such as for evaluation and treatment. Critical pathways can be beneficial to health professionals as well as to the patient. Development of a critical pathway first requires a team to define and agree upon current practice in relation to a specific diagnosis. This process requires us to reexamine tacit assumptions we may have made about approaches to care for a subset of our patients. Other benefits of the use of critical pathways cited have included: (1) increased multidisciplinary collaboration, (2) education and orientation of staff, patients and families, (3) reduced length of stay and (4) reduced variation in the care process (The American Occupational Therapy Association Managed Care Project Team, 1996). Critical pathways may also be utilized as a marketing tool in a managed care environment by allowing the institution to estimate the cost of a particular pathway and sharing this information with potential managed care contractors (Abreu, 1996).

Downsizing

During the 1980s and early 1990s, occupational therapy experienced a dramatic increase in the number of professionals entering the market and continued growth and expansion of services was predicted. The growth in educational programs continues as evidenced by 21 new programs entering the Accreditation Council for Occupational Therapy Education

(ACOTE) accreditation process in the first three quarters of 1995. This represents an increase of 8% in entry level OTR and COTA programs (ACOTE, 1995). The number of occupational therapy practitioners providing services in skilled nursing facilities and intermediate care facilities increased by 170% from 1991 to 1995. However, as noted by the American Occupational Therapy Association's (AOTA) recently released report *Health Care and Market Reform: Workforce Implications for Occupational Therapy*, reductions in the number of occupational therapy practitioners were also seen in some practice settings (such as a decrease of 48.8% in psychiatric hospitals and 20.2% in general hospitals) during the same period (AOTA, 1996). In addition, many hospitals and health care providers both public and private have undergone major reorganizations. The results of these efforts have included "downsizing" and for the first time occupational therapy practitioners are experiencing layoffs similar to those experienced in other industries throughout this decade (Wolf, 1995). According to a 1995, survey by the American Hospital Association, an increasing number of hospital managers (27%) plan workforce reductions (Association of Academic Health Centers, 1995). One impact of these layoffs has been to require remaining staff to carry higher caseloads and to cause facilities to encourage the use of therapists as generalists rather than in specialty staffing patterns. General hospitals have begun to require staff to "cross-train" to other areas of practice within the field of occupational therapy. While this challenge has led to some dissatisfaction among staff at these facilities, it has also caused these staff to reinvestigate the nature of their practice and to focus on the evaluation and treatment of occupational dysfunction. While reinventing oneself as a therapist who works in occupational dysfunction rather than "psych" or "rehab" may be frustrating in the short term; it may prove to be the most beneficial effect of managed care on the profession of occupational therapy.

SURVIVAL SKILLS FOR THE NEW ENVIRONMENT

Systems Thinking

Occupational therapy practitioners in many settings have, historically, often enjoyed the luxury of remaining insulated from larger policy and organizational issues. After all, most occupational therapy personnel entered the profession to focus on direct patient care. However, as the rate of change in the environment has increased, having a limited understanding of the process for establishing organizational and public policy has placed us at risk of having others decide where and when organizations feel they can afford to provide occupational therapy services. In order to anticipate future change, occupational therapy practitioners must gain an understanding of the larger health care arena and the factors influencing it. This applies not only to those fulfilling the primary role of occupational therapy manager, but also those whose primary role is the delivery of direct care. Gaining an understanding of the public policy-making process at the local, state, and national levels, and the impact of such policies on our practice provides occupational therapy practitioners with a view that will empower them to understand how national level decisions can affect day-to-day service delivery (Baum, 1991). For example, proposals to reform health insurance are currently pending and may impact eligibility for services and reimbursement limitations. Changes in Medicare and Medicaid reimbursement guidelines have a major impact on organizations, including rehabilitation departments.

In addition, a basic awareness of forces influencing the health care marketplace is essential. It has become apparent that massive system-wide change can occur rapidly, without changes in federal regulation. The growth in managed care, for example, has been fueled by nongovernmental entities and market forces. Being aware of the trends which contribute to this type of change can be helpful in anticipating change, preparing for change, and advocating for change. This knowledge can be gained from following the national and local news, attending the American Occupational Therapy Political Action Committee's annual legislative conference or the Health Policy Forum presented annually at AOTA national conference, reading pertinent occupational therapy publications, and becoming part of the AOTA ActionLine Network which receives direct mailings on current legislative issues and the need for advocacy. There are currently a number of new workshops on managed care that are available, as well as new publications which focus on the impact of managed care on occupational therapy (The American Occupational Therapy Association Managed Care Project Team, 1996). These resources help one to learn the terms and concepts that are part of managed care, and to translate them to one's practice setting. Discussing these concepts and issues, whether in a classroom or clinic environment, facilitates understanding and allows individuals to gain this larger perspective.

Advocating for Ourselves and Others

Occupational practitioners are probably most comfortable in the role of advocate when we are acting as an advocate for our patients. As reimbursement systems have changed, many occupational therapy practitioners have had to become more active in communicating with third party payers to advocate for coverage of services. In the environment of the 1990s and beyond, occupational therapy personnel will also need to continually advocate for themselves as individuals and for the profession in their organizations as well as in the legislative arena. The American Occupational Therapy Political Action Committee and some state occupational therapy associations have developed materials to assist occupational therapy practitioners in advocacy activities (AOTPAC, 1993). There are many examples of how occupational therapy practitioners have assumed the role of advocate including the efforts in the 1980s and 1990s which resulted in all 50 states now having some form of licensure or regulation of practice. In addition, occupational therapy practitioners have had a role in advocating for the inclusion of occupational therapy in recent legislation related to school system practice. Grass roots lobbying is essential for legislators to be familiar with the benefits of occupational therapy. Advocacy in the future may also include the need to advocate to maintain or increase the level of services provided to an individual or group of patients. As organizations seek to lower costs to allow them to remain competitive, and as we continue to move away from a fee-for-service model, organizations may seek to limit the amount of occupational therapy service provided. As tools such as critical pathways are utilized, we must become active in their development and in the development of our own critical pathways, which reflect our knowledge and experience (Foto, 1995). While it will be necessary (and wise) for us to collaborate and cooperate with those responsible for cost-cutting in organizations, we must also maintain a strong ethical base to avoid compromising care beyond acceptable levels. As Sabin (1994) suggested, clinicians must learn how to care for clients while acting as stewards of society's resources; must recommend the least costly treatments, unless there is strong evidence that a more expensive intervention is clearly superior; and must advocate for justice in the health care system in addition to advocating for clients.

By the year 2000, it is estimated that 65% of health care will be provided outside of hospitals (MacLaren, 1994). As the provision of care continues to move from in-patient environments to ambulatory care environments, we will need to be active in developing new models of service delivery and advocating for their implementation. Finally, we should remain strong advocates for our personal views within the profession. We must remember the personnel who work within the American Occupational Therapy Association work for, and must answer to its membership. The elected representatives who sit in the Representative Assembly, a primary decision-making body for the American Occupational Therapy Association, are there to represent the views of their respective constituencies. Each of us can assume an active role within our profession by communicating with the staff of the AOTA, our representatives in the Representative Assembly and by participating in state associations or pursuing and accepting leadership roles within our state and national associations.

Increasing Your Centrality in the Organization

Edgar Sol (1987) described a model of career development which included not only the traditional career move of "moving up the corporate ladder," but, also used the word "centrality" to describe how an individual may advance his or her career by consciously becoming more "central" to the organization. Individuals may become more central to the organization in which they work by actively pursuing, volunteering for and accepting responsibilities outside their occupational therapy department or beyond their standard role. Such

activities may include participating on organization-wide task forces or committees. It is not necessary to assume that these committees must be focused on completing the "serious" work of the organization in order to assist with making oneself more central to one's organization. Participation in the planning of organizational social activities or employee reward or recognition programs can also be effective. Attending and being vocal at open forums which are offered are effective means of establishing credibility as an employee who is concerned and willing to look beyond oneself to the larger organizational community. In doing so, we must be careful to align ourselves as allies for change with organizational administrations rather than being obstructionists.

Assuming New Roles

The changing environment has created new opportunities for both hospital-based practitioners and those practicing in the community. Both OTRs and COTAs will be doing more supervision of aides for the more routine aspects of care, and this expanded role will be challenging for some individuals. This change requires department staff to come to consensus on guidelines for determining what levels of personnel are required for various patient groups and services, what type of personnel is adequate to provide the type of services required, how to evaluate if an individual patient is an exception to the general guidelines, and how to insure quality care and outcomes when service is provided by others. Competencies and training programs for aides must be developed to insure they can adequately carry out their expanded responsibilities (The American Occupational Therapy Association Managed Care Project Team, 1996). Given the need for all occupational therapy practitioners to provide supervision to others, this requires therapists to develop skills in assessing competency, delegating and instructing others, giving constructive feedback, and evaluating performance. These skills can be learned through role modeling from one's own supervisor, attending a seminar on supervision which may be provided by the organization's human resources department, attending a university course on human resource management, and reading pertinent resources by human resources personnel.

As cost considerations influence service delivery to a greater extent, consultation skills will become a valuable commodity (Jaffe, 1996). More therapists are moving into community-based consultation roles, as the job market for hospital-based therapists shifts. These opportunities offer multiple rewards for therapists with the requisite skills and personal attributes. One can learn these skills by reading one of the texts that are oriented specifically to occupational therapy consultation (Jaffe & Epstein, 1992; Hanft & Place, 1996), attending one of the workshops being offered by consultation experts, and seeking supervision and mentoring from an experienced consultant.

The changing health care system has created opportunities for occupational therapists as case managers for employers or insurance companies. Case management is an integral part of managed care, and provides coordination and evaluation of services provided to an individual. This area of specialized practice includes professionals with a variety of backgrounds, and allows for voluntary credentialing as a Certified Insurance Rehabilitation Specialist. The demand for case managers is expected to grow, as managed care expands (Fisher, 1996).

Learning how to gain satisfaction from these new and expanded roles and gaining the skills necessary to perform them allows therapists to redefine their roles within their organizations or to be more prepared for roles outside of their organizations. There are many opportunities in non-hospital-based settings, which view these roles as essential and required for the job.

Working with Others

The increased expectations for productivity without compromising quality challenge therapists to work more effectively with others. Payers are not going to reimburse identical services that are provided by more than one discipline. Areas of unnecessary redundancy must be identified and eliminated and areas of overlap must be explicitly defined and responsibility assigned. The interdisciplinary team, whose members work with patients independently but have ongoing communication and shared decision-making, may define areas of multi-skilling which may facilitate the patient's achievement of functional outcomes. Although multi-skilling is a term that is now frequently used, often with controversy, the transdisciplinary team, whose professionals cross the lines of their own traditional expertise and are familiar with the goals and methods of the other professionals, has been utilized for a long time in early intervention settings (Woodruff & Hanson, 1987). With the demand increasing for multiskilled therapists, it is important for a team to decide what is appropriate within the context of their setting. For example, is it appropriate for the speech and language pathologists to know how to do proper toilet transfers from the wheelchair, so that they don't have to interrupt their sessions for toileting, and so they can use this essential task as a medium for facilitating communication (Foto, 1996)? Is it appropriate for the occupational therapy practitioner to know how to use cuing to promote attainment of vocabulary as identified by the speech therapist. Each setting and team must work together to answer these types of questions, which will maximize rehabilitation progress and team functioning.

The functioning of the interdisciplinary team is becoming more important than ever with the emphasis on product line management. Occupational therapy practitioners can use their skills in group dynamics and active listening to facilitate team meetings and informal communication (Kane, 1975). Skills in assertiveness and conflict management are also valuable in helping the team work through difficult tasks and issues. Confidence in one's own professional role, in addition to knowing and respecting the roles of others, creates a more valuable team member.

With the push for more cross-training among occupational therapy practitioners within a diversified department, an individual therapist may be called upon to train another occupational therapy practitioner in his or her area of competence. Likewise, the therapist may be expected to become familiar with an area of practice that he or she may not have experience with. Learning new skills advances the expertise of the individual therapist, while making him or her more valuable to the organization by allowing for greater flexibility in staffing patterns (Christiansen, 1996). New graduates often value jobs where they can rotate between different areas within the occupational therapy department, so they can learn to apply their knowledge with a variety of patients. Encouraging that perspective will allow them to continue to grow professionally and be better prepared for the demands of current practice settings. Staff with expertise in one particular area may find it more difficult to work with a new patient population or program. Provision of continuing education, shadowing an experienced practitioner, and providing time for clinical supervision during the initial phase will assist the experienced therapist in becoming comfortable and proficient with the role expectations in a new area. Maximizing cross-training possibilities within an occupational therapy department requires the therapists to develop skills in collaboration and to work together in new and rewarding ways.

Understanding the Bottom Line

Traditional occupational therapy education has included, at best, only a basic review of accounting and budgetary principles. Some practitioners have remained resistant to incorporating fiscal concerns into their day-to-day practice. Success in today's managed care environment requires a much more advanced understanding of financial factors which influence how care will be delivered. As payers begin to profile our employer's track record for quality and cost outcomes, our employers will also begin to demand such monitoring from their therapists. Job requirements will entail not only clinical excellence but also the ability to exert fiscal control over limited resources (Foto, 1995). Understanding what influences payer mix and cost per unit of care is essential to plan and implement services that are in sync with the organization's capabilities and priorities. Understanding simple concepts such as revenue, operating expenses, and capital expenses will help support the department manager in budget planning and implementation to manage existing services efficiently and in planning proposals for new services. Direct care clinicians must understand how the day-to-day and hour-to-hour decisions they make regarding how care is delivered will impact the cost of that care to our patients and payers. As Foto (1995) has written, "We share a responsibility as a partner with the payers, policy makers, employers, and patients; a partner who has an equal stake in the evolution of effective cost and quality management tools. The increased utilization of technical and support staff and the increased scrutiny of utilization of services which may result in the provision of fewer treatment sessions may be of concern for some occupational therapists." Being aware of community resources which provide low or no-cost treatment and equipment is particularly important with reduced lengths of stay and and the number of patients without health care insurance. This knowledge can be valuable to both the patient and the institution, as these services can provide alternatives for patients who do not have reimbursement available for therapy. Therapists can consult social workers or social service directories to locate these services. Therapists can also organize to provide "pro bono" or free services on a limited basis to those in need. Some facilities have programs which refurbish and recycle used adaptive equipment and wheelchairs for those with limited resources. These types of services can help to augment the limited capabilities of institutions to provide unlimited uncompensated care.

Justifying Occupational Therapy Intervention

Managed care requires us to be accountable and to be prepared to justify our services. This requires therapists to determine expected outcomes for patient groups, through the use of critical pathways and similar tools. Making the link between what we can actually accomplish in the limited time we have for treatment and the desired outcome is a challenging but an essential task. We must be prepared to justify the necessary components of treatment as verified by research and accepted clinical practice. We must link our treatment activities with the desired outcome, and be prepared to justify it in a cost-effective manner. For example, interventions which reduce hospital length of stay and prevent rehospitalization are valued more than ever in a managed care environment. Assisting patients and families to transition to the next level of care becomes a more important priority as lengths of stay decrease. Justifying the continuation of outpatient treatment to an insurance company case manager requires one to be able to make an argument for the cost-effectiveness of increased functional independence with reduced need for paid assistance at home. Increasing a patient and family's ability to manage with residual disability without requiring crisis-oriented medical services due to a fall or impaired problem-solving is a powerful argument for continuing services on a short-term basis to accomplish specific goals. Measurement of achievement of outcomes and quality of care provided is expected in a managed care environment (Ellenberg, 1996). A recent flurry of workshops and publications on functional outcomes (Forer, 1996; Mayhan, 1994; Rogers & Holm, 1994) are available to assist therapists in becoming more knowledgeable and skilled in this area. These skills may also be gained by pursuing graduate education or an advanced degree in occupational therapy or a related field.

Embracing Change

Joel Barker (1992), a noted futurist, has observed that, "When a paradigm shifts, everyone goes back to zero." The meaning that we might find in this observation is that each time the paradigms regarding how health care services are delivered change, new challenges, new expectations and new opportunities arise. "Going back to zero" means that we all start off on equal footing. As Barker states, "The practitioners of the new paradigm have a chance not just to compete with but defeat the titans of the old paradigm." Those who are unable to make the sometimes rapid changes in thinking which are required to adapt to new paradigms risk being left behind as the competition reorganizes to respond to the new environment. Ann Grady, Past-President of AOTA stated, "If change is to be successful, we must consider preparation for the process of change to be at least as important as change itself" (Grady, 1991). As changes in skill mix occur, we must prepare for change by becoming fully informed and comfortable in managing the roles of OTR, COTA and aides in multiple practice environments. This may also mean the willingness to accept new responsibilities, treat patients with a wider range of diagnoses, work in new environments, and to prioritize activities on a daily, and sometimes an hourly basis. As Foto (1996) notes, "We must make choices, sometimes difficult ones, as well as changes—changes in our perception of ourselves as well as how we perceive our customers (patients, families, and payer), and changes in our practice." Remaining flexible yet bound by the basic philosophical and theoretical tenets which guide our profession will also assist us in maintaining a healthy perspective on managing change. Change, even when ultimately beneficial, can create stress, and in the current climate of almost feverish change, stress is inevitable. Maintaining interests outside of work provides a means for satisfying unmet needs for creativity and personal relationships. Developing stress management strategies such as exercise, relaxation and doing enjoyable leisure activities may help to offset physical and psychological tension.

All therapists should be continually appraising the match between their values and priorities and those of the institution in which they work. It is smart to be proactive and to anticipate changes in one's position before they actually occur. This allows one to either prepare for the change or explore other options. Networking with other therapists in similar positions can provide additional knowledge and strategies, as well as a support group for the particularly trying times. Occupational therapists are familiar with the process of assessing the occupational environment of clients to facilitate their adaptation. As Brayman (1996) notes, an appreciation of the relationship between the changing occupational environment in which we work as occupational therapy practitioners and work performance will be helpful in facilitating our own adaptation.

PREPARING OCCUPATIONAL THERAPY STUDENTS FOR CURRENT AND FUTURE ENVIRONMENTS

Educators and fieldwork supervisors can greatly impact the occupational therapist's ability to survive and thrive in this changing environment. This mandates that those individuals who educate and supervise others learn about the changes in the health care system and keep abreast of ongoing developments through reading, attending workshops and networking. Students will be better prepared for the new environment if survival skills are integrated into curricula content. This may require added emphasis on developing supervisory skills, consultation skills, organizational analysis, teamwork, and knowledge of critical pathways and outcomes research. These components will assist students to acquire the knowledge, skills, and attitudes which will assist them in adapting to, and influencing this environment.

CONCLUSION

Futurists predict that efforts to control costs through managed care initiatives will continue, as will the emphasis on cost-effectiveness and functional outcomes (Christiansen, 1996). Organizations will continue initiatives to meet the priorities of this new system. This compels us to be knowledgeable about and prepared for the challenges and opportunities that the managed care environment will hold for occupational therapy practitioners.

REFERENCES

Abreu, B. C., Seale, G., Podlesak, J., & Hartley L. (1996). Development of critical paths for post-acute brain injury rehabilitation: Lessons learned. *American Journal of Occupational Therapy, 50*(6), 417-427.

Accreditation Council on Occupational Therapy Education. (1995). *The American Occupational Therapy Association roster of accreditation evaluators newsletter.* Fall, 5.

American Occupational Therapy Association. (1996). Use of multiskilled personnel. *OT Week,* 18.

American Occupational Therapy Association. (1996). *Health care and market reform: Workforce implications for occupational therapy.* Bethesda, MD: The American Occupational Therapy Association.

erican Occupational Therapy Association Managed Care Project Team. (1996). *Managed care: An occupational therapy sourcebook.* Bethesda, MD: The American Occupational Therapy Association.

American Occupational Therapy Association Political Action Committee. (1993). *1993 AOTPAC National Legislative Conference Handbook.* Bethesda, MD: American Occupational Therapy Association.

Association of Academic Health Centers. (1995). Hospitals cut back staff. *Synergy, 1*(2),1.

Barker, J. A. (1992). *Paradigms: The business of discovering the future.* New York, NY: Harper Collins Publishers.

Baum, C. (1991). Professional issues in a changing environment. In C. Christiansen & C. Baum (Eds.), *Occupational therapy: Overcoming human performance deficits* (pp. 805-817). Thorofare, NJ: SLACK Incorporated.

Brayman, S. J. (1996). Managing the occupational environment of managed care. *American Journal of Occupational Therapy, 50*(6), 442-443.

Christiansen, C. (1996). Nationally speaking managed care: Opportunities and challenges for occupational therapy in the emerging systems of the 21st century. *American Journal of Occupational Therapy, 50*(6),409-412.

Conrad, D. A. & Dowling, W. L. (1990). Vertical integration in health services: Theory and managerial implications. *Health Care Management Review, 15*(4), 9-22.

Fisher, T. (1996). Roles and functions of a case manager. *American Journal of Occupational Therapy 50*(6), 452-453.

Forer, S. (1996). *Outcome Management and Program Evaluation Made Easy—A Toolkit for Occupational Therapy Practitioners.* Bethesda, MD: American Occupational Therapy Association

Foto, M. (1996). Nationally speaking-multiskilling: Who, how, when and why? *American Journal of Occupational Therapy, 50*(2), 7.

Foto, M. (1995). Nationally speaking-new president's address: the future challenges, choices and changes. *American Journal of Occupational Therapy, 49*(10), 955.

Grady, A.P. (1991). Directions for the future: Opportunities for leadership. *American Journal of Occupational Therapy, 45*(1), 9.

Hanft, B. E. & Place, P. A. (1996). *The consulting therapist.* San Antonio, TX: Therapy Skill Builders.

Jaffe, E. (1996). Occupational therapy consultation in a managed care environment. *OT Practice,* 26-31.

Jaffe, E., & Epstein, C. (1992). *Occupational therapy consultation: Theory, principles, and practice.* St. Louis, MO: Mosby.

Kane, R. A. (1975). The interprofessional team as a small group. *Social Work in Health Care, 1*(1),19-32.

Landry, C. & Knox, J. (1996). Managed care fundamentals: implications for health care organizations and health care professionals. *American Journal of Occupational Therapy, 50*(6), 413-416.

Lumsdon, K. (1994). Want to save millions? *Hospitals & Health Networks, 11,* 24-28.

MacLaren, E. (1994). Basics of managed care. *Nurseweek, 7*(13), 10-11.

Mayhan, A. D. (1994). The importance of outcomes measurement in managed care. *The American Occupational Therapy Association Administration & Management Special Interest Section Newsletter, 10*(4), 2-4.

Rogers, J. & Holm, M. (1994). Nationally Speaking—Accepting the challenge of outcome research: Examining the effectiveness of occupational therapy practice. *American Journal of Occupational Therapy, 48*(3), 871-876.

Sabin, J. (1994). A credo for ethical managed care in mental health practice. *Hospital and Community Psychiatry, 45,* 859-860.

Schein, E. G. (1987). *Career dynamics: Matching individual and organizational needs.* Reading, MA: Addison-Wesley Publishing Company.

Sinnott, M. C. (1994). Critical pathways to success. *PT Magazine,* 55-62.

Wolf, M. (1995). Surviving in health care. *Advance for Directors of Rehabilitation, 9,* 11.

Wolford. G. R., Brown, M., & McCool, B. P. (1993). Getting to go in managed care. *Health Care Management Review, 18*(1), 7-19.

Woodruff, G. & Hanson, C. (1987). *Project KAI.* 77B Warren Street, Brighton, MA 02135.

Yerxa, E. J. (1994/1996). Dreams, dilemmas, and decisions for occupational therapy in a new millennium: An American perspective. *American Journal of Occupational Therapy, 48*(7), 586. (Reprinted in Cottrell, R. P. (Ed.). (1996). *Perspectives on purposeful activity: Foundation and future of occupational therapy* (pp. 613-616). Bethesda, MD: AOTA.)

CHAPTER SIXTY-EIGHT

Now That We Have Managed Care, Shall We Inspire It?

Suzanne M. Peloquin

This chapter was previously published in American Journal of Occupational Therapy, 30*, 455-459. Copyright ©* *1996, The American Occupational Therapy Association, Inc.*

We knew it, but Mary Foto said it: "Managed care 'is here to stay'" (as quoted by Hettinger, 1995, p. 19). It seems apt, then, that we come to terms with managed care—literally. And coming to terms is a process with which occupational therapists are familiar. Parham (1987) said that reflective practitioners name and frame their realities, using language and logic to first explain what they see (name) and then to spell out a course of action (frame). Although Parham discussed this process in the context of treatment, therapists might benefit from a reflection that names and frames managed care. This (chapter) aims to prompt such reflection while making this point we have *managed* care, but we must continue to *inspire* it—to keep caring for the health of others central to our practice.

Before turning to this discussion, I will speak of my intent. Some readers may argue that an educator who is removed from clinical realities has no grounds for commenting on managed care. The argument has logic, but it does not consider that people can support one another from different vantage points. What therapists offer patients is an empathic but divergent perspective on their realities; we sometimes name it *hope*. This reflection has a similar aim. My purpose is to salute those who grapple with managed care and to offer suggestions that make sense from where I practice.

THE LANGUAGE AND LOGIC OF MANAGED CARE

Some may argue that *managed care* is the ultimate oxymoron because it names an incongruence larger than *grateful dead*. More typically, descriptions of a different kind associate with the term *care*. Some descriptors name those who will receive care—child, elder, patient, and others name the types of care that will be given—critical, intensive, quality. The odd juxtaposition of managed care causes one to ask how manage-ment applies to care. Usually a person is said to manage a budget or a household. Does care warrant such management?

Interestingly, the first dictionary definitions for manage-ment associate with the training and handling of horses. From these earlier meanings came the more familiar one of skilled handling, direction, or control. (*Merriam Webster's Collegiate Dictionary,* 1993). Given this understanding, one can better grasp the thinking of those who named managed care. A delivery system gone wild needed taming. Those who named the problem framed a congruent action. Unbridled excesses, runaway costs, and a galloping use of procedures invited management.

Syndicated columnist Dave Barry (1994) saw humor in the health care system's extravagance before managed care. He told the story of 8-year-old Natalie who modified a children's board game by putting the gamepieces in her nose. When one gamepiece accidentally went in the wrong direction during an intake breath, Natalie's parents took her to the hospital. Although the gamepiece was already in her digestive tract, the total bill was $3,200. Barry suggested that stool searches done at home are far cheaper.

Certainly, the cost of health care delivery needs to be man-aged, and a logical approach to managing cost is to control both access and use. Management extends beyond cost, however. As a business, health care delivery warrants accountability; as a human service, it needs ethical responsibility. Productivity, measurability of outcome, reasonableness of cost, efficiency of effort, quality of service, and justification of effectiveness are con-cepts fundamental to the practice of good business *and* ethical service. It is unfair to assume that the managed care industry has pressed practitioners toward functions that *oppose* good care.

Early in our profession's history, when a reconstruction aide named Ora Ruggles (Carlova & Ruggles, 1946) took leave from practice, Eleanor Clarke Slagle asked her to return, say-ing, "Get behind the effort and push!" (p. 113) Ruggles did so, starting occupational therapy departments in many places. More currently, Foto argued this need relative to managed care (Hertinger, 1995). Good management is an effort therapists can push. If over the years, occupational therapists failed to tend to good business, thus adding to the extravagance of health care delivery, they invited the redirection inherent in managed care. Therapists will always need to be good managers who are accountable for business and responsible for service, and in this context, managed care makes sense.

MANAGED CARE: NAMING THE INCONGRUENCE

Boisaubin (1994) took a more serious look at runaway costs than Barry (1994) did, noting the larger implications of cost-containment:

The Kaiser Permanente System found that it would save $3.5 million if it stopped using an expensive non-ionic x-ray agent, even though the cheaper alternative caused more patient reactions. Most reactions have been mild and nonfatal; is it worth $3.5 million to avoid those reactions, However, in this trade-off an occasional patient will encounter discomfort, morbidity, or even mortality. Ideally, the $3.5 million would be better spent on health screening to prevent 35 breast cancer deaths, 100 cervical cancer deaths, or 105 heart attacks. The once rhetorical debate focusing on the worth of a human life becomes all too realistic in this new calculus. (p. 1)

The management of extravagance is a powerful function; it can change the ways in which helpers offer care and patients receive it.

Occupational therapists have described the effects of managed care on their therapies. Noting the restrictions on access that have followed capitation, Kornblau (1995) asked:

Is this legal? Yes. Health care is not a right. It is something agreed to in a contract between a coverage provider company and a policy purchaser... Although the behavior is legal, I cannot help asking myself whether it is ethical. Is it right to give physicians monetary incentives to sacrifice care which would improve the quality of one's life? (p. 4).

Occupational therapists have described far-reaching outcomes of managed care, including shorter lengths of stay, cross-training, augmentation of revenues by raising patient volume, interdisciplinary treatment, fewer and shorter outpatient and home health services, and "one-stop shopping" where patients can access many services in one place (Joe & Hettinger, 1995). Some therapists note that the managed care system has compromised care by turning it into a bureaucracy that forces poor treatment, misunderstanding of patient needs, disregard for therapists' opinions, delays in authorization, increased paperwork, and compromised reimbursement (Hettinger, 1995). Years before the introduction of the term managed care, many therapists cautioned against a growing press for productivity, efficiency, and profit that threatened humane practices (Baum, 1980; Boyle, 1990; Burke & Cassidy, 1991/1996; Dickerson, 1990; Grady, 1992; Howard, 1991/1996;

Kari & Michels, 1991/1996; Peloquin, 1993/1996; Yerxa, 1980). The far-reaching controls of managed care, aimed first at excess, have limited care. How should therapists frame a response?

We might recall the appeals for reform of the health care system that invited a greater change than management. Many persons proposed a broader action with several aims, including universal access to adequate health care (Council on Ethical and Judicial Affairs, American Medical Association, 1995), comprehensive and affordable (quality) care by competent providers (Boisaubin, 1994), and a hope to focus on prevention and to personalize delivery (Boisaubin, 1994; Peloquin, 1993). This call to action transcends any response named management. Ron Anderson, a physician and administrator, said it well in his interview with PBS personality Bill Moyers (1993):

You try to bring healing to a person and help them [sic] heal themselves. Many times, if they have information and if they're empowered through a caring milieu, they will be better able to function. The doctors and nurses won't be going home with them, so it is very important that we get them to the highest plane of function that we can. We have a saying in our geriatric ward that we've never met a patient we couldn't care for. We've met many we couldn't cure (p.26)

Management—skillful handling, direction, and control, is a function of good care but only a part of good care. Even in the realm of horse training where the term management originated, trainers have suggested other actions:

We shall have to give up our inclination to control our horse by force. Instead we shall have to try to learn to respect the way he wants to do things....And, instead of trying to impose on our particular animal our idea of what he should be able to achieve, we must first seek to learn what his capabilities really are...we shall have to add to our analytical capability an equal capacity for intuitive thought... Without this, our relationship with our horse will be one of spiritual warfare instead of harmony and beauty. (Hassler, 1994, p. 163)

In health care, when management issues preempt all other concerns, the ethics of caring and the art of practice are at risk.

There is much logic to the language of managed care, but that language seems inadequate to the task of caring. As Hayakawa (1969) noted, any one instrument has its limitations. A thermometer, made to read temperature, will not read color, weight, or odor. Every language," said Hayakawa, "like the language of the thermometer, leaves work undone for other languages to do" (pp. 8). Attention to sound management principles, one valid approach to reforming health care delivery, leaves work undone; it needs to be part of a larger vision and responsivity.

NAMING AND FRAMING ANOTHER RESPONSE

In his rejections about education, Davies (1991) said much that may help this discussion. From his position on a state

governing board, Davies concluded that the regulatory function of those on state boards is mere background; their essential function is to inspire education. A question that he
thought board members must ask is this: "Are we helping to
create an environment in which teaching and learning are
honored and can flourish?" (p. 58). He said that the making of
that environment is a call to (a) engender a restlessness
throughout the system, (b) disturb complacency, and (c) insist
that rules be broken when there is good and sufficient reason.

The health care system invites a similar effort.
Occupational therapists must see their business functions as
a vial background to good practice. Because they have high
stakes in health care delivery, therapists must manage themselves well. They must get behind the management effort.
But they must also ask whether they are making an environment that nourishes care for the health of others. They might
then name and frame a more essential action: inspire care.

Why should occupational therapists inspire health care
delivery? To inspire is to exert a livening influence, to animate or hearten the spirit (*Merriam-Webster Collegiate
Dictionary*, 1993). To inspire is to make something happen—
to build something, from the inside out. Inspiration is a form
of edification. The various systems within which therapists
practice need inspiration if they will emerge reformed. And
occupational therapists are immersed in the kind of making
that inspires.

Since its origins, occupational therapy has made inspiration a basic function. The strong link between occupation
and the human spirit is well-portrayed by Petersen (1976):

> There is a shouting SPIRIT
> deep inside me:
> TAKE CLAY, it cries,
> THE PEN AND INK,
> TAKE FLOUR AND WATER,
> TAKE A SCRUB BRUSH,
> TAKE A YELLOW CRAYON,
> TAKE ANOTHER'S HAND—
> AND WITH ALL THESE SAY YOU,
> SAY LOVING.
> So much of who I am
> is subtly spoken
> in my making. (p. 61)

Meaningful occupation, the core of our therapy, animates
and extends the human spirit.

The founders of the profession often spoke of its spiritual
aims. Barton (1920) named occupational therapy a *making* –
not of a product, but of a person stronger physically, mentally, and spiritually than before. The inspiring action of occupational therapy is well described by Ruggles (Carlova & Ruggles, 1946): "it is not enough to give a patient something to
do with his hands. You must reach for the heart as well as the
hands. It's the heart that really does the healing" (p. 69).

On a systemic level, occupational therapists are also ani-
mators. Whether they practice in hospitals or schools, prisons or community programs, therapists hear comments that
note their singularity in livening the settings within which

they work. Occupational therapy clinics are alive; therapists
make life worlds that inspire and empower.

Inspiration is a function of occupational therapy; it is
familiar and basic. It seems fitting that we stand among those
who manage responsibly while also inspiring care for the
health of others.

INSPIRING CARE: MOVING PAST THE RHETORIC

The features of managed care — efficiency, accountability,
and cost containment —have become familiar, and we recognize in them the actions of good business. But how shall we
recognize the actions that inspire care? As long as they shape
an environment in which caring for the health of others is
central, these actions may take many forms. And whether this
shaping occurs on a large or small scale, its function might,
as Davies (1991) suggested, engender a restlessness throughout the system, disturb complacency, and cause any rules
that compromise health care to be broken with good reason.

Therapists might consider the following example a large
action aimed at the rules of managed care. *OT Week* ran part
of an article from *The Washington Post* about the bills spear-
headed by physicians and passed by five legislatures (Doctors
Take on Managed Care, 1995). These bills restricted managed
care business practices "in the name of patient protection".
(p. 12). The Arkansas law, for example, requires that every
health maintenance organization allow patients to see any
physician who will accept the HMO rate, thereby increasing
access. Occupational therapists can launch like efforts. At
the very least, they can lend support to those who inspire the
system politically.

Therapists might consider the following to be an action
that challenges the rules but on a smaller scale. Many persons
spend time writing letters to justify treatment or advocate
therapy, the letters propose a broader view of health.
Whenever caring for a person's health becomes more central
to payers as a result of these letters, the therapists who wrote
them can claim to have inspired health care.

As I considered the smaller actions that inspire, I saw a
woman walking briskly down my street. Although walkers are
common in my neighborhood, she caught my attention
because she carried a brown bag and moves from one side of
the road to the other, grabbing up curbside litter. I was
inspired. Nested within her personal routine (exercise) was an
action that launched a larger effort (neighborhood cleanup).

Persons can inspire most of the systems within which they
function. In 2 to 3 minutes, sales cashiers can liven someone's day. If a form of inspiration can occur within such short
time frames, there is cause to believe that therapists can, over
longer periods, make caring for health a more central concern among patients, coworkers, administrators, and
third-party payers.

One of our founders named the inspiration that can edify
our practice as he spoke to a group of graduating students:

May you realize in increasing measure the value of certain spiritual things which are the real making of life, but which we call by many common names. Kindness, humanity, decency, honor, good faith—to give these up under any circumstances whatever would be a loss greater than any defeat, or even death itself. (Kidner, 1929, p. 385)

The call to manage and inspire care is a plea to bring to life forms of health care delivery that manage the system and animate the act of caring about health.

ACTIONS THAT INSPIRE: A SAMPLING

The following are general suggestions for inspiring the health care delivery system. Each has a background managerial function within which nests a more essential and inspiring function (Abreu, personal communication, October 15, 1995). These suggestions make sense within the context of this reflection, and they seem sound to clinicians with whom I have shared them. Admittedly, they lack the particularity of application that persons who enact them might provide. I offer them to those who seek possibilities.

1. Infuse competent treatment with kindness, decency, honor, and good faith.

   Managerial function. This action makes a good "package deal" for patients, payers, and referral sources.

   Inspirational function. We do the right thing for our clients.

2. Introduce, research, and publicize clinical improvements, flexible approaches, and creative managing techniques.

   Managerial function. This action establishes our efficacy as therapists, our artistry as practitioners, and our skill as managers.

   Inspirational function. We promote practice by showing what we do and telling how it works.

3. Include in clinical pathways and practice guidelines the protocols and critical outcomes that address physical and mental health in the broad sense.

   Managerial function. This measure is cost-effective in the long run.

   Inspirational function. We retain our holistic heritage.

4. Speak with logic and passion for patients whose health depends on longer stays and more therapy.

   Managerial function. This action reclaims consumers at risk and offers good service.

   Inspirational function. We temper limited access with advocacy.

5. Educate clients with a knowledge that leads them to prevent dysfunction and manage themselves.

   Managerial function. This action taps a new market and supports a goal of managed care.

   Inspirational function. We enact our ethos of helping others to help themselves.

6. Declare boldly and widely (at local, sate, and national levels) the links between human occupation and health.

   Managerial function. This action touts our unique position in health care systems.

   Inspirational function. We promote the profession's core function, values, and standards.

7. Open channels that foster dialogue with managed care personnel.

   Managerial *function.* This action affirms our worth as players in the system.

   Inspirational function. We declare aims for reform broader than cost containment.

8. Assume leadership roles (e.g., members of quality improvement councils, case managers, case reviewers) in the systems within which we practice.

   Managerial function. This action shows systems personnel that we are savvy leaders.

   Inspirational function. We take positions from which to argue a vision of health that includes occupation.

9. Monitor and support larger political actions (e.g., legislation, coalitions).

   Managerial function. This action helps us shape policy.

   Inspirational function. We press for health care delivery that is managed, caring, and ethical.

10. Apply sound problem-solving approaches to paperwork and business tasks.

    Managerial function. This action jostles the sluggishness of reimbursement.

    Inspirational function. We make more time for caring.

11. Cultivate among practitioners a respect for business principles.

    Managerial function. This action supports quality-process models (i.e., total quality management, continuous quality improvement).

    Inspirational function. We include in process monitoring the actions that meet high standards.

12. Collaborate with those whose vision (i.e., caring for the health of others) supports our own.

    Managerial function. This action gains us strength in numbers and conveys our faith in teams.

    Inspirational function. We cause deeper and better reform.

When Hall (1922) spoke about the task faced by the Society for the Promotion of Occupational Therapy, he could have been noting the challenge we face today: "It seems reasonable to assert that here is a work of national importance, a human reclamation service touching vitally on matters of vast social and economic consequence". (p. 164). We have begun to manage health care delivery, and there is logic in our getting behind that effort. But we can reclaim more.

Health care reform is a building from the inside that calls for a greater responsivity than any form of management that shapes from the outside in. Health care reform, in its truest sense, is an edification through actions large and small—it is the making of an environment in which caring for the health of others is central. When it comes to health care delivery, the issue goes past the logic that we must manage care to this question: Shall we inspire it?

REFERENCES

Barry, D. (1994). *The world according to David Barry.* New York, NY: Wing.

Barton, G. E. (1920). What occupational therapy may means to nursing. *Trained Nurse and Hospital Review, 64,* 304-310.

Baum, C M. (1980). Eleanor Clarke Slagle lecture—Occupational therapies put care in the health system. *Anglican Journal of Occupational Therapy, 34,* 505-516.

Boisaubin, E. V. (1994, May). Ethical and legal dilemmas in managed care. *Medical Humanities Rounds, 11,* 1-2.

Boyle, M. (1990). The Issue Is — The changing face of the rehabilitation population: A challenge for therapists. *American Journal of Occupational Therapy, 44,* 941-945.

Burke, J. P., & Cassidy, J. C. (1991/1996). The Issue Is —Disparity between reimbursement driven practice and humanistic values of occupational therapy. *American Journal of Occupational Therapy, 45,* 173-176. (Reprinted in Cottrell, R. P. (Ed.). (1996). *Perspectives on purposeful activity: Foundatin and future of occupational therapy* (pp. 595-598). Bethesda, MD: AOTA.)

Carlova, J., & Ruggles, O. (1946). *The healing heart.* New York, NY: Julian Messner.

Council on Ethical and Judicial Affairs, American Medical Association. (1995). Ethical issues in managed care. *Journal of the American Medical Association, 273,* 331-335.

Davies, G. K (1991). Teaching and learning: What are the questions? *Teaching Education, 4*(1), 57-61.

Dickerson, A. (1990). Evaluating productivity and profitability in occupational therapy contractual work. *American Journal of Occupational Therapy, 44,* 133-137.

Doctors take on managed care. (1995, September 14). *OT Week, 9*(37), 12.

Grady, A. P. (1992). Nationally Speaking—Occupation as vision. *American Journal of Occupational Therapy, 46,* 1062-1065.

Hall, H. J. (1922). Editorial—American Occupational Therapy Association. *Archives of Occupational Therapy, 1,* 163-165.

Hassler, J. K (1994). *Beyond the mirror—The study of mental and spiritual aspects of horsemanship.* Quarryville, PA: Goals Unlimited.

Hayakawa, S. I. (1969). Introduction. In G. Kepes (Ed.), *Language of vision* (pp. 1-11). Chicago, IL: Paul Theobald.

Hertinger, J. (1995, September 7). Hand therapy in the grip of managed care. *OT Week, 9*(36), 18-20.

Howard, B. S. (1991/1996). How high do we jump? The effect of reimbursement on occupational therapy. *American Journal of Occupational Therapy, 45,* 875-881. (Reprinted in Cottrell, R. P. (Ed.). (1996). *Perspectives on purposeful activity: Foundation and future of occupational therapy* (pp. 587-594). Bethesda, MD: AOTA.)

Joe, B., & Hettinger, J. (1995, July 27). Hand therapy in the grip of managed care. *OT Weekly 9*(30), 18-20.

Kari, N., & Michels, P. (1991). The Lazarus Project: The politics of empowerment. *American Journal of Occupational Therapy, 44,* 719-725. (Reprinted in Cottrell, R. P. (Ed.). (1996). *Perspectives on puposeful activity: Foundation and future of occupational therapy* (pp. 209-216). Bethesda, MD: AOTA.)

Kidner, T. B. (1929). Address to graduates. *Occupational Therapy and Rehabilitation, 8,* 379-385.

Kornblau, B. (1995, July). Capitation could kill commitment. *Advance for Occupational Therapists, 4.*

Merriam-Webster's collegiate dictionary (10th ed.). (1993). Springfield, MA: Merriam-Webster.

Moyers, B. (1993). *Healing the mind.* New York, NY: Doubleday.

Parham, D. (1987). Nationally Speaking—Toward professionalism: The reflective therapist. *American Journal of Occupational Therapy, 41,* 555-561.

Peloquin, S. M. (1993). The patient-therapist relationship: Beliefs that shape care. *American Journal of Occupational therapy. 47,* 935-942. (Reprinted in Cottrell, R. P. (Ed.). *Perspectives on purposeful activity: Foundation and future of occupational therapy* (pp. 373-381). Bethesda, MD: AOTA.)

Petersen, J. (1976). *The book of yes.* Niles, IL: Argus.

Yerxa, E. J. (1980). Occupational therapy's role in creating a future climate of learning. *American Journal of Occupational Therapy, 34,* 529-534.

CHAPTER SIXTY-NINE

Occupation as Means to Mental Health: A Review of the Literature, and a Call for Research

Karen L. Reberio

This chapter was previously published in the Canadian Journal of Occupational Therapy, 65, *12-19, and is reprinted here with permission of CAOT Publications ACE © 1995.*

ABSTRACT

Occupational therapy is a profession which is based upon many beliefs about occupation. One belief is that engagement in occupation can promote physical and mental health. This belief appears to support the profession's jurisdictional claim to the use and application of occupation in psychosocial practice. A review of the psychosocial occupational therapy literature yielded few empirical studies which addressed the use of occupation-as-means to mental health. A discrepancy exists between what the profession theoretically advances about occupation and the research conducted in this area. This discrepancy is highlighted as a possible explanation for the lack of recognition of the value of occupational therapy in mental health and is forwarded as a potential risk to the profession's jurisdictional claim to the use and application of occupation. A call to research is advanced to develop a knowledge base on occupation, to empirically support the use of occupation as therapy and to secure a unique role for occupational therapy in psychosocial practice.

The profession of occupational therapy has historically claimed the use and application of occupation-as-means as the core of professional practice. The profession contends that it is the use of occupation which distinguishes occupational therapy from other health care professions (Rogers, 1984; Yerxa, 1991a). In addition, it is the use and application of occupation which forms the basis of the profession's jurisdictional claim (Abbott, 1988) in health care. The construct of occupation has been ascribed several purposes over the years, including the promotion of human health and well-being. A review of the occupational therapy literature was conducted with two purposes in mind: first, to examine the theoretical literature and the assumptions which have supported the use of occupation as therapy, and second, to examine the empiri-cal research literature for evidence in support of the use of occupation as therapy and the beliefs that the profession holds about occupation. The theoretical literature suggests that occupational therapy, values and is committed to, the use of occupation as the basis of therapy. However, the literature revealed few research studies which support this commitment. In the psychosocial area of practice, few studies were located which directly investigated occupation-as-means to mental health.

This purpose of this paper is twofold. The first purpose is to forward the position that the profession of occupational therapy appears to be firmly committed to claiming the jurisdiction (Abbott, 1988) over the use and application of occupation as therapeutic means and that this claim is largely grounded in professional beliefs and assumptions. The second purpose is to argue that despite the importance of occupation to the profession of occupational therapy, therapists have not actively pursued exploration of the construct in psychosocial research. A discrepancy exists between what we say, what we scientifically know, and what we pursue in research. This discrepancy may contribute to a lack of recognition of the value of occupational therapy in psychosocial practice, to a reluctance by therapists to practice in this area, and ultimately, may jeopardize any jurisdictional claim of occupational therapy in mental health. A call for research is advocated.

LITERATURE REVIEW

The profession of occupational therapy has its historical roots in psychosocial practice (Barris, Kielhofner, & Hawkins Watts, 1983). In Meyer's (1922/1977/1996) philosophical essay, he described the value of occupation as therapy for the mentally ill. Meyer discovered that engaging his patients in a variety of occupations provided a positive focus for their faulty thinking, developed habits and rhythms of a normal lifestyle and provided a means of developing skills which would be useful to earn a livelihood. In addition, Meyer (1922/1977/1996) believed that engaging in occupation could promote the mental health of his patients.

Barris et al., (1983, p. 289) stated that "the oldest and most central role of occupational therapists is that of directly engaging people in occupations as treatment." In early professional conceptualizations, occupation was described as both therapeutic means and a therapeutic end. The literature suggested that the use of occupation provided a means to divert psychic and physical energies away from worrisome thoughts and anxieties, and to channel them into a more purposeful and positive focus. Therapists, educators and physicians (Dunton, 1918; Howland, 1944; LeVesconte, 1935; Meyer, 1922/1977/1996; Menzel, 1947) believed that diversion of focus was the key to the rehabilitation of any neuropsychiatric patient and that this diversion allowed the patient to begin to focus on their potential. Engagement in occupations served as a means to correct the faulty thinking habits created by an industrialized society and to reestablish rhythms of sleeping, waking, eating and resting (Meyer 1922/1977/1996). Menzel (1947) suggested that man [sic] was at his best when directly engaged in occupations. Occupation was largely described as a process of therapeutic engagement over and beyond any therapeutic end.

The literature also describes the importance of occupation as end. Occupation as a goal of therapy, the attainment of employment and reestablishment of the patient within mainstream society were valued by early writers (LeVesconte, 1935; Meyer, 1922/1977/1996). Dunton (1918), LeVesconte (1935) and Meyer (1922/1977/1996) all speculated as to how occupation as therapy could contribute to a satisfying and productive therapeutic end within the community. The reestablishment of the patient in paid employment and in being a productive member of society was deemed to be evidence of successful treatment Ambrosi and Barker-Schwartz (1995) suggested that the rehabilitation of individuals into productive employment was highly valued by society and was a therapeutic end upon which occupational therapy did not capitalize.

In early descriptions of the use of occupation as therapy, authors recognized the larger systems which appeared to impact health and well-being. The literature described the influences of sleep and wake cycles, nutrition, psychological and physical states and of social and economic situations as contributing to human health. In the early literature, authors did not specify any one particular aspect of human function or the reduction of impairment as rationale for the application of therapeutic occupation. Instead, they considered the whole person and described the potential of the occupation as means/end to address human physical/biological states, psychological distress and social/productivity needs. LeVesconte (1935), for example, described a vision of the creation of occupational opportunities within mainstream society as a means to the fulfillment of individual goals, creativity and talents of all persons. LeVesconte (1935) believed in the value of occupa-

tion for all individuals, not just for the disabled and its capacity to influence total human health needs. In her opinion, industrialized society and its focus upon production had limited the capacity of vocational occupations to be wholesome and satisfying, and that piecework greatly curtailed individual creativity and potential. Similarly, Meyer (1922/1977/1996) lamented what he perceived to be a valuing by society of the end products of work, with the emphasis on work as a means to monetary ends, rather than the actual process and benefits of engaging in occupation. Therapists of this time clearly advanced that the attainment of an occupation in society and the development of skills and habits towards this goal was a favorable outcome of occupation therapy.

Over the next two decades, this holistic conceptualization of occupation temporarily faded. In lieu, a focus on the use of occupation in the development of physical skills and abilities (Mosey, 1971) or as a means to express the unconscious psyche prevailed (Soloman, 1947). Therapists came to question their primary belief that it was good for humans to engage in occupations as a basis for therapy and began to borrow philosophies and methods of other disciplines (Levine & Brayley, 1991). Therapists began to use activities as a means to restore lost function and to reduce impairment created by the effects of war. In addition, therapists began to use occupation as an adjunct to therapy, whereby the occupation served as means to uncover unconscious conflict and sublimations which Freudian theory contended were the basis of mental illness (Soloman, 1947; Burton, 1954). Kielhofner and Burke (1977) and Rerek (1971) provided excellent discussions of the factors which contributed to this philosophical shift during the depression years.

Occupation, in its earliest conceptualizations, was believed to be an ideal means of exercising both the mind and body towards health. In the thirties, forties and fifties, there was a dichotomous emphasis upon either the mind or the body with the goal of reducing impairments. Intervention was directed to either the mind or the body. Human health became categorically isolated to mental health or physical health. This division was a departure from earlier beliefs and observations of the uniting links between mental and physical health. The benefits of process or actual engagement in occupation-as-means to treating the whole person was relinquished to a focus on measurable outcomes and the goal of functional ability (Casio, 1971; Johnson, 1971; Mosey, 1971).

The literature describes a variety of means to promote functional ability, the least of which was by engagement in therapeutic occupation. Instead, activities and adjunctive therapeutic techniques (splinting, sensory integration, projective tests, etc.) became the topic of professional discussion for several decades and the means by which functional ability was to be achieved. Pragmatically, any therapeutic technique which could result in better function could theoretically fall under the auspices of occupational therapy during this time. Subsequently, the focus and identifying links to occupation therapy became "submerged" (Thorner, 1991) and "confusing" (Christiansen, 1991). The ideas once germane to practice became lost to the greater cause of efficacy

(Primeau, Clark, & Pierce, 1990) and to the development of technology (Kielhofner & Burke, 1977).

In 1962, Reilly called attention to the untapped and unproven promise of occupation as therapy. Reilly challenged therapists to be cautious in using adapted, simulated activities and adjunctive techniques given the evolutionary and historical evidence in support of occupation. According to Reilly (1962/1996), occupation is an innate human need which addresses both physical and mental health. Reilly (1962, p. 1/1996, p. 66) spoke directly of this integrating effect when she stated that "man [sic] through the use of his hands as they are energized by his mind and will, can influence the state of his own health".

A reconceptualization of holism and of the capacity of occupation to meet innate human needs has been a topic of ongoing philosophical discussion (Rogers, 1984; Wilcock, 1993; Yerxa, 1995). Christiansen (1994, p .5) stated that until recently, the profession has paid "only modest attention ...to defining occupation or describing it in a manner that would capture its structural complexity and reduce the ambiguity associated with the term". Kielhofner and Burke (1977) postulated that a professional focus on reductionism left few professional resources for the development of and research on occupation. Similarly, Primeau et al. (1990) suggested that therapists focused largely on efficacy to the demise of research which validated a place for occupation as therapy and a knowledge base to support its use. Why is it then, that a construct so integral to the practice of occupational therapy and to its jurisdictional claim remains largely "esoteric" (Rogers, 1984), "ambiguous" (Christiansen, 1994) and rarely researched" (Trombly, 1995/1996).

Barris et al. (1983, p. 311) suggested that past criticisms that occupational therapy is primarily diversional (particularly in psychosocial practice), "has led therapists away from our original mission and to adopt tools and methods more like others" (e.g., verbal groups with no occupational basis or goal. Fidler (1992, p. 567) suggested that "it is truly ironic that we continue to devalue the essence of occupational therapy, that we struggle to look more like others and less like ourselves...while all the while these others are discovering the efficacy of authentic occupational therapy and striving to own it. These observations are reflective of a growing discontent within the profession about the continued use of occupation as an adjunct to therapy, other than the central focus of therapy. By reducing people to their physical or mental parts, the profession indirectly proposed the person as part of the whole and occupation as an either-or phenomenon. In addition, the earlier conceptualizations about occupation and health became secondary to substantiating a role for occupational therapy within health care.

The literature suggests that therapists focused more on defining, debating and defending the practice of occupational therapy at the cost of generating empirical knowledge on occupation as a therapeutic means. This focus ultimately contributed to occupational therapy looking more like the other disciplines and less like occupational therapy (Fidler, 1992).

The literature is highly suggestive that the construct of occupation is important to the profession of occupational

therapy. However, Barris et al (1983, p. 319) suggested that "occupational therapy has failed to fulfill the broad mandate earlier conceptualized" and has not fulfilled "the promise of being one of the great ideas of 20th century medicine". They suggested that occupational therapy has "been slow to operationalize [the] hypothesis that occupation can influence health"(p. 311). Subsequently, professional practice has continued to be based on professional belief and assumptions rather than empirical evidence.

OCCUPATIONAL THERAPY BELIEFS ABOUT OCCUPATION

Occupational therapists uphold many beliefs about the potential of human occupation. One belief is that occupation is a basic human need which is directly related to the meaning and quality of one's life. Wilcock (1993) suggested that the evolution of occupation is linked not only to sustenance of basic survival needs, but also that occupation is the primary means by which physical and mental abilities are exercised and kept sharp. According to Wilcock (1993), occupation is not only the medium through which humankind develops, but it is also the opportunities and options that humans pursue to realize meaning, purpose and self-actualization throughout the lifespan.

OCCUPATION IS A BASIC HUMAN NEED

Occupational therapists believe that occupation is a basic human need (Reilly, 1962/1996; Trombly 1995/1996). Occupation has been postulated to be the means by which individuals not only procure the basic essentials of life (eg., food, safety and shelter), but is also an essential element to existence (Wilcock, 1993). Occupation is believed to be innately-driven. Individuals act upon their environment both as a means of adaptation, and as a means of making an impact upon one's world (Breines, 1989/1996). Wilcock (1993) stated that engagement in occupation allows humans to act upon and master the environment in ways which allow for both the individual and the species to prosper.

Wood's review (1993) of the primatology literature suggests that the presence of occupational opportunities is related to adaptive and life supporting behaviors on the part of the primates. Wood (1993) noted that an absence of occupational opportunities appeared to be "related to an increase in maladaptive behaviors, including self-abusive acts and not caring for their [the primates] young" (p. 518). These findings parallel Meyers (1922/1977/1996) observations of individuals with mental illness who were engaged in occupations. Meyer noted that humans appeared to be driven to doing something, and that this drive was expressed in a variety of idiosyncratic ways, for example, picking at the wool of a loom or picking up debris from the floor. Meyer noted that humans need to do something and what they do is directly tied to the meaning of their day.

OCCUPATION GIVES MEANING TO LIFE

A second belief held about occupation concerns its relationship to the meaning and purpose of one's life (Breines, 1989/1996; Fidler and Fidler, 1978/1996; Meyer, 1922/1977/1996; Polatajko, 1992; Reilly, 1962/1996; Wilcock, 1993; Yerxa et al., 1990). Meyer (1922/1977/1996) wrote that "it is the use that we make of ourselves that gives the ultimate stamp to our every organ" (p. 640). Adler & Adler (1978) stated that "it is through such action (engagement in occupation) with feedback from both humans and non-human objects that an individual comes to know the potential and limitations of self and the environment and achieves a sense of competence and intrinsic worth... it is through doing that one becomes"(p. 306). Breines (1989/1996) suggested that humans are driven to make a difference in their lives and the lives of others and that occupation provides the means for accomplishing this difference. The belief that occupation gives meaning to life speaks to the essence of everyday doing. What people do gives one a sense of purpose each day, contributes to the meaning which individuals ascribe to their lives and contributes an organization of behavior and a measure of time.

OCCUPATION ORGANIZES BEHAVIOR

A third belief about occupation is that it organizes behavior (Kielhofner & Burke, 1977; Meyer, 1922/1977/1996; Polatajko, 1992; Primeau et al, 1990; Slagle, 1928). Meyer (1922/1977/1996) observed that patients who were engaged in occupation tended to exhibit a general rhythm to their daily routine, a balance to work, rest, play and sleep activities and display more organized thoughts and actions. Slagle (1928) based her habit training program upon a belief that a balance in time and activity would contribute to a healthy lifestyle and better reintegration within the community. In discussing the occupational therapy view on mental illness, Barris et al. (1983) noted that "the majority of the clients seen by occupational therapy... suffer from an inability to occupy themselves in a productive and self-fulfilling manner... they lack the skills for action, the habits for an organized life style and the roles that give them identity and make them acceptable to society"(p. 279).

OCCUPATION HAS SOCIOCULTURAL AND CONTEXTUAL DIMENSIONS

The literature also recognizes that what one does has both personal and societal value. Grady (1995) challenged thera-

pists to not only be aware of the unique culture and community of each client, but also "to work actively to create occupational opportunities for individuals with disability to enable them to develop their capabilities in community settings of the client's choice"(p. 300). The American Occupational Therapy Association's position paper on occupation (1995) stated that "social or group conformity may be a compelling drive towards occupation and that the social meaning ascribed to any given occupation will be established by the societal culture in which the individual resides" (p. 1015). Occupational therapists, (Ambrosi & Baker-Schwartz, 1995; Meyer, 1922/1977; Reilly, 1962/1996; Suto & Frank, 1994) and others (Anthony & Liberman, 1986; Leete, 1989; Scheid & Anderson, 1995) have advanced that society values occupation and that the enablement of occupation-as-end will contribute to greater societal acceptance for those with a mental illness.

However, it has also been recognized that this very social context may create handicap "when disabilities put an individual at a social disadvantage relative to others in society" (Anthony & Liberman, 1986, p. 548). Leete (1989) clearly illustrated the experience of social disadvantage through the eyes of a consumer: "We are subjected ..to the misunderstanding, distrust, and ongoing stigma we experience from the community... where one is discounted" (p. 199) and "...progress is measured by professionals with concepts like 'consent' and 'cooperate' and 'comply instead of 'choose'"(p. 200). Similarly, a study by Scheid and Anderson (1995), on the perceptions of the work experience by consumers with severe and persistent mental illness, identified that rehabilitation efforts must not define a positive outcome only in terms of vocational readiness or the attainment of a job, e.g., occupation-as-end. They suggested that the effects of psychotropic medications, the perceived threat to one's disability pension and stigma all contribute to the perception of work as stressful (p. 163). Similarly, Goffman (1963) and Estroff (1989) have alerted mental health professionals to the impact of social stigma upon successful community integration. Suto and Frank (1994) suggested that therapists need to be alert not only to the constraints within the individual, but also "to the sociocultural reality that influences occupation, and phenomenon in the external environment that may handicap one's efforts"(p. 16).

SUMMARY OF THE THEORETICAL LITERATURE

The theoretical literature suggests that the profession is committed to occupation as the common core of practice. However, Rogers (1984) reminds us that our ideas will remain esoteric if they cannot be substantiated in science. How well has occupational therapy grounded its beliefs about occupation in science? In particular, have therapists conducted scientific studies which support occupation as a determinant of mental health? Yerxa (1991a, 1991b, 1995) has frequently alerted therapists to the fact that our jurisdictional claim (Abbott, 1988) as a profession will be won or lost on the basis of scientific inquiry which substantiates our beliefs. Yerxa, et al (1990) stated "that one of the greatest challenges society faces today is understanding the relationship between engagement in occupation and health" (p. 13). Has occupational therapy met this challenge? Has occupational therapy generated a knowledge base in support of our beliefs about occupation and which substantiates our jurisdictional claim in health care? A review of psychosocial research casts considerable doubt upon both our knowledge of how occupation promotes mental health and upon our jurisdictional claim.

PSYCHOSOCIAL OCCUPATIONAL THERAPY RESEARCH

A review of the psychosocial occupational therapy literature yielded a variety of studies which considered activity therapy and its effectiveness in practice. For example, Kremer, Nelson and Duncombe (1984) conducted a randomized post-test experimental design to see how individuals with a psychiatric illness would rate three traditional occupational therapy groups—(cooking, crafts and sensory awareness)—after completion of the activity. Using the Osgoode Semantic Differential Scale, clients rated cooking highest in terms of power and action followed by sensory awareness and then craft activities. In 1985, DeCarlo and Mann conducted a pre and post-test experiment to ascertain if there would be differences between an activity-based, a verbal-based, and a control group on clients' perceived interpersonal communication skills. The authors concluded that a significant increase in communication skills for those involved in the activity-based group occurred compared to the verbal group and that there was a non-significant increase for the activity based group over the control group.

Klyczek and Mann (1986/1996) conduced a descriptive study to see if individuals who participated in twice as much activity than verbal therapy would demonstrate differences in symptomology, community tenure or relapse rate compared with individuals who participated in twice as much verbal therapy. The authors found inconsistent findings. Clients who participated in mostly activity-based therapy showed a 4x decrease in symptoms, equal community tenure and 3.5x increase in relapse rate. Unfortunately, the sample size for the activity group was more than twice the size of the verbal group, and both groups received activity and verbal therapy further confounding the results.

In 1988, Cole and Green used a descriptive study to determine the response of two groups of clients (individuals with psychotic versus borderline disorders) to activity versus psychotherapy groups. The authors concluded that both subject groups responded more favorably to the occupational therapy groups. However, they failed to describe the intervention (other than it being activity-based), and did not clarify whether responding more favorably resulted in enhanced mental health.

In 1992, Webster and Schwartzberg concluded a post group ranking of curative factors of occupational therapy groups using the Yalom's Q-Sort questionnaire. They found that occupational therapy groups were ranked similar to psychotherapy groups and were believed to be strong in cohesiveness, interpersonal, altruistic, hope, and cathartic factors. The authors suggested that further study was indicated to understand why occupation-based groups were rated this way.

In a qualitative study examining the future time perspective of 50 individuals in a room and care lodging, Suto and Frank (1994) identified that limited future time perspective appeared to be related to less activity by the participants. This study emphasized the impact of occupational deprivation for individuals with a severe and persistent mental illness and the impact of limited occupational opportunity on future goal planning.

A qualitative study by Strong (1995), which explored the experiences of individuals with persistent mental illness working in an affirmative business, found that work was perceived as a powerful influence on participants' self-concept and self-efficacy. Based on in-depth interviews with 15 participants and 15 months of participant action research, Strong affirmed the central occupational therapy belief "that people need to engage in meaningful activity and by 'doing' we influence our health and sense of self"(p. 198).

Similarly, a recent qualitative study (Rebeiro, 1997), which explored the experience of occupational engagement for eight participants involved in an occupation-based mental health group, identified that occupation served as means to enhanced perceived self-confidence and self-competence. In this study, in-depth interviews and participant observation were utilized to explore the experience of engaging in occupations. Participants suggested that occupations served as a means to define and redefine self, and enhanced subjective well-being. Further, the participants stated that ongoing engagement in occupations served as means to sustain their redefined sense of self and subjective well-being over time. In this study, a supportive, safe environment was essential to both initial and continued occupational engagement. Rebeiro (1997) suggested that therapists need to consider both the environment and the provision of occupational opportunities in order to fully understand any mental health impact on the person.

SUMMARY OF THE RESEARCH LITERATURE

The empirical research literature offered few studies which directly examined the use of occupation-as-means to mental health. Most studies explored consumer perceptions of activity-based groups, the use of independent variables other than occupation (e.g., stress management, (Stein & Smith, 1989), and the use of dependent variables other than mental health (e.g., interpersonal communication skills, recidivism). Ironically, those variables which best explicate a unique role for occupational therapy in mental health were least utilized in the various research studies reviewed.

DISCUSSION

The preceding review of the literature is important to the profession of occupational therapy for two reasons. The first concerns an internal matter for the profession. The examination of our practice is essential to gain a bearing of where we are, who we are and what we claim to be. As a profession, we uphold firm convictions about the value of occupation in promoting mental health. Yet, few of the research studies notated within the literature identified occupation as the means or as the end of the intervention. Most of the studies reviewed attempted to isolate and measure variables that had little to do with occupation and which subsequently inform the reader of new knowledge or substantiate our beliefs and jurisdictional claim. If we are to lay claim to the use and provision of occupation for therapeutic purposes as a profession, greater attention is required in the area of research to empirically support our beliefs and our assumptions. It is reasonably correct to assume that a reconciliation between what we say and what we do in psychosocial practice is not only indicated, but perhaps, essential to lifting our 'identity confusion' and creating the cohesive, professional focus that Kielhofner and Burke (1977) suggest is requisite for a successful paradigm shift towards occupation.

The second reason concerns matters external to the profession which are directly related to the success of our jurisdictional claim (Abbott, 1988). External matters concern the continued confusion within the public arena of the role of the profession of occupational therapy, the contributions to knowledge that the profession generates within the academic arena and the future role of occupational therapy in the workplace arena in a changing health care system. Abbott (1988, p. 71) suggested that full jurisdictional claims require that "legitimization within the culture by the authority of the profession's knowledge, be established within the law and shaped by the very public idea of the tasks that the profession does." In his book, Abbott (1988, p. 81) stated that "it is unclear whether we should identify professions by the group claims ...or by the functional realities." What might be the functional reality of the profession of occupational therapy? What is the image that we project to the public arena? What contribution has occupational therapy made to the universe of knowledge in psychosocial practice?

Part of our reality is that we appear to be firmly committed to the construct of occupation and to a belief that occupation can promote and maintain mental health. This reality is not so much grounded in fact and scientific proof, as it is within our beliefs These beliefs appear to be the threads which have united occupational therapy since its inception in the early part of this century. Our beliefs purport that occupation may be a reasonable means to promote mental health. However it must be argued that our 80 some odd years of

beliefs have merely led therapists to assume that a relationship exists between occupation and health, but without sufficient data to substantiate this claim (Fossey, 1992). If this review is at all indicative of the evidence that we present to the academic and public arenas, our jurisdictional claim may in fact be at risk. Given the fierce competition within the present health care system, one needs to ask, how can occupational therapy successfully compete? How can our jurisdictional claim be differentiated from that of others?

The answer to these questions and to the reconciliation of internal confusion lies within an enhanced knowledge of the construct of occupation. If the profession of occupational therapy stakes its jurisdictional claim to the therapeutic use of and the enablement of occupation, this focus should be reflected in our workplace arenas. There should be little doubt in either the clients' or other disciplines' minds as to the role and purpose of occupational therapy in mental health. Single case studies could be conducted within the clinic which tap and document the insider's experience and perceptions of engaging in occupations. Collectively, single case studies can contribute to a growing body of empirical data and subsequently contribute to what we know about occupation-as-means to mental health and well being. Creative and collaborative partnerships with consumers which examine the meaning of engaging in occupations and of the greater societal influences to engaging in occupations are essential to understanding the importance of human occupation to mental health and the reality of accessing occupation beyond the confines of the clinic.

Dunton (1918) stated that occupation requires expression in the "insane as well as the sane". The theoretical literature suggested that occupation is an ideal medium for funneling one's talents into a greater purpose and for realizing meaning in one's life. However, the empirical literature revealed that occupational therapy has not actively investigated this relationship in science.

If occupational therapists aspire to reflect a unique occupation approach to client care and desire to distinguish themselves from other professions, then we need to seriously reconcile what we say and publicly declare, and what we research and do in the clinic. Qualitative research, which seeks to understand better the construct of occupation and its importance to the mental health needs of the consumer, is recommended as the first step. By examining why occupation is helpful to an individual with mental illness, occupational therapists may not only substantiate their belief but also, identify how occupation-as-means can be utilized to promote mental health.

CONCLUSION

In this (chapter), the professional literature was examined in order to identify if there is a good fit between what we say about occupation, what we know and what we pursue in research. Occupational therapy's claim to the use of occupation-as-means to mental health does not appear to be well supported by research studies. This position is substantiated by an observed discrepancy between the formal declarations about occupation by the profession and the reality of the research initiatives within psychosocial practice. The research studies failed to substantiate our beliefs about occupation, and subsequently, have not contributed to a successful jurisdictional claim in the workplace, public or academic arenas. A reconciliation between the profession's beliefs and the reality of clinical practice and research endeavors may have both internal and external benefits. A broader conceptualization of occupation-as-means and as-end most clearly reflects what Meyer told us about occupation and most clearly looks like occupational therapy. Such a conceptualization will open up both qualitative and quantitative research opportunities to explore, to discover and to better understand if and how occupation-as-means contributes to mental health, and if and how the enablement of occupation-as-end maintains the health cycle and furthers the "means" by which individuals with severe and persistent mental illness can find meaning and purpose in their lives.

ACKNOWLEDGEMENT

I would like to thank Dr. J.U. Cook for her assistance with this paper and for challenging my complacency and acceptance of the 'status quo'.

REFERENCES

Abbott, A. (1988). *The system of professions.* Chicago, Ill: University of Chicago Press.

Ambrosi, E., & Barker Schwartz, K. (1995). The profession's image 1917-1925, part II: Occupational therapy as represented by the media. *American Journal of Occupational Therapy, 49,* 828-32.

American Occupational Therapy Association. (1995). Position paper on occupation. *American Journal of Occupational Therapy, 49,* 1015-1018.

Anthony, W. A., & Liberman, R. W. (1986). The practice of psychiatric rehabilitation: Historical, conceptual, and research base. *Schizophrenia Bulletin, 12,* 542-559.

Barris, R., Kielhofner, G., & Hawkins Watts, J. (1983). *Psychosocial occupational therapy: Practice in a pluralistic arena* (pp. 289-311). Laurel, MD: RAMSCO Publishing.

Breines, E. (1989). The issue is: Making a difference: A premise of occupation and health. *American Journal of Occupational Therapy, 43,* 51-52. (Reprinted in Cottrell, R. P. (Ed.). (1996). *Perspectives on purposeful activity: Foundation and future of occupational therapy* (pp. 245-247). Bethesda, MD: AOTA.)

Burton, A. (1954). The occupational therapist as therapist. *American Journal of Occupational Therapy, 8,* 78-79.

Christiansen, C. (1991). Occupational therapy intervention for life performance (pp. 1-43). In C. Christiansen & C. Baum (Eds.), *Occupational therapy: Overcoming human performance deficits.* Thorofare, NJ: SLACK Incorporated.

Christiansen, C. (1994). Classification and study in occupation. A review and discussion of taxonomies. *Journal of Occupational Science, 1*(3), 3-21

Cole, M. B., & Green, L. R. (1988). A preference for activity: A comparative study of psychotherapy groups versus occupational therapy groups for psychotic and borderline inpatients. *Occupational Therapy in Mental Health, 8*(3) 53-67.

DeCarlo, J. J., & Mann, W. C. (1985). The effectiveness of verbal versus activity groups in improving self-perceptions of interpersonal communication skills. *American Journal of Occupational Therapy, 39,* 20-27.

Diasio, K. (1971). The modern era—1960 to 1970. *American Journal of Occupational Therapy, 25,* 237-242.

Dunton, W. R. (1918). *Occupation therapy: A manual for nurses.* Philadelphia, PA: W. B. Saunders.

Estroff, S. E. (1989). Self-identity and subjective experiences of schizophrenia: In search of the subject. *Schizophrenia Bulletin, 15,* 189-196.

Fidler, G. (1992/1996). Against use of physical agent modalities. [Letter to Editor]. *American Journal of Occupational Therapy, 46,* 567.

Fidler, G., & Fidler, J. W. (1978). Doing and becoming: Purposeful action and self-actualization. *American Journal of Occupational Therapy, 32,* 305-310. (Reprinted in Cottrell, R. P. (Ed.). (1996). *Perspectives on purposeful activity: Foundation and future of occupational therapy* (pp. 75-80). Bethesda, MD: AOTA.)

Fossey, E. (1992). The study of human occupations: Implications for research in occupational therapy. *British Journal of Occupational Therapy, 55,* 148-152.

Goffman, E. (1963). *Stigma: Notes on the management of spoiled identity.* New York, NY: Simon & Schuster.

Grady, A. (1995/1996). Building inclusive community: A challenge for occupational therapy. *American Journal of Occupational Therapy, 49,* 300-310. (Reprinted in Cottrell, R. P. (Ed.). (1996). *Perspectives on purposeful activity: Foundation and future of occupational therapy* (pp. 229-240). Bethesda, MD: AOTA.)

Howland, G. W. (1944). Occupational therapy across Canada. *Canadian Geographical Journal, 28*(1), 32-40. Reprinted in 1986. *Canadian Journal of Occupational Therapy, 53,* (commemorative issue), 18-26.

Johnson, I. (1971). Consideration of work as therapy in the rehabilitation process. *American Journal of Occupational Therapy, 25,* 303-308.

Kielhofner, G., & Burke, J. P. (1977). Occupational therapy after 60 years: An account of changing identity and knowledge. *American Journal of Occupational Therapy, 32,* 675-689.

Klyczek, J. R., & Mann, W. C. (1986). Therapeutic modality comparisons in day treatment. *American Journal of Occupational Therapy, 40,* 606-611. (Reprinted in Cottrell, R. P. (Ed.). (1996). *Perspectives on purposeful activity:Foundation and future of occupational therapy* (pp. 545-550). Bethesda, MD: AOTA.)

Kremer, E. R. H., Nelson, D. L, & Duncombe, L. W. (1984). Effects of selected activities on affective meaning in psychiatric patients. *American Journal of Occupational Therapy, 38,* 522-528.

Leete, E. (1989). How I perceive and manage my illness.. *Schizophrenia Bulletin, 25,* 197-200.

LeVesconte, H. R. (1935). Expanding fields of occupational therapy. *Canadian Journal of Occupational Therapy, 3,* 4-12.

Levine, M. E. & Brayley, C. R. (1991). Occupation as a therapeutic medium. In C. Christiansen & C. Baum (Eds.), *Occupational Therapy: Overcoming human performance deficits* (pp. 596-598). Thorofare, NJ: SLACK Incorporated.

Menzel, M. (1947). Methods and techniques used in occupational therapy for the imbecile. *American Journal of Occupational Therapy, 1,* 137-145.

Meyer, A. (1922). The philosophy of occupation therapy. Archives of Occupational Therapy, 1, 1-10. Reprinted in 1977. *American Journal of Occupational Therapy, 32,* 639-642. (Reprinted in Cottrell, R. P., (Ed.). (1996). *Perspectives on purposeful activity: Foundation and future of occupational therapy* (pp. 27-30). Bethesda, MD: AOTA.)

Mosey, A. (1971). Involvement in the rehabilitation movement— 1942-1960. *American Journal of Occupational Therapy, 25,* 234-236.

Polatajko, H. (1992). Muriel Driver Lecture. Naming and framing occupational therapy: A lecture dedicated to the life of Nancy B. *Canadian Journal of Occupational Therapy, 59,* 189-200.

Primeau, L. A., Clark, F., & Pierce, D. (1990). Occupational therapy alone has looked upon occupation: Future applications of occupational science to pediatric occupational therapy. In J. A. Johnson & E. J. Yerxa (Eds.), *Occupational science: The foundation for new models of practice* (pp. 19-32). New York, NY: The Haworth Press.

Rebeiro, K. L. (1997). *Opportunity, not prescription: An exploratory study of the experience of occupational engagement.* Unpublished master's thesis. London, Ontario: The University of Western Ontario.

Reilly, M. (1962). Occupational therapy can be one of the great ideas of 20th century medicine. *American Journal of Occupational Therapy, 16,* 1-9. (Reprinted in Cottrell, R. P. (Ed.). (1996). *Perspectives on purposeful activity: Foundation and future of occupational therapy* (pp. 65-73). Bethesda, MD: AOTA.)

Rerek, M. (1971). The Depression Years—1929 to 1941. *American Journal of Occupational Therapy, 25,* 231-233.

Rogers, J.C. (1984). Why study human occupation? *American Journal of Occupational Therapy, 38,* 47-49.

Scheid, I. L., & Anderson, C. (1995). Living with chronic mental illness: Understanding the role of work. *Community Mental Health Journal, 31,* 163-176.

Slagle, E. C. (1928). Handicrafts used as treatment: The handicrafter. *Archives of Occupational Therapy, 1,* 26-27.

Soloman, A. R. (1947). Occupational therapy, a psychiatric treatment. *American Journal of Occupational Therapy, 1,* 1-9..

Stein, F., & Smith, J. (1989). Short-term stress management program with acutely depressed in-patients. *Canadian Journal of Occupational Therapy, 56,* 185-191.

Strong, S. (1995). *An ethnographic study examining the experiences of persons with persistent mental Illness working at an affirmative business.* Unpublished masters thesis. Hamilton, OH: McMaster University.

Suto, M. & Frank, G. (1994). Future time perspectives and daily occupations of persons with chronic schizophrenia in a board and care home. *American Journal of Occupational Therapy, 48,* 7-18.

Thorner, S. (1991). The essential skills of an occupational therapist *British Journal of Occupational Therapy, 54,* 222-223.

Trombly, C. (1995). Occupation: Purposefulness and meaningfulness as therapeutic mechanisms. *American Journal of Occupational Therapy, 49,* 960-972. Reprinted in Cottrell, R. P. (Ed.). (1996). *Perspectives on purposeful activity: Foundation and future of occupational therapy* (pp. 99-111). Bethesda, MD: AOTA.)

Webster, D., & Schwartzberg, S.L (1992). Perception of curative factors and occupational therapy groups. *Occupational Therapy in Mental Health, 12*(1), 3-7.

Wilcock, A. (1993). A theory of the human need for occupation. *Occupational Science: Australia, 1*(1), 17-24.

Wood, W. (1993). Occupation and the relevance of primatology to occupational therapy. *American Journal of Occupational Therapy, 47,* 515-522.

Yerxa, E. J. (1991a). Occupational Therapy: An endangered species or an academic discipline in the first century. *American Journal of Occupational Therapy, 45,* 680-685.

Yerxa, E. J. (1991b). Seeking a relevant, ethical, and realistic way of knowing for occupational therapy. *American Journal of Occupational Therapy, 45,* 199-204.

Yerxa, E. J. (1995). Who is the keeper of occupational therapies practice and knowledge? *American Journal of Occupational Therapy, 49,* 295-299.

Yerxa, E. J., Clark, F., Frank, G., Jackson, J., Parham, D., Pierce, D., Stein, C., & Zemke, R. (1990). An introduction to occupational science: A foundation for occupational therapy in the 21st century. In J. A. Johnson & E. J. Yerxa (Eds.), *Occupational science: The foundation for new models of practice* (pp. 1 17). New York, NY: Haworth Press.

APPENDIX A

Position Paper:
The Psychosocial Core of Occupational Therapy

Gail S. Fidler

This appendix was previously published in the American Journal of Occupational Therapy, 49, *1021-1022.* *Copyright © 1991, The American Occupational Therapy Association, Inc.*

Central to the study and practice of occupational therapy are those concepts and principles the attest to the inexorable union of body and mind and to the inherent significance of purposeful activity in the quest for health, self-actualization, and social efficacy (American Occupational Therapy Association, 1979; Christiansen, 1991). Occupational therapy has historically viewed human performance from a broad, holistic perspective. The doctrine of Moral Treatment in the late 17th and early 18th centuries employed many of the beliefs and concepts that became the foundation of occupational therapy. This philosophy of humane treatment was built on a set of beliefs attesting to the value of human relationships; the importance of a pleasant, humane environment; and the value of daily purposeful activity.

From its inception, occupational therapy has viewed the human being as a complex mix of internal physical, psychologic, social, and cultural variables living within an equally-dynamic environmental mixture of social, cultural, interpersonal, economic, and political variables (Kielhofner, 1985). Human performance, the ability "to do," has come to be understood from the perspective of the dynamic interrelationship of the person and the environmental context. Any intervention, any restorative or rehabilitative effort acknowledged as occupational therapy, must address and skillfully accommodate the interrelatedness of these internal and external variables for each unique individual (Fidler, 1996; Fidler & Fidler, 1983.)

The profession has continued to develop from a deeply rooted belief in the critical importance of "doing," of active engagement in purposeful activity as a catalyst in the development of self, and in fulfillment of social membership. This conviction is supported by the concept that the innate human drive to explore and master the environment is essential to human existence and adaptation, not only to ensure survival, but also to enable the process of humanization. Such a process can be understood as motivation toward achieving a sense of competence, self-reliance, social role learning, and societal contribution.

Occupational therapy seeks to engage an individual's motivation to undertake those activities that minimize disability, encourage compensating behaviors, and/or establish a new activity repertoire to fulfill basic personal needs and meet social role requirements. A fundamental principle that underlies this goal is that an individual's motivation is triggered and sustained when there is a congruence between the characteristics of an activity and the biopsychosocial characteristics of the person (Fidler, 1981, 1996).

Seen from these perspectives, the psychosocial dimensions of the discipline become clearly evident. To speak of independence, competency, self-development, motivation, social membership, and the like, is to accept and respond to the construct that says what touches the body touches the mind, and what touches the mind affects the body. The efficacy of occupational therapy intervention is measured by its considered inclusion of these principles and beliefs, regardless of the nature or acuteness of a disability (Yerxa, 1967).

These psychosocial concepts and postulates are addressed in the developing science on which occupational therapy is based. This evolving body of knowledge seeks to explain how purposeful activity relates to physical integrity, psychologic structure, social relatedness, and the cultural meanings of activities (Fidler, 1988). Such study also investigates how these interrelationships may generate and sustain the motivation and ability to cope with and manage relevant roles and activities of living in ways that are more satisfying than not to self and significant others (Fidler, 1981).

Any injury, illness, or disability elicits a variety of psychosocial responses on the part of the individual and that person's family. Such reactions may be characterized, for example, by a hindering lack of motivation, refusal to participate, an expressed sense of hopelessness, anger, over-concern or protectiveness, or denial. Although such psychologic reactions are not the primary diagnosis, they must be understood and dealt with by the occupational therapy practitioner if intervention goals are to be achieved. An appreciation for and accommodation to the impact of the family's expectations and reactions is a significant aspect that must shape any occupational therapy intervention. Understanding the complex psychosocial dimensions of human performance, knowing which activities can best be expected to elicit the desired adaptive response, and possessing the artful skill of enabling fruitful, reciprocal relationships are integral aspects of all occupational therapy practice.

The therapeutic use of self characterizes the interpersonal dynamic of a helping relationship and is therefore an essential feature of a professional skills repertoire (Mosey, 1986; Peloquin, 1989/1996). The importance of this skill extends well beyond the parameters of the therapeutic dyad. The development and display of an interpersonal competence is a significant component in team membership, collaboration, collegial engagement, family relationships, supervision, teaching, and mentoring. Interpersonal competence is a crucial variable in the occupational therapy practitioner's role of agent for growth and change in self and others.

The psychosocial dimensions of human performance are acknowledged as fundamental in all aspects of occupational therapy, whether practice occurs in settings such as the classroom, rehabilitation center, hospital, nursing home, or community. Such perspectives comprise the context within which occupational therapy practitioners view and address the dynamics of individual performance. These are the psychologic and sociologic foundations from which all occupational therapy specialization develops and matures.

There is a difference between the psychosocial foundations of occupational therapy and the specialty of mental health practice. Like other areas of specialization, mental health practice is grounded in the psychosocial core concepts of the profession, but, like other specialties in occupational therapy, it reaches beyond this core to develop a specialized knowledge and expertise that is applicable to a particular population or disability.

Thus, mental health as a specialty practice in occupational therapy is the application of both core and specialized knowledge to those individuals with a diagnosis of mental illness. This area of expertise encompasses knowledge of how psychopathologies (e.g., faulty perceptions, aversions to interpersonal encounters, cognitive dysfunctions, pathologic affective states, aberrant social behavior) affect the ability to cope with and manage daily living roles and activities. It includes the skillfull application of occupational therapy principles, procedures, and interpersonal processes to assess, remediate, and/or compensate for the disabilities of a mental illness and to enjoy a more satisfying level of performance (Mosey, 1986). These processes call upon a specialized knowledge and skill of engaging the individual with a mental illness

in selected individual and group activities that can be expected to have a remedial effect on given psychopathologies, and at the same time be congruent with those activities of daily living that are relevant to that person's lifestyle.

Occupational therapy is a profession committed to making it possible for individuals to attain a way of living that gains for them and for those with whom they share living, a mutual sense of satisfaction, achievement, and contribution. This mission requires vigorous pursuit of an educational process and research endeavors focused on the development and refinement of knowledge about the multidimensional aspects of human occupation, the crucial meanings and roles of purposeful activity, and the skillful application of such knowledge. This endeavor thus includes a continuing incentive to reach a sophisticated appreciation of the psychodynamics of human performance and an artful skill in interpersonal engagement.

It is such study and learning that shapes and enables internalization of an identity of a professional self. These goals can be realized to the extent of our abiding commitment to demonstrate in our education and daily practice a profound understanding of the unity of mind and body.

Prepared by Gail S. Fidler, OTR, FAOTA, for the Commission on Practice (Linda Kohlman Thomson, MOT, OT(C), FAOTA, Chairperson). Adopted by the Representative Assembly April 1995; edited 1997.

REFERENCES

American Occupational Therapy Association. (1979). The philosophical base of occupational therapy. *American Journal of Occupational Therapy, 33*, 785.

Christiansen, C. (1991). Occupational therapy intervention for life performance. In C. Christiansen & C. Baum (Eds.), *Occupational Therapy: Overcoming human performance deficits* (pp. 1-43). Thorofare, NJ: SLACK Incorporated.

Fidler, G. (1981). From crafts to competence. *American Journal of Occupational Therapy, 35*, 567-573.

Fidler, G. (1988). *Examining the knowledge base of occupational therapy.* Unpublished paper.

Fidler, G. S. (1996). Lifestyle performance: From profile to conceptual model. *American Journal of Occupational Therapy, 50*, 139-147.

Fidler, G., & Fidler, J. (1983). Doing and becoming: *The occupational therapy experience.* In G. Kielhofner (Ed.), *Health through occupation* (pp. 267-280). Philadelphia, PA: F. A. Davis.

Kielhofner, G. (1985). *A model of human occupation: Theory and application.* Baltimore, MD: Williams & Wilkins.

Mosey, A. (1986). *Psychological components of occupational therapy.* New York, NY: Raven.

Peloquin, S. (1989/1996). Sustaining the art of practice in occupational therapy. *American Journal of Occupational Therapy, 43*, 219-226. (Reprinted in Cottrell, R. P. (Ed.). (1996). *Perspectives on purposeful activity: Foundation and future of occupational therapy* (pp. 605-612). Bethesda, MD: AOTA.)

Yerxa, E. (1967). Authentic occupational therapy, 1966 Eleanor
   Clarke Slagle lecture. *American Journal of Occupational
   Therapy, 21,* 1-9.

50 Simple Things You Can Do To Promote Occupational Therapy In Mental Health

American Occupational Therapy Association

Regardless of your area of practice, there *are* easy things you can do that will make a difference in the degree to which people know about, understand, and ultimately advocate for occupational therapy in mental health. The following suggestions were compiled from over 200 made by 40 occupational therapists from 21 states...

We hope you will find these suggestions helpful. *As the first simple thing you can do, xerox this and pass it on to another occupational therapist in mental health!*

COMMUNICATE CLEARLY TO OTHERS ABOUT WHAT YOU DO

1. Don't wait until someone asks about occupational therapy. Delineate for yourself two clear sentences: one about what occupational therapy in mental health is and another about what you specifically do within it. When you use these sentences, make sure they are relevant to the listener; i.e., clinician, insurance company, employer, client.
2. Many facilities have a newsletter of some kind. Volunteer to write a human interest article about occupational therapy and some issue, client, event, or accomplishment. Once they see you as a resource, they will come to you in the future.
3. Suggest that your program hold an event sponsored by a non-profit organization with similar goals, such as NAMI (National Alliance for the Mentally Ill). Advertise the event in part through public service announcements (PSAs). They are very simple to write, and expose the name "Occupational Therapy" to the public. AOTA-Public Relations Department can help in learning to write these.
4. Place visual media in your workplace that defines or promotes, in consumer language, the process and outcome of occupational therapy services.
5. AOTA publishes some mental health booklets. Have these available for your clients and/or families of clients.
6. Use communication media that "de-stigmatizes" mental illness, such as sending Christmas cards from NARSAD (National Alliance for Research on Schizophrenia and Depression).
7. Make sure your name tag at work says Occupational Therapist or Psychiatric Occupational Therapist, not simply the name of your position. For example, "Arlene Jones, OTR; Program Director" is not enough. The value of spelling out the name "Occupational Therapy"and having people see it every time they look at your name tag is enormous.
8. Business cards and stationery should emphasize and communicate something about occupational therapy. Use "Occupational Therapy" or "Occupational Therapy in Mental Health" and at the bottom, add "A vital link to productive living."
9. Communicate an occupational therapy message by wearing logos on shirts, pins, pens, totes. Wear occupational therapy sweatshirts and T-shirts to games, exercise programs, and be prepared to use the two sentences about occupational therapy that you have developed (from #1).
10. Introduce yourself to family members of clients as an occupational therapist, not just by your role in the program. Explain what occupational therapists in mental health do in general and in your program.
11. Title groups with therapeutic names and process the purpose and outcomes of occupational therapy in specific groups with the clients. For example, "Occupational Therapy Problem Solving Skills Group, Occupational Therapy Communication Skills Groups".

12. Do not refer to yourself as an activities therapist. There really is no such thing from a professional standpoint. Many people call themselves this and say they do occupational therapy. If you see this happening, bring it to the attention of the program director in a positive and non-defensive way. Suggest ways to delineate roles while giving respect to other disciplines.

13. Keep outcome records for your clients. These can be the basis for developing local norms for tests you are using for assessment. AOTA/AOTF can assist with this process.

14. If you are an independent contractor, it is essential to list yourself in the yellow pages. This not only promotes occupational therapy but is one informal way which government agencies use to determine if you are an independent contractor or really an employee.

EDUCATE OTHERS

Educate others about occupational therapy in mental health and educate yourself about current trends in the field of psychiatry in general.

15. Physicians and other professionals in physical medicine often have no idea that occupational therapists work in mental health. Occupational therapists in physical disabilities may not be clear about what occupational therapists in mental health do. Twice a year take a doctor or physical disablities occupational therapist to lunch. Discuss what we do. (This may also apply to psychiatrists who do not work around occupational therapy, for example in private practice).

16. Once a year volunteer to speak at a community center, church, or local business about mental health care and how occupational therapy fits into productive living. Facilities and corporations often have departments that arrange for speakers on various topics.

17. Contact your local occupational therapy school and volunteer to speak once each semester on clinical practice in mental health, or other pertinent topic. You might also volunteer to "mentor" a student who shows special interest in mental health. Set this up with occupational therapy school faculty, and agree to try it for one semester to start. Contact AOTA Products Department for the "Find a Mentor or Be One" packet.

18. Provide regular ongoing in-service training sessions for new employees and students of other disciplines if you work in a hospital or community-based program setting.

19. Once a year, write a letter to the editor of a local, state, or national publication, (not just in the mental health or occupational therapy fields) in response to a health related article. Write to Newsweek, Time, etc. and sign your name as an Occupational Therapist in mental health. If possible, use research and statistics to back up your comments.

20. When you read an article about function that does not mention occupational therapy, write to the author and educate him/her about the vital role that occupational therapy has been playing for decades in this arena.

21. Once a year, take the time to write to someone who should know about occupational therapy or occupational therapy in mental health, but doesn't. For example, the movie "Gorillas in the Mist" misrepresented Diane Fossey as a physical therapist. Write a non-defensive but helpful letter to educate him/her about what occupational therapy is and what we do.

22. Once a year, offer to speak at local occupational therapy meetings about mental health. This suggestions came from an occupational therapists who was part of a panel that addressed similarities and differences experienced by therapists working in state, county and private psychiatric facilities.

23. Contact your local school district and volunteer to speak at a career day and/or host a student visit to your facility or community-based practice, or offer to provide a guest lecture on the role of occupational therapy in mental health to health related classes in local community colleges, adult education classes or universities.

EDUCATE YOURSELF

24. Consider attending continuing education classes sponsored by AOTA or other groups that may not specifically target mental health, but in which much of the information may be transferable. For example, reimbursement issues, long term care.

25. Once a year, tour another facility that has an occupational therapy program to get ideas and to conceptualize for yourself the "state of the art" of occupational therapy in mental health.

26. Read *AJOT* and *OT Week*, but also allow time to follow up on articles. Once a year, write a letter to the editor, or respond directly to authors about mental health content.

27. Read SIS newsletters from the SIS with whom you most identify, and others. Ideally, a facility should arrange for one person to belong to each SIS, so the literature available reflects the broad range of practice. (An example is a recent article on Sensory Integration and Affective Disorders in the SISIS Newsletter.)

28. Read one non-mental health journal, either occupational therapy or nonoccupational therapy. Identify trends and niches where occupational therapy in mental health might make inroads. For example, Hospital and Community Psychiatry.

29. At conferences, attend at least one session outside of your area of interest to see what is happening outside of mental health. You may gain ideas that are applicable to mental health arenas.

30. If you know an occupational therapist who is doing something innovative in mental health, suggest that he/she present the program or ideas at a local conference or group meeting. *Also inform AOTA.*

31. Belong to one SIS in additon to the one with whom you most identify. Assume an active role on committee or task force of one or the other SIS.

32. When attending presentations, ask questions and identify yourself as an occupational therapist in mental health. If you are shy about asking questions during the presentation, approach speakers after the presentation. Introduce yourself as an occupational therapist practicing in mental health and ask questions, compliment the speaker on the talk, or clarifiy issues about OT. If appropriate, follow up with a letter.

33. Send a copy of your CV to the MHSIS at AOTA letting her know your interests, availability for special projects, and/or involvement in innovative areas of mental health.

34. Invite people from administration to lunch with you at least once a year, if you work in a hospital or other large setting. Let them know what OT is doing on an informal level even if you see them in various meetings throughout the week.

35. Make an effort to meet the "problem people" and the "power people" in your environment. These are the key people with whom to develop a positive relationship.

36. On whatever regular basis is possible, arrange to meet or have lunch with people from a variety of disciplines both inside and outside of your immediate setting. For example, people who are involved with legal aspects of mental health, insurance claims representatives, other direct service providers.

37. Encourage your local OT group or special interest section to collaborate with a local AMI (Alliance for the Mentally Ill) or other consumer oriented group to introduce or promote various community projects.

38. Try to meet other OTs who are pioneering programming in non-traditional areas. Get ideas for your own future directions in mental health.

39. If the MHSIS is not meeting a specific need, call the mental health liason for your state (AOTA can give you this information), or the chairperson or the Mental Health Special Interest Section and discuss the possibility of becoming involved in evaluating and being part of the solution to this problem.

Have a Positive Attitude!

40. Know the language of the people you are dealing with and adapt your language and terms so that people are comfortable with the information you provide. Do not use language above or below the level of the people with whom you communicate. Especially make sure you are not talking down to people.

41. Convey enthusiasm about mental health to your affiliating students. Inform them of the challenges in the area of mental health. Do *not* tell them not to go into mental health because it is a dying area of practice. This happens much more often than we think!

42. Realize that your positive message about occupational therapy in mental health will have to be heard or read many times. The average person needs to hear a message at least seven times before really hearing it.

43. Remember that first impressions count. Your dress, manners, tone of voice, and smile go a long way toward building an impression of occupational therapy that will be remembered.

44. When approaching others about occupational therapy in mental health, find out from them if there is anything you can do to make their job easier. A "canned speech" will not target their needs. Ask yourself: What itch can I scratch?

45. Apply what you know about clinical reasoning and group dynamics to multidisciplinary teams, SIS group meetings, etc.

46. Do not blame AOTA for past problems. Be realistic about what AOTA or any national association can provide. Don't always expect answers. Be part of the solution.

47. Do *not* be defensive. Display a positive, energetic, open, and nonjudgmental attitude, even when faced with conflict and crisis. Be open to learning from other rehabilitation professionals such as art, dance, music, and recreation therapists. We all contribute something unique and different to the arena of treatment interventions available to the person with emotional disabilities.

48. Do NOT be apologetic about practicing psychiatric occupational therapy, but be prepared to discuss what we do as occupational therapy and what you do specifically in your position.

49. Stop using language that contributes to the stigma against mental illness, i.e., "crazy." Sometimes we as professionals use this language without thinking what impressions we may be making on others. Politely point out to others who may do this the negative effects of this practice.

50. Do not complain in general about your job in mental health around students or people in other disciplines. Be realistic about the challenges involved in mental health in your position, but do not discourage others from going into mental health based on your own experiences.

50 Not-So-Simple-But-Very-Worthwhile Things You Can Do to Promote Occupational Therapy in Mental Health

Educators are Key Players

1. Successful occupational therapists in mental health may be able to "mentor" promising students before they come to their internships. Set this up with local occupational therapy school faculty.

2. Consider presenting at COE {Committee on Education)

2. Consider presenting at COE {Committee on Education) if you are an educator.

3. Introduce level I and II students to doctors, nurses, social workers and others and if possible arrange to have students tell them what role they will be playing in the program.

4. Focus on what you can do to help with the fieldwork site shortage. Volunteer to help the school develop new sites, agree to supervise a student in non-traditional setting, or introduce pre-occupational therapy students to occupational therapy and mental health.

5. Arrange for students in hospital-based settings to visit community sites and vice-versa to promote continuity of care and promote various roles that occupational therapy can play.

6. Masters programs are needed along with more opportunity to attend mental health seminars (suggestion from Alaska). Write to AOTA and/or COE about local needs for masters programs or mental health seminars.

7. Communicate to educators the need to increase emphasis on psychiatry in occupational therapy programs in universities, especially in communication, psychopathology and function.

8. Develop recruitment strategies, such as occupational therapy as a recession-proof career, to attract psychology majors in college to consider occupational therapy school rather than graduate school in psychology. Doctoral programs are glutted. Offer another option.

9. Make sure that mental health components are integrated throughout the curriculum, e.g. in research, pediatrics. Volunteer to help the school develop the mental health components of their program.

10. Encourage students to attend workshops on function and outcomes in mental health so they can see first hand how challenging and interesting working in mental health can be.

11. Explore the possibility of taking more than one student per time slot. Take more students using different training models. Foster independence. Do not cling to ideas of constant 1:1 student/supervisor relationship. Call your regional fieldwork consultant or AOTA for assistance in designing a program.

12. Consider placing students in sites where there are no occupational therapists working. Centers having occupational therapy departments or occupational therapists in private practice may be willing to offer supervisory seminars to students in non-traditional settings where there is no occupational therapist Contact AOTA or local occupational therapy school to establish this program.

13. Rather than insisting on hiring an experienced therapist, consider hiring a recent graduate and asking therapists in the community to assist with supervision. Begin local peer support and supervision groups.

14. Develop psychiatric affiliations in rehabilitation and physical medicine settings. Work with the occupational therapist in physical disabilities to develop mental health fieldwork objectives that can be achieved in their settings. (An example is the high percentage of clients with a substance abuse-related physical disability.)

15. Develop a non-traditional fieldwork setting in which you work as the supervisor and consultant. Mental health expertise can be developed in homeless shelters, after school programs, long-term care, and/or residential settings.

AOTA STRUCTURES: IDEAS ABOUT WHAT AOTA CAN DO FOR US AND US FOR THEM.

16. We need additional brochures about occupational therapy in mental health from which we can get ideas and which can be used to provide information to clients and their families. AOTA will be developing brochures about different aspects of occupational therapy in mental health. Volunteer ideas for a brochure to AOTA and suggest program sites where photographs may be taken.

17. Call AOTA. Public Relations and request promotional materials for your workspaces that have interesting visuals and pertinent information about occupational therapy.

18. We need more videotapes on mental health for students to watch and evaluate. Contact various schools with audiovisual departments and volunteer your site as one which students may use for videotaping projects, or volunteer to "role play" in a video.

19. It would be helpful to have groups that serve as "connection groups", for both students and therapists. SIS groups may not meet this need. (Texas Women's University has done this very successfully.)

20. SIS groups can be disappointing and may not feel as if they function to empower practitioners. Programs should be established for mutual support and education. You can establish, even on the local level, peer support groups and mutual supervision groups. Get involved. Join the MHSIS.

21. Therapists who are just beginning, or on their own, need a network of therapists with whom to consult. Volunteer to be a mental health liaison for your state by contacting your state association president. If you are a new therapist, or practicing alone, contact a local facility with a large psychiatric staff and begin a peer support group.

22. Develop telephone trees to inform people about legislative activities. Write letters to congressmen and congresswomen. The Legislative and Political Relations Department of AOTA can assist in helping to present testimony and write effective letters.

23. Contact the Public Relations Department at AOTA for resource materials which can be helpful in terms of promoting occupational therapy. They can also assist with developing strategies for your particular situation.

24. Ask what you can do for AOTA or your state association: be a resource person, consultant, liaison, etc.
25. AOTA needs to compile a list of all occupational therapy in mental health, not just those who are members of the MHSIS. It should be organized by area of interest and published annually. Send your name, address and specialty areas.
26. Find out what AOTA considers key groups to affiliate with such as NAMI, NIMH, IAPSRS. Join one and become involved.
27. Local SIS groups can "adopt" a facility that doesn't have occupational therapy and provide free consultation to help increase the awareness and outcomes of occupational therapy.
28. Local chapters of the MHSIS can take on special initiatives, similar to wheelchair races. Plan activities during Mental Illness Awareness Week. It is always the second full week in October.
29. AOTA can help you determine what state, federal, and local regulations for licensing and accreditation exist in your area. Learn how to use these and the functional outcomes of occupational therapy to justify occupational therapy services in mental health.

Develop Jobs in Non-occupational Therapy Areas

30. Develop relationships with people doing occupational therapy related services. Discuss with them how occupational therapy would approach various problems, challenges, etc. Do not be defensive or territorial.
31. Clearly delineate the potential role of occupational therapy in non-traditional mental health settings as well as the potential prophylactic role occupational therapy can play in promoting wellness and early intervention programs.
32. Market the role of occupational therapy in mental health to insurance companies. Give brief and understandable scenarios and case examples. Use statistics and research on decreased length of stays for inpatient settings and the role of vocational training for community settings in increasing consumer self-sufficiency. Call AOTA Payment Program Manager for more information on the Expanding Payment Network.
33. Apply to ads addressed to other professional disciplines that you feel an occupational therapist could fill. Often ads are more specific than the mind set of the individual placing them. Promote the skills you have as an occupational therapist that appear to meet the needs described in the ad.
34. In job interviews, emphasize the breadth of our profession in areas such as cognitive and behavioral assessment, as well as leisure skill development. This can be an asset in today's job market where there are decreasing numbers of jobs to meet varied needs. For example,

you may be able to supervise professionals from a variety of fields more satisfactory than could someone from other disciplines.
35. Given the basic skills of occupational therapy, human relations departments and employee assistance programs of corporations are logical arenas in which to develop jobs. Approach them with information about occupational therapy and how your skills may be able to assist them with their needs.
36. Be willing to simply provide information. A corporation or organization may not be able to use you or any occupational therapist right now, but if you leave information, resumes, etc. they will have the possibility of using an occupational therapist when the next opportunity arises.

Become Consumer Oriented

37. Encourage mental health consumers to talk about how occupational therapy has impacted them lives. Develop partnerships with consumers to promote occupational therapy together on a local state, and national level.
38. Co-present at occupational therapy or non-occupational therapy conferences with consumers. Stress your role as an occupational therapist in mental health by using laymen's terms. AOTA can assist in developing ways to promote the consumer orientation.
39. Assist consumers to develop the language to clearly define what the outcome of occupational therapy was to them and how it impacted their illness and/or how it compared to other professional interventions made during their illness. Encourage them to advocate occupational therapy when appropriate.
40. Donate two hours a week to a homeless shelter or other community service in your neighborhood. Find out how problems are perceived by consumers and see if you can help change structures that will improve situations.
41. If your community doesn't have a shelter, find out why. Volunteer to be involved in helping to start one.
42. Be active in local drop-in centers. Develop partnerships with people involved in staffing these centers and with others concerned about mental health.
43. Plan consumer-oriented activities for occupational therapy month (APRIL) Ask AOTA Public Relations for resources and let them know what you did

For the Experienced Therapist

44. Help promote a symposium at which papers that were not accepted for publication at various conferences could be presented. This could be done in conjunction with local MHSIS groups.
45. Help organize, in collaboration with your local occupational therapy department, workshops on psy-

chopathology, theory and clinical skills reviews for therapists who have been working for several years. Volunteer to mentor a re-entry therapist. AOTA has information on re-entry programs.

46. Promote pilot and research projects with clinicians and professors as directors. Outcome research is especially needed and not as difficult to accomplish as some beginning therapists imagine. It can be done with some mentoring and surprisingly little time, assuming you are already doing some kind of program evaluation and quality assurance checks. AOTF can offer support and research suggestions.

47. Do not be afraid to learn about the status of "independent contractor". It has some advantages and some requirments, but provides enormous flexibility and opportunity to expand into nontraditional areas.

48. Consider the possibility of learning about and starting a non-profit corporation which enable tax exampt status for an organization that provides services to disabled people. Do not be afraid of organizational structures with which you are not familiar.

49. Assist in developing a certification exam review course that strongly represents psychiatric considerations.

50. Develop multi-disciplinary inservices for students and other staff at your facility or community center.

Author Index

Index

BUILD *Your Library*

This book and many others on numerous different topics are available from SLACK Incorporated. For further information or a copy of our latest catalog, contact us at:

Professional Book Division
SLACK Incorporated
6900 Grove Road
Thorofare, NJ 08086 USA
Telephone: 1-856-848-1000
1-800-257-8290
Fax: 1-856-853-5991
E-mail: orders@slackinc.com
www.slackbooks.com

We accept most major credit cards and checks or money orders in US dollars drawn on a US bank. Most orders are shipped within 72 hours.

Contact us for information on recent releases, forthcoming titles, and bestsellers. If you have a comment about this title or see a need for a new book, direct your correspondence to the Editorial Director at the above address.

Thank you for your interest and we hope you found this work beneficial.